H A N D B O O K

# *Primary Care Procedures*

LIPPINCOTT WILLIAMS & WILKINS
A **Wolters Kluwer** Company

Philadelphia • Baltimore • New York • London
Buenos Aires • Hong Kong • Sydney • Tokyo

## STAFF

**Publisher**
Judith A. Schilling McCann, RN, MSN

**Editorial Director**
David Moreau

**Clinical Director**
Joan M. Robinson, RN, MSN

**Senior Art Director**
Arlene Putterman

**Clinical Editors**
Jana L. Sciarra (project manager), RN, MSN, CRNP; Joyce G. McDonnell, RN, CCRN

**Editors**
Julie Munden (senior editor),
Ty Eggenberger, Patricia Wittig

**Copy Editors**
Kimberly Bilotta, Tom DeZego,
Shana Harrington, Judith Orioli,
Carolyn Petersen, Dorothy Terry,
Peggy Williams, Pamela Wingrod

**Designers**
Lesley Weissman-Cook (book design),
Susan L. Sheridan (design project manager),
Donna S. Morris

**Electronic Production Services**
Diane Paluba (manager), Joyce Rossi Biletz
(senior desktop assistant), Richard Eng

**Manufacturing**
Patricia K. Dorshaw (senior manager),
Beth Janae Orr (book production
coordinator)

**Editorial Assistants**
Danielle J. Barsky, Beverly Lane, Linda Ruhf

**Librarian**
Catherine M. Heslin

**Indexer**
Karen C. Comerford

**Library of Congress
Cataloging-in-Publication Data**
Handbook of primary care procedures.
    p. ; cm.
Includes bibliographical references and index.
    1. Nurse practitioners—Handbooks, manuals, etc. 2. Primary care (Medicine)—Handbooks, manuals, etc.
    [DNLM: 1. Primary Health Care—Handbooks. W 49 H2368 2003] I.Lippincott Williams & Wilkins.
    RT82.8 .H36 2003
    616—dc21
    ISBN 1-58255-183-9 (pbk. : alk. paper)
                                    2002010330

# CONTENTS

# CONTRIBUTORS AND CONSULTANTS

**Peggy D. Baikie, RN, MS, CNNP, CPNP**
Senior Instructor and Nurse Practitioner
University of Colorado School of Nursing — Gilliam Youth Center
Denver

**Cheryl L. Brady, RN, MSN**
Adjunct Faculty
Kent State University
East Liverpool, Ohio

**Michael Calvin, PA-C, MPAS**
Physician Assistant
Colorado Allergy and Asthma Centers
Wheat Ridge

**Michael A. Carter, DNSc, FAAN, FNP**
University Distinguished Professor
The University of Tennessee Health Science Center
Memphis

**Janice T. Chussil, RN,C, MSN, ANP, DNC**
Nurse Practitioner
Dermatology Associates, P.C.
Portland, Ore.

**Diane Dixon, PA-C, MA, MMSc**
Assistant Professor
Department of Physician Assistant Studies
University of South Alabama
Mobile

**James B. Doody, PA-C, MS**
Assistant Clinical Professor
University of Colorado Health Sciences Center
Denver

**Joseph L. DuFour, RN, MS, CS, FNP**
Lecturer
State University of New York at New Paltz

**Linda Fuhrman, MSN, ANCC, ANP**
Nurse Practitioner
San Francisco VA Medical Center

**Kenneth R. Harbert PA-C, PhD, CHES**
Professor and Chair
Philadelphia College of Osteopathic Medicine

**Clifford D. Korf, RN, PA-C, MPAS**
Clinical Director Physician Assistant Program
Union College
Lincoln, Nebr.

**Francie Likis, MSN, CNM, FNP**
Faculty
Frontier School of Midwifery and Family Nursing
Hyden, Ky.

**Dawna Martich, RN, MSN**
Clinical Trainer
American Healthways
Pittsburgh

**Richard O. Nenstiel, PA-C, MBA**
Assistant Professor and Chairman
Department of Physician Assistant
    Studies
University of South Alabama
Mobile

**Virginia Richardson, RN, DNS, CPNP**
Assistant Dean for Student Affairs
Indiana University School of Nursing
Indianapolis

**Ronni H. Rothman, MPH, MSN,
    CNM**
Certified Nurse Midwife
Private Practice
Philadelphia

**Lourdes "Cindy" Santoni-Reddy,
    NP-C, MEd, MSN, FAAPM**
Associate Professor
Mercer County Community College
Trenton, N.J.
Faculty
Frankford Hospital School of Nursing
Philadelphia

**Barbara L. Sauls, PA-C, EdD**
Clinical Director
Physician Assistant Program
King's College
Wilkes-Barre, Pa.

**Sylvia J. Smith, RNC, CRNP**
OB/GYN Nurse Practitioner
Rosedale Women's Care, P.C.
Pottstown, Pa.

**Arlene M. Sperhac, RN, PhD,
    CPNP, CS**
Coordinator
Pediatric Nurse Practitioner Program
Rush University
Chicago

**Allison J. Terry, RN, MSN**
Staff Development Coordinator
Beverly Healthcare — Tyson
Montgomery, Ala.

**Dan Vetrosky, PA-C, MEd**
Assistant Professor
Department of Physician Assistant
    Studies
University of South Alabama
Mobile

**Gail A. Viergutz, RN, MS, ANP-C**
Nurse Practitioner — Urgent Care and
    Emergency
St. Michael's Hospital and Ministry
    Corporation
Stevens Point, Wis.

**Marilyn J. Vontz, RN, MA, MSN, BS,
    PhD**
Nurse Educator
Bryan School of Nursing
Lincoln, Nebr.

# FOREWORD

"The times, they are a-changin'," sang Bob Dylan nearly 40 years ago. At the time, he was most likely referring to the tumultuous social changes of the 1960s that were occurring in the United States. I doubt he had any inkling how appropriate his comment would be with regard to the medical profession at the beginning of the third millennium.

As a practicing family physician, I'm well aware of the numerous changes in medicine. For starters, the various ways in which financial coverage is provided — via health maintenance organizations, preferred provider organizations, independent practice organizations, point-of-service plans — and the numerous other mechanisms designed to affect the delivery of health care are changes I know all too well. What's more, physicians, nurse practitioners (NPs), and physician assistants (PAs) face steadily increasing pressure to maintain their bottom lines because of reduced payments by insurance companies for services. We're also challenged with the unavailability of major vaccines for our pediatric and elderly patients, the glut of direct marketing to patients by pharmaceutical compa-

nies, and the increasing necessity of personal computers.

The most important change of all, however, is the dramatic explosion in knowledge. Today, it requires more effort to keep up with all of the advances in medicine and provide our patients with the quality care they deserve. After all, that's the reason why most of us went into medicine in the first place — to care for patients.

Computers are helpful tools for accessing the information we need to provide better patient care, from the latest journal articles to treatments of choice for a specific condition. However, if a patient requires a specific procedure, it isn't always that easy to find concise information quickly about how to perform a particular procedure. More than ever, students, as well as NPs and PAs could benefit from a resource that provides a better understanding of procedures.

Look no further — *Handbook of Primary Care Procedures* is your resource for performing the simplest to the most complex of procedures. This book combines well-organized content in an easy-to-read format with start-to-finish instructions for over 150 procedures you'll need to know as a busy health care professional. Do you need to know how to remove an imbedded fishhook? Perform a postcoital test? Fit a cervical cap? Reduce a rectal prolapse? All of these — and more — are fully explained in detail, accompanied by numerous illustrations and photos that provide step-by-step views of the procedure and the equipment involved. In addition, you'll find out what equipment is needed and how to prepare it as well as tips to make the procedure go more smoothly. There's even a section that identifies the proper CPT codes to use to ensure reimbursement. Each procedure is presented in a format that allows you to quickly find the information you need, including description and purpose, indications, contraindications, equipment, preparation, essential steps, patient teaching, complications, and special considerations.

Furthermore, important icons appear throughout the book to highlight *clinical tips,* procedures that require an *informed consent* form, and *collaboration* situations that tell you when referrals or consultations are necessary. Finally, you'll benefit from the helpful appendices that include Medical English-Spanish translations, obtaining informed consent, and 12-lead electrocardiogram interpretation.

I won't be surprised when *Handbook of Primary Care Procedures* quickly becomes a standard reference on the shelves of most primary care providers in the United States. But there's no need to wait. With the aid of this book, you can share your wealth of information and knowledge with the patients you care for now, as "the times they are a-changin'."

**Philip Zazove, MD**
Clinical Professor of Family
   Medicine and Associate Medical
   Director of Ambulatory Care
University of Michigan Health
   System
Ann Arbor

## ABSCESS INCISION AND DRAINAGE

### CPT codes
10060  *Incision and drainage of abscess, single or simple*
10061  *Incision and drainage of abscess, multiple or complicated*
10080  *Incision and drainage of pilonidal cyst, simple*
10081  *Incision and drainage of pilonidal cyst, complicated*

### Overview

An abscess is a local collection of pus in a cavity formed by tissue breakdown and surrounded by inflamed tissue. The pressure, tissue damage, and pain can be relieved by incising and draining the abscess. Abscesses typically result from *Staphylococcus aureus* or a streptococcal infection. Males and children have a higher incidence of abscess formation than adult females.

Specific types of abscesses include furuncles, pilonidal cysts, and perianal cysts. Furuncles, or boils, occur in hair follicles and sweat glands. Pilonidal cysts result from ingrown hairs close to the anus and may have sinus openings. Perianal cysts typically result from a rectal fistula.

### Indications

■ To relieve the pressure and pain associated with an abscess (furuncle, pilonidal cyst, perianal cyst) that doesn't resolve with application of warm compresses

### Contraindications
**RELATIVE**
■ Cellulitis
■ Coagulopathies
■ Facial furuncles located within the triangle of the nose and the corners of the mouth
■ Diabetes
■ Immunosuppression

### Preprocedure patient preparation

■ Tell the patient that he can expect immediate pain relief when the abscess is drained.
■ Advise him of alternatives to abscess incision and drainage such as application of warm compresses.

## Equipment

Antiseptic skin cleaner (such as povidone-iodine) ◆ topical anesthetic (such as ethyl chloride or a tissue freezing kit) ◆ 1% to 2% lidocaine with or without epinephrine ◆ 3- to 10-ml syringe ◆ 25G to 30G ½″ needle ◆ 16G to 18G needle ◆ 4″ × 4″ sterile gauze pads ◆ #11 scalpel ◆ sterile drape ◆ sterile gloves ◆ sterile curved hemostat ◆ iodoform gauze ◆ culture swab (optional) ◆ tape ◆ protective eyewear (optional)

## Procedure

■ Explain the procedure to the patient, and address any questions or concerns that he may have.

**☑ OBTAIN
INFORMED CONSENT**

■ Wash your hands.
■ Position the patient comfortably, with the abscess exposed.
■ Verify that the patient isn't allergic to iodine.
■ Clean the site and surrounding area with an antiseptic skin cleaner.
■ Put on protective eyewear if abscess contents appear under pressure.
■ Apply the sterile drape, and put on sterile gloves.
■ Anesthetize the area by spraying the surface with a topical anesthetic until it appears frosted or by injecting the perimeter with lidocaine solution, using a small (25G to 30G ½″) needle on a 3-ml syringe.
■ With the scalpel, make an incision deep and wide enough to allow purulent material to drain easily and to prevent premature closure.
■ Insert the culture swab deep into the wound to collect material for culturing, if culture is indicated. (You also may use a 16G or 18G needle and a syringe to withdraw fluid for culturing before incising.)
■ Use a curved hemostat to explore the cavity and break down membranes leading to other fluid-filled compartments.
■ After expressing all purulent material, pack the cavity with iodoform gauze, leaving at least ¼″ (0.5 cm) of gauze extending outside the wound.
■ Dress the wound with sterile gauze and tape.
■ Prescribe broad-spectrum antibiotic prophylaxis, such as cephalexin or cefadroxil.
■ Prescribe a narcotic analgesic (such as Tylenol with Codeine No. 3) the first day.
■ Prescribe a nonsteroidal anti-inflammatory drug (such as ibuprofen) to be used after the first day.

## Postprocedure patient teaching

■ Emphasize the importance of thorough hand washing and appropriate changing of the site dressing.
■ Have the patient return for a follow-up visit in 2 days.
■ Explain that healing can take up to 3 weeks.
■ Instruct the patient with a pilonidal cyst to take a sitz bath four times per day. Tell him to clean

and irrigate the area with a flexible shower hose or water from a squeeze bottle and to leave the wound open to air to promote drainage and healing. Explain that the wound must heal from the inside outward, which can take an additional 2 months.

■ Urge the patient to notify you promptly if he experiences signs and symptoms of infection, including increasing redness, swelling, pain, and warmth; cloudy yellow, green, or brown drainage; opening of the wound; foul odor; a red streak from the wound area; or fever.

## Complications

■ Pain and scarring are minimized by the use of pain medications, antibiotics, aseptic technique, and skilled wound closure.

 **COLLABORATION**
*Recurrence or worsening of symptoms, cellulitis, and gangrene warrant collaboration with or referral to a physician, a surgeon, or an infectious disease specialist. Extensive debridement and I.V. antibiotics may be required.*

 **COLLABORATION**
*Chronic anal fistula is common after perianal abscess incision and drainage and requires referral to a surgeon for fistulectomy.*

 **COLLABORATION**
*Hand, joint, or facial involvement as well as an abscess close to blood vessels, nerves, or tendons warrants referral to a specialist.*

## Special considerations

■ Don't inject lidocaine into the abscess; lidocaine loses its effectiveness in an acidic environment.

■ Breast abscesses, excluding those in the subareolar area, are rare and should be biopsied to rule out malignancy. Local breast infection introduced through the nipple during breast-feeding is the only common cause of subareolar abscess.

■ For paronychia under the nail, use a hot needle to bore through the nail and facilitate drainage. Partial removal of the nail may be necessary.

■ For a pilonidal cyst, position the patient in the left lateral or lithotomy position. Probe the sinus tracts with a cotton-tipped applicator. If the abscess is more than 5 mm deep, refer the patient to a surgeon. For a pilonidal cyst less than 5 mm in depth, perform elliptical excision.

■ Certain patient populations require more stringent observation after the procedure. A history of diabetes, a compromised immune system, or a debilitating disease indicates a need for increased vigilance. Consider sending an aspiration or a swab specimen for culture and sensitivity testing to help you detect and efficiently treat unusual organisms.

## Documentation

■ Before performing abscess incision and drainage, document any abnormal physical findings on the consent form. Have the patient initial the comments and sign the form to signify acknowledgment of preprocedural abnormalities. In the chart, the preprocedural and postprocedural notes must include an evaluation of potentially affected function, range of motion, and neurosensory testing (such as two-point discrimination).

■ Note whether a culture was sent to the laboratory.

■ Describe the site before and after the procedure, the type and amount of anesthetic used, the characteristics of the drainage, the patient's reaction to the procedure, medications ordered, the time frame for follow-up evaluation, and any instructions given to the patient.

## ACNE THERAPY

### CPT codes
10040  *Acne surgery, opening of multiple cysts, comedones, or pustules*
11900  *Intralesional injection of up to 7 lesions*
11901  *Intralesional injection of more than 7 lesions*
17340  *Cryotherapy (CO$_2$ slush) for acne*

### Overview

Acne vulgaris is an inflammatory disease of the sebaceous follicles. A closed comedo, or whitehead, occurs if the acne plug doesn't protrude from the follicle and is covered by the epidermis. An open comedo, or blackhead, occurs if the acne plug does protrude and

isn't covered by the epidermis. Rupture or leakage of an enlarged plug into the dermis produces inflammation and characteristic acne pustules, papules, and acne cysts or abscesses (severe). Chronic, recurring lesions produce acne scars.

Treatment for acne includes a variety of oral and topical agents. However, when these medications fail, treatment options for the primary care provider include comedo removal, cryotherapy with CO$_2$ slush (a mixture of solid carbon dioxide and acetone), intralesional corticosteroid injection, and acne surgery for pustules and cysts.

Using a comedo extractor instrument, the plug of an acne lesion may be removed. The removal of open comedones may prevent the development of inflamed acne lesions, promote healing, and enhance physical appearance.

The use of cryotherapy has been advocated by some physicians as a way to treat acne. Cryotherapy produces superficial erythema and desquamation that can result in reduced pustules, redness, and scarring after healing has occurred. Facial cryotherapy has become less popular as newer therapies have evolved.

Intralesional injection of a corticosteroid can dramatically decrease the size of nodular or cystic acne lesions. This is a relatively painless, effective procedure that takes little time, and multiple cysts can be treated at one time.

The surgical drainage of acne pustules and cysts may facilitate the resolution of the lesions, prevent subdermal rupture, and enhance cosmetic appearance. Surgical drainage can also be done to closed comedones to prevent progression to inflammatory lesions.

## Indications
■ To treat acne when medications fail

### For comedo removal
■ To remove the plug of a closed or open comedo

### For intralesional corticosteroid injection
■ To decrease the size of nodular or cystic acne lesions

### For acne surgery
■ To surgically drain contents of acne pustules and cysts

## Contraindications
### ABSOLUTE
### For intralesional corticosteroid injection
■ Skin atrophy from previous corticosteroid injections
■ Persistent skin depression from previous corticosteroid injections

### RELATIVE
■ Tendency of the patient to develop hypertrophic scarring
■ Inability of the patient to tolerate redness, scabbing, or mild atrophic scarring

## Preprocedure patient preparation
■ Discuss with the patient why and how the procedure will be

performed, including instruments that will be used (for example, a comedo retractor or a syringe with a needle), associated discomforts that may be experienced (for example, pressure, burning, throbbing, stinging, or sharp pain from a needle stick or scalpel point), and potential complications (such as a small amount of bleeding, increased redness or swelling, mild atrophic scarring, or skin depression).

## Equipment
### For comedo removal
Comedo extractor ◆ gloves ◆ alcohol pads or normal saline–soaked gauze pads ◆ #11 scalpel blade ◆ cool compresses

### For cryotherapy
Cryotherapy agent ($CO_2$ slush, cryogenic spray, or liquid nitrogen) ◆ gloves ◆ cotton-tipped applicator ◆ alcohol pads

### For intralesional corticosteroid injection
Corticosteroid (such as triamcinolone acetonide) ◆ gloves ◆ sterile normal saline solution ◆ 3-cc or tuberculin syringe ◆ 30G needle ◆ 22G or larger needle ◆ alcohol pad or dry gauze pad ◆ adhesive bandage (optional) ◆ small dressing (optional)

### For acne surgery
25G needle or #11 scalpel blade ◆ gloves ◆ alcohol pad or gauze soaked with normal saline solution ◆ comedo extractor (optional)

## Using a comedo extractor

A comedo extractor is needed to remove the plug of a comedo. Depending on the size of the comedo, hold the small or large end of the extractor and encircle the pore. Apply uniform, smooth pressure to remove the plug.

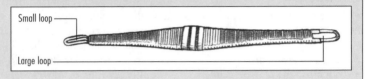

Small loop

Large loop

## Procedure

- Explain the procedure to the patient, and address any questions or concerns he may have.

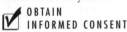
**OBTAIN INFORMED CONSENT**

- Wash your hands, and put on gloves.
- Assist the patient to a comfortable position.
- Clean the site with an alcohol pad.

### For comedo removal

- Closed comedones (whiteheads) need to be gently opened with the tip of a #11 scalpel blade or needle tip before using the comedo extractor.
- Place the comedo extractor with the loop encircling the pore. (See *Using a comedo extractor.*)
- Apply uniform, smooth pressure to the comedo extractor to remove the plug. A large amount of sebaceous material may be found beneath the plug.

▶ **CLINICAL TIP**
*Open comedones (blackheads) that offer resistance can sometimes*

be loosened and removed with a #11 scalpel blade or needle tip. Use a blade, extractor tip, or needle to stretch the walls of the pore opening without cutting into tissue. Insert the scalpel tip 1 mm into the comedo along the angle of the follicle opening. Angle the tip to push the plug upward through the enlarged pore opening.

- Clean the area with an alcohol pad or normal saline–soaked gauze.
- Apply cool compresses to the area immediately after comedo removal to prevent swelling and to enhance comfort.

### For cryotherapy

- Apply the cryotherapy agent. For cryotherapy slush, lightly paint the slush on the affected area. For cryogenic spray, spray the area for 2 to 3 seconds. For liquid nitrogen, dip a cotton-tipped applicator into the liquid nitrogen and then swab on the affected area.

▶ **CLINICAL TIP**
*Longer contact with the liquid nitrogen, either from extended*

*spraying times or repeated applications with cotton-tipped applicator, will increase the depth of the freeze and may be required in deeper, cystic acne.*

### For intralesional corticosteroid injection

■ Shake the corticosteroid vial to disperse the suspension.

■ Using the 22G or larger needle, draw saline into the 3-ml or tuberculin syringe, followed by steroid solution to obtain the desired concentration.

➤ **CLINICAL TIP**
*Saline is the preferred diluent for injection; injections with local anesthetics, such as lidocaine, can be painful.*

■ Carefully remove the 22G or larger needle, and place the 30G needle onto the syringe.

■ Insert the 30G needle through the thinnest portion at the roof of the cyst, and inject 0.1 ml to 0.3 ml of the saline/steroid mixture. Inject into the upper portion of the cyst. The injection will usually blanche the cyst.

➤ **CLINICAL TIP**
*Skin atrophy is more common if the steroid is injected below the cyst or if the steroid concentration is too high.*

■ Clean the area with an alcohol pad or dry gauze.

■ If drainage is present, cover the area with an adhesive bandage or a small dressing.

### For acne surgery

■ Place the 25G needle or the tip of the #11 scalpel blade into the head of a white pustule. Using lateral pressure or with the assistance of an extractor, drain the pustule.

■ For superficial cysts that have thin roofs and easily palpated fluid, make a small incision, less than 4 mm long, and drain the contents using lateral pressure with fingers or a comedo extractor.

■ Clean the area with an alcohol pad or normal saline–soaked gauze.

## Postprocedure patient teaching

■ Reinforce the importance of not picking at acne lesions or wearing tight clothing that may traumatize acne lesions.

■ Instruct the patient to wash his face once or twice daily with a mild soap.

■ For patients who use makeup and moisturizers, emphasize the importance of choosing oil-free products or those labeled as nonacnegenic or noncomedogenic.

■ For patients who received cryotherapy, inform them that they may experience redness and scabbing from 2 to 4 weeks after freezing.

■ For patients who received intralesional corticosteroid injection, inform them that skin depression may occur but will usually resolve in 4 to 6 months. If their acne is severe, it may require repeated injections every 2 to 3 weeks.

■ Consider prescribing tretinoin cream or gel to prevent the recurrence of comedones.

## Complications

- Small amounts of bleeding usually resolve minutes after the procedure is completed.
- Increased redness, swelling, and inflammation at the site of treatment may persist for several days after the procedure.

✦ COLLABORATION
*Hypertrophic scarring, pigmentary changes, and skin atrophy may occur and require referral to a dermatologist or a plastic surgeon, if indicated.*

## Special considerations

- The feelings of discomfort the patient experiences during the procedure may be most intense in the first several minutes following the procedure and usually resolve within 1 hour.
- Comedo removal shouldn't be done on patients with cystic acne. This method could worsen these lesions.

## Documentation

- Record the number of acne lesions treated.
- Document the method of acne treatment and, if applicable, whether the plugs or contents of pustules or cysts were successfully removed.
- Chart the degree of redness, swelling, or inflammation that occurs postprocedure.
- Record the patient's tolerance of the procedure and the follow-up instructions he was given.

# ＡLLERGY INJECTIONS (IMMUNOTHERAPY)

## CPT codes

*95115 to 95199   Specific code will depend on the number of injections and the type of allergenic extract or immunotherapy administered.*

## Overview

The best therapy for allergic disease is avoidance of the allergen. Allergy injections are indicated in cases where avoidance of the allergen is unfeasible, allergic manifestations are immediately life threatening, or patient response to optimal drug therapy is limited. For example, allergy injections, or immunotherapy, are an effective and safe treatment for allergic asthma, allergic rhinitis, and insect venom allergy. They involve repeated administration of specific allergens to a patient with documented immunoglobulin E (IgE)-mediated conditions. Their purpose is to provide protection against the allergic symptoms and inflammatory reactions associated with natural exposure to the allergens.

## Indications

- To prevent life-threatening venom sensitivity, allergic rhinitis, and allergic conjunctivitis that's unresponsive to optimal drug therapy
- To control asthma specifically triggered by allergens

## Contraindications

**ABSOLUTE**
- Extreme sensitivity to the specific allergen
- Exacerbation of chronically unstable asthma
- Current use of oral or topical beta-adrenergic blockers or of monoamine oxidase inhibitors
- Unstable angina, recent myocardial infarction or significant arrhythmias, or uncontrolled hypertension
- Infection or flu, accompanied by fever
- Failure of a major organ system (such as renal failure)

**RELATIVE**
- Immunotherapy shouldn't be initiated during pregnancy unless the risk of not doing so outweighs the risk to the fetus; however, it may be maintained during pregnancy if the patient doesn't have a history of systemic reactions.
- Defer if the patient has had any of the following within the past 24 hours: another injection (such as a flu vaccine or measles-mumps-rubella vaccine), a local anesthetic used in dental work, or a bee, wasp, hornet, or yellow jacket sting.

## Preprocedure patient preparation

- Confirm the patient's medical history, including whether he's presently well or ill, if there were any problems with his last set of shots, and if he has had any changes in medications.

- Instruct the patient to avoid heavy exercise 1 hour before and after immunotherapy.
- Tell the patient that 6 months to 1 year of immunotherapy may be needed before symptoms diminish.

## Equipment

Antigen vial, as appropriate ◆ 27G ¼″ needle ◆ tuberculin syringe ◆ alcohol pad or cotton ball soaked with 70% isopropyl alcohol ◆ gloves (preferably latex free) ◆ resuscitative equipment (such as stethoscope and sphygmomanometer, tourniquet and large-bore needles, aqueous epinephrine hydrochloride [1:1000], equipment to administer oxygen by mask, I.V. fluid set-up, self-inflating bag valve and mask apparatus, oral airway, diphenhydramine or similar antihistamine, aminophylline, corticosteroids, vasopressor, and bronchodilator for inhalation therapy)

## Procedure

- Explain the procedure to the patient, and address any questions or concerns he may have.

☑ **OBTAIN INFORMED CONSENT**
- Verify the patient's name on the chart, his treatment record, the allergen treatment set box, and the antigen vial.
- Check the expiration date on the antigen vial.
- Review the typed dosage and frequency instructions, any handwritten orders, and the three most recent allergy injections (date, di-

lution, dose, and any reaction) to determine the current dose.

■ Document the current dose and the site of the injection, and initial them with your credentials.

■ Wash your hands. Gloves aren't required for administering allergy injections unless the patient's skin is abraded or he has a known infectious disease such as hepatitis B per Occupational Safety and Health Administration guidelines.

■ Roll the antigen vial gently to mix.

■ Clean the top of the vial with an alcohol pad or isopropyl alcohol–soaked cotton ball, and withdraw the appropriate dose into the syringe.

■ Clean the injection site with an alcohol pad or isopropyl alcohol–soaked cotton ball. Give the injection subcutaneously (S.C.) to the posterolateral surface of the middle-third upper arm at a 90-degree angle, avoiding joint and muscle.

◥ **CLINICAL TIP**
*Always pull back on the plunger before the antigen is administered. If blood returns, withdraw the needle and discard it. Redraw the dose and deliver in the opposite arm.*

■ To lessen unduly rapid absorption of the antigen, avoid massaging the injection site. Patients with a history of local reactions may prefer to apply an ice pack to the site.

■ The patient must wait in the medical facility for 20 minutes after receiving the injection. After 20 minutes, inspect the injection site to observe for any local reactions, such as erythema, wheal formation, or induration.

### Postprocedure patient teaching
■ Instruct the patient to call your office with any signs or symptoms of a systemic reaction (see complications below).

## Complications
■ Local reactions, such as local tissue edema or itching, can be expected after allergy injections, especially during the build-up period. An antihistamine or ice application will help to relieve these reactions. Wheal formation should be handled according to its size:
– equal to or less than 25 mm: progress with the injection course
– from 25 to 30 mm: repeat the same dose on the next visit for injections
– greater than 30 mm but less than a tennis ball: reduce the dose by one-half the current volume on the next visit
– greater than a tennis ball: confer with an allergist.

■ Mild systemic reactions, such as rhinorrhea, nasal congestion, nasal itching, sneezing, eye tearing, eye itching, or mild conjunctival edema, may be treated with an oral antihistamine. The patient will require observation.

■ Moderate or severe systemic reactions, such as urticaria, angioedema, generalized itching, erythema, airway obstruction (coughing, wheezing, stridor, hoarseness, or throat pain or tightness), anxiety, abdominal symptoms (nausea, vomiting, or pain), or diaphoresis, need to be treated as a medical emergency:

– Give an injection of aqueous epinephrine hydrochloride (1:1000) S.C. into the opposite arm. Repeat at 20-minute intervals as needed.

– Give an additional 0.1-ml dose of epinephrine into the allergy injection site to retard allergen absorption.

– Administer diphenhydramine and a corticosteroid.

– Consider placing a tourniquet above the injection site; remove briefly every 10 minutes.

– Administer I.V. fluids and vasopressors if the patient shows signs of shock, and bronchodilators if the patient exhibits respiratory symptoms.

– Administer oxygen as needed.

## Special considerations

✳ COLLABORATION

*If the patient has had previous moderate or severe systemic reactions, don't administer further allergy injections without consulting with an allergist.*

■ If the patient has missed a scheduled allergy injection, his next dose may need to be adjusted according to the length of time from the last injection. This is also the case for build-up doses as well as maintenance doses.

## Documentation

■ Document the patient's medical history, physical assessment, and results of diagnostic testing that justify the need for allergy injections.

■ Record the date, time, and site of injection. Include the type of antigen and the dosage given.

■ Document any reaction to the injection and treatment given.

■ Chart patient teaching that was done and the date for the next scheduled injection.

## ALLERGY TESTING

**CPT codes**
95004 to 95078   *Allergy testing (Specific code will depend upon the type of testing.)*

## Overview

Allergy diagnostic testing by prick/puncture skin tests and intradermal tests are a method for detecting allergen-specific immunoglobulin E (IgE). These tests are considered the most convenient, least expensive, and most specific screening methods for detecting the presence of IgE antibodies in patients with appropriate histories. Based on their results correlated with the patient's history and physical examination, a treatment plan can be initiated. An appropriate plan includes avoidance of the allergen, environmental controls, drug therapy and, possibly, immunotherapy (allergy injections).

## Indications

■ To confirm immediate hypersensitivity induced by a wide variety of naturally occurring inhalant and food allergens

## Contraindications

**ABSOLUTE**

- The use of beta-adrenergic blockers or monoamine oxidase inhibitors
- Current severe allergic symptoms
- Unstable asthma
- Active dermatitis at the test site
- Certain drug use, such as first-generation antihistamines in the past 24 to 72 hours, hydroxyzine in the past 96 hours, nonsedating antihistamines within the past week, tricyclic antidepressants within the past 7 to 14 days, or daily topical corticosteroid applied to the test site 2 to 3 weeks prior to the skin test

**RELATIVE**

- History of unusually severe allergic reactions, particularly when associated with minimal allergen exposure
- Pregnancy
- Severe lung disease
- Unstable angina

## Preprocedure patient preparation

- Before the scheduled visit, advise the patient about taking medications appropriately.
- Explain why and how the procedure will be performed. To decrease the patient's anxiety, allow him to inspect the equipment that will be used.

## Equipment

*For prick/puncture skin testing*
Positive control: aqueous histamine phosphate 2.75 mg/ml ◆ negative control: 50% glycerin/50% buffered saline ◆ allergenic extract (1:20 weight per volume, 50% glycerin) ◆ bifurcated needle or similar lancet

*For intradermal skin testing*
26G or 27G ¼" safety needle with syringe ◆ allergenic extract dilution from 1/100 to 1/1000 of the concentrate ◆ positive control: aqueous histamine phosphate 0.275 mg/ml ◆ negative control: 50% glycerin/50% buffered saline

*For both procedures*
Alcohol pad or cotton ball soaked in 70% isopropyl alcohol ◆ resuscitative equipment (such as stethoscope and sphygmomanometer, tourniquet and large-bore needles, aqueous epinephrine hydrochloride [1:1000], equipment to administer oxygen by mask, I.V. fluid setup, self-inflating bag valve and mask apparatus, oral airway, diphenhydramine or similar antihistamine, aminophylline, corticosteroids, vasopressor, and bronchodilator for inhalation therapy)

## Procedure

- Explain the procedure to the patient, and address any questions or concerns he may have.

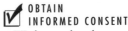 **OBTAIN INFORMED CONSENT**

- Wash your hands.

## Performing prick/puncture skin testing

The purpose of pricking the skin through a drop of allergen is to expose sensitized mast cells to the allergen. Place the needle bevel up on the skin through the allergen drop (first illustration), and then gently prick the needle on the skin in the direction shown (second illustration). There should be no bleeding from the skin prick; however, some redness around the test site is common.

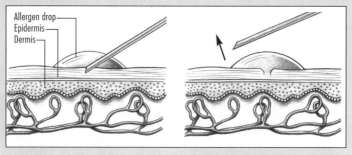

Allergen drop
Epidermis
Dermis

### *For prick/puncture skin testing*

■ Determine the injection site. For a large number of tests, use the back; for a small number of tests, use the volar surface of the forearm.

■ Assist the patient to a comfortable position if using the arm. Have the patient disrobe from the waist up and lie down on his stomach or straddle a chair and lean forward if using the back.

■ Clean the test site with an alcohol pad or a cotton ball soaked with isopropyl alcohol.

■ Number the test site area. Numbers should be 2″ (5 cm) apart. Utilize all of the back area, staying 1″ to 2″ (2.5 to 5 cm) away from the spine, no lower than mid-kidney level, and no higher than the shoulders.

■ Apply drops of the specific extract next to each number. Then apply the histamine and saline controls.

■ Apply downward pressure with a bifurcated needle or lancet, and prick the skin. This shouldn't draw blood but should lightly chafe the skin. (See *Performing prick/puncture skin testing.*)

■ Wipe the needle after each prick with an alcohol pad or a cotton ball soaked in isopropyl alcohol or, if using disposable needles, discard each needle appropriately after each prick.

■ After all of the pricks have been done, you may blot the test site with a paper towel so the patient may sit up.

■ Instruct the patient not to touch, scratch, or rub the test site.

■ Read the histamine control at 10 minutes. If negative or inadequate (a wheal that's less than 3 to 5 mm), then perform intradermal skin testing.

■ Read the test at 15 minutes. Record all reactions according to the following grading schedule:
– grade 1: erythema only, less than or equal to 10 mm
– grade 2: a wheal that's less than 3 mm and erythema
– grade 3: a wheal that's 3 to 5 mm and erythema
– grade 4: a wheal that's greater than 5 mm and erythema with or without pseudopods.

■ Gently wash the numbers off with soap, water, and a paper towel.

### For intradermal skin testing

■ Assist the patient to a comfortable position. Clean his upper arms with an alcohol pad or a cotton ball soaked in isopropyl alcohol. Number sites on the outer extensor surface of the middle third of the upper arm.

■ Inject, with the bevel of the needle facing up, intradermally 0.02 ml to 0.05 ml of extract and observe for a "bleb" made by the injection.

■ The histamine result from the prick/puncture skin test is your control. If you don't have this result, perform a prick/puncture histamine skin test.

■ Read the test in 15 minutes, with grading assigned as follows:
– grade 1: a wheal that's 3 mm to 4 mm and erythema
– grade 2: a wheal that's 4 mm to 8 mm and erythema
– grade 3: a wheal that's 8 mm to 12 mm and erythema
– grade 4: a wheal that's greater than 12 mm and erythema with or without pseudopods.

■ Discard each needle and syringe after performing each test.

■ Wash the site with soap and water after testing.

## Postprocedure patient teaching

■ Review your findings with the patient. Instruct the patient to call you if he experiences such signs or symptoms as increased allergic rhinitis, itching, urticaria, or asthma.

■ Inform the patient that positive skin reactions will usually resolve spontaneously.

■ Provide the patient with his treatment plan, and schedule a follow-up visit within the next 4 weeks.

## Complications

■ Adverse systemic reactions, although rare, may occur within minutes after the testing. These reactions consist primarily of allergic symptoms, such as generalized itching, urticaria, erythema, angioedema, or airway obstruction. (See "Allergy injections [Immunotherapy]," page 8, for management of these reactions.)

## Special considerations

■ Intradermal testing should be performed for any result of a prick/puncture test that's grade 3 or less.

## Documentation

- Document the results of the allergy testing in the patient's chart, including any reactions and treatment, if applicable.
- Document patient teaching done and any follow-up appointments that were made.
- Provide the patient with a written copy of his skin test results.

# AMBULATORY BLOOD PRESSURE MONITORING

## CPT codes

93784 *Ambulatory blood pressure monitoring for 24 hours or longer, including recording, scanning analysis, interpretation, and report*
93786 *Recording only*
93788 *Scanning analysis with report*

## Overview

Ambulatory blood pressure monitoring (ABPM) allows for the measurement of blood pressure over a period of time, without confining a patient to a facility. ABPM records the variations that occur in a patient's blood pressure as well as his average blood pressure during normal activity. Such monitoring more readily allows diagnosis of sustained hypertension and response to treatment than do isolated blood pressure measurements taken in a facility. During monitoring, the patient needs to maintain an accurate log of activities and associated symptoms he may experience.

## Indications

- To identify those who don't require pharmacotherapy
- To rule out a diagnosis of sustained hypertension
- To determine the range of variability in labile hypertension
- To monitor the effectiveness of therapy and to evaluate drug-resistant hypertension
- To determine diurnal blood pressure variations in patients with diabetes or autonomic insufficiency
- To evaluate discrepancies between blood pressure measurements in and out of a facility

## Contraindications

**ABSOLUTE**
- Hypertensive crisis that requires immediate intervention

## Preprocedure patient preparation

- Tell the patient that he'll feel no pain from the procedure but that the tape and monitor may cause mild discomfort.
- Tell the patient that he'll need to wear a small microprocessor and blood pressure cuff for 24 hours after activation of the monitor. Tell him not to remove the blood pressure cuff or microprocessor unless told to do so. Explain that he'll have a carrying case with a strap to carry the 2-lb monitor.

■ Tell the patient he'll need to maintain an activity log during the 24-hour monitoring period. He should record the time, activities he performs, and any symptoms (such as headache, dizziness, light-headedness, palpitations, or chest pain) that may occur. Explain the importance of maintaining his usual routine, including working, eating, sleeping, using the bathroom, driving, and taking his medication. He should be sure to record the time medications are taken.

■ Suggest wearing a watch to make it easier to keep an accurate log.

■ Encourage the patient to wear loose-fitting clothes with tops that open in the front.

■ Tell the patient that he can sponge bathe but that he should keep the equipment from getting wet.

■ Tell the patient to take the usual steps for medical emergencies, such as taking nitroglycerin and going to the emergency department for chest pain.

■ Show the patient how to use tape to secure the microphone on the brachial area of his arm in case the microphone becomes loose.

■ To ensure that measurements are accurate, tell the patient to keep the cuff arm still and free from extraneous noise when he feels the cuff inflating and deflating.

■ Tell the patient to avoid activities — such as mowing the lawn, golfing, running, and tennis — that call for isometric use of the upper extremities, to help avoid erroneous blood pressure measurements during such activities.

■ Tell the patient to call your facility if any problems or questions arise.

## Equipment

Monitor with new battery that contains a cuff, microphone, and microprocessor that pumps the cuff and records measurements ◆ carrying case with strap ◆ 1″ adhesive tape ◆ logbook or diary

## Procedure

■ Explain the procedure to the patient, and address any questions or concerns that he may have.

■ Ask the patient whether he has any allergies to adhesive tape.

■ Wash your hands.

■ Place the equipment into the carrying case, and connect the neck strap.

■ Position the microphone over the brachial artery on the inner aspect of the nondominant arm, just above the elbow. Secure the microphone with tape. Then choose an appropriately sized blood pressure cuff. Manufacturers supply regular adult, obese adult, and pediatric sizes.

■ Calibrate the monitor while the patient both sits and stands by measuring simultaneous blood pressure readings, using the ABPM unit and a mercury sphygmomanometer attached to the monitor with a T-tube device.

■ Place the strap over the patient's neck, and position the unit comfortably. Make sure there isn't too much slack or pull on the cables because artifact may occur.

## Postprocedure patient teaching

■ Tell the patient that he'll need a follow-up appointment to review results 48 to 72 hours after removal of the monitor.

## Complications

■ None known

## Special considerations

■ If the patient can't return to your facility immediately after the monitoring period, show him how to remove the equipment and store the monitor, blood pressure cuff, and log.

## Documentation

■ Document the indications for monitoring.
■ Note the date and time the monitor was applied.
■ Record the patient's medication regimen and blood pressure before monitoring.
■ Include the patient's event log in documentation, including the date and time the monitor was removed.
■ Document postprocedure results and actions taken.

# *ANAPHYLAXIS MANAGEMENT*

***CPT code***
*No specific code has been assigned.*

## Overview

Anaphylaxis is a dramatic, acute atopic reaction marked by the sudden onset of rapidly progressive urticaria and respiratory distress. A severe reaction may precipitate vascular collapse, leading to systemic shock and, possibly, death. Rapid assessment and intervention is essential.

The source of anaphylactic reactions is systemic exposure (for example, through ingestion) to sensitizing drugs or other substances. Such substances may include serums (usually horse serum), vaccines, allergen extracts, enzymes (L-asparaginase), hormones, penicillin and other antibiotics, sulfonamides, local anesthetics, salicylates, polysaccharides, diagnostic chemicals (sulfobromophthalein, sodium dehydrocholate, and radiographic contrast media), foods (especially legumes, nuts, berries, seafood, and egg albumin) and sulfite-containing food additives, insect venom (honeybees, wasps, hornets, yellow jackets, fire ants, mosquitoes, and certain spiders) and, rarely, ruptured hydatid cyst.

An anaphylactic reaction produces sudden physical distress within seconds or minutes (although a delayed or persistent reaction may occur for up to 24 hours) after exposure to an allergen. The severity of the reaction is inversely related to the interval between exposure to the allergen and the onset of signs and symptoms.

Initial signs and symptoms include feeling of impending doom or fright, weakness, sweating, sneezing, shortness of breath, nasal pruritus, urticaria, and angioedema. These initial signs and symptoms are followed rapidly by symptoms in one or more target body systems, including cardiovascular (hypotension, shock, and cardiac arrhythmias), respiratory (nasal mucosa edema, profuse watery rhinorrhea, itching, nasal congestion, sudden sneezing attacks, and edema of the respiratory tract), and GI and genitourinary (severe stomach cramps, nausea, diarrhea, and urinary urgency and incontinence) symptoms.

## Indications

- To treat anaphylactic reactions

## Contraindications

- None known (anaphylaxis requires immediate treatment)

## Preprocedure patient preparation

- Attempt to relieve the patient's anxiety by speaking calmly while briefly explaining your actions.

## Equipment

Crash cart or commercially available emergency kit containing emergency drugs, respiratory equipment, and I.V. supplies and solutions ◆ gloves

## Procedure

- Determine that the patient is experiencing anaphylactic reaction by observing for signs and symptoms.
- Wash your hands if time permits because life-threatening symptoms may be occurring. Put on gloves.
- Obtain vital signs.
- For mild reactions, treatment with diphenhydramine (I.V., I.M., or by mouth) or a systemic corticosteroid may be all that's necessary, along with close observation.
- For severe reactions, immediately inject epinephrine 1:1,000 aqueous solution, 0.1 to 0.5 ml, and repeat every 5 to 20 minutes as necessary. If in the early stages of anaphylaxis, when the patient hasn't lost consciousness and is normotensive, administer the epinephrine I.M. or subcutaneously (S.C.). If the patient has lost consciousness and is hypotensive, give the epinephrine I.V.

 **CLINICAL TIP**
*After I.M. or S.C. injections, help the epinephrine move into circulation faster by massaging the site of injection.*
- Assess and maintain airway patency. Observe for early signs of laryngeal edema (hoarseness, stridor, and dyspnea), which will probably require endotracheal tube insertion or tracheotomy and oxygen therapy.
- Assess circulation. In case of cardiac arrest, begin cardiopulmonary

resuscitation. Establish large vein venous access lines (preferably two). Sodium bicarbonate may be indicated. Watch for hypotension and shock, and maintain circulatory volume with volume expanders (plasma, plasma expanders, saline, and albumin), as needed. Use blood pressure and urine output as a response index.

■ Arrange for transportation to an acute care facility.

## Postprocedure patient teaching

■ To prevent anaphylaxis, teach the patient to avoid exposure to known allergens. A person who is allergic to certain foods or drugs must learn to avoid the offending food or drug in all its forms. A person who is allergic to insect stings should avoid open fields and wooded areas during the insect season.

■ Instruct the patient with known severe allergic reactions to carry an anaphylaxis kit (epinephrine, antihistamine, and tourniquet) whenever he goes outdoors.

■ Instruct the patient to seek medical attention if he experiences further signs or symptoms of a reaction, such as shortness of breath, edema, a feeling of swelling in his throat, or urticaria.

■ Encourage the patient prone to anaphylaxis to wear a medical identification bracelet identifying his allergies.

## Complications

■ Death can occur if anaphylaxis is unrecognized and untreated. However, most patients survive if the condition is identified and treated promptly. Other severe complications include myocardial ischemia and brain injury caused by prolonged hypoxia.

■ Airway or chest trauma may result from resuscitative effort and may require further evaluation.

## Special considerations

■ Patients who are taking beta-adrenergic blockers may be resistant to the effects of epinephrine and may require larger than usual doses.

■ If a patient must receive a drug to which he's allergic, prevent a severe reaction by making sure he receives careful desensitization with gradually increasing doses of the antigen or advance administration of steroids. Ensure that a person with a known allergy history receives a drug with a high anaphylactic potential only after cautious pretesting for sensitivity is performed. Closely monitor the patient during testing, and make sure you have resuscitative equipment and epinephrine ready.

## Documentation

■ Record the allergen (if known), the patient's reaction, treatment or resuscitative efforts needed, the patient's response to treatment, and the follow-up care or the patient's condition prior to transportation to an acute care facility.

■ Document patient teaching and written materials given to the patient.

## *A*NESTHESIA: TOPICAL, LOCAL, AND DIGITAL NERVE BLOCK

### *CPT code*
*Usually included in the CPT code of the procedure with which it's being performed.*

## Overview

Anesthesia causes loss of sensation and is beneficial in a variety of procedures, from removal of a small skin lesion to surgery. Factors that affect the type, amount, and duration of anesthetic needed include the local blood supply, the presence of infection, the effects of certain chronic diseases, the size of the affected area, the diameter and conduction of nerve fibers, and psychological factors (such as anxiety and pain threshold).

Topical anesthesia involves applying an anesthetic agent directly to the area where inhibition of sensory conduction is desired. Needles are usually not used. Local anesthesia involves injecting an anesthetic agent into the site where inhibition of sensory conduction is desired. Digital nerve block, also known as saddle block, involves injecting an anesthetic

agent near the branch of the nerve that innervates the digit where the inhibition of sensory conduction is desired. Knowledge of the anatomy of the fingers and toes is essential to successfully performing a digital nerve block.

## Indications

■ To render the patient incapable of feeling pain during surgical repair (such as incision and drainage), laceration repair, biopsy, foreign-body removal, and dislocation reduction

### *Topical*
■ To anesthetize for small, uncomplicated, and superficial areas requiring procedures

### *Local*
■ To anesthetize for minor procedures such as suturing

### *Digital nerve block*
■ To anesthetize when broad areas of anesthesia are required (such as for a finger or toe); when distortion of the local anatomy would compromise the procedure; or when the area requiring anesthesia is infected

## Contraindications
### ABSOLUTE
■ Allergy (to a specific anesthetic)
■ History of hypersensitivity reaction to a specific anesthetic

### *Local and digital nerve block*
■ Septicemia
■ Injecting through infected tissue

■ Profound bleeding tendencies

**RELATIVE**
■ Cellulitis
■ Compromised circulation

## Preprocedure patient preparation

■ Inform the patient about the duration of the anesthesia to be used.

### *Local and digital nerve block*
■ If the procedure is planned, eutectic mixture of local anesthetic (EMLA) may be applied to the injection site 1 hour prior to the procedure to reduce pain.

## Equipment

Anesthetic (such as EMLA, ice, or ethyl chloride) ◆ antiseptic skin cleaner (such as povidone-iodine solution) ◆ normal saline solution ◆ gloves ◆ soap (optional) ◆ acetone or rubbing alcohol (optional) ◆ occlusive dressing (optional)

### *For local anesthesia*
Anesthetic (such as 1% to 2% lidocaine with or without a vasoconstricting agent) ◆ appropriate-sized syringe for site ◆ 18G needle to draw up the anesthetic ◆ 25G to 30G ½″ to 1″ needle

### *For digital nerve block*
Anesthetic without a vasoconstricting agent ◆ sterile gloves ◆ sterile drape ◆ sterile 4″ × 4″ gauze pads ◆ appropriate-sized syringe for site ◆ 18G needle to

draw up the anesthetic ◆ 25G to 30G ½″ to 1″ needle

> **CLINICAL TIP**
> *A vasoconstrictor is contraindicated for use in extremities (such as the digits, nose, ear, and penis); in patients with vascular disorders, diabetes, or thyrotoxicosis; and in areas with compromised blood flow (such as a skin flap).*

## Procedure

■ Explain the procedure to the patient, and address any questions or concerns he may have.

> **OBTAIN INFORMED CONSENT**

■ Verify that the patient isn't allergic to iodine, topical medications, or local anesthetics.
■ Wash your hands.
■ Place the patient in a comfortable position with the affected area fully exposed.
■ Put on gloves.
■ Remove visible debris by irrigating the area with normal saline solution.
■ Clean the site and surrounding area with povidone-iodine solution.

### *For topical anesthesia of intact skin*
■ Remove oils from the skin with soap, acetone, or rubbing alcohol.
■ Apply EMLA and an occlusive dressing for 1 to 2 hours.

### *For topical short-term anesthesia of intact skin*
■ Rub the skin firmly with ice for 10 seconds, or spray with ethyl chloride for no longer than 2 sec-

onds (to reduce the risk of blistering).

### For local anesthesia

■ Draw up the anesthetic into the appropriate-sized syringe, using the 18G needle. Then replace the needle with a 25G to 30G needle.

■ Identify the appropriate injection site.

■ If EMLA hasn't been applied, freeze the injection site by spraying with ethyl chloride.

■ Insert the needle at a 45-degree angle.

■ Ask the patient whether he notices any change in sensation. If he reports pain, indicating direct contact with the nerve, withdraw the needle 1 mm.

■ Aspirate to make sure there's no blood return. If there is, the needle is in a blood vessel. Withdraw the needle slightly and reinsert it in another area.

■ Inject 1 to 2 ml of lidocaine while partially withdrawing the needle. Then redirect the needle across the surface, advance it, and inject another 0.5 ml while withdrawing the needle. This method distributes the anesthetic uniformly, providing the optimal effect.

■ Wait for the local anesthetic to work before beginning the procedure. The maximum effect should occur in 5 to 15 minutes.

### For digital nerve block

■ Draw up the anesthetic into the appropriate-sized syringe (5 ml for fingers; 10 ml for toes) using an 18G needle.

■ Identify the appropriate injection site. Use the anterior and posterior web spaces of the digit, close to the bone.

■ Prepare the area using 4″ × 4″ gauze pads and povidone-iodine solution, and let it dry; repeat this three times.

■ Using sterile technique, drape the area with a sterile drape.

■ If EMLA hasn't been applied, freeze the injection site by spraying with ethyl chloride.

■ Put on sterile gloves.

■ Insert the needle and advance at a 90-degree angle.

■ Ask the patient whether he notices any change in sensation. If he reports pain, indicating direct contact with the nerve, withdraw the needle 1 mm.

■ Aspirate to make sure there's no blood return. If there is, the needle is in a blood vessel. Withdraw the needle slightly and reinsert it in another area.

■ For the toe, insert needle into the skin adjacent to the base of the metatarsal, advancing it along the lateral aspect until you just begin to tent the skin on the plantar surface. (See *Choosing injection sites for a digital nerve block of the toe.*) Withdraw the needle approximately 1 cm so that you're at the level of the plantar aspect of the metatarsal head; then inject 2 ml of anesthetic. Withdraw the needle, slowly injecting another 2 ml along the lateral aspect of the toe. Lastly, inject another 1 ml over the dorsal surface of the toe to ensure anesthesia of the dorsal sensory nerve. Repeat the procedure on the opposite side of the toe.

■ For the finger, insert the needle into the web space adjacent to the

## Choosing injection sites for a digital nerve block of the toe

The illustration below shows the injection sites for a digital nerve block of the toe. Appropriate injection sites include the web spaces adjacent to the base of the toe.

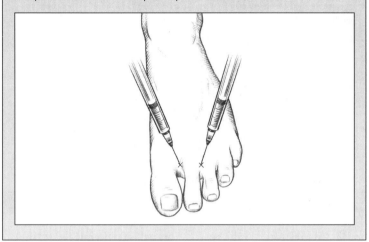

base of the first metacarpal and inject 1cc of anesthetic. (See *Choosing injection sites for a digital nerve block of the finger,* page 24.) Advance the needle almost to the palmar skin and inject another 1 ml. Lastly, bring the needle to the dorsal surface and inject another 1 ml of anesthetic. Repeat the procedure on the opposite side of the finger.

■ Wait for the nerve block to work before beginning the procedure. The maximum effect should occur in 5 to 15 minutes.

### Postprocedure patient teaching

■ Tell the patient that full sensation usually returns within 2 hours.

■ Urge the patient to contact you if he experiences changes in sensation lasting longer than 2 hours or notices signs or symptoms of infection, including increasing redness, swelling, pain, and warmth; cloudy yellow, green, or brown drainage; opening of the wound; foul odor; a red streak from the wound area; or fever.

### Complications

■ Ice or ethyl chloride blistering is prevented by avoiding excessive freezing.

■ After a digital nerve block, necrosis is extremely rare but may occur if epinephrine is used or if a circumferential block is administered. If the digit turns blue or black or becomes cold to the

## Choosing injection sites for a digital nerve block of the finger

The first illustration below shows the positions of the digital nerves around the bone in the finger. The second illustration shows the injection sites for a digital nerve block of the finger. Appropriate injection sites include the web spaces adjacent to the base of the metacarpal bone of the finger.

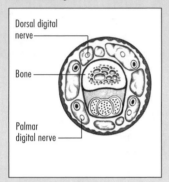

Dorsal digital nerve

Bone

Palmar digital nerve

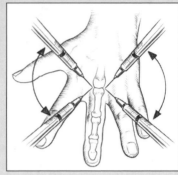

touch, have the patient call your facility immediately.

### Special considerations

■ EMLA is indicated for use on intact skin when required penetration is less than or equal to 5 mm. EMLA penetrates more quickly in diseased tissues and is contraindicated for use on mucous membranes and genitalia. The duration of action of EMLA is 2 hours after removal of the agent.

■ Ice or ethyl chloride is useful for quick procedures, such as skin tag clipping and before injecting a local anesthetic, because its duration of action is less than 3 seconds.

■ An anesthetic without a vasoconstrictor is used for poorly vascularized, infected areas and for immunocompromised patients. The addition of sodium bicarbon-

ate will significantly reduce the anesthetic's initial burning sensation.

■ An anesthetic with a vasoconstrictor, such as epinephrine, is best used for a clean wound in a highly vascular area to reduce bleeding and systemic absorption.

■ Topical anesthesia is indicated for nosebleeds and eye injuries and before painful procedures on mucous membranes.

■ Topical lidocaine starts working in under 5 minutes. Ophthalmic tetracaine is indicated before examination of an eye injury and has an onset of action of 5 to 8 minutes. These drugs readily penetrate mucous membranes. Topical phenylephrine can also cause vasoconstriction. Most topical anesthetics have a duration of action of 30 to 45 minutes.

- Duration of anesthesia for a nerve block is 30 minutes to 1 hour.

## Documentation

- Before performing topical, local, or digital nerve block anesthesia, document any abnormal physical findings or prior nerve damage on the consent form. Have the patient initial the comments and sign the form to signify acknowledgment of preprocedural abnormalities. In the chart, the preprocedural and postprocedural notes must include an evaluation of potentially affected function, range of motion, and sensation.
- Record the type and amount of anesthetic used and a summary of the procedure.

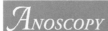

## ANOSCOPY

*CPT code*
46600  *Anoscopy*

## Overview

Anoscopy is the direct visualization of the anus with the use of a speculum. This procedure is performed to diagnose and evaluate diseases of the perianal and distal anal canal. Anoscopes are tubular metal or plastic instruments about 2¾″ (7 cm) long and ¾″ (2 cm) in diameter. Some have built-in fiberoptic light sources; others require an external light source.

## Indications

- To evaluate perianal or anal pain, hemorrhoids, rectal prolapse, rectal bleeding, or abnormality in the anal canal on digital examination
- To identify perianal abscess or condyloma

## Contraindications

### ABSOLUTE

- Acute cardiovascular problems (anoscopy may stimulate a vasovagal response)
- Anal canal stenosis
- Severe rectal pain

## Preprocedure patient preparation

- Inform the patient that he may feel fullness in the rectal area during the examination.
- Tell the patient that he can resume normal activity after the procedure.

## Equipment

Anoscope with obturator ◆ gloves ◆ drape ◆ water-soluble lubricant or anesthetic ointment (such as 2% lidocaine) ◆ large cotton-tipped applicators

## Procedure

- Explain the procedure to the patient, and address any questions or concerns he may have.

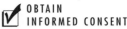
OBTAIN INFORMED CONSENT

- Wash your hands.

- Position the patient in the left lateral decubitus position with knees bent up toward the chest.
- Drape him so that only the perianal area is exposed, to promote privacy.
- Put on gloves.
- Inform the patient that you're going to touch his rectal area.
- Spread the gluteal fold, and examine the external anal structure; observe for fissures, bleeding, or pus.
- Instruct the patient to bear down as if having a bowel movement; observe for hemorrhoids or prolapse of rectal tissue.
- Apply lubricant to your index finger, and perform a digital rectal examination. Rotate your finger inside the rectum, and note irregularities in the contour of the vault.
- Lubricate the anoscope.
- Instruct the patient to take slow, deep breaths to relax the anal sphincter.
- Insert the anoscope, gently angling it toward the umbilicus.
- Remove the obturator.
- Visualize the rectal mucosa (normal mucosa appears pink with visible vessels).
- If fecal matter obstructs the view, remove it with a large cotton-tipped applicator.
- Remove the anoscope gently, and observe the mucosa on withdrawal for abnormalities and potential trauma from the anoscope.

## Postprocedure patient teaching

- If the patient feels light-headed or nauseous, instruct him to remain in the left lateral position for several minutes before sitting up.
- Inform him that slight bleeding is normal because of the possibility of trauma from an abrasion, tearing of the mucosa, or hemorrhoids.
- Urge him to notify you if bleeding lasts for more than 2 days or becomes heavy with clots.
- Advise him that sitz baths twice daily relieve rectal pain and swelling.

## Complications

- Bleeding can occur if a fissure or thrombosed hemorrhoid is irritated during the procedure. Such bleeding warrants ice application, analgesics, and follow-up care to ensure resolution.

✺ COLLABORATION
*Heavy bleeding or other unresolved symptoms may require collaboration with a physician or gastroenterologist.*

## Special considerations

- Use a topical anesthetic lubricant, such as 2% lidocaine, if the patient has evidence of a fissure or can't tolerate the discomfort of anoscope insertion.

## Documentation

- Record the date and time of the anoscopy, the depth of visualization, the appearance of mucosa and abnormalities (such as pus, hemorrhoids, and fissures), and the patient's tolerance of the procedure.

- Use clock referents (such as 12:00 for ventral midline and 6:00 for dorsal midline) to describe abnormal findings.

# ARTHROCENTESIS

### CPT codes
20600 *Arthrocentesis, aspiration, or injection of small joint or bursa (for example, fingers or toes)*
20605 *Arthrocentesis, intermediate joint or bursa (for example, temporomandibular; acromioclavicular; wrist, elbow, or ankle; or olecranon bursa)*
20610 *Arthrocentesis, major joint or bursa (for example, shoulder, hip, knee joint, or subacromial bursa)*

## Overview

Arthrocentesis, a joint puncture, is used to collect fluid for analysis to identify the cause of pain and swelling and to relieve painful joints by draining effusions or instilling medication. When done correctly, it's a simple, safe procedure that causes few complications.

Joint fluid analysis allows differentiation of nontraumatic joint disease (septic joint or crystal-induced arthritis), ligamentous or bony injury (blood or fat globules, or both, in the joint), and hemarthrosis.

Commonly performed simultaneously with arthrocentesis, intra-articular corticosteroid injection can provide immediate relief from pain and swelling in the affected joint. Such injections typically provide only temporary symptomatic relief. The underlying cause of the problem still needs to be identified and treated. Corticosteroids used for injection include betamethasone, hydrocortisone, methylprednisolone, and triamcinolone. No one corticosteroid has proven more effective than another in joint infection. Medication is dependent on prescriber's preference, cost, and previous injection history. High corticosteroid doses and repeated injections cause serious local and systemic complications; therefore, judicious use of the procedure for purposes of corticosteroid administration is essential.

## Indications
- To analyze joint fluid
- To treat overuse injuries and rheumatoid arthritis
- To relieve painful, swollen joints

## Contraindications
### ABSOLUTE
- Bleeding diathesis
- History of fracture, joint surgery, osteoporosis, or sickle cell anemia
- Infection or broken skin present in the overlying area
- Sepsis
- Unavailability of emergency equipment

### RELATIVE
- Anticoagulant therapy
- Age (children or adolescents)
- Diabetes

- Lack of response to previous injections
- Prosthetic joints
- Recent joint injury (unless infection must be ruled out)

## Preprocedure patient preparation

- Explain to the patient that arthrocentesis is typically performed in an office or emergency department and that he can go home after the procedure.
- Reassure the patient that pain is minimal after the procedure is completed. Pain relief may be immediate because of decreased fluid pressure or may occur 12 hours later with steroid injection.

## Equipment

Povidone-iodine and alcohol pads ◆ sterile gloves ◆ sterile drapes ◆ 1% or 2% lidocaine solution without epinephrine or vasocoolant spray ◆ sterile syringes (3, 5, 10, 20, or 30 ml [up to 50 ml for larger joints]) ◆ 25G ⅝" needle ◆ 18G, 20G, or 22G needle ◆ hemostat ◆ sterile 4" × 4" gauze pads ◆ appropriate laboratory collection tubes ◆ corticosteroid

## Procedure

- Explain the procedure to the patient, and address any questions or concerns he may have.

☑ **OBTAIN INFORMED CONSENT**
- Ask the patient whether he has any allergies.
- Wash your hands.

- Place the patient in a comfortable position that allows you to easily access the involved joint, and tell him to slightly flex the joint to be aspirated. Carefully identify landmarks, and mark the exact injection site by indenting the skin with the blunt end of a ballpoint pen or a deeply embedded fingernail—ensuring a marking that won't readily wash away. (See *Choosing an intra-articular injection site*.)
- Prepare the area using 4" × 4" gauze pads and povidone-iodine solution, and let it dry; repeat this three times. Just before injection, wipe the area with an alcohol pad. Povidone-iodine solution in the joint can cause a local inflammatory response.
- Put on gloves.
- Using sterile technique, drape the area and anesthetize it with vasocoolant spray. If appropriate, use the 25G ⅝" needle to infiltrate the subcutaneous skin with the lidocaine solution. Lidocaine may distort landmarks in smaller joints, making aspiration more difficult.
- After applying a local anesthetic, quickly insert the needle through the skin to minimize patient discomfort. Avoid moving the needle from side to side as it enters the joint. For smaller joints, use a 22G needle with a 3- to 5-ml syringe. For larger joints, use an 18G needle and as many large syringes as necessary.
- Aspirate as the needle advances into the joint space or bursal sac until fluid flows freely. Continue aspirating fluid until the joint is empty.

## Choosing an intra-articular injection site

To avoid injury to adjacent structures during intra-articular injection, you need to identify an appropriate injection site at the target joint. Appropriate sites for finger (A) and toe (B) joints include lateral, medial, or dorsal aspects of the joint.

Before puncturing the joint, flex it slightly to open the joint space. Then direct the needle to enter just medial or lateral to the extensor tendon. Avoid deep lateral or medial penetration of the joint to avoid damaging the nerves or blood vessels.

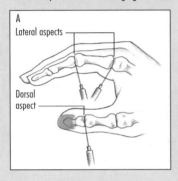

A
Lateral aspects
Dorsal aspect

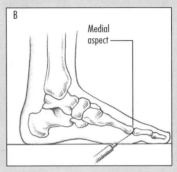

B
Medial aspect

■ To change syringes for continued aspiration or for joint injection, use the two-syringe technique. (See *Using the two-syringe technique,* page 30.) Attach the hemostat at the needle hub, and stabilize the needle while removing the first syringe (to prevent needle rotation while detaching or attaching a syringe). When you've finished collecting fluid, remove the first syringe, replace it with the second syringe that contains the corticosteroid, and inject into the joint space.

■ Place the fluid in the appropriate laboratory tubes and send them for analysis. (See *Understanding synovial fluid analysis,* page 31.)

■ When you've finished, remove the needle and apply pressure and a sterile dressing.

■ As appropriate, perform passive range-of-motion (ROM) exercises on the joint to help distribute the corticosteroid throughout the joint space.

■ Immobilize the joint, and provide adequate analgesia to control pain.

### Postprocedure patient teaching

■ Tell the patient to apply ice, compress the area with an elastic wrap, and elevate the joint to reduce swelling and pain.

■ Remind him to take acetaminophen and anti-inflammatory analgesics as prescribed.

## Using the two-syringe technique

When you're performing joint injection with arthrocentesis, the two-syringe technique can prove valuable. Insert a syringe into the joint and aspirate joint fluid (top illustration). Then attach a hemostat at the needle hub and stabilize the needle while removing the syringe (middle illustration). Replace the syringe containing the joint aspirate with a second syringe containing a corticosteroid (bottom illustration), and inject the drug into the joint space. When the injection is finished, remove the needle and apply pressure and a sterile dressing.

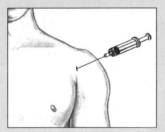

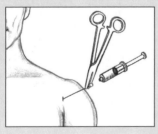

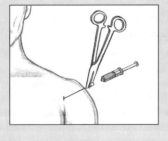

■ Instruct him to rest and immobilize the joint for 24 hours after treatment. Tell him that he can remove the dressing and elastic bandage 24 hours after the procedure. Providing an immobilization device and crutches may encourage him to avoid overuse and weight-bearing activities on the affected joint.

■ Urge the patient to report signs of infection (increasing redness, swelling, pain, and warmth; unusual drainage; opening of the wound; foul odor; a red streak from the wound area; or fever) and warmth or increased pain and stiffness within the joint.

■ Instruct him to return for a follow-up visit within 1 week.

## Complications

■ Infection, the most serious complication, may occur if aseptic technique isn't followed or if the needle passes through an infected area. The patient shouldn't receive a corticocosteroid injection if you suspect infection. Repeated intra-articular corticosteroid injections also can result in necrosis of the joint space and the juxta-articular bone, with subsequent joint destruction and instability. Other complications include tendon rupture, local soft-tissue atrophy, hemarthrosis (bleeding into the joint), and transient nerve palsy. High-dose or repeated corticosteroid injections might have long-term systemic effects.

■ Trauma to the joint may produce hemarthrosis. Arthrocentesis can help identify this condition,

## Understanding synovial fluid analysis

Analysis of synovial fluid helps identify the underlying cause of pain and swelling in a joint. This chart outlines various tests conducted on synovial fluid, common observations or results of those tests, and what each observation or result indicates.

| TEST | OBSERVATIONS | INDICATIONS |
|------|-------------|-------------|
| Color and clarity | ◆ Clear (straw-colored) | ◆ Normal finding or degenerative joint disease |
| | ◆ Cloudy | ◆ Inflammation |
| | ◆ Purulent | ◆ Infection |
| | ◆ Bloody | ◆ Traumatic injury |
| Mucin clot test for viscosity | ◆ Good mucin clot | ◆ Normal |
| | ◆ Denatured mucin | ◆ Inflammation |
| Gram stain | ◆ Positive | ◆ Septic arthritis |
| White blood cell count | ◆ 2,000 to 50,000 cells/$\mu$l | ◆ Inflammation |
| | ◆ More than 50,000 cells/$\mu$l | ◆ Septic joint |
| Glucose level | ◆ Decreased | ◆ Inflammation |
| Microscopy | ◆ Strong negative birefringence (quality of transmitting light unequally in different directions) with needle-shaped crystals (monosodium urate) | ◆ Gout |
| | ◆ Weakly positive birefringence with box-shaped crystals (calcium pyrophosphate dihydrate crystals) | ◆ Pseudogout |
| Culture | ◆ Positive culture | ◆ Infection |

but it can also cause it (rarely) in a patient with a bleeding disorder such as hemophilia. A small amount of blood-tinged fluid may result when the joint has been emptied. Grossly bloody arthrocentesis requires further investigation.

■ Improper needle placement, obstruction of the needle lumen, or misdiagnosis may result in failed arthrocentesis, or dry tap. If a needle is improperly placed, try repositioning it without removing it from the joint. If this doesn't help, you will need to insert the needle in another site. If debris or anatomic structures obstruct the needle lumen, limiting access to fluid, try adjusting the position of the needle or injecting a small amount of the synovial fluid back into the joint to dislodge the obstructing material. Purulent fluid from an infected joint may be too thick to pass through the lumen, requiring the use of a large-lumen needle. Misdiagnosis of an effusion can occur when a chronically inflamed joint undergoes fat replacement and appears distended.

■ An allergic reaction may result from the local anesthetic; a complete history can reduce this risk.

■ Fluid may re-collect in the joint space (arthrocentesis can only provide temporary relief for an acute condition); identification and treatment of the underlying condition can reduce flare-ups.

■ Corticosteroid arthropathy, a condition in which relief from symptoms results in the patient's overuse of the joint, can cause further injury.

## Special considerations

■ Drain the joint completely. If the flow stops, the joint may be empty or the needle lumen obstructed. To ensure the joint is empty, retract the needle slightly, decrease the pressure applied for aspiration and, if you suspect obstruction, reinject a small amount of fluid into the joint to remove obstruction from the needle lumen itself.

■ The patient shouldn't receive corticosteroid injections more than three times per year; more frequent injections may cause cartilage damage, systemic effects, and avascular necrosis.

■ When performing arthrocentesis for culture and sensitivity studies, make sure you don't introduce lidocaine into the joint space because it kills bacteria, possibly altering test results. Change needles between lidocaine injection and joint penetration.

■ If the patient may have gouty arthritis, examine the fluid for crystals under polarized light.

■ The presence of fat cells in joint fluid indicates a fracture.

■ For corticosteroid injection, avoid direct contact with the skin or subcutaneous tissue to prevent skin atrophy. For an intrabursal injection, inject the corticosteroid around — not into — the tendon or ligament. Because direct injection can lead to tendon or ligament rupture, reposition the needle if it meets resistance.

## Documentation

■ Before performing arthrocentesis, document any abnormal physical findings on the consent form and have the patient initial the comments and sign the form to signify acknowledgment of preprocedural abnormalities. In the chart, the preprocedural and postprocedural note must include an evaluation of function, ROM, and neurosensory testing (such as two-point discrimination).

■ Provide a detailed description of the site before and after the procedure, and record the name of the anesthetic used as well as the dosage administered, the appearance and amount of fluid removed, whether a culture was sent, the patient's reaction to the procedure, medications ordered, the time frame for follow-up evaluation, and instructions given to the patient.

# $\mathcal{A}$UDIOMETRY TESTING

***CPT codes***
92551 *Audiologic screening test, pure tone, air only*
92552 *Audiometry, threshold test, pure tone, air only*

## Overview

A hearing screening is simply a pass or fail test that gives a general idea of whether a patient has some type of hearing loss. In audiometry testing, hearing thresholds are also recorded. It's used for most age-groups older than age 6 months as an important screening tool, considering that one in every 15 people in the United States experiences some degree of hearing loss. Audiometry uses a standard pure-tone audiometer to present stimuli through earphones (air conduction testing) or through a bone conduction vibrator (bone conduction testing). The pure-tone threshold measurement finds the lowest level that the person can hear each tone about 50% of the time and uses this data to form an audiogram. By quantifying the patient's ability to hear various intensities and frequencies, the audiogram assists the health care provider in determining the type of hearing disorder that exists and assesses the degree of impairment. Audiometry requires specialized training, an audiometer, and the cooperation of the patient.

## Indications

- To evaluate hearing loss
- To screen patients who are exposed to environmental factors that contribute to hearing loss, such as those working in a noisy setting (for example, with loud machinery or explosives), those who listen to music at a high volume, and those with allergies or who smoke
- To assess complaints of tinnitus
- To assess speech and language developmental delays in children and infants
- To assess children who are experiencing poor academic progress
- To assess elderly patients with unexplained behavior changes
- To assess infants at high risk for a hearing deficit

## Contraindications

**ABSOLUTE**
- Cerumen obstruction
- Otitis externa

**RELATIVE**
- Children younger than age 6 months

## Preprocedure patient preparation

- Tell the patient that there should be no discomfort associated with this procedure.

## Equipment

Otoscope ◆ appropriately sized earphone speaker or earplug ◆ audiometry tool with a minimal decibel frequency range of 500 to 4,000 Hz ◆ quiet room

## Procedure

■ Explain the procedure to the patient or his parents, and address any questions or concerns they may have.

■ Wash your hands.

■ Perform the screening in a quiet area with the patient sitting comfortably upright but not looking at you or the audiometer.

■ Have the patient remove any jewelry or glasses that could interfere with earphone application.

■ Instruct the patient to indicate when a tone is heard by raising a hand.

■ Using an otoscope, inspect the ear for evidence of infection or obstruction.

■ Place an earphone speaker over the external os, and check to be certain that nothing (including the tragus) covers the opening. The earphone or earplug must have a tight seal.

■ If using a handheld audiometry tool, obtain a good seal by gently pulling the pinna back for children and up and back for adults.

■ If one ear is known to have better hearing, begin testing with that ear.

■ Observe for each tone indicator and the patient's response. Repeat the test in the opposite ear.

■ Testing is typically repeated four times, until the patient reproduces the same response at least 50% of the time. This is the result entered on the audiogram. *Note:* Some audiometers require the results to be

sent to the company and analyzed by specially trained personnel. Typical results are as follows:
– Less than or equal to 20 dB is normal hearing.
– 21 to 40 dB is a mild hearing loss.
– 41 to 55 dB is a moderate hearing loss.
– 56 to 70 dB is a moderately severe hearing loss.
– 71 to 90 dB is a severe hearing loss.
– Greater than or equal to 91 dB signifies a profound hearing loss.

■ Record and interpret the results.

✿ **COLLABORATION**
*If results aren't within normal limits, ask the patient to return for repeat testing. If results aren't persistently within normal limits at that time, refer the patient to an audiologist.*

■ Review the results and implications with the patient or his parents.

## Postprocedure patient teaching

■ Explain the results of audiometry testing and the epidemiology if a problem is present. Discuss choices for therapeutic interventions and expected resolution, including a time frame. Instruct the patient or his parents of the need for follow-up care and evaluation. Be sure to specify the date and health care provider's name, phone number, and address for each needed referral or follow-up evaluation.

■ Teach the patient how to avoid overexposure to loud noise.

■ Instruct the patient to call you if any problems develop, although none are expected.

## Complications
■ None known

## Special considerations
■ Review environmental variables that affect hearing, such as allergies, smoke, and exposure to loud noises, with the patient or his parents.
■ *Note:* Audiometers range from semiautomatic to fully automatic. Some models (such as the Castle RA500 audiometer) repeat frequencies that evoke an inconsistent response, analyze data as the test is performed, and even provide categorized results to guide the health care provider.

## Documentation
■ Record the reason for audiometry testing.
■ Provide the number, type, and frequency of problems reported.
■ Note previous treatment modalities.
■ Record audiogram findings.

### *A*URICULAR HEMATOMA EVACUATION

*CPT codes*
69000 *Draining external ear, abscess, or hematoma, simple*

69005 *Draining external ear, abscess or hematoma, complicated*

## Overview
Auricular hematoma evacuation is the drainage of a blood collection in the pinna followed by compression to prevent further bleeding. An auricular hematoma may result from direct or indirect trauma to the external ear. Early intervention prevents further damage to the ear tissue, the infection process, and preventable permanent ear deformities. If the hematoma site is too large, a referral to a plastic surgeon may be considered.

## Indications
■ To alleviate local pressure or discomfort
■ To assess vascular compromise causing a blue tint and swelling of the auricle

## Contraindications
ABSOLUTE
■ Laceration or complex injury

## Preprocedure patient preparation
■ Inform the patient that the procedure may produce some discomfort and that it's crucial for him to stay still during the procedure.
■ Explain to the patient that full recovery from this procedure may take up to 2 weeks.

## Applying an auricular pressure dressing

If you're unable to apply a pressure dressing with tape alone, consider suturing it in place. To do this, first apply the antibiotic ointment to the incision. Form two rolls, using 2″ gauze, each rolled to ½″ (1.3 cm) thickness. Then take a straight suture needle and 4-0 or 5-0 nylon suture material, and pass it through the anterior roll and then through the ear (close to the incision) in an anterior-to-posterior direction. Pass the needle back and forth through the posterior roll twice before piercing the ear in the posterior-to-anterior direction.

After again passing through the anterior roll, ensure that both rolls are snug against the ear and tie the suture in place to form a pressure dressing on the anterior and posterior surfaces of the auricular hematoma site.

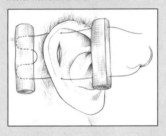

## Equipment

1% lidocaine anesthetic ◆ #15 scalpel blade with handle ◆ 18G or 20G needle and 3-ml syringe ◆ 30G needle and 3-ml syringe ◆ curved hemostat ◆ sterile towels or drape ◆ povidone-iodine topical antiseptic ◆ gloves (sterile and unsterile) ◆ 4″ × 4″ gauze pads ◆ 2″ gauze roll ◆ nonadherent gauze ◆ antibiotic ointment (such as bacitracin) ◆ protective eyewear ◆ tape

◆ 4-0 or 5-0 nylon sutures with a straight suture needle (optional)

## Procedure

■ Explain the procedure to the patient, and address any questions or concerns he may have.

☑ OBTAIN INFORMED CONSENT

■ Wash your hands.

■ Remind the patient that it's crucial that he remain still during the procedure.

■ Position the patient in the supine position with the injured ear accessible.

■ Drape the patient's head to expose the injured ear only.

■ Assess the ear and hematoma site for size, consistency, tenderness, drainage, and color.

■ Put on unsterile gloves and protective eyewear.

■ Clean the ear site using 4″ × 4″ gauze pads and antiseptic solution.

■ Dispose of gloves, and put on sterile gloves.

■ Inject the hematoma site anteriorly, posteriorly, and directly with 1% lidocaine anesthetic using a 30G needle and a 3-ml syringe.

■ Insert an 18G or 20G needle attached to a 3-ml syringe into the hematoma, and aspirate.

■ If unable to aspirate with the syringe and needle, make a 4- to 5-mm incision into the hematoma site with #15 scalpel with a handle. The more time that has passed since the trauma, the greater the likelihood of needing multiple incisions for evacuation.

■ Use a curved hemostat and manual pressure to probe, release, and expel remaining fluid and clots.

■ When the area is fully evacuated, cover the incision site with antibiotic ointment, then a nonadherent gauze, and apply a dry sterile auricular pressure dressing (with 2″ gauze and roll to ½″ [1.3 cm] thickness) on each side of the ear and tape securely.

■ Prescribe analgesics and antibiotics (such as cephalexin or cefadroxil) as indicated, for 5 to 7 days.

■ Keep the pressure dressing in place for 48 to 72 hours postprocedure.

■ Reevaluate the hematoma site in 48 to 72 hours.

## Postprocedure patient teaching

■ Tell the patient that some bleeding can be expected for 24 hours.

■ Instruct the patient to follow up with you in 48 hours for reevaluation of the site and further postprocedure instructions.

■ Tell the patient to contact you immediately if he experiences bleeding or drainage from the site, a foul odor, fever, or an increase in pain or discomfort.

■ Tell the patient to use cool compresses or ice on the surrounding area for comfort.

■ Inform the patient that Tylenol with Codeine No. 3 may be taken if necessary for the first day. After that, regular acetaminophen should be adequate. If pain persists, he should call you.

■ Provide dressing instructions to the patient, and emphasize that

pressure must be maintained to prevent bleeding and scarring.

## Complications

■ Cosmetic scarring or auricular deformity may occur, depending on the size of the hematoma, procedure difficulties, or inadequate postprocedure site care.

■ Infection risk is minimized by aseptic technique and prophylactic antibiotics as needed.

## Special considerations

■ If you're unable to apply a pressure dressing with tape, place 4-0 or 5-0 nylon sutures through the dressing and the pinna and tie to hold the pressure dressing in place. (See *Applying an auricular pressure dressing.*)

## Documentation

■ Document the indications for auricular hematoma evacuation.

■ Record an assessment of the ear preprocedure and postprocedure, including changes in function or appearance.

■ Document the type of procedure used and postprocedure patient status (site evaluation, pain tolerance, and temperature).

■ List any instructions given to the patient and any medications prescribed.

■ Document the patient's understanding of postprocedure instructions, such as dressing change procedure and when to schedule an appointment.

# $\mathcal{B}$

## $\mathcal{B}$ACTERIAL ENDOCARDITIS PROPHYLAXIS

**CPT code**
*No specific code has been assigned.*

## Overview

Bacterial endocarditis prophylaxis is prescribing or administering antibiotics before certain procedures to minimize a patient's risk of contracting bacterial endocarditis, an infection that results in vegetative growths on the heart valves or the wall of the endocardium. Prophylaxis may be necessary before surgery or dental work that increases the chance of bacteria entering the bloodstream. Patients who are at high risk for the disease should also receive prophylactic treatment. (See *Conditions that increase the risk of endocarditis.*) The recommendations listed here are from the American Heart Association as revised in 1997.

The disease can occur in acute or subacute forms. Acute endocarditis typically affects functional valves and results from infection with staphylococci; subacute endocarditis tends to occur in a previously damaged endothelium and typically results from infection with *Streptococcus viridans.* Appropriate therapy usually reduces such signs as fever and results in a return to negative blood cultures.

Bacterial endocarditis can also be classified as native or prosthetic valve. (A form of the disease can also develop in I.V. drug abusers, but the infecting organism in these cases isn't clear, and such patients generally don't receive endocarditis prophylaxis.) Native valve endocarditis affects the mitral valve more often than the aortic valve. It typically results from infection with streptococci, although staphylococci, enterococci, and (rarely) fungi can also cause this form of the disease. Only 60% to 80% of patients with native valve endocarditis have identified cardiac lesions. Prosthetic valve endocarditis can develop in any patient who has an intravascular prosthesis such as a prosthetic valve. The incidence is highest during the first 6 to 12 months after valve replacement. Regardless of whether the patient has a mechanical or bioprosthetic valve or has the prosthe-

## Conditions that increase the risk of endocarditis

Certain cardiac conditions increase the risk of endocarditis as well as the likelihood of a poor outcome from the disease. Patients at high risk include those with:

◆ a prosthetic cardiac valve (bioprosthetic or homograft)
◆ previous bacterial endocarditis
◆ complex cyanotic congenital heart disease (single ventricle malfunction states, such as tricuspid atresia, transposition of the great vessels, or tetralogy of Fallot)
◆ a surgically constructed systemic-pulmonary shunt or conduit

◆ mitral valve prolapse with murmur present or mitral insufficiency (or both)
◆ hypertrophic cardiomyopathy.
    Patients at moderate risk include those with:
◆ many congenital cardiac malformations not included in the high-risk categories
◆ acquired valvular dysfunction
◆ cardiomyopathy
◆ mitral valve prolapse with insufficiency or thickened redundant leaflets.

sis in the mitral or aortic position, the infection rate typically remains constant. However, the prosthesis makes curing the disease more difficult, increasing the importance of prevention.

## Indications

■ To prevent infection during traumatic procedures, particularly those involving epithelial surfaces colonized by flora (such as the oropharynx, the GI and genitourinary tracts, and the skin)
■ To prevent infection during procedures that involve the prostate or female reproductive tract (such as cystoscopy, urethral dilatation, and catheterization)
■ To prevent infection during procedures that can cause transient bacteremia, such as certain dental, diagnostic, and therapeutic procedures (See *When to administer endocarditis prophylaxis,* page 40.)

## Contraindications

ABSOLUTE
■ Allergy or hypersensitivity to any component of the antibiotic (an alternative drug should be used)

## Preprocedure patient preparation

■ Explain to the patient his specific risks for endocarditis, the seriousness of the disease, and the usefulness of prophylactic treatment.

## Procedure

■ Obtain a complete history from the patient, including any past or present heart disease, previous cardiac surgery, and drug allergies.
■ Perform a comprehensive cardiovascular examination, including special maneuvers to elicit heart murmurs.
■ Review available records for results of echocardiograms, electrocardiograms, and operations.

# When to administer endocarditis prophylaxis

Endocarditis prophylaxis is recommended for many — but not all — dental, respiratory, genitourinary, and GI procedures. Listed below are procedures that call for prophylaxis and those that don't.

## PROPHYLAXIS RECOMMENDED

### Dental*
◆ Dental extractions
◆ Periodontal procedures
◆ Dental implant placement and reimplantation of avulsed teeth
◆ Endodontic instrumentation or surgery beyond the apex
◆ Subgingival placement of antibiotic fibers or strips
◆ Initial placement of orthodontic bands (but not brackets)
◆ Intraligamentary local anesthetic injections
◆ Prophylactic teeth cleaning or implants in which bleeding is expected

### Genitourinary
◆ Prostatic surgery
◆ Cystoscopy
◆ Urethral dilatation

### GI**
◆ Sclerotherapy for esophageal varices
◆ Esophageal stricture dilation
◆ Endoscopic retrograde cholangiography with biliary obstruction
◆ Biliary tract surgery
◆ Surgery that involves the intestinal mucosa

### Respiratory
◆ Tonsillectomy or adenoidectomy
◆ Surgery that involves respiratory mucosa
◆ Rigid bronchoscopy

## PROPHYLAXIS NOT RECOMMENDED

### Dental
◆ Restorative dentistry
◆ Local anesthetic injections (nonintraligamentary)
◆ Intracanal endodontic treatment
◆ Placement of rubber dams
◆ Postoperative suture removal
◆ Placement of removable prosthodontic or orthodontic appliances
◆ Oral impressions
◆ Oral radiographs
◆ Orthodontic appliance adjustment

### Cardiovascular
◆ Implanted cardiac pacemakers, defibrillators, and coronary stents
◆ Cardiac catheterization and angioplasty

### Genitourinary
◆ Vaginal hysterectomy***
◆ Vaginal delivery*** or cesarean delivery
◆ Urethral catheterization, uterine dilatation and curettage, therapeutic abortion, sterilization procedures, and insertion or removal of intrauterine devices (in uninfected tissue)

### GI
◆ Transesophageal echocardiogram
◆ Endoscopy***

### Respiratory tract
◆ Endotracheal intubation
◆ Flexible bronchoscopy***
◆ Tympanostomy tube insertion

---

\* Prophylaxis is recommended for high- and moderate-risk cardiac conditions.
\*\* Prophylaxis is recommended for high-risk patients and is optional for moderate-risk patients.
\*\*\* Prophylaxis is optional for high-risk patients.

Source: *Prevention of Bacterial Endocarditis* (1997). American Heart Association.

- Determine the patient's risk for developing endocarditis by evaluating the risk of the procedure coupled with the nature of the existing heart disease.
- Discuss the risk of developing endocarditis and the benefits of antibiotic prophylaxis with the patient.
- Prescribe the appropriate antibiotic regimen based on the type of procedure the patient will undergo. (See *Endocarditis prophylaxis regimens,* pages 42 and 43.)

## Postprocedure patient teaching

- Tell the patient to take the complete prescribed dosage of medication within the prescribed time before the procedure.
- Discuss the signs and symptoms of an allergic reaction to the prescribed antibiotic, and instruct the patient to notify you if any occur.
- Instruct the patient to carry a wallet card from the American Heart Association that will notify other health care providers of his risk of bacterial endocarditis.

## Complications

- Instruct the patient that if he develops an allergic reaction to the prescribed antibiotic, he should stop taking the medication and contact you at once.

## Special considerations

- For genitourinary procedures, consider the most likely pathogen and prescribe an antibiotic specific to that pathogen.

- Consider prescribing antibiotics prophylactically for low-risk procedures involving the lower respiratory, GI, or genitourinary tract for patients with prosthetic heart valves, surgically constructed cardiac shunts, or a history of endocarditis.
- The 1997 revision of the guidelines of the American Heart Association states that patients with certain conditions are no longer considered to be at increased risk and don't need prophylactic measures beyond those for the general population. These patients include those with isolated atrial defect; surgical repair of atrial septal defect, ventricular septal defect, or patent ductus arteriosus (without residual effects beyond 6 months); previous coronary artery bypass graft surgery; mitral valve prolapse without valvar regurgitation; benign heart murmurs; previous Kawasaki syndrome or rheumatic fever without valvar dysfunction; or cardiac pacemakers or implanted defibrillators.

## Documentation

- Document the type of procedure and the patient's risk factors for endocarditis.
- Thoroughly document the cardiac examination, including a description of heart murmurs.
- List the type and amount of antibiotic prescribed.
- Note the patient's response to teaching.
- Document the procedure and follow-up assessment, noting the presence or lack of infection.

# Endocarditis prophylaxis regimens

This table details the type of medication and regimen for various types of patients requiring endocarditis prophylaxis. Note that the total children's dose shouldn't exceed the adult dose, and cephalosporins shouldn't be used in patients with immediate-type hypersensitivity reaction (such as urticaria, angioedema, or anaphylaxis) to penicillins.

| PATIENT TYPE | MEDICATION | REGIMEN |
|---|---|---|
| **For dental, oral, respiratory tract, and esophageal procedures (no follow-up dose recommended)** | | |
| Requires standard prophylaxis | amoxicillin | Adults: 2 g; children: 50 mg/kg P.O. 1 hour before procedure |
| Can't take medications by mouth | ampicillin | Adults: 2 g I.M. or I.V.; children 50 mg/kg I.M. or I.V. within 30 minutes before procedure |
| Allergic to penicillin | clindamycin OR cephalexin or cefadroxil OR azithromycin or clarithromycin | Adults: 600 mg; children: 20 mg/kg P.O. 1 hour before procedure Adults: 2 g; children: 50 mg/kg P.O. 1 hour before procedure Adults: 500 mg; children: 50 mg/kg P.O. 1 hour before procedure |
| Allergic to penicillin and can't take medications by mouth | clindamycin OR cefazolin | Adults: 600 mg; children: 20 mg/kg I.V. within 30 minutes before procedure Adults: 1 g; children: 25 mg/kg I.M. or I.V. within 30 minutes before procedure |
| **For genitourinary and GI (excluding esophageal) procedures** | | |
| High risk | ampicillin plus gentamicin | Adults: ampicillin 2 g I.M. or I.V. plus gentamicin 1.5 mg/kg (not to exceed 120 mg) within 30 minutes of starting procedure; 6 hours later, ampicillin 1 g I.M. or I.V. or amoxicillin 1 g P.O. Children: ampicillin 50 mg/kg I.M. or I.V. (not to exceed 2 g) plus gentamicin 1.5 mg/kg within 30 minutes of starting procedure; 6 hours later, ampicillin 25 mg/kg I.M. or I.V. or amoxicillin 25 mg/kg P.O. |

**Endocarditis prophylaxis regimens** *(continued)*

| PATIENT TYPE | MEDICATION | REGIMEN |
|---|---|---|
| **For genitourinary and GI (excluding esophageal) procedures** *(continued)* | | |
| High risk and allergic to ampicillin or amoxicillin | vancomycin plus gentamicin | Adults: vancomycin 1 g I.V. over 1 to 2 hours and gentamicin 1.5 mg/kg I.M. or I.V. (not to exceed 120 mg) completed within 30 minutes of starting procedure<br>Children: vancomycin 20 mg/kg I.V. over 1 to 2 hours plus gentamicin 1.5 mg/kg I.M. or I.V. completed within 30 minutes of starting procedure |
| Moderate risk | amoxicillin<br><br>OR<br><br>ampicillin | Adults: amoxicillin 2 g P.O. 1 hour before procedure<br>Children: amoxicillin 50 mg/kg P.O.1 hour before procedure<br>Adults: ampicillin 2 g I.M. or I.V. within 30 minutes of starting procedure<br>Children: ampicillin 50 mg/kg I.M. or I.V. within 30 minutes of starting procedure |
| Moderate risk and allergic to ampicillin or amoxicillin | vancomycin | Adults: vancomycin 1 g I.V. over 1 to 2 hours completed within 30 minutes of starting procedure<br>Children: vancomycin 20 mg/kg I.V. over 1 to 2 hours completed within 30 minutes of starting procedure |

Source: *Prevention of Bacterial Endocarditis* (1997). American Heart Association.

# BARTHOLIN'S GLAND ABSCESS INCISION AND DRAINAGE

***CPT code***
56420 *Incision and drainage of Bartholin's gland abscess*

## Overview

A Bartholin's cyst forms when the gland duct is occluded. The cause of ductal occlusion is unknown, but sources suggest that congenital stenosis or atresia, thickened mucus, or trauma may contribute to accumulated secretions. Small, asymptomatic cysts require no therapy. However, the dilated gland may become infected. Common organisms cultured from infected cysts include *Escherichia coli, Bacteroides* species, *Proteus, Peptostreptococcus,* and *Chlamydia trachomatis;* however, 10% are caused by *Neisseria gonorrhoeae.* Because a sexually transmitted disease (STD) may be the source of the Bartholin's gland abscess, tests for chlamydia and gonorrhea should be performed before treatment is initiated.

Conservative therapy for an acute Bartholin's gland abscess may be sitz baths for 72 hours, although the patient must be informed that spontaneous rupture is commonly accompanied by recurrence. Broad-spectrum antibiotics may be used in early bartholinitis; however, this therapy may delay maturation of the abscess.

After incising and draining a Bartholin's gland abscess, Word catheter insertion is commonly done. The purpose of using the Word catheter is to create a temporary fistulous tract from the Bartholin's gland to the vaginal vestibule to facilitate drainage of the abscess.

## Indications

■ To treat acute, symptomatic Bartholin's gland or abscess
■ To assess tenderness, pain and throbbing of the labia, dyspareunia, and pain when walking or sitting

## Contraindications

### RELATIVE

■ Pregnancy (refer to a gynecologist)

## Preprocedure patient preparation

■ Advise the patient that although the procedure may be uncomfortable, pain relief typically accompanies initial evacuation of purulent fluid.
■ Inform the patient of the alternatives for treatment; show her the Word catheter if incision and drainage will be done.

## Equipment

Disposable scalpel with pointed knife blade ◆ Word catheter ◆ syringe with 2 to 4 ml sterile water ◆ lidocaine 1% and 10-ml syringe ◆ povidone-iodine solution or a dilute Hibiclens solution ◆ 4″ × 4″ gauze sponges ◆ drape ◆ curved hemostat ◆ 25G needle ◆ sterile gloves ◆ cotton-tipped applicator with transport medium ◆ irrigant (peroxide and normal saline mixed 1:1, #16 angiocatheter with inserter needle removed, 5-ml syringe (optional)

### *Equipment preparation*

■ Set up a sterile field with gauze, scalpel, needle, and syringes.
■ Using the 10-ml syringe and 25G needle, draw up 5 to 10 ml of lidocaine.
■ Inflate the Word catheter with 2 to 4 ml of sterile water to ensure that the catheter bulb functions. Deflate the catheter and leave the

syringe attached to the catheter port to lessen manipulation after the catheter is placed.

## Procedure

■ Explain the procedure to the patient, and address any questions or concerns she may have.

☑ **OBTAIN INFORMED CONSENT**

■ Instruct the patient to empty her bladder. Have her undress from the waist down.
■ Wash your hands.
■ Assist the patient to the lithotomy position, and drape the perineum appropriately.
■ Put on sterile gloves; maintain strict asepsis throughout the procedure.
■ Verify that the patient isn't allergic to iodine, and clean the skin near the Bartholin's gland abscess and vaginal introitus with povidone-iodine and 4″ × 4″ gauze in a circular manner from the site outward.
■ Anesthetize with lidocaine along a vertical line at the medial aspect of the abscess by inserting the needle and then slowly infusing as the needle is withdrawn.
■ Stab the scalpel tip into the abscess near the duct opening (usually between the hymenal ring and labia majora at 4:00 or 8:00, near the fourchette). Successful incision will result in the spontaneous release of purulent drainage and be just large enough to allow catheter insertion.
■ Obtain a specimen for culture at this time, if indicated, using the cotton-tipped applicator. Place it in a plastic transport tube, and crush the tip to release the culture medium.
■ Insert a gloved finger into the vaginal opening, positioning your finger medial to the abscess and applying gentle pressure to express all material possible.
■ Gently insert a curved hemostat to aid inspection and to break any septa leading to fluid-filled cavities. Grasp the cyst wall with the hemostat to stabilize the tract opening.
■ Irrigate the cyst cavity with a 1:1 solution of normal saline and peroxide, using the 5-ml syringe with a needleless angiocatheter to perform the irrigation, if necessary.
■ Insert the tip of the Word catheter into the cyst, and inflate the retention balloon with sufficient water (from 2 to 4 ml) to retain the catheter tip inside the cyst. Remove the syringe from the Word catheter's self-sealing port.

➤ **CLINICAL TIP**
*Be sure to maintain pressure on the syringe while verifying that the catheter is inflated enough to stay in place. Without adequate pressure, the catheter will eject fluid into the syringe and slip out of place.*
■ Tuck the catheter tip into the vagina.

## Postprocedure patient teaching

■ Inform the patient that the Word catheter remains in place for 4 to 6 weeks while the cavity heals and that the expected outcome is drainage from the site for up to 6 weeks until complete resolution of the abscess and infection occurs.

- Instruct the patient to return in 1 week for Word catheter and abscess examination.
- Advise the patient to take over-the-counter pain medications, such as ibuprofen (Advil) and acetaminophen (Tylenol), every 4 to 6 hours as necessary to relieve pain. Sitz baths also provide pain relief. Three or four sitz baths a day promote healing while cleaning the area.
- Tell the patient that sexual intercourse may be resumed when tenderness subsides.
- Discuss the etiology and nature of acute abscess with the patient. Advise her that there's an association between abscesses and STDs. Review the necessity for safer-sex practices. Suggest that the patient's partner be examined for STDs before resuming intercourse. Inform the patient of confidential testing options. such as public health clinics and self-testing, as appropriate.
- Instruct the patient to contact the facility if pain increases, discharge increases or changes in color, fever is greater than 100.4° F (38° C), or bleeding from cavity or catheter occurs.

## Complications

COLLABORATION
*Overinflation of the Word catheter bulb may cause pressure necrosis of the cyst wall with formation of a chronic defect and requires referral to a gynecologist.*

COLLABORATION
*Recurrence of Bartholin's gland cyst or abscess is an indication for referral to a gynecologist.*

## Special considerations

- When expressing material from the cyst, use gentle pressure only.
- Deflate the catheter bulb only if drainage has stopped or if the bulb is causing discomfort. Reinsertion is difficult after the catheter becomes dislodged.
- For cyst incision and drainage (without inserting a Word catheter), pack the site with iodoform gauze, making sure you leave at least ¼" (0.5 cm) of iodoform gauze protruding from the cavity to allow for easy removal of the gauze later. Half the gauze is generally removed at 24 hours, and half at 48 hours.

COLLABORATION
*Primary Bartholin's cyst in a woman older than age 40 may indicate a neoplastic process and should be referred to a gynecologist for treatment.*

## Documentation

- Record any subjective indications for the procedure, including unilateral swelling of the labia, tenderness, dyspareunia, pain (especially when walking or sitting), and a previous history of Bartholin's cyst or abscess.
- Note all objective findings, such as erythema, acute tenderness, edema, a fluctuant mass located lateral to the vestibule, purulent drainage, and tender and enlarged inguinal nodes.
- Document all physical findings that indicate Bartholin's gland cyst or abscess, carcinoma of Bartholin's gland, STDs, inclusion

cyst, sebaceous cyst, lipoma, or fibroma.

■ Chart the procedure as performed, medications used (amount of lidocaine injected), and how the procedure was tolerated. Record the plan for subsequent follow-up or referral, including the health care provider's name, address, and phone number, and a specific time frame for follow-up.

■ Document patient teaching and the patient's understanding.

## *B*IOPSY, ELLIPTICAL EXCISION

### CPT codes
*Note:* Precise code depends on lesion size.

11400 to 11406 *Excision of benign lesions on trunk, arms, or legs*
11420 to 11426 *Excision of benign lesions on scalp, neck, hands, feet, or genitalia*
11600 to 11606 *Excision of malignant lesions on trunk, arms, or legs*
11620 to 11626 *Excision of malignant lesions on scalp, neck, hands, feet, or genitalia*

### Overview
In an elliptical excision (also called fusiform excision), the health care provider can remove a skin lesion too large for a cutaneous punch and then suture the area closed, leaving behind a linear scar (larger lesions require a different form of

excision and require skin flaps or grafts for closure). The location of the incision usually depends on the location of natural skin tension lines, which correspond with wrinkle lines. If such lines aren't readily apparent, gently pinching the skin in several directions should bring them out (this technique may not work with children and adolescents).

The goal of such surgery is to remove the lesion and leave as small a cosmetic defect as possible by following skin tension lines and, for lesions on the face, facial expressions. When deciding where to make the excision, the health care provider must consider the depth of the skin; the impact of the excision on adjacent structures; the length, width, and orientation of the resulting scar; and the scar's effect on function. Placement of a shoulder incision, for example, depends more on creating a scar that won't pull apart than on appearance. Ideally, the procedure will transform the oval-shaped wound left by the excision into a thin-line closure.

### Indications
■ To excise suspected melanoma
■ To remove lesions too large for punch biopsy

### Contraindications
**ABSOLUTE**
■ Lesion on eyelid, lip, face, or genitalia
■ Suspected infection

**RELATIVE**

■ Tension on the incision line (such as on joint or scalp wounds)
■ Coagulopathy impairing hemostasis
■ Deep lesions
■ Allergy to anesthetic

## Preprocedure patient preparation

■ Discuss the procedure with the patient, including the location of the excision and what the resulting scar may look like.

## Equipment

Marker ♦ sterile gloves ♦ sterile drape ♦ mask ♦ protective eyewear ♦ antiseptic solution ♦ 2″ × 2″ or 4″ × 4″ gauze pads ♦ anesthetic such as lidocaine ♦ #11 scalpel ♦ straight or curved iris scissors ♦ forceps or hook ♦ specimen container with 10% formalin ♦ electrocautery unit ♦ sutures ♦ suture needles (see *Indications for suture materials*) ♦ 3-ml syringe ♦ 25G or 27G needle ♦ antibiotic ointment ♦ nonadherent dressing ♦ tape

## Procedure

■ Explain the procedure to the patient, and address any questions or concerns he may have.

☑ **OBTAIN INFORMED CONSENT**

■ Note the area to be excised in a circle at its clinical margins. Imagine a concentric circle around the first circle that includes the margin for normal skin. Use the marker to draw a final ellipse that's three times as long as it is wide.

■ Wash your hands, put on sterile gloves and a mask, and use protective eyewear.

■ Verify that the patient isn't allergic to local anesthetics and iodine.

■ Clean the area in a circular motion from the site outward with antiseptic solution.

■ Draw up the anesthetic for injection.

■ Using a syringe and a 25G to 27G needle, inject in a ring to obtain field anesthesia. Insert the needle with the anesthetic agent at a 45-degree angle.

■ Ask the patient whether he notices any change in sensation. If he reports pain, indicating direct contact with the nerve, withdraw the needle 1 mm.

■ Aspirate to make sure there's no blood return. If there is, the needle is in a blood vessel. Withdraw the needle slightly, and redirect it in another area.

■ Inject 1 to 2 ml of lidocaine while partially withdrawing the needle. Then redirect the needle across the surface, advance it, and inject another 0.5 ml while withdrawing the needle. This method distributes the anesthetic uniformly, providing the optimal effect. Make sure that you anesthetize beyond the demarcated margins in anticipation of undermining.

■ Massage the area gently, and wait 5 to 15 minutes for the optimal effect to occur.

■ Use a gauze pad to apply antiseptic to the area, starting at the center and spiraling outward. Then drape the area to allow a clear view of the surgical site.

## Indications for suture materials

Sutures can be absorbable or nonabsorbable. Absorbable sutures eventually dissolve. Because the body is unable to dissolve nonabsorbable sutures, they must be removed. The chart below outlines various types of suture material and their indications for use.

| TYPE OF SUTURE | INDICATIONS FOR USE |
|---|---|
| **Absorbable** | |
| Plain gut | Superficial vessels and rapid-healing subcutaneous tissues (rarely used due to its high tissue reactivity) |
| Chromic catgut | Oral mucosa, vermilion border |
| Polyglycolic acid | Superficial closure of skin and mucosa |
| **Nonabsorbable** | |
| Silk | Tying off blood vessels |
| Nylon | Use and size of suture vary with location of wound: <br>◆ 6-0 for eyelids and face <br>◆ 5-0 for forehead, neck, and other delicate skin <br>◆ 4-0 for neck, scalp, extremities, and back <br>◆ 3-0 for running suture of scalp. |

■ Hold the scalpel like a pencil at a 90-degree angle, with the anterior belly of the blade in contact with the previously marked line. Apply three-point traction with the other hand, using firm, confident, vertical pressure at the corner of the ellipse. (See *Using three-point traction*, page 50.)

■ Press down gently with the scalpel, and draw it through the skin in one firm, constant stroke, keeping the blade perpendicular to the skin surface (to avoid beveling the wound and margins). You don't have to cut through the skin's full thickness with a single stroke, but make sure you can see upper subcutaneous fat before trying to remove the specimen.

■ Rarely, you may encounter a highly active blood vessel. If this happens, remove the blade and cauterize the affected site before continuing.

■ After making the incisions, use straight or curved iris scissors and a forceps or hook, and gently elevate one end of the fusiform ellipse.

■ Insert the scissors through the subcutis, and complete the incision through the subcutis along both sides of the specimen. Undermine the base completely and elevate the specimen. (See *Mastering the undermining technique*, page 51.)

■ Place the specimen in a specimen container.

### Using three-point traction

Making an elliptical incision requires that you maintain firm traction to the skin surface in more than one direction. The illustration below shows how to apply three-point traction to maintain multidirectional traction when making an elliptical incision.

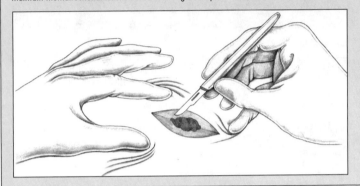

- Cauterize as needed to stop bleeding, but don't cauterize too much or the wound won't heal as quickly.
- Suture the wound closed.
- Apply a thin layer of antibiotic ointment, a nonadherent dressing, and 4″ × 4″ gauze pads; tape securely.

## Postprocedure patient teaching

- Caution the patient to keep the sutures dry.
- Tell him to remove the initial dressing in 24 hours and to replace it with a smaller gauze bandage. Advise him not to place the gauze itself directly over the wound — fibers in the gauze can get trapped in the wound edge, become matted, and delay healing.
- Teach him to clean the site twice per day with soap and water (no rubbing or scrubbing, just pat on and rinse off) and to cover it with antibiotic ointment and a three-layer dressing (triple antibiotic ointment, nonadherent dressing, and gauze followed by tape covering).
- Instruct him to limit his sun exposure, particularly to the affected area, by wearing sunscreen, covering up with protective clothing, and avoiding outdoor activities when the sun is strongest (between 10 a.m. and 3 p.m.).
- Inform the patient that he must return for suture removal. Have him return in 3 to 6 days for a face wound, 7 to 10 days for an ear wound, or 5 to 10 days for a trunk or an extremity wound.
- Urge the patient to notify you promptly if he experiences signs and symptoms of infection, including increasing redness, swelling, pain, and warmth; cloudy yellow, green, or brown drainage; wound opening; foul

## Mastering the undermining technique

Undermining, the technique of freeing the skin from underlying tissues, can decrease tension on the wound edge and is critical for obtaining acceptable cosmetic results after wound repair. Proper undermining minimizes scarring and keloid formation.

The level of undermining that you should perform depends on the location and natural plane of the wound. In general, you'll undermine an area about the size of the widest part of the wound.

### BLUNT UNDERMINING
In blunt undermining (as shown below), advance the scissors with the tips closed and then force them open. This causes blunt dissection of the underlying tissues.

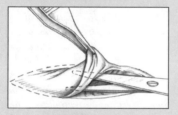

### SHARP UNDERMINING
In sharp undermining (as shown top right), a less frequently used technique, use short, cutting strokes with a scalpel to separate the skin from underlying tissues.

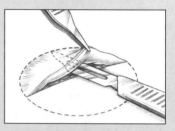

### UNDERMINING LEVEL
The proper undermining level (as shown below) is achieved when the skin is carefully separated from the subcutaneous fat.

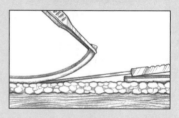

### UNDERMINING TIPS
◆ Keep in mind that undermining increases bleeding. Make sure you can see the source of bleeding before cauterizing it. Cauterizing blindly may damage the surrounding tissue without stopping the bleeding.
◆ Treat the wound edge gently and stay within the subcutaneous fat layer.

odor; a red streak from the site; or fever after 24 hours.

## Complications
■ Infection may be treated with local or systemic antibiotics or antiseptic soaks. It may also require consultation with a physician, a dermatologist, or an infectious disease specialist.

■ Scarring and keloids are minimized with gentle handling and the use of such techniques as undermining and layered suturing.

## Special considerations
**COLLABORATION**
*Refer the patient to a plastic surgeon for facial lesions greater*

*than ¼" (0.5 cm); refer him to a dermatologist for deep lesions.*

■ Tools for marking the lesion before excision include a skin marker (such as the Devon skin marker). It doesn't leave a very dark mark, however, and tends to dry out when the cap is left off. Because of these drawbacks, many health care providers prefer using an indelible marker, although this can leave a permanent mark if the ink isn't completely removed before wound closure.

■ Keep in mind that wounds closed by approximation of the skin edges heal by primary intention.

■ To speed healing and prevent crust formation, cover the wound with an occlusive or a semiocclusive dressing (particularly important for wounds created by a procedure).

## Documentation

■ Before performing an elliptical excision biopsy, document any abnormal physical findings on the consent form. Have the patient initial the comments and sign the form to signify acknowledgment of preprocedural abnormalities. In the chart, the preprocedural and postprocedural notes must include an evaluation of potentially affected function, range of motion, and sensation.

■ Note whether you sent a culture to the laboratory for analysis.

■ Record indications for and details of the procedure. Describe the site before and after the procedure, the type and amount of anesthetic used, the patient's reaction to the procedure, medications ordered, the time frame for follow-up evaluation, and any instructions given to the patient.

# Biopsy, punch

## CPT codes
*Note:* Precise code depends on lesion size.
11200  *Removal of skin tags or multiple fibrocutaneous tags on any area less than or equal to 15 lesions*
11201  *As above, for each additional 10 lesions after the first 15 lesions (code may be listed as many times as needed)*
11400 to 11406  *Excision of benign lesions on trunk, arms, or legs*
11420 to 11426  *Excision of benign lesions on scalp, neck, hands, feet, or genitalia*
11600 to 11606  *Excision of malignant lesions on trunk, arms, or legs*
11620 to 11626  *Excision of malignant lesions on scalp, neck, hands, feet, or genitalia*

## Overview
A skin biopsy is performed to obtain material for pathologic evaluation or to remove a precancerous lesion or one causing the patient discomfort. It can be either incisional (removing only part of a lesion) or excisional (removing the entire lesion). The entire lesion is generally removed if doing so will permit proper healing and an aesthetically acceptable outcome.

For a punch biopsy, a specialized instrument is used to remove a cylindrical, full-thickness skin specimen. It's performed to obtain material for pathologic evaluation and to remove small cutaneous lesions quickly and effectively. Punches are available in sizes ranging from 1.5 to 10 mm and can be permanent or disposable. Disposable punch biopsy instruments are preferable because they're sterile and inexpensive and they don't get dull from repeated use. Because the instrument can only go as deep as the length of the cylinder, a biopsy that must include deeper fat or fascia may require two complete punches. The resulting wound may require suturing. Punch biopsies generally produce an acceptable cosmetic result, provide a deep specimen, and heal rapidly when sutured. However, they require sterile technique and local anesthesia, specimen size is limited by the width and depth of the punch, and the wound may require extra time for suturing.

## Indications

■ To remove a precancerous skin lesion or one causing discomfort
■ To obtain material for pathologic evaluation

## Contraindications

**ABSOLUTE**

■ Suspected cancerous lesion
■ Unknown diagnosis
■ Infection at the biopsy site

## Preprocedure patient preparation

■ Prior to the procedure, obtain from the patient a detailed history and perform a physical examination.

## Equipment

Antiseptic such as 70% isopropyl alcohol or povidone-iodine ◆ gloves ◆ sterile drape ◆ local anesthetic ◆ 25G to 30G ½″ to 1″ needles and 3- to 5-ml syringe ◆ punch, skin hook, blade (such as P2 or P3 blade), or needle ◆ sterile sharp scissors ◆ suture equipment ◆ sterile adhesive strips, such as Steri-Strips or monofilament nylon sutures ◆ three-layer pressure dressing with triple antibiotic ointment ◆ nonadherent pad ◆ gauze ◆ adhesive dressing

## Procedure

■ Explain the procedure to the patient, and address any questions or concerns he may have.

✓ **OBTAIN INFORMED CONSENT**

■ Wash your hands.
■ Verify that the patient isn't allergic to iodine preparations or local anesthetics.
■ Place the patient in a comfortable position that leaves the skin lesion and surrounding area easily accessible.
■ Clean the skin lesion and a 3″ (7.6 cm) area around it with antiseptic solution.
■ Place a sterile drape over the area.
■ Put on gloves.

- Inject the local anesthetic under the lesion, using the 25G or 30G needle to create a wheal.
- Position the punch vertically over the area. Using your non-dominant hand, apply perpendicular tissue traction. This results in an oval rather than a circular defect. (A circular defect may result in a redundant cone of skin, called a "dog-ear," on closure.)
- Push the punch against the skin with firm, steady pressure, and simultaneously twist it clockwise. Continue this until you feel the punch advance slightly, indicating the descent of the punch into the fat layer.
- Withdraw the punch with the column of tissue. Remove the specimen gently to avoid histologic artifacts.
- Use a skin hook or local anesthesia needle to elevate the plug of tissue, and transect the base with a pair of sharp scissors.
- To obtain the best cosmetic result and fastest healing, suture the biopsy site using simple interrupted or vertical mattress sutures. Typically, a 2-mm punch requires one suture; a 4- to 6-mm punch, two sutures; and a 7- to 10-mm punch, three to four sutures. Using 4-0 monofilament nylon sutures and a P2 blade is best for wounds on the extremities and trunk, and using 5-0 and 6-0 monofilament nylon sutures with a P3 blade is best for biopsies taken from the face and anterior neck. If necessary, reinforce the sutures on a wound under tension with sterile adhesive strips.
- Place a three-layer pressure dressing that contains triple antibiotic ointment (Polysporin) on the wound, followed by a nonadherent pad, gauze, and an adhesive dressing overlay.

## Postprocedure patient teaching

- Advise the patient how long the pain will last and how long the wound will take to heal. Pain may be minimal to moderate, and resolution of pain varies with the size of the wound and progression of healing. Tell him to expect bloody to clear yellow drainage in the first 24 to 48 hours.
- Teach the patient how to care for the wound. He should gently clean the biopsy site daily with tap water and soap (with no rubbing or scrubbing) and then apply a small amount of antibiotic ointment, preferably Polysporin rather than an ointment that contains neomycin, which carries a higher risk of allergic reaction. Tell him to continue wound care until the area completely heals.
- Explain that the wound will appear uniformly pink or red when epithelialization is complete. Emphasize that keeping the wound covered and occluded promotes rapid healing and reduces the risk of scarring.
- Advise the patient to minimize activity to prevent bleeding and wound dehiscence, if the punch biopsy site is in an area of tension.
- Teach the patient to examine his skin frequently to detect new or changing lesions.
- Instruct the patient to make a follow-up appointment in 5 to 7 days to remove sutures from the

face or 10 to 14 days to remove sutures from the trunk or extremities. You can also evaluate wound healing and conduct a neurosensory examination, as indicated by depth of injury. Emphasize that even superficial wounds must be evaluated.

■ Instruct the patient to notify you promptly if he develops signs of infection, including increasing redness, swelling, pain, and warmth; cloudy yellow, green, or brown drainage; opening of the wound; foul odor; a red streak leading from the site; or fever after 24 hours. He should be seen in a facility for evaluation.

## Complications

■ Infection may be treated with local or systemic antibiotics and antiseptic soaks. You also may need to refer the patient to a physician, a dermatologist, or an infectious disease specialist.

■ Scarring can be minimized with gentle handling and with the use of skin adhesives and techniques such as undermining.

■ Pain is minimized with local anesthesia and over-the-counter medications, such as acetaminophen or ibuprofen.

## Special considerations

### COLLABORATION
*For deeper lesions, suspected neoplasms, and facial or penile lesions, consult with a dermatologist or refer the patient to one.*

■ If the patient has an atypical-appearing melanocytic lesion, obtain a good specimen for pathology

by performing a deep punch biopsy. If unsure of the diagnosis, consider referral before biopsy to minimize the cost and the number of painful procedures that the patient will experience.

■ Don't keep removing the punch from the biopsy site to check your progress; if you do, the specimen may have histologic artifacts.

■ The pathologist needs an adequate specimen for diagnosis (for example, a specimen that includes the dermis for a dermal lesion). If the pathologist also needs a portion of adjacent normal skin (for example, if the patient has a more complex skin disease such as panniculitis), a wedge-shaped section can provide the larger and deeper specimen needed. You should also provide as much detail about the site as possible.

■ If you can't identify a lesion or don't plan to treat it, don't biopsy it. Instead, refer the patient to someone who may be able to recognize the lesion, possibly saving the patient the discomfort and cost of biopsy.

### COLLABORATION
*If a patient has a lesion that you suspect is skin cancer, refer him to a dermatologist. The dermatologist has the background needed to choose the most appropriate treatment (including excision, radiation therapy, and chemotherapy).*

## Documentation

■ Before performing a punch biopsy, document any abnormal physical findings on the consent form. Have the patient initial the comments and sign the form to signify acknowledgment of preprocedural abnormalities. In the chart, the preprocedural and postprocedural note must include an evaluation of potentially affected function, range of motion, and sensation.

■ Record the indications for the procedure as well as its details, including a thorough description of the site before and after the procedure, the patient's reaction to the procedure, medications ordered, patient instructions given, and the time frame for follow-up evaluation.

## ℬIOPSY, SCISSOR

### CPT codes
*Note:* Precise code depends on lesion size.
11200  *Removal of skin tags or multiple fibrocutaneous tags on any area less than or equal to 15 lesions*
11201  *As above, for each additional 10 lesions after the first 15 lesions (code may be listed as many times as needed)*
11400 to 11406  *Excision of benign lesions on trunk, arms, or legs*
11420 to 11426  *Excision of benign lesions on scalp, neck, hands, feet, or genitalia*
11600 to 11606  *Excision of malignant lesions on trunk, arms, or legs*
11620 to 11626  *Excision of malignant lesions on scalp, neck, hands, feet, or genitalia*

## Overview

A skin biopsy is performed to obtain material for pathologic evaluation or to remove a precancerous lesion or one causing the patient discomfort. It can be either incisional (removing only part of a lesion) or excisional (removing the entire lesion). The entire lesion is generally removed if doing so will permit proper healing and an aesthetically acceptable outcome.

The scissor biopsy, a variant of the shave biopsy, allows removal of small, superficial growths, such as skin tags and filiform warts. It usually doesn't require local anesthesia.

## Indications

■ To remove a precancerous skin lesion or one causing discomfort
■ To obtain material for pathologic evaluation

## Contraindications

**ABSOLUTE**
■ Suspected cancerous lesion
■ Unknown diagnosis
■ Infection at the biopsy site

## Preprocedure patient preparation

■ Prior to the procedure, obtain from the patient a detailed history and perform a physical examination.

## Equipment

Antiseptic such as 70% isopropyl alcohol or povidone-iodine ◆

gloves ◆ forceps ◆ sterile sharp scissors ◆ aluminum chloride (20% to 40%) ◆ triple antibiotic ointment with adhesive dressing

## Procedure

- Explain the procedure to the patient, and address any questions or concerns he may have.

☑ **OBTAIN INFORMED CONSENT**

- Wash your hands.
- Verify that the patient isn't allergic to iodine preparations or local anesthetics.
- Place the patient in a comfortable position that leaves the skin lesion and surrounding area easily accessible.
- Clean the skin lesion and a 3″ (7.6 cm) area around it with antiseptic solution.
- Put on gloves.
- Use forceps to gently grasp and apply traction to the lesion.
- Using sterile sharp scissors, cut the lesion at its base.
- Apply aluminum chloride and pressure to control bleeding.
- Apply triple antibiotic ointment and an adhesive dressing.

## Postprocedure patient teaching

- Advise the patient how long the pain will last and how long the wound will take to heal. Pain may be minimal to moderate, and resolution of pain varies with the size of the wound and progression of healing. Tell him to expect bloody to clear yellow drainage in the first 24 to 48 hours.

- Teach the patient how to care for the wound. He should gently clean the biopsy site daily with tap water and soap (no rubbing or scrubbing) and then apply a small amount of antibiotic ointment, preferably Polysporin rather than an ointment that contains neomycin, which carries a higher risk of allergic reaction. Tell him to continue wound care until the area completely heals.
- Explain that the wound will appear uniformly pink or red when epithelialization is complete. Emphasize that keeping the wound covered and occluded promotes rapid healing and reduces the risk of scarring.
- Teach the patient to examine his skin frequently to detect new or changing lesions.
- Instruct the patient to make a follow-up appointment in 2 days to evaluate wound healing and conduct a neurosensory examination, as indicated by depth of injury. Emphasize that superficial wounds also must be evaluated.
- Instruct the patient to notify you promptly if he develops signs of infection, including increasing redness, swelling, pain, and warmth; cloudy yellow, green, or brown drainage; opening of the wound; foul odor; a red streak leading from the site; or fever after 24 hours. He should be seen in a facility for evaluation.

## Complications

- Infection may be treated with local or systemic antibiotics and antiseptic soaks. You also may need to refer the patient to a physician, a dermatologist, or an infectious disease specialist.

■ Scarring can be minimized with gentle handling and with the use of skin adhesives and techniques such as undermining.

■ Pain is minimized with over-the-counter medications, such as acetaminophen or ibuprofen.

## Special considerations

**COLLABORATION**

*For deeper lesions, suspected neoplasms, and facial or penile lesions, consult with or refer the patient to a dermatologist.*

■ The pathologist needs an adequate specimen for diagnosis (for example, a specimen that includes the dermis for a dermal lesion). If the pathologist also needs a portion of adjacent normal skin (for example, if the patient has a more complex skin disease such as panniculitis), a wedge-shaped section can provide the larger and deeper specimen needed. You should also provide as much detail about the site as possible.

■ If you can't identify a lesion or don't plan to treat it, don't biopsy it. Instead, refer the patient to someone who may be able to recognize the lesion, possibly saving the patient the discomfort and cost of biopsy.

**COLLABORATION**

*If a patient has a lesion that you suspect is skin cancer, refer him to a dermatologist. The dermatologist has the background needed to choose the most appropriate treatment (including excision, radiation therapy, and chemotherapy).*

## Documentation

■ Before performing a scissor biopsy, document any abnormal physical findings on the consent form. Have the patient initial the comments and sign the form to signify acknowledgment of preprocedural abnormalities. In the chart, the preprocedural and post-procedural note must include an evaluation of potentially affected function, range of motion, and sensation.

■ Record the indications for the procedure as well as its details, including a thorough description of the site before and after the procedure, the patient's reaction to the procedure, medications ordered, patient instructions given, and the time frame for follow-up evaluation.

## *B*IOPSY, SHAVE

### *CPT codes*

*Note:* Precise code depends on lesion size.

11200 *Removal of skin tags or multiple fibrocutaneous tags on any area less than or equal to 15 lesions*

11201 *As above, for each additional 10 lesions after the first 15 lesions (code may be listed as many times as needed)*

11300 to 11303 *Shaving of epidermal or dermal lesion on trunk, arms, or legs*

11305 to 11308 *Shaving of epidermal or dermal lesion on scalp, neck, hands, feet, or genitalia*

## Overview

A skin biopsy is performed to obtain material for pathologic evaluation or to remove a precancerous lesion or one causing the patient discomfort. It can be either incisional (removing only part of a lesion) or excisional (removing the entire lesion). The entire lesion is generally removed if doing so will permit proper healing and an aesthetically acceptable outcome.

In a shave biopsy, the specimen doesn't extend deep into the dermis. It's a quick, easy way to remove superficial lesions and is ideal for raised lesions in the epidermis or superficial dermis; if necessary, the procedure can extend down to the subcutis. The procedure is faster than a punch biopsy, generally requires only local anesthesia and topical aluminum chloride to control bleeding, has a favorable cosmetic outcome, and can provide a relatively large specimen. However, a shave biopsy can leave a depressed scar if the biopsy goes too deep.

Most health care providers remove lesions with a sterilized razor blade; some prefer a surgical blade such as the #15 Bard-Parker blade. The inexpensive, sharp, flexible razor blade allows you to curve the blade to match the surface of the lesion by applying pressure with your index finger and thumb. You can then advance the blade across the base of the lesion with a steady sawing motion.

## Indications

- To remove a precancerous skin lesion or one causing discomfort
- To obtain material for pathologic evaluation

## Contraindications

**ABSOLUTE**
- Suspected cancerous lesion
- Unknown diagnosis
- Infection at the biopsy site

## Preprocedure patient preparation

- Prior to the procedure, obtain from the patient a detailed history and perform a physical examination.

## Equipment

Antiseptic such as 70% isopropyl alcohol or povidone-iodine ◆ gloves ◆ sterile drape ◆ local anesthesia ◆ 25G to 30G ½″ to 1″ needles and 3- to 5-ml syringe ◆ razor blade or surgical blade such as #15 Bard-Parker blade ◆ aluminum chloride (20% to 40%) or electrocautery unit ◆ cotton-tipped applicators ◆ triple antibiotic ointment with adhesive dressing

## Procedure

- Explain the procedure to the patient, and address any questions or concerns he may have.

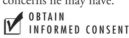 OBTAIN INFORMED CONSENT

- Wash your hands.

## Performing a shave biopsy

When performing a shave biopsy, hold the scalpel so that it's almost parallel to the skin surface, as shown below.

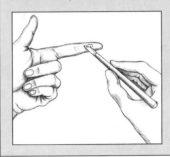

■ Verify that the patient isn't allergic to iodine preparations or local anesthetics.

■ Place the patient in a comfortable position that leaves the skin lesion and surrounding area easily accessible.

■ Clean the skin lesion and a 3″ (7.6 cm) area around it with antiseptic solution.

■ Place a sterile drape over the area.

■ Put on gloves.

■ Inject the local anesthetic under the lesion, using the 25G or 30G needle to create a wheal.

■ Secure the lesion and the surrounding tissue with your nondominant hand while passing the razor blade or scalpel under the lesion. Control the depth of the biopsy with the appropriate angle of entry. (See *Performing a shave biopsy.*)

■ To control bleeding, apply 20% to 40% aluminum chloride directly to the wound with a cotton-tipped applicator or use electrocautery.

■ Apply triple antibiotic ointment and an adhesive dressing.

## Postprocedure patient teaching

■ Advise the patient how long the pain will last and how long the wound will take to heal. Pain may be minimal to moderate, and resolution of pain varies with the size of the wound and progression of healing. Tell him to expect bloody to clear yellow drainage in the first 24 to 48 hours.

■ Teach the patient how to care for the wound. He should gently clean the biopsy site daily with tap water and soap (no rubbing or scrubbing) and then apply a small amount of antibiotic ointment, preferably Polysporin rather than an ointment that contains neomycin, which carries a higher risk of allergic reaction. Tell him to continue wound care until the area completely heals.

■ Explain that the wound will appear uniformly pink or red when epithelialization is complete. Emphasize that keeping the wound covered and occluded promotes rapid healing and reduces the risk of scarring.

■ Teach the patient to examine his skin frequently to detect new or changing lesions.

■ Instruct the patient to make a follow-up appointment in 2 days to evaluate wound healing and conduct a neurosensory examination, as indicated by depth of injury. Emphasize that even superficial wounds must be evaluated.

■ Instruct the patient to notify you promptly if he develops signs of infection, including increasing redness, swelling, pain, and warmth; cloudy yellow, green, or brown drainage; opening of the wound; foul odor; a red streak leading from the site; or fever after 24 hours. He should be seen in the facility for evaluation.

## Complications

■ Infection may be treated with local or systemic antibiotics and antiseptic soaks. You also may need to refer the patient to a physician, a dermatologist, or an infectious disease specialist.

■ Scarring can be minimized with gentle handling and with the use of skin adhesives and such techniques as undermining.

■ Pain is minimized with over-the-counter medications, such as acetaminophen or ibuprofen.

## Special considerations

✿ **COLLABORATION**
*For deeper lesions, suspected neoplasms, and facial or penile lesions, consult with or refer the patient to a dermatologist.*

■ Deeper shave biopsies can result in a permanent depression at the biopsy site.

■ If the patient has an atypical-appearing melanocytic lesion, don't remove it with the shave procedure. Instead, obtain a good specimen for pathology by performing a deep punch biopsy. If unsure of the diagnosis, consider referral before biopsy to minimize the cost and the number of painful

procedures that the patient will experience.

■ The pathologist needs an adequate specimen for diagnosis (for example, a specimen that includes the dermis for a dermal lesion). If the pathologist also needs a portion of adjacent normal skin (for example, if the patient has a more complex skin disease such as panniculitis), a wedge-shaped section can provide the larger and deeper specimen needed. You should also provide as much detail about the site as possible.

■ If you can't identify a lesion or don't plan to treat it, don't biopsy it. Instead, refer the patient to someone who may be able to recognize the lesion, possibly saving the patient the discomfort and cost of biopsy.

✿ **COLLABORATION**
*If a patient has a lesion that you suspect is skin cancer, refer him to a dermatologist. The dermatologist has the background needed to choose the most appropriate treatment (including excision, radiation therapy, and chemotherapy).*

## Documentation

■ Before performing a shave biopsy, document any abnormal physical findings on the consent form. Have the patient initial the comments and sign the form to signify acknowledgment of preprocedural abnormalities. In the chart, the preprocedural and postprocedural note must include an evaluation of potentially affected function, range of motion, and sensation.

■ Record the indications for the procedure as well as its details, including a thorough description of the site before and after the procedure, the patient's reaction to the procedure, medications ordered, patient instructions given, and the time frame for follow-up evaluation.

## BLOOD CULTURE

### CPT codes
87040 *Blood culture, bacterial, with isolation and presumptive identification of isolates (includes anaerobic culture, if appropriate)*
87103 *Blood culture, fungi, with presumptive identification of isolates*

### Overview
Normally bacteria-free, blood is susceptible to infection from many sources, including contaminated infusion lines, infected shunts, thrombophlebitis, bacterial endocarditis, and local tissue infections. Bacteria can also invade through the lymphatic system and thoracic duct. Blood cultures allow the detection of such bacterial invasion (bacteremia) and the systemic spread of such infection (septicemia) through the bloodstream. Patients at greater risk, including febrile patients with rigors, other seriously ill patients, immunosuppressed patients, and patients suspected of having endocarditis, should have blood samples collected for culturing.

After collection, blood samples are placed in two blood culture bottles. One contains an anaerobic medium; the other, an aerobic medium. An alternative single-tube system, the Isolator system, is also available. (See *Isolator blood-culturing system.*)

The bottles are then incubated, encouraging any organisms in the sample to grow in the medium. These cultures allow identification of about 67% of pathogens within 24 hours and up to 90% within 72 hours. For the most accurate results, some authorities recommend drawing three samples at least 1 hour apart, with the first drawn at the first signs of bacteremia or septicemia (other authorities consider the timing of culture specimens debatable). In cases of suspected bacterial endocarditis, three or four blood samples taken from different sites at 5- to 30-minute intervals before starting antibiotic therapy may produce more positive test results.

### Indications
- To diagnose bacterial invasion
- To rule out systemic spread of infection
- To detect infection, regardless of age, in febrile patients with rigors, seriously ill patients, high-risk patients, patients who present in shock, immunosuppressed patients, or patients with unexplained ill appearance
- To assess effectiveness of current or recent antibiotic treatment

### Contraindications
**RELATIVE**
- Coagulopathies

## Isolator blood-culturing system

A single-tube blood-culturing system, the Isolator uses lysis and centrifugation to help detect septicemia and monitor the effectiveness of antibacterial drug therapy. It's indicated for fungus and mycobacterium isolation; however, it's very costly and not readily available.

The Isolator tube used to collect the blood sample contains a substance that lyses red blood cells. Then centrifugation concentrates bacteria and other organisms in the sample onto an inert cushioning pad; the concentrate can then be applied directly onto four agar plates.

The Isolator has several advantages over conventional blood-culturing methods. This system:

◆ eliminates the bottle method's lengthy incubation period, providing faster results
◆ improves bacterial survival
◆ yields more valid positive results through direct application onto agar plates, which dilutes any antibiotic present in the sample to a greater degree and detects more yeast and polymicrobial infections
◆ improves the laboratory's ability to detect organisms that are difficult to grow
◆ facilitates use at the patient's bedside and during transport because blood is drawn directly into the Isolator tube.

## Preprocedure patient preparation

■ Tell the patient that he should feel only minimal pain during the procedure.

## Equipment

Tourniquet ◆ gloves ◆ alcohol pads ◆ povidone-iodine pads ◆ 10-ml syringe (for adult) or 6-ml syringe (for child) ◆ 20G ½″ needles ◆ adhesive bandage ◆ 2″ × 2″ gauze pads ◆ two blood culture bottles (50-ml for adult or 20-ml bottles for infant or child), one aerobic and one anaerobic ◆ labels

### Equipment preparation

■ Check the dates on the culture bottles to make sure they haven't expired.

## Procedure

■ Tell the patient that you need to collect a series of blood samples to check for infection. Explain the procedure to the patient, and address any questions or concerns he may have.

■ Wash your hands, and put on gloves.

■ Tie a tourniquet 1″ (2.5 cm) proximal to the collection site.

■ Clean the site with just an alcohol pad, or use an alcohol pad followed by a povidone-iodine pad. Start at the site and work outward in a circular motion. Allow the site to dry thoroughly.

**CLINICAL TIP**
*If you're using povidone-iodine as well as alcohol, use the alcohol first. Using alcohol after povidone-iodine cancels the effect of the povidone-iodine.*

- Perform a venipuncture, drawing 10 ml of blood from an adult or 2 to 6 ml from a child.
- Apply pressure to the venipuncture site with a 2″ × 2″ gauze pad. When hemostasis is achieved, apply an adhesive bandage.
- Wipe the diaphragm tops of the culture bottles with an alcohol pad.
- Replace the needle on the syringe with a new sterile needle. Use a large-gauge needle to prevent hemolysis.
- Inject 5 ml of blood into each 50-ml culture bottle or 2 ml into a 20-ml pediatric culture bottle; fill the aerobic bottle first (bottle size may vary, but the sample dilution should never be less than 1:5).
- Label the culture bottles with the patient's name and identification number, the site, and the date and time of collection. Indicate the patient's temperature, and note any recent antibiotic therapy.
- Immediately send the samples to the laboratory.

## Postprocedure patient teaching

- Tell the patient that you should have the results in 24 to 72 hours.
- Instruct the patient to remove the bandage when bleeding stops.
- Describe hematoma formation to the patient, and instruct him to apply a warm compress to the area if a hematoma develops.

## Complications

- Place a warm soak over the site, and apply pressure to prevent hematoma formation.

## Special considerations

- Obtain each set of cultures from different sites. Ideally, you should take the samples 1 hour apart, but this isn't necessary in emergencies or if the patient is febrile.
- Don't take a sample for culturing from an existing line unless you draw the sample when the line is initially inserted. In suspected line sepsis, draw a set of blood cultures from the catheter but also draw a set from a venipuncture site at the same time.
- Don't use the femoral vein for blood culture samples because of the difficulty of adequately disinfecting the skin.
- Inform the laboratory if you suspect that the patient may have an unusual cause of infection, such as viremia, fungemia, brucellosis, tularemia, or leptospirosis.
- If the patient is currently on antibiotic therapy, obtain the blood sample right before administering the next dose so that the sample has a low level of the antibiotic.
- Notify the laboratory that the patient is taking antibiotics so that the laboratory can allow for extra dilution or use of an antibiotic removal device. Alternatively, you can use special culture bottles that have resin in the medium, which absorbs antibiotics from the blood; however, these bottles are very expensive.
- Keep in mind that sample contamination can occur even with careful skin preparation.

## Documentation

- Document the indications for drawing the cultures.
- Record the site, date, and time of blood sample collections; the number of bottles used; the patient's temperature; and any adverse reactions to the procedure.
- Record intervening antibiotic or other therapy.
- Note the results of the cultures (when available) and any changes or response to therapy.

# BLOOD GLUCOSE TESTING

### CPT codes
82947 *Glucose, quantitative, blood (except reagent strip)*
82948 *Glucose, blood, reagent strip*
82962 *Glucose, blood by glucose monitoring devices cleared by the Food and Drug Administration specifically for home use*

## Overview

Rapid, easy-to-perform reagent strip tests (such as Glucostix, Chemstrip bG, and Multistix) use a drop of capillary blood obtained by fingerstick, heelstick, or earlobe puncture as a sample. They can be performed in the hospital, a facility, or the patient's home.

In blood glucose tests, a reagent patch on the tip of a handheld plastic strip changes color in response to the amount of glucose in the blood sample. Comparing the color change with a standardized color chart provides a semiquantitative measurement of blood glucose levels; inserting the strip in a portable blood glucose meter (such as Glucometer II, Accu-Chek II, and One Touch) provides quantitative measurements that compare in accuracy with other laboratory tests. Some meters store successive test results electronically to help determine glucose patterns.

You may be performing the procedure in a facility or teaching the patient how to perform the procedure at home.

## Indications

- To screen for hypoglycemia and hyperglycemia
- To confirm blood glucose level in patients with symptoms of hypoglycemia or hyperglycemia
- To screen for diabetes, gestational diabetes, and neonatal hypoglycemia
- To monitor blood glucose levels for the management of patients with diabetes, including pregnant women

## Contraindications
### ABSOLUTE
- Raynaud's disease or other severe arteriospastic disorders

### RELATIVE
- Anemia or polycythemia, which can lead to inaccurate test results
- Physical or mental disabilities or vision disturbances, such as color blindness, which can make this procedure difficult for the patient

to perform in the home setting without assistance

## Preprocedure patient preparation

■ Explain to the patient the importance of monitoring blood glucose level and his disease process as necessary.

■ If the patient's extremities are cool, it may be necessary to dilate the capillaries by applying warm, moist compresses to the area for about 10 minutes prior to the procedure.

## Equipment

Reagent strips ◆ gloves ◆ portable blood glucose meter, if available ◆ alcohol pads ◆ gauze pads ◆ disposable lancets or mechanical blood-letting device ◆ small adhesive bandage ◆ watch or clock with a second hand

## Procedure

■ Explain the procedure to the patient or his parents, and address any questions or concerns they may have.

■ Select the puncture site, usually the fingertip or earlobe for an adult or child.

**CLINICAL TIP**
*For an infant, the heel or great toe should be utilized for a site.*

■ Wash your hands, and put on gloves.

■ Wipe the puncture site with an alcohol pad and dry it thoroughly with a gauze pad.

■ Position the lancet on the side of the patient's fingertip, perpendicular to the lines of the fingerprints. Pierce the skin sharply and quickly to minimize the patient's anxiety and pain and to increase blood flow. You may also use a mechanical blood-letting device such as an Autolet, which uses a spring-loaded lancet.

■ After puncturing the fingertip, don't squeeze the puncture site, to avoid diluting the sample with tissue fluid.

■ Touch a drop of blood to the reagent patch on the strip; make sure you cover the entire patch.

■ After collecting the blood sample, briefly apply pressure to the puncture site. Hold a gauze pad firmly over the puncture site until bleeding stops.

■ Make sure you leave the blood on the strip for exactly 60 seconds, referring to a watch or a clock.

■ Compare the color change on the strip with the standardized color chart on the product container. If you're using a blood glucose meter, follow the manufacturer's instructions. Meter designs vary, but they all analyze a drop of blood placed on a reagent strip that comes with the unit and provide a digital display of the resulting glucose level.

■ After bleeding has stopped, apply a small adhesive bandage to the puncture site.

## Postprocedure patient teaching

■ If the patient will be using the reagent strip system at home, teach him the proper use of the lancet or Autolet, reagent strips and color chart, and portable blood glucose meter as necessary (following instructions provided by the manufacturer). Also, provide him with written guidelines. Include when and how often he should check his blood glucose level. Instruct him on how to keep a log of his blood glucose levels.

## Complications
■ None known

## Special considerations
■ To help detect abnormal glucose metabolism and diagnose diabetes mellitus, other blood glucose tests may be needed, such as an oral or I.V. glucose tolerance test.
■ Before using reagent strips, check the expiration date on the package and replace outdated strips. Check for special instructions related to the specific reagent. The reagent area of a fresh strip should match the color of the "O" block on the color chart. Protect the strips from light, heat, and moisture.
■ Before using a blood glucose meter, calibrate it and run it with a control sample. Follow the manufacturer's instructions for calibration.
■ To ensure an accurate result, avoid selecting cold, cyanotic, or swollen puncture sites for the sample. If you can't obtain a capillary sample, perform venipuncture and place a large drop of venous blood on the reagent strip. If you want to

test blood from a refrigerated sample, allow the blood to return to room temperature before testing it.

## Documentation
■ Record the date and time of the blood glucose test.
■ Record the reading from the reagent strip (using a portable blood glucose meter or color chart) in the appropriate location of the patient's chart.

# *B*URN *CARE*

**CPT codes**
16000 *Initial treatment, first-degree burn, when no more than local treatment is required*
16020 *Dressings and/or debridement, initial or subsequent; without anesthesia, office or hospital, small*

## Overview
Burns are one of the most common injuries to the skin. They can be thermal, caused by fire, automobile accidents, or playing with matches; chemical, resulting from the contact, ingestion, inhalation, or injection of acids, alkalis, or vesicants; or electrical, occurring after contact with faulty electrical wiring or high-voltage power lines.

The goals of burn care are to maintain the patient's physiologic stability, repair skin integrity, prevent infection, and promote maximal functioning of the affected area.

Burn severity is determined by the depth and extent of the burn and the presence of other factors, such as age, complications, and co-existing illnesses. (See *Estimating burn surfaces in adults and children,* pages 70 and 71, and *Evaluating burn severity,* page 72.)

A correlation of the burn's depth and size permits an estimate of its severity, as follows:

◆ *Major:* third-degree burns on more than 10% of body surface area (BSA); second-degree burns on more than 25% of adult BSA (more than 20% in children); burns of hands, face, feet, or genitalia; burns complicated by fractures or respiratory damage; chemical burns; electrical burns; all burns in poor-risk patients

◆ *Moderate:* third-degree burns on 2% to 10% of BSA; second-degree burns on 15% to 25% of adult BSA (10% to 20% in children)

◆ *Minor:* third-degree burns on less than 2% of BSA; second-degree burns on less than 15% of adult BSA (10% in children).

For moderate and major burns, the patient should be transferred to an emergency department or a burn center. The patient may require stabilization of airway, breathing, and circulation. Bleeding should be controlled. The burn should be covered with a dry, sterile sheet until the patient is transported.

The following procedure is for care of the minor burn. If debridement of the burn wound is necessary, please refer to "Mechanical debridement," pages 309 to 311.

## Indications

■ To provide care to a minor or first-degree burn

## Contraindications

### ABSOLUTE

■ Any moderate or major burn or a burn suspected of being moderate or major (refer to an emergency department or a burn center)

■ Any burn suspected of involving tendon, muscle, or bone (refer to an emergency department or a burn center)

## Preprocedure patient preparation

■ Discuss with the patient the expected course of illness based on the extent of the burn.

■ Administer pain medication as appropriate prior to the procedure to prevent excessive pain.

## Equipment

Normal saline solution ◆ sterile bowl ◆ sterile blunt scissors ◆ sterile tissue forceps ◆ topical medication such as silvadene ◆ burn gauze ◆ roller gauze ◆ elastic netting or tape ◆ pain medication ◆ sterile gloves ◆ 4″ × 4″ gauze pads
*Note:* All equipment and supplies used in the dressing should be sterile.

### Equipment preparation

■ Warm normal saline solution by immersing unopened bottles in warm water.

- Assemble equipment, and open using aseptic technique.
- Arrange supplies on a sterile field in order of use.

## Procedure

- Explain the procedure to the patient, and address any questions or concerns he may have.
- Pour warmed normal saline solution into the sterile bowl in the sterile field.
- Wash your hands, and put on sterile gloves.

### Applying a dry dressing with a topical medication

- Clean the wound using 4″ × 4″ gauze pads moistened with normal saline solution, and gently remove any exudates.
- Apply the topical medication to the wound in a thin layer (about 2 to 4 mm thick) with your sterile gloved hand. Then apply several layers of burn gauze over the wound to contain the medication but allow exudate to escape.
- Remember to cut the dry dressing to fit only the wound areas; don't cover unburned areas.
- Cover the entire dressing with roller gauze, and secure it with elastic netting or tape.

### Providing arm and leg care

- Apply the dressings from the distal to the proximal area to stimulate circulation and prevent constriction. Wrap the burn gauze once around the arm or leg so the edges overlap slightly. Continue wrapping in this way until the gauze covers the wound.

- Apply a dry roller gauze dressing to hold the bottom layers in place. Secure with elastic netting or tape.

### Providing chest, abdomen, and back care

- Apply the topical medication to the wound in a thin layer. Then cover the entire burned area with sheets of burn gauze.
- Wrap the area with roller gauze or apply a specialty vest dressing to hold the burn gauze in place.
- Secure the dressing with elastic netting or tape. Make sure the dressing doesn't restrict respiratory motion, especially in very young or elderly patients or in those with circumferential injuries.

## Postprocedure patient teaching

- Teach the patient signs and symptoms of infection, and instruct him to notify your facility if infection is suspected.
- Provide the patient with aftercare instructions, such as keeping the dressing dry and clean, elevating the burned extremity for the first 24 hours, performing range-of-motion exercises to the affected body area at least three times per day, and taking analgesics for pain relief.
- Have the patient scheduled to return to the facility for a wound check in 1 to 2 days.

## Complications

- Infection, the most common complication, can result if aseptic technique isn't followed. Topical or

*(Text continues page 72.)*

# Estimating burn surfaces in adults and children

You need to use different formulas to compute burned body surface area (BSA) in adults and children because the proportion of BSA varies with growth.

### RULE OF NINES

You can quickly estimate the extent of an adult patient's burn by using the Rule of Nines. This method quantifies BSA in percentages either in fractions of nine or in multiples of nine. To use this method, men- tally assess your patient's burns by the body chart shown below. Add the corresponding percentages for each body section burned. Use the total — a rough estimate of burn extent — to calculate initial fluid replace- ment needs.

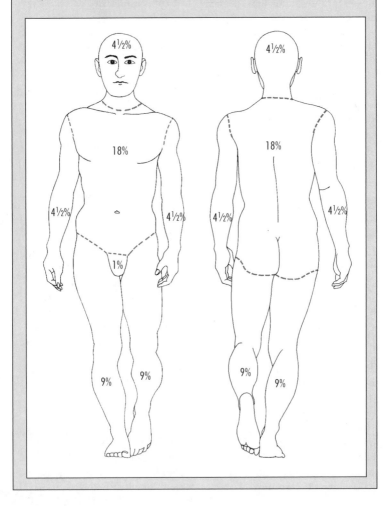

## Estimating burn surfaces in adults and children *(continued)*

### LUND AND BROWDER CHART

The Rule of Nines isn't accurate for infants and children because their body shapes differ from those of adults. An infant's head, for example, accounts for about 17% of his total BSA, compared with 7% for an adult. Instead, use the Lund and Browder chart shown here.

### PERCENTAGE OF BURNED BODY SURFACE BY AGE

| | AT BIRTH | 0 TO 1 YR | 1 TO 4 YR | 5 TO 9 YR | 10 TO 15 YR | ADULT |
|---|---|---|---|---|---|---|
| A: Half of head | $9\frac{1}{2}\%$ | $8\frac{1}{2}\%$ | $6\frac{1}{2}\%$ | $5\frac{1}{2}\%$ | $4\frac{1}{2}\%$ | $3\frac{1}{2}\%$ |
| B: Half of one thigh | $2\frac{3}{4}\%$ | $3\frac{1}{4}\%$ | $4\%$ | $4\frac{1}{4}\%$ | $4\frac{1}{2}\%$ | $4\frac{3}{4}\%$ |
| C: Half of one leg | $2\frac{1}{2}\%$ | $2\frac{1}{2}\%$ | $2\frac{3}{4}\%$ | $3\%$ | $3\frac{1}{4}\%$ | $3\frac{1}{2}\%$ |

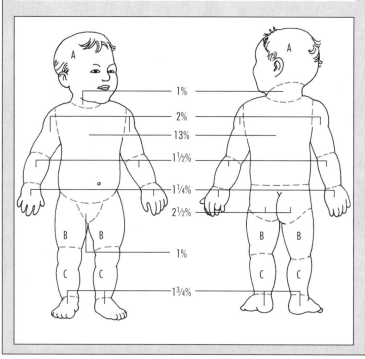

## Evaluating burn severity

To judge a burn's severity, assess its depth and extent as well as the presence of sensitivity, pain, color, and hair.

### SUPERFICIAL PARTIAL-THICKNESS (FIRST-DEGREE) BURN

Does the burned area appear pink or red with minimal edema? Is the area sensitive to touch and temperature changes? If so, your patient most likely has a superficial partial-thickness, or first-degree, burn affecting only the epidermal skin layer.

### DEEP PARTIAL-THICKNESS (SECOND-DEGREE) BURN

Does the burned area appear pink or red, with a mottled appearance? Do red areas blanch when you touch them? Does the skin have large, thick-walled blisters with subcutaneous edema? Does touching the burn cause severe pain? Is the hair still present? If so, the person most likely has a deep partial-thickness, or second-degree, burn affecting the epidermal and dermal layers.

### FULL-THICKNESS (THIRD-DEGREE) BURN

Does the burned area appear red, waxy white, brown, or black? Does red skin remain red with no blanching when you touch it? Is the skin leathery with extensive subcutaneous edema? Is the skin insensitive to touch? Does the hair fall out easily? If so, your patient most likely has a full-thickness, or third-degree, burn that affects all skin layers.

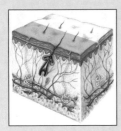 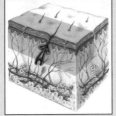 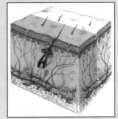

oral antimicrobials may be indicated.

## Special considerations

■ Because blisters protect underlying tissue, leave them intact unless they impede joint motion, become infected, or cause the patient discomfort.

## Documentation

■ Record the date and time of all care provided. Be sure to include a detailed description of the wound's appearance and condition.
■ Record any pain or topical medications administered or prescribed and the patient's tolerance of the procedure.

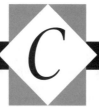

## Casting

### CPT codes
29049 *Application of cast, figure eight*
29065 *Application of long arm cast*
29075 *Application of short arm cast*
29085 *Application of gauntlet cast*
29345 *Application of long leg cast*
29405 *Application of short leg cast*
29425 *Application of short leg cast, walking or ambulatory type*
29730 *Windowing of cast*

### Overview

Casts are applied for fracture immobilization, to allow ambulation or semi-use of limb while injured, and to maintain the position of a reduced fracture. Stabilizing these injuries allows healing to take place. A variety of materials may be used in casting such as synthetic fiberglass; however, plaster of paris remains a popular choice.

To avoid causing joint deformities, the cast should be applied by a trained health care provider with experience in applying casts. In addition, whenever casting is done,

the affected extremity should be held in its proper functioning position. Casting should be done in an orderly sequence every time to avoid skipping any essential steps. (See *Layers of a cast,* page 74.)

### Indications

■ To treat closed fractures, dislocations, or deformities that are either acquired or congenital
■ To treat closed or open fracture reductions

### Contraindications
**ABSOLUTE**
■ Unstable fractures that require surgical pinning or hardware introduction
■ Angular deformities
■ Large areas of broken skin integrity

**RELATIVE**
■ Uncooperative patients

### Preprocedure patient preparation
■ Explain the need for casting, how long the cast will be in place, and any limitations that may need

## Layers of a cast

The illustrations below depict the three layers of a cast.

**1.** First, stockinette is placed over the extremity so that it covers and extends past the intended casting area.

**2.** Next, soft cast padding is applied by wrapping from one end of the extremity to the other. Each layer of the padding should overlap half the width of the previous layer.

**3.** Finally, the casting material is applied by rolling it on in the same direction as the cast padding. Like the padding, each new layer should overlap half the width of the previous layer. The number of layers of casting material applied depends on the casting material used.

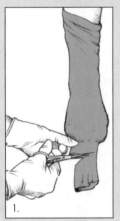
1.

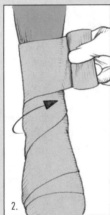
2.

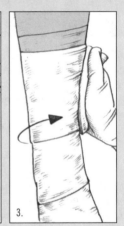
3.

to be placed on daily activity such as non-weight bearing on the extremity.

■ Provide the patient with adequate pain relief as necessary.

## Equipment

Stockinette ◆ cotton cast padding ◆ casting material of choice (plaster of paris or a synthetic such as fiberglass) ◆ room temperature or warm water (depending on casting material) ◆ bowl or basin for water ◆ cast file ◆ heavy duty bandage scissors

### *Equipment preparation*

■ Assemble the equipment. Place the water, which will be used to activate the plaster of paris or synthetic casting material, in a bowl or basin.

## Procedure

■ Explain the procedure to the patient, and address any questions or concerns he may have.

 **OBTAIN INFORMED CONSENT**

■ Wash your hands.

■ Wash and thoroughly dry the skin that will be covered with the cast. Inspect the area for lacerations, abrasions, or any other signs of broken skin integrity.

■ Position the patient so that he can hold the injured extremity in place throughout the procedure. You may need an assistant to accomplish this. The extremity should be casted in a position that will prevent contractures.

■ Apply the stockinette to the affected extremity. Make sure it lies smoothly and won't bunch up under the cast; wrinkled areas can become pressure points that lead to skin breakdown. The stockinette layer should extend past the area to be casted so that it can be folded down later in the procedure.

■ Next, apply the layer of soft cast padding. Begin at one end of the extremity and roll toward the other, overlapping each roll by one-half the width of the padding roll. Like the stockinette, make sure the padding lies smoothly and without wrinkles.

**CLINICAL TIP**

*Limit padding to no more than two layers. Overpadding can lead to a loose cast, which may allow the patient to move the extremity into misalignment. However, extra padding may be placed over bony prominences, prominent nerves, or any area where there may be increased pressure.*

■ Apply the third and final layer, the casting material.

### For plaster casting material

■ Place the plaster roll into a bowl of warm water, and remove it from the water after the bubbles cease. To remove excess water and air,

gently squeeze the roll on both sides.

■ Following the direction of the cast padding, apply the plaster roll using gentle pressure. Like the padding, overlap each roll by one-half and smooth using the palm of your hand. To accommodate limb tapering, the plaster roll may be folded over, or tucked, and then smoothed. Start additional rolls where the last one ended.

■ Apply approximately five layers of plaster, following the same direction for each. Before applying the last layer, fold down the extra stockinette and smooth it into the previous layer for a smooth finish.

■ Smooth the cast after all of the layers have been applied, making sure it fits the anatomy appropriately.

■ Recheck the casted area for proper positioning before the cast hardens. Also, perform a neurovascular check, noting movement and warmth of digits, and palpable pulses.

### For synthetic casting material

■ Place the synthetic roll into a bowl of room temperature water, and apply immediately after gently squeezing out any excess water or air.

■ Application is the same as working with plaster material, except only three layers are needed. Tucking of the rolls may not be needed as synthetic materials are stretchable and more conforming, but make sure you don't pull the rolls too tight. Smooth out the casting material between each layer.

- Unlike plaster casts, the rough edges of a synthetic cast may need to be trimmed using a file or bandage scissors.
- Recheck the casted area for proper positioning before the cast hardens. Also, perform a neurovascular check, noting movement and warmth of digits, and palpable pulses.

## Postprocedure patient teaching

- Instruct the patient to avoid weight bearing on the casted extremity for the first 48 hours after casting to allow the cast to cure. For synthetic casts, this time is cut in half.
- The casted extremity may be elevated to help reduce edema. Ice may be applied as necessary.
- Instruct the patient on proper cast care, including avoiding getting the cast wet by covering with plastic bags and securing closed or using commercial products for cast protection in water; not placing any objects inside the cast to relieve an itch; and to follow limitations in daily activities as necessary.
- Explain how to relieve itching by using a hair dryer (set on cool) at the cast edges; this also decreases dampness from perspiration.
- Tell the patient to notify you immediately if there appears to be any circulatory compromise to the casted area or distal extremity, such as pain, burning, skin color changes, skin breakdown, loss of feeling, tingling, numbness, or cast odor.

- Instruct the patient on the use of crutches or slings, as appropriate. Make sure the crutches are properly fitted to the patient.
- Discuss the need for follow-up and physical therapy appointments as necessary.

## Complications

- Compartment syndrome typically results from crush injuries or fractures that require casting. It occurs when the pressure within the muscle compartment, resulting from edema or bleeding, increases to the point of interfering with circulation. Treatment involves removing the constricting forces such as taking off the cast.
- Other complications include skin breakdown, joint deformity, thrombus formation, and nerve damage with sensory loss.

## Special considerations

- Be sure to provide the patient with written discharge instructions to take home with him.
- Comparison X-rays taken before and after the casting may be done.

## Documentation

- You should record the indications for the casting, pertinent X-ray findings, informed consent, and a brief summary of the procedure.
- Document neurovascular evaluation performed after cast application.
- Also document patient education, including written materials

given to the patient, instruction on using crutches or slings, and follow-up appointments as appropriate.

## CAUTERY FOR LESION REMOVAL

### CPT codes

17000 *Destruction by any method, including laser, curettage, or electrodesiccation of one lesion not including skin tags (use code 11200) or vascular lesions (code depends on exact diagnosis).*

*Add code 17003 if treating 2 to 14 lesions. Some codes depend on type, size and location of the lesions and can be quite complex. Refer to the current CPT code manual.*

## Overview

There are several methods used to treat skin lesions; one of these is electrocautery, also known as electrosurgery and electrodesiccation. In this method, heat is used to destroy the lesion and the base layer of skin, which commonly helps to prevent recurrence. A benefit of this treatment method is that it also cauterizes blood vessels that are disrupted during the procedure so minor bleeding is controlled. Depigmentation or hypertrophic scars may result in some areas, such as the upper lip and deltoid, especially if the area treated is deep.

## Indications

- To remove skin lesions, such as skin tags, verruca, actinic and seborrheic keratoses, squamous and basal cell carcinoma, benign nevi, condyloma, mucosal lesions, some hemangiomas, and telangiectasias

## Contraindications

### ABSOLUTE

- Allergy to anesthetic solution
- A significantly uncooperative patient

## Preprocedure patient preparation

- Topical, local, or digital nerve block anesthesia may be needed for larger lesions.

## Equipment

Antibacterial cleaning solution ◆ electrocautery unit ◆ needle tips of various sizes and shapes, depending on location and type of lesion to be removed ◆ sterile 4″ × 4″ gauze pads ◆ antibiotic ointment ◆ equipment to administer topical or local anesthesia or a digital nerve block

### Equipment preparation

- Sterilize the tip of the needle of the electrocautery unit.

## Procedure

- Explain the procedure to the patient. Answer all questions and address any concerns he may have.

**☑ OBTAIN INFORMED CONSENT**

■ Wash your hands.

■ Clean the lesion and the skin surrounding it (at least a 3″-diameter area) with antibacterial cleansing solution and pat dry.

■ Anesthetize the lesion being treated using topical or local anesthesia or a digital nerve block. (See "Anesthesia: topical, local, and digital nerve block," page 20.)

**◤ CLINICAL TIP**
*Epinephrine in the anesthetic solution isn't needed because cautery controls bleeding.*

■ If laboratory analysis is necessary for identification, obtain a specimen first. Use the punch, shave, scissor, or elliptical excision biopsy method to obtain the sample. (See separate entries under "Biopsy," pages 47 to 62.)

■ If the lesion is large and bulky, "debulk" it before destroying the remaining tissue with cautery. The biopsy procedures noted above may be used to debulk the lesion.

■ Touch the tip of the cautery unit to the lesion, and step on the power switch. Be sure to hold the insulated handle or you'll receive significant burns.

**◤ CLINICAL TIP**
*Use the lowest cautery level that produces the desired result. Thick or keratotic lesions usually require a higher setting, but start low.*

■ Move the tip around the lesion so that all areas are destroyed.

■ It may be necessary to burn part of the lesion and then remove the dead tissue with forceps or by wiping with gauze.

■ Continue to burn tissue until the entire lesion has been destroyed down to the base.

■ If treating verruca, be sure to burn into the cores of the lesion. Verruca may require several treatments to completely eradicate the lesion.

■ When cautery is complete, wipe the area with sterile gauze, and apply a topical antibiotic ointment. Dress the site with gauze and tape.

## Postprocedure patient teaching

■ Instruct the patient to keep the area clean and dry until it's healed. Some lesions may need to be kept covered.

■ Application of antibiotic ointment may help to control eschar formation and prevent secondary bacterial infection, which are uncommon complications.

■ Follow-up isn't necessary unless the patient develops signs of infection, such as redness, edema, increase in temperature, or foul-smelling, yellow or green drainage at the site, in which case the patient should return to the facility. However, if a large area is involved, instruct the patient to return for follow-up in 1 to 2 weeks to assess healing.

## Complications

■ A secondary bacterial infection can develop at the procedure site, but this isn't common. Treatment consists of topical or oral antibiotics.

■ Occasionally, too much tissue is destroyed, causing a scar to form.
■ Excessive bleeding may occur in a patient on anticoagulation therapy.

## Special considerations

■ Redness, swelling, and blister formation are part of the normal response to this procedure, and usually start immediately after the procedure is performed and lasting 3 to 7 days. The wound will heal from the outside inward; some wound weeping is normal for up to 8 weeks.

## Documentation

■ Because cautery is a surgical procedure, document that you obtained informed consent.
■ Record the preprocedure location and size of the lesion.
■ Document the anesthesia used.
■ Document whether specimens were taken from the lesion or whether it was debulked. Document the methods that were used.
■ Chart the postprocedure care, such as any topical medications or dressings applied.
■ Record patient teaching and any follow-up.

## Overview

The goal of cerumen impaction removal is to mobilize and evacuate cerumen from the external ear canal. Although cerumen is an ear canal lubricant and protector, it may become dried and hardened, causing pain and decreased hearing. If ceruminolytic eardrops are ineffective in removing cerumen, manual disimpaction is most commonly done by irrigation. Irrigating the ear involves washing the external auditory canal with a stream of solution to clean the canal of discharges, to soften and remove impacted cerumen, or to dislodge a foreign body. Sometimes, irrigation aims to relieve localized inflammation and discomfort. The procedure must be performed carefully to avoid causing the patient discomfort or vertigo and to avoid increasing the risk of otitis externa. Because irrigation may contaminate the middle ear if the tympanic membrane is ruptured, an otoscopic examination always precedes ear irrigation. If visualization of the tympanic membrane is impaired due to cerumen buildup, an ear curette is used to remove it.

## Indications

■ To remove symptomatic cerumen impaction (pain, dizziness, hearing loss)

# *C*ERUMEN IMPACTION REMOVAL

***CPT code***
69210  *Removal of impacted cerumen (one or both ears)*

## Contraindications

**ABSOLUTE**
- Suspected tympanic membrane perforation
- Infectious process present

**RELATIVE**
- Recent ear or head trauma
- Large foreign body present
- Tympanic membrane or ear canal deformities present

## Preprocedure patient preparation

- Tell the patient that he should notice immediate relief from ear pressure or fullness and restoration of hearing after complete evacuation of impacted cerumen.

## Equipment

Otoscope with aural speculum ◆ tuning fork ◆ prepackaged or sterile ear curette ◆ ear irrigation syringe ◆ emesis basin and irrigation reservoir setup ◆ towel or absorbent drape ◆ cotton-tipped applicator ◆ gloves ◆ warm water (body temperature) ◆ mineral oil or ceruminolytic agent such as triethanolamine polypeptide oleate-condensate (Cerumenex)

### Equipment preparation

- Select the appropriate syringe, and obtain the prescribed irrigant.
- Put the container of irrigant into the large basin filled with hot water to warm the solution to body temperature: 98.6° F (37° C). An irrigant that's too warm or cold can af-

fect inner ear fluids, causing nausea and dizziness.
- Test the temperature of the solution by sprinkling a few drops on your inner wrist.
- Inspect equipment (syringe or catheter tips) for breaks or cracks; inspect all metal tips for roughness. Ensure adequate lighting is available.

## Procedure

- Explain the procedure to the patient, and address any questions or concerns he may have.
- Assist the patient to a sitting position. Cover him with an absorbent clean towel or drape.
- Wash your hands, and put on clean gloves.
- With the patient seated, assess the external ear canal with the otoscope. (Remember to pull the pinna up and back on an older child and adult; pull the pinna back on an infant or child younger than age 3.) Look for consistency, amount, and color of ear canal matter as well as the condition of the surrounding ear canal wall tissue. Perform Weber's and Rinne test for hearing status.
- Fill the ear irrigation syringe with body-temperature, warm water.
- Tilt the patient's head to the side. Have him participate by instructing him to hold the reservoir or emesis basin to the ear being irrigated. (See *How to irrigate the ear canal*.)
- Remove the equipment from the ear, and dry the external area.

■ Assess the external ear canal with an otoscope.

■ If necessary, use an ear curette to remove existing cerumen.

■ If the cerumen remains hardened, instill a commercial preparation or mineral oil to soften it. Wait approximately 5 to 10 minutes for the preparation to soften the cerumen.

■ Reassess the external ear with the otoscope.

■ Gently flush the ear canal again with warm water. Observe and assess debris eliminated. Don't use more than 500 ml of irrigating solution during this procedure.

■ Repeat ear curette usage if necessary.

■ Reassess the ear canal with the otoscope. Inspect the ear canal walls for redness, bleeding, and irritation. Assess the tympanic membrane for infections, perforations, and landmarks. Perform postprocedure Weber's and Rinne hearing tests.

■ If the cerumen remains hardened, it may be necessary to instill cerumen softening products into the ear canal over a period of time (1 to 2 days), then instruct the patient to return for proper irrigation.

■ Dry the pinna and outer ear canal area with a cotton-tipped applicator.

■ Properly dispose of debris material and solutions.

## Postprocedure patient teaching

■ Instruct the patient to contact you if any abnormal discharge,

## How to irrigate the ear canal

Follow these guidelines for irrigating the ear canal.

■ Gently pull the pinna up and back to straighten the ear canal. (For a child, pull the pinna back.)

■ Have the patient hold an emesis basin beneath the ear to catch returning irrigation fluid. Position the tip of the irrigating syringe at the meatus of the auditory canal. Don't block the meatus because you'll impede backflow and increase pressure in the canal.

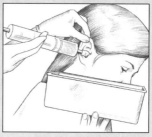

■ Tilt the patient's head toward you and point the syringe tip upward and toward the posterior ear canal. This angle prevents damage to the tympanic membrane and guards against pushing debris further into the canal.

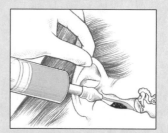

■ Direct a steady stream of irrigation fluid against the upper wall of the ear canal and inspect returned fluid for cloudiness, cerumen, blood, and foreign matter.

pain, vertigo, or hearing problems ensue. Instruct him to follow up with you in 1 to 2 days to evaluate hearing and check for infection.

■ Instruct the patient in proper ear care to prevent future cerumen impaction. This may include the use of over-the-counter earwax preparations at regular intervals and the avoidance of self-irrigation and the insertion of foreign objects into the ears for self-evacuation.

## Complications

■ Trauma to mucous membranes is minimized by gentle handling and careful aiming of the stream of fluid into the ear. Bleeding is handled with pressure to the site.

■ Infection is treated on a case-by-case basis and may result from a foreign body or the extraction. Options include local or systemic antibiotics or consultation with the collaborating physician or an ear, nose, and throat (ENT) specialist.

■ Inability to remove the impacted cerumen requires consultation with or a referral to a physician, ENT specialist, or an acute care facility.

■ Nausea and vomiting typically resolve within a few hours.

■ Tinnitus may result from stimulation of the vestibular system with cold water. This can be minimized by using warm water, but will resolve spontaneously without treatment.

## Special considerations

■ If the canal begins to bleed, or become irritated or swollen, stop the procedure to avoid an external ear infection. The procedure should also be stopped if the patient complains of increasing discomfort as this may indicate tympanic membrane rupture.

■ If signs of infection are present, irrigation may cause the infection to spread inward. In this case, remove cerumen plugs with a cerumen spoon.

■ Avoid dropping or squirting irrigant on the tympanic membrane. This may startle the patient and cause discomfort. If you're using an irrigating catheter instead of a syringe, adjust the flow of solution to a steady, comfortable rate with a flow clamp. Don't raise the container more than 6″ (15.2 cm) above the ear. If the container is higher, the resulting pressure could damage the tympanic membrane.

■ If you place a cotton pledge in the ear canal to retain some of the solution, pack the cotton loosely. Tell the patient when he can remove it.

■ If irrigation doesn't dislodge the impacted cerumen, instruct the patient to instill several drops of glycerin, carbamide peroxide (Debrox), or a similar preparation two to three times daily for 2 to 3 days, and then have the ear irrigated again.

## Documentation

■ As indicated, document the reason for not performing disimpaction and if the patient was referred to an ENT specialist for further evaluation.

■ Record preprocedure and postprocedure hearing results (including Weber's and Rinne testing) and otoscope assessment.

■ Document the type of procedure performed and irrigant used.

■ Record the patient's response to the procedure and assessments, such as hearing status changes and comfort level, as well as the type and amount of ear canal debris removed.

■ Document the instructions given to the patient and his understanding of them.

# CERVICAL CAP FITTING

### CPT code
57170 *Diaphragm or cervical cap fitting with instructions*

## Overview

A cervical cap is a barrier method of contraception with an efficacy rate of about 80%. The cervical cap is a thimble-shaped soft rubber cup that the patient places over the cervix. It's similar to a diaphragm, but smaller. The cervical cap may be worn by women who aren't suited for the diaphragm. The cap requires less spermicide, is less likely to become dislodged during coitus, and doesn't require refitting with a change in weight. For parous women, the cap is less effective than the diaphragm or the female condom. For nulliparous women, the cap and diaphragm provide similar contraceptive efficacy during typical use. Failure of the cervical cap is commonly due to neglect to use the device or inappropriate use of the device.

## Indications

■ To provide contraceptive protection during sexual intercourse

## Contraindications

### ABSOLUTE

■ Perpendicular cervical angle
■ Unusually long or short cervix
■ Allergy to latex or spermicides
■ Vaginal stenosis or pelvic abnormalities
■ Personal factors that interfere with insertion and removal
■ History of toxic shock syndrome, cervical warts, or polyps

## Preprocedure patient preparation

■ Discuss birth control options with the patient, including the benefits, risks, and efficacy rate of each, to help her select the method that's right for her.
■ Explain the insertion and removal procedures necessary for cervical cap use.

## Equipment

Cervical cap fitting set ◆ gloves

## Procedure

■ Explain cervical cap fitting to the patient, and address any questions or concerns she may have.
■ Check the patient's history for allergies, especially to latex.
■ Instruct the patient to undress

below the waist, and assist her into a dorsal lithotomy position.

■ Wash your hands, and put on gloves.

■ Perform a bimanual pelvic examination and Papanicolaou (Pap) test as indicated.

■ During the bimanual examination, assess the degree of vaginal tone and estimate the length, diameter, and symmetry of the cervix:

– The length of the cervix must be at least ½" (1 cm), and the width of the cervix must be ⅓" to 1" (1 to 2.5 cm).

– The cervix must be fairly symmetrical, without extensive laceration or scarring that may interfere with proper fit.

– The cervix should be in the same angle as the vagina, and fairly distal to the introitus.

– Vaginal tone should be good, and vaginal length should be adequate to minimize dislodgment of the cap and partner complaints.

■ Determine the appropriate cap size:

– Caps come in four sizes: 22, 25, 28, and 31 mm.

– The cap diameter is measured across the cap rim.

– The cap depth increases with the diameter.

– The internal ring creates a "suction" seal on the cervix.

■ Insert the best-estimated cap size (try at least two):

– With cap rim dry, hold cap in the middle and squeeze fingers together, separate labia, and insert cap.

– Once inside the vagina, reposition fingers to either side of the cap rim.

– Move cap opening toward the cervix, and cover cervix completely.

■ Assess the fit. (See *Fitting a cervical cap*.)

■ Trace the entire upper rim of the cap to determine that the cervical base is fully covered.

■ Ensure that the cap rim fits completely against the vaginal fornices. The dome of the cap should be deep enough so that it doesn't rest on the cervical os.

■ After a minute or two, assess the cap's suction.

■ Assess the ability of the cap to relocate itself to the cervix when dislodged—an indicator of good fit.

■ Involve the patient before and during the fitting:

– Allow her to view her cervix (a plastic speculum offers the best unobstructed view).

– Instruct her to check the cap's placement by tracing the entire upper rim (360 degrees) around her cervix.

■ Remove the cap:

– Insert fingers and push cap rim to one side to dislodge.

– Remove the cap sideways with one or two fingers.

■ Facilitate the patient's comfort level with cap insertion and removal by allowing her to practice:

– Ask the patient to feel her cervix and note where the cap was.

– Review cap placement and removal techniques.

– Ask her to insert the cap. This may be best accomplished in a

## Fitting a cervical cap

With the proper fit, the "gap" or space between the base of the cervix and the inside of the cap ring should be 1 to 2 mm (to reduce the possibility of dislodgement), and the rim should fill the cervicovaginal fornix. Leave the cap in place for a minute or two. Then with the cervical cap in place, pinch the dome until there is a dimple.

A dimple that takes about 30 seconds to resume a domed appearance indicates good suction and a good fit. If the cap is too small, the rim leaves a gap where the cervix remains exposed. If the cap is too large, it isn't snug against the cervix and is more easily dislodged.

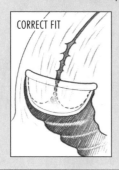

CORRECT FIT

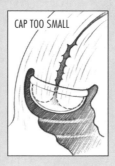

CAP TOO SMALL

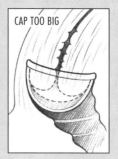

CAP TOO BIG

squatting position or lying down. Leave her to practice in private, then return to assess proper insertion.

– Ask her to remove the cap by pushing the rim to one side to dislodge and removing it with one or two fingers.

■ Demonstrate how to properly clean the cap with warm soapy water and pay special attention to the groove on the inside rim.

### Postprocedure patient teaching

■ Tell the patient to make sure her hands are clean and dry and that the cervical cap is clean and dry prior to insertion.

■ Before insertion, instruct her to fill the cap one-third full with a

spermicidal cream or jelly. Overfilling the cap may interfere with its suction.

■ Teach the patient to always check for proper placement. She should trace the entire upper cap rim. If it's correctly positioned, she won't feel her cervix (it's inside the cap and feels similar to a nose).

■ Instruct the patient about the following:

– Slightly turning the cap by a quarter- to half-turn may improve its suction and fit. This is done by pushing the rim up and to the side.

– If the cap is dislodged during intercourse, it shouldn't be moved or removed. Instead, the patient should insert an applicator full of spermicide into her vagina and re-

main in a reclining position for at least 30 minutes.
– The cap must remain in place at least 8 hours following intercourse, and it may safely remain in place up to 48 hours at one time.
– The cap must not be worn during menses because menstrual flow will interfere with the fit.
– The cap may be inserted up to 1 day before intercourse.
– Additional spermicide isn't necessary with repeated intercourse.
– The cap shouldn't be reinserted for at least 8 hours after removal.
■ Teach the patient how to properly care for the cervical cap. After removal, wash the cap with warm, soapy water and be careful to clean the groove on the inside rim. Allow it to air dry completely, and store the cap in its plastic container in a cool, dry place. Never apply powder, oil-based lubricants, or medications to the cap. Inspect the cap at least once a month for any holes or damage to the latex.
■ Tell the patient to return in 3 months to reassess fit and her skill and comfort level with the cap.
■ Tell the patient that the cap should be replaced every 2 years, and may require refitting following any delivery or cervical surgery.
■ Advise the patient to notify you and temporarily discontinue use of the cap if she suspects she has a vaginal, urinary, or pelvic infection; if pain is associated with use of the cap; if the cap repeatedly dislodges; if she suspects she's pregnant; if she has abnormal Pap test results; if she suspects she has toxic shock syndrome; or if she has

continued problems associated with the cap.
■ Emphasize the importance of using the cap every time she and her partner have intercourse. Reinforce that this birth control method doesn't prevent sexually transmitted diseases.

## Complications

**COLLABORATION**
*Pregnancy, leukoplakia, endometriosis, urinary tract infection (risk is less than with a diaphragm), toxic shock syndrome (a theoretical risk), and cervical dysplasia are all indications for referral to a gynecologist.*

## Special considerations

■ Standard precautions must be observed during fitting, cleaning, and disinfecting cervical caps. Because caps come into contact with intact mucous membrane, fitting caps are classified as semicritical devices that require processing with a high-level disinfectant according to Occupational Safety and Hazard Administration guidelines. Following disinfection, allow the caps to air dry, and then store them in a disinfected container.

## Documentation

■ Preprocedure, document that patient education and counseling has taken place. Note that a history and physical examination has been performed and reflects no absolute or relative contraindications to the patient using the cervical cap.

■ Postprocedure, record the size of the cervical cap fitted and the patient's demonstrated ability to properly insert and remove the cervical cap properly. Note that the patient was instructed to schedule a return visit for 3 months postprocedure.

## CERVICAL RIPENING

### CPT code
59200 *Insertion of cervical dilator (such as prostaglandin)*

## Overview

Cervical ripening is the softening, effacement, and dilation of the cervix before the onset of active labor. When the cervix is fully ripened, the chance of having a successful labor induction is much greater. Elective induction for the patient's or health care provider's convenience is never justified. Methods of induction and augmentation of labor are used only when the benefits to either the patient or the fetus outweigh the benefits of continuing the pregnancy. Labor is induced most commonly for postdates, which occur in more than 13% of deliveries in the United States. In the event that induction or augmentation of labor becomes necessary, nonpharmacologic advances (such as sexual intercourse and stripping the membranes) and recent phar-

macological advances may facilitate a vaginal birth.

Cervical ripening with prostaglandin $E_2$ ($PGE_2$) or dinoprostone (such as Cervidil or Prepidil) is the most common pharmacological method of induction or augmentation of labor. $PGE_2$ may prove beneficial if the cervix is unfavorable for induction. The application of $PGE_2$ gel into the endocervical canal has the effect of ripening (or softening) the cervix and provides an oxytoxic effect. This method of action directly stimulates the collagenase of the cervix, breaking down the collagen network and softening it for induction. The gel can be applied via an intracervical route with greater efficacy. Alternatively, a vaginal insert (Cervidil) is available and provides a lower rate of release of medication than the gel and is single dose only, removed upon onset of active labor or 12 hours after insertion. Should hyperstimulation occur, Cervidil also has the added advantage of easy removal.

Likewise, Prepidil (up to three doses) may be applied at 6-hour intervals. Following the placement of $PGE_2$ and the recommended waiting time after the last dose (12 hours), administration of intravenous oxytocin can be initiated.

Recently, misoprostol, a prostaglandin $E_1$ analog, has been used for preinduction cervical ripening and labor induction. Although the U.S. Food and Drug Administration hasn't approved its use for these indications, it's being used more frequently. Misoprostol is less expensive and is stable at room temperature. Be sure to follow your facility's protocol for use of misoprostol.

## Indications

- To induce a patient with premature rupture of membranes if maternal temperature is rising, if the patient is at term with a positive cervical culture for group B beta-hemolytic streptococci, or if the management plan is to impose a limited number of hours before delivery
- To induce a patient with chorioamnionitis, severe pregnancy-induced hypertension, maternal diabetes mellitus, polyhydramnios (the accumulation of an excessive amount of amniotic fluid), oligohydramnios (too little amniotic fluid), or Rh incompatibility (fetus is being sensitized due to blood type incompatibility between the mother and fetus)
- To induce a patient who is post-term with gestational age past 42 weeks
- To induce a patient in which fetal demise has occurred
- To induce labor when the biophysical profile score is less than eight (See *Understanding the biophysical profile score.*)

## Contraindications

### ABSOLUTE

- Patients with low-lying or marginal placentas or with any vaginal bleeding
- Patients in whom oxytocic drugs

are contraindicated or where prolonged contractions of the uterus are considered inappropriate
- History of cesarean delivery or major uterine surgery
- A clinical suspicion or definite evidence of fetal compromise where delivery isn't imminent
- Known hypersensitivity to prostaglandins
- Evidence of cephalopelvic disproportion
- A history of six or more term pregnancies
- Active herpes genitalis
- Patients receiving oxytoxic drugs
- Nonvertex presentations
- History of difficult labor or traumatic delivery

### RELATIVE

- Fetal demise after 28 weeks gestation
- With fetal demise, $PGE_2$ is contraindicated in the case of maternal cyanotic or ischemic cardiac disease, or severe asthma
- Use of $PGE_2$ with a history of asthma, glaucoma, or increased intraocular pressure, renal, or hepatic dysfunction

## Preprocedure patient preparation

- Explain the risks and benefits of cervical ripening to the patient.

## Equipment

$PGE_2$ administered with a 20-mm endocervical catheter if the cervix isn't effaced or a 10-mm endocervical catheter if the cervix is 50% effaced ◆ sterile speculum ◆ sterile

## Understanding the biophysical profile score

A biophysical profile is a real-time ultrasound performed for a maximum of 30 minutes. In conjunction with a nonstress test (NST), a biophysical score is used to identify a healthy or compromised fetus and to aid the development of rational management schemes. Frequency of biophysical profiling should be based on the clinical circumstances for each individual case.

Parameters included in the biophysical profile are:

■ fetal tone (fisted hand, fat folds in the neck, flexion of extremities)
■ fetal movement
■ fetal breathing
■ amniotic fluid volume
■ fetal heart rate activity (28 to 32 weeks gestation) usually performed by an NST.

Each parameter is given either two points or zero, with a healthy score being ten points. Amniotic fluid volume is the most profound criteria. It's measured in quadrants of the uterus. An amniotic fluid volume less than 5 ml indicates oligohydramnios, and induction should be considered. This finding receives a score of zero in the biophysical profile. A volume greater than 23 ml indicates polyhydramnios and requires careful observation, as it may lead to preterm labor.

In understanding the management with relation to the biophysical profile, the risk of asphyxia is extremely rare in scores of:

■ 10 out of 10
■ 8 out of 10
■ 8 out of 8 when an NST is not done.

**ALERT**
A test result of 8 out of 10 (with abnormal amniotic fluid volume) is a strong indication for intervention. Chronic fetal compromise is probable.

---

gloves ◆ external electronic fetal monitor ◆ linen-saver pads

## Procedure

■ Explain the procedure to the patient and address any questions or concerns she may have.

**☑ OBTAIN INFORMED CONSENT**

■ Have the patient empty her bladder prior to the examination.
■ Identify and record the fetal heart rate (FHR) with an external fetal monitor. Continue to monitor the FHR throughout the procedure and after the procedure following your facility's protocol.
■ Help the patient into the lithotomy position with slight elevation, placing the patient's legs in stirrups with her buttocks near the end of the table as for a vaginal examination.

■ Place a linen-saver pad under the buttocks.
■ Wash your hands, and put on the sterile gloves. Using a sterile speculum, locate the cervix.
■ Apply the $PGE_2$ preparation.
■ After the procedure, return the patient to a supine or semi-Trendelenburg position for 15 to 30 minutes to minimize leakage. Then return the patient to a more comfortable position while monitoring the FHR and contractions following your facility's protocol. At a minimum, the FHR should be monitored by the external fetal monitor for at least 30 minutes, and for up to 2 hours, after the

PGE$_2$ is placed in the endocervical canal.

## Postprocedure patient teaching

■ Tell the patient that the dosage can be repeated in 6 hours for a maximum of three doses.
■ Tell the patient that labor will usually ensue within 12 hours.

## Complications

■ If uterine hyperstimulation occurs, the patient should be placed on her left side and oxygen should be administered. If uterine hyperstimulation persists, a tocolytic agent may be used to reverse the action of the prostaglandin.
■ Hypertonus or maternal fluid overload can occur, and the patient should be vigilantly observed.

## Special considerations

■ Oxytocin may be started 12 hours after the last dose of prostaglandin.
■ If PGE$_2$ gel is to be used in the case of fetal demise after 28 weeks gestation, use caution due to the risk of uterine rupture.
■ An interval of 6 hours before repeating the dose or 12 hours before starting intravenous oxytocin or a maximum cumulative dose of 1.5 mg (0.5 mg of gel in three applications) in 24 hours is recommended to avoid hyperstimulation.
■ Gel shouldn't be placed above

the internal cervical os because this may lead to hyperstimulation.

## Documentation

■ Record that informed consent was obtained.
■ Document the indication for cervical ripening, along with the date and time and how the patient tolerated it.
■ Record the FHR and establish a baseline prior to the administration of prostaglandin. Record maternal vital signs and fetal response to the administration of the medication. Document the contraction pattern hourly, or more frequently, as conditions warrant.

# Chalazion and Hordeolum Therapy

***CPT code***
*No specific code has been assigned.*

## Overview

A chalazion is a local inflammation of the meibomian glands, which are sebaceous follicles located between the tarsi and the conjunctiva of the eyelid. This may result from a chronic hordeolum or a chronic granuloma from an obstructed meibomian gland. A chalazion is a nontender, firm, discrete swelling with overlying skin that's freely movable. A hordeolum, also called a stye, is usually caused by the *Staphylococcus aureus* organism. It's a localized, purulent, inflammatory infection that plugs one or more sebaceous glands of the eyelids and usually projects from or localizes on the lid border; it's usually painful, red, and swollen.

When a patient presents with an inflammatory disorder that affects the eye, prompt assessment, diagnosis, and treatment is imperative along with an ophthalmic referral (if necessary) for incision and drainage. However, in general, asymptomatic chalazia and hordeoli normally resolve with periodic application of warm moist compresses in under a week's time and don't require invasive treatment.

### Indications
■ To treat the presence of chalazia or hordeoli

### Contraindications
**RELATIVE**
■ Suspected infection

### Preprocedure patient preparation
■ Inform the patient that temporary pain relief should be noted with the application of the warm compresses. Most discomfort should fully resolve within 7 to 10 days of therapy.

### Equipment
Ophthalmoscope ◆ Snellen's chart ◆ topical antibiotics (such as gentamycin, tobramycin, or ciprofloxacin) ◆ warm, moist 4″ × 4″ compresses ◆ eye patch ◆ sterile swab with medium (optional)

### Procedure
■ Explain the procedure to the patient, and address any questions or concerns he may have.
■ Wash your hands.
■ Assess the external and internal eye structures using the ophthalmoscope and visual fields examination.
■ Assess the external structure for any abnormal masses of the eyelid or eyelash borders. Look for any redness, swelling, drainage, or pustular areas. If desired, obtain a culture specimen at this time with a sterile swab with medium. If these signs are present, apply warm 4″ × 4″ compresses for 15 minutes to provide comfort and clean the eyelid and eyelash area.
■ Assess visual acuity with the Snellen's chart.
■ Reassess the external and internal eye structures.
■ Prescribe an antibiotic ointment, such as gentamicin, tobramycin, or ciprofloxacin, if indicated.

✺ **COLLABORATION**
*If palliative treatment isn't successful and the patient complains of severe pain, if a large pustule is present, or if vision is impaired, refer the patient to an ophthalmologist*

*for chalazion removal or incision and drainage.*

- Apply an eye patch before discharge for comfort, if necessary.

## Postprocedure patient teaching

- Tell the patient to follow up with you in 7 to 10 days if no relief is noted, otherwise in 2 to 3 weeks.
- Inform the patient that pain relief can also be achieved by systemic analgesics, such as acetaminophen, if necessary.
- Teach the patient that eye makeup shouldn't be used until the chalazion or hordeolum is clinically resolved. Instruct her to discard old eye makeup to prevent reinfection.
- Instruct the patient to use an eye patch over a gauze pad between compress applications to collect any drainage and promote comfort until the eye feels better.
- Tell the patient to apply warm compresses several times per day (four to five) for approximately 15 to 20 minutes at a time. Also tell the patient not to squeeze the site but to allow it to open and drain spontaneously.
- If you prescribe antibiotics, instruct the patient to apply a thin layer to the affected area with a cotton swab.

## Complications

- Cellulitis or corneal abrasion may occur if a chronic chalazion is large enough or grows to a large

size. An induced astigmatism may persist until the nodule is removed. An ophthalmology consult should be obtained for evaluation and treatment of these cases.

- Recurrent infections may indicate immunocompromise and require systemic evaluation.

## Special considerations

✿ COLLABORATION
*Consider referral to an ophthalmologist, as up to one-half of adults with chalazia may have rosacea. In addition, meibomian gland carcinoma presentation is similar to that of chalazia.*

- Topical antibiotics (such as gentamycin, tobramycin, or ciprofloxacin) may be prescribed for 7 to 10 days to eliminate any microorganisms.

## Documentation

- Document the pretreatment ophthalmic assessment.
- Record the visual acuity results obtained using Snellen's chart.
- Note the appearance, color, and amount of wound drainage.
- Record the patient's understanding of instructions given.
- Document if an ophthalmic referral is necessary. When referring a patient, include the name, address, and phone number of the ophthalmologist and that you discussed at length the patient's need to go for further evaluation and treatment.

# CHEST PERCUSSION

### CPT code
97124 *Therapeutic procedure, one or more areas, each 15 minutes; massage, including tapotement (stroking, compression, percussion)*

## Overview
Chest percussion can mobilize and eliminate secretions, reexpand lung tissue, and promote efficient use of respiratory muscles. Candidates in the ambulatory setting for chest percussion include patients who expectorate large amounts of sputum, such as those with bronchiectasis and cystic fibrosis.

Percussing the chest with cupped hands mechanically dislodges thick, tenacious secretions from the bronchial walls. Vibration can be used with percussion or as an alternative to it in a patient who is frail or in pain.

## Indications
■ To assist the patient in expectorating excess sputum from the bronchial tree

## Contraindications
**ABSOLUTE**
■ Active pulmonary bleeding with hemoptysis
■ Fractured ribs
■ Unstable chest wall, lung contusions, acute asthma or bronchospasm, or recent myocardial infarction

## Preprocedure patient preparation
■ Perform a physical examination to assess the patient's baseline respiratory status.

## Equipment
Emesis basin ◆ suction equipment ◆ sterile specimen container (optional)

## Procedure
■ Explain the procedure to the patient, and address any questions or concerns he may have.
■ Wash your hands.
■ Assist the patient to a comfortable sitting position, or have him lie down.
■ Perform percussion and vibration. (See *Performing percussion and vibration,* page 94.)
■ After percussion and vibration, instruct the patient to cough to remove loosened secretions. First, tell him to inhale deeply through his nose and then exhale in three short huffs. Then have him inhale deeply again and cough through a slightly open mouth. Three consecutive coughs are highly effective. An effective cough sounds deep, low, and hollow; an ineffective one, high-pitched. Have the patient perform these exercises for about 1 minute, and then rest.
■ The patient can expectorate secretions into the emesis basin, or a

## Performing percussion and vibration

To perform percussion, instruct the patient to breathe slowly and deeply, using the diaphragm, to promote relaxation. Hold your hands in a cupped shape, with fingers flexed and thumbs pressed tightly against your index fingers. Percuss each segment for 1 to 2 minutes by alternating your hands against the patient in a rhythmic manner. Listen for a hollow sound on percussion to verify correct performance of the technique.

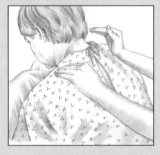

To perform vibration, ask the patient to inhale deeply and then exhale slowly through pursed lips. During exhalation, firmly press your fingers and the palms of your hands against the chest wall. Tense the muscles of your arms and shoulders in an isometric contraction to send fine vibrations through the chest wall. Vibrate during five exhalations over each chest segment.

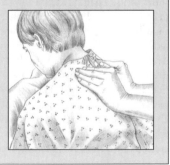

sterile specimen container if necessary. If the patient has difficulty coughing, use suction equipment to remove secretions.
- Reevaluate the patient's respiratory status.

## Postprocedure patient teaching

- Explain to the patient that he can perform the coughing and deep breathing exercises at home, gradually progressing to 10 minute exercise periods 4 times daily. Stress the importance of these activities to aid the lungs in healing after pneumonia or bronchitis.

## Special considerations

- Be aware that chest percussion can cause bronchospasm. The patient may need nebulizer therapy before or after the procedure if his lungs are extremely reactive.
- Refrain from percussing over the spine, liver, kidneys, or spleen to avoid injury to the spine or internal organs. Also avoid performing percussion on bare skin or the female patient's breasts. Percuss over soft clothing (but not over buttons, snaps, or zippers), or place a thin towel over the chest wall. Remember to remove jewelry that might scratch or bruise the patient.

## Complications

- Vigorous percussion or vibration could cause rib fracture, especially in the patient with osteoporosis.

■ Coughing could lead to pneumothorax in the patient with blebs due to emphysema.

## Documentation

■ Record the date and time of chest percussion, the position of the patient, locations on the chest that were percussed, and the color, amount, odor, and viscosity of secretions produced, including the presence of any blood.
■ Document the patient's toleration of the procedure.
■ Document the patient instructions given and that the patient can properly perform coughing and deep breathing.

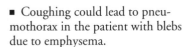

# CHILD RESTRAINT TECHNIQUES

### *CPT code*
*No specific code has been assigned. Restraint techniques, if needed, are considered part of the examination or procedure for which they are utilized; they receive no separate charge.*

## Overview

When performing examinations and procedures with younger children, often the child is restless or uncooperative, leading to difficulty or failure in obtaining the necessary information. Utilizing various methods of restraint may help the health care provider in obtaining the most accurate and thorough

### How to use the parent-assisted supine restraint

The illustration below shows how to use the parent-assisted supine restraint. Lay the child down on his back and ask the parent to hold the child's arms down beside his head. While you examine the child, ask the parent to comfort the child by talking to him. If necessary, a second assistant may hold down the child's legs.

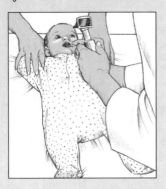

information while ensuring the safety of the child.

## Indications

■ To safely and quickly perform examinations and procedures on an infant or uncooperative younger child
■ To properly position an infant or child for an examination or procedure
■ To minimize movement and discomfort during an examination or procedure

## Contraindications

■ The method of restraint should

## How to perform the hug restraint

The illustration below shows how to perform the hug restraint. Ask the parent to sit the child on his lap and place one arm around the child's waist, holding the exposed arm securely, and one arm around his head in a hug position. The child's arm that's against the parent should be tucked under the parent's arm so the parent can hold it there securely.

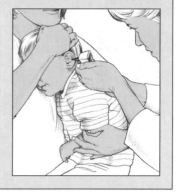

have no effect on the child's respiratory, cardiovascular, or musculoskeletal system.

## Preprocedure patient preparation

■ Calm the child as much as possible to prevent the need for restraint. Games are a helpful adjunct in preparing a child for cooperation with an examination or procedure.
■ Explain the need for and method of restraint to the parents, without criticism of the child.
■ Utilize the parents or other support staff as much as possible.

> **CLINICAL TIP**
> *Assess the value of utilizing the parents as an assistant during an uncomfortable procedure or examination. Some parents and children may need to see the parent as the "good" person and the health care provider as the "bad" person.*

## Equipment

Blanket or towel (if mechanically restraining the child)

## Procedure

■ Gather as much information as possible regarding the child's behavior to aid in choosing the most appropriate method of restraint.
■ Explain the restraint procedure to the parents, and address any questions or concerns they may have.
■ Wash your hands.

### Parent-assisted supine restraint

■ Place the child in a supine position with arms extended.
■ Have assisting parent hold the arms alongside the head, keeping both from moving.
■ If necessary, a second assistant may need to hold the child's legs. (See *How to use the parent-assisted supine restraint,* page 95.)

### Hug restraint

■ Sit the child on the parent's lap with the child's legs to one side.
■ Tuck one of the child's arms under the parent's arm, and have the parent hold it securely.

■ With the parent's same arm, hug the child holding his other arm securely.

■ With the parent's other arm, hold the child's head securely. (See *How to perform the hug restraint.*)

*Leg restraint*
■ Follow the procedure for a hug restraint.
■ Have the parent hold the child's legs securely between his legs.

*Mummy restraint (papoose)*
■ Place a blanket on a safe, secure surface.
■ Fold down one corner of the blanket so the tip is approximately halfway to the midsection of the blanket.
■ Place the child on the blanket with his head halfway off the folded part of the blanket.
■ Bring one side of the blanket over the child's straightened arm, and tuck the blanket securely underneath the opposite arm, around the back.
■ Tightly wrap the other side of the blanket, again over the child's straightened other arm, across to the other side and securely tuck the blanket underneath his back.
■ If also swaddling the legs, bring the bottom of the blanket up in between his legs prior to tucking the second side of the blanket underneath his back. (See *Applying a mummy restraint.*)
■ For all of these techniques, release the restraint as quickly as possible, and praise the child for cooperating with the examination.

## Applying a mummy restraint

The illustration below shows the application of a mummy restraint, or papoose, using a blanket.

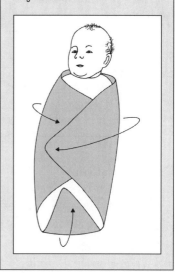

## Postprocedure patient teaching

■ Explain the findings of the examination, or the results of the restraint procedure, to the parents.

## Complications

■ The child may become less cooperative as the restraints are applied. Examine him as quickly, safely, and efficiently as possible.

## Special considerations
■ Use caution when utilizing child

restraint techniques; other alternatives might be more appropriate.

■ Often, infants and children will allow examinations without needing to utilize restraints. Establishing a rapport with the parents and child prior to the examination, and saving the most uncomfortable procedures until the end may prevent the need for restraint techniques.

■ Utilizing toys, games, and techniques that the child may be more familiar and comfortable with may help the examination go more smoothly.

## Documentation

■ Document the method of restraint used and the patient's toleration of it.

■ Document findings of the examination, or results of the restraint procedure, in the patient's chart.

# CIRCUMCISION

### CPT code
54150 *Circumcision, using clamp or other device; neonate*

## Overview

Steeped in controversy and history, circumcision — the removal of the penile foreskin — is thought to promote a clean glans and to minimize the risk of phimosis (tightening of the foreskin) in later life. It's also thought to reduce the risk of penile cancer and the risk of cervical cancer in sexual partners, although the American Academy of Pediatrics (AAP) has contended since 1971 that no valid medical reason exists for routine circumcision. Currently, the AAP is continuing its studies on the effects of circumcision.

In Judaism, circumcision is a religious rite (known as a bris) performed by a mohel on the 8th day after birth, when the neonate officially receives his name. Because most neonates are discharged before this time, the bris rarely occurs in the hospital.

One method of circumcision involves removing the foreskin by using a Yellen clamp to stabilize the penis. With this device, a cone that fits over the glans provides a cutting surface and protects the glans penis. Another technique uses a plastic circumcision bell (Plastibell) over the glans and a suture tied tightly around the base of the foreskin. This method prevents bleeding. The resultant ischemia causes the foreskin to slough off within 5 to 8 days. This method is thought to be painless because it stretches the foreskin, which inhibits sensory conduction.

## Indications

■ To satisfy religious requirement
■ To fulfill parental choice
■ To treat phimosis, balanoposthitis, and paraphimosis if other treatment modalities fail

## Contraindications

### ABSOLUTE

- Neonates who are ill or who have bleeding disorders
- Ambiguous genitalia
- Congenital anomalies of the penis, such as hypospadias, epispadias, or chordee (because the foreskin may be needed for later reconstructive surgery)

## Preprocedure patient preparation

- Tell the parents that feedings should be withheld 1 hour prior to the circumcision.
- Discuss the selected pain control option.

## Equipment

Sterile circumcision tray (contents vary but usually include circumcision clamps, various-sized cones, scalpel, probe, scissors, forceps, basin, towel, and drapes) ◆ povidone-iodine solution ◆ restraining board with arm and leg restraints ◆ gloves ◆ sterile gloves ◆ sterile petroleum gauze ◆ sterile 4″ × 4″ gauze pads ◆ tuberculin syringe ◆ 27G needle ◆ local anesthetic such as lidocaine without epinephrine ◆ alcohol swabs ◆ sutures, plastic circumcision bell, antimicrobial ointment, topical anesthetic, and overhead warmer (optional)

### *Equipment preparation*

*For circumcision using a Yellen clamp*

- Assemble the sterile circumci-

sion tray and other equipment in the procedure area.

- Open the tray and pour povidone-iodine solution into the basin.
- Using aseptic technique, place sterile 4″ × 4″ gauze pads and petroleum gauze on the tray.
- Arrange the restraining board and direct adequate light on the area. Turn on overhead warmer, if necessary.

*For circumcision using a plastic circumcision bell*

- Although you won't need to assemble a circumcision tray, do assemble sterile gloves, sutures, restraining board, petroleum gauze and, if necessary, antibiotic ointment. Turn on the overhead warmer, if necessary.

## Procedure

- Explain the procedure to the parents, and address any questions or concerns they may have.

☑ **OBTAIN INFORMED CONSENT**

- Withhold feeding for at least 1 hour before the procedure to reduce the possibility of emesis and aspiration.
- Wash your hands.
- Place the neonate on the restraining board, and restrain his arms and legs. Don't leave him unattended.
- Comfort the neonate as needed, using soft talking, a pacifier, or other calming methods.
- Put on gloves. Inspect the penis for abnormalities and identify the

## Penile anatomy

Being aware of penile anatomy can help prevent trauma to internal structures, such as the urethra, or resecting too much prepuce.

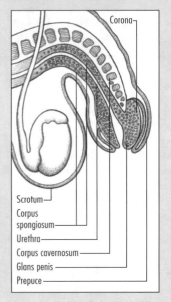

Corona

Scrotum

Corpus spongiosum

Urethra

Corpus cavernosum

Glans penis

Prepuce

location of the meatus on the glans. Drape the neonate. (See *Penile anatomy*.)

■ If no abnormalities are detected, you may anesthetize the penis. First, clean the insertion site with an alcohol swab. Prepare a tuberculin syringe with a 27G needle and lidocaine without epinephrine. Insert the needle around the midpoint of the penile shaft. Infiltrate in a band or ring pattern as you withdraw the needle. (See *Performing local anesthesia*.)

■ After putting on sterile gloves, clean the penis and scrotum with povidone-iodine, moving from the tip of the glans toward the body, covering an area approximately 3″ (7.5 cm) in diameter around the base of the penis as well as the entire penis.

### Using a Yellen clamp

■ Apply a Yellen clamp to the penis. Then loosen the foreskin and insert the cone under it to provide a cutting surface and protect the penis. Next, remove the foreskin. (See *Performing a circumcision*, pages 102 and 103.)

■ Alternatively, a plastic bell may be used. (See *Using a plastic bell*, page 104.)

■ Cover the wound with sterile petroleum gauze to prevent infection and control bleeding.

■ Remove the neonate from the restraining board, and check for bleeding.

■ Show the neonate to his parents or caregivers to reassure them.

■ Write instructions for his care postcircumcision:

– Place the neonate on his back to minimize pressure on the excisional area.

– Leave him diaperless for 1 to 2 hours to observe for bleeding and to reduce possible chafing and irritation.

– After the neonate is rediapered, his diaper should be changed as soon as he voids. If the dressing falls off, clean the wound with warm water to minimize pain from urine on the circumcised area. Don't remove the original dressing until it falls off (usually after the first or second voiding).

– Check for bleeding every 15 minutes for the 1st hour and then every hour for the next 24 hours. If bleeding occurs, apply pressure with sterile gauze pads. You should be notified if bleeding continues.

– Avoid leaving the neonate under the radiant warmer after placing petroleum gauze on the penis because the area might burn.

– Apply diapers loosely to prevent irritation. At each diaper change, apply antimicrobial ointment, petroleum jelly, or petroleum gauze until the wound appears healed.

– Watch for drainage, redness, or swelling. Don't remove the thin, yellow-white exudate that forms over the healing area within 1 to 2 days. This normal incrustation protects the wound until it heals in 3 to 4 days.

– Don't discharge the neonate until he has voided.

## Postprocedure patient teaching

■ Inform the parents or caregivers that the circumcision site may appear yellow in light-skinned neonates and lighter than the surrounding skin in dark-skinned neonates. Tell them that this signifies healing and isn't a cause for concern.

■ Instruct the parents or caregivers to observe the circumcision site regularly for pus or bloody discharge, which may indicate delayed healing or infection. If these signs occur, the parents or caregivers should notify you.

■ Tell the parents or caregivers that the rim of the device used for

## Performing local anesthesia

The neonate does experience pain during circumcision. The neural pathways that relay pain, the cortex and subcortex that perceive pain, and the neurotransmitters are all functioning before birth. Research has shown that neonatal circumcision produces increases in heart rate, blood pressure, plasma cortisol levels, crying, wakefulness, and irritability, and decreases in the transcutaneous partial pressure of oxygen for up to an hour after the procedure. Local anesthesia reduces or eliminates these changes.

To perform local penile anesthesia, draw up the anesthetic (such as 1% lidocaine without epinephrine) into a tuberculin syringe with a 27G needle. Insert the needle halfway along the penile shaft on each side.

Infiltrate the lidocaine in a band or ring around the penis.

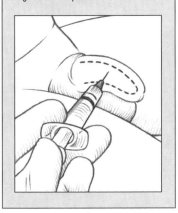

circumcision may remain in place after discharge from the hospital. Reassure them that the rim will fall off harmlessly in 3 or 4 days. However, if the rim doesn't fall off after 1 week, tell them to notify

## Performing a circumcision

When performing a circumcision, you may find it helpful to use clock positions as reference points. Place hemostats on very small segments of the prepuce (be sure not to clamp onto the glans) at the 3 o'clock and the 9 o'clock positions, and assert gentle traction. Gently insert a straight hemostat between the prepuce and the glans to the depth of the corona (the rounded proximal border of the glans penis). Open the hemostat, and gently sweep it in both directions in a circumferential motion. Avoid going deeper than the corona or traumatizing the urethra.

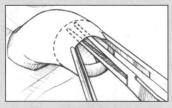

Raise the hemostat away from the glans, forming a tent. Inspect underneath the tented area to ensure that no part of the glans is in the way.

Take the straight hemostat and carefully clamp the dorsal aspect of the prepuce in the vertical line of the penis from one-third to one-half of the total distance to the corona. Wait 1 minute for hemostasis to occur and then remove the straight hemostat.

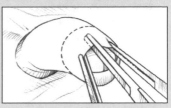

Immediately tent the skin again with straight scissors and cut along the center of the indentation left by the clamped hemostat, making a dorsal slit. Be careful not to cut past the indentation, as this will result in excessive bleeding.

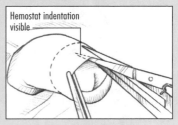

Hemostat indentation visible

Gently retract the prepuce from the glans and lyse any adhesions with a 4″ × 4″

you, since a retained rim may lead to infection.

## Complications

■ Infection and bleeding may occur after circumcision and are treated locally. If they don't resolve, a further evaluation and work-up are indicated.

■ Scarring or fibrous bands may result when the skin of the penile shaft adheres to the glans. The most severe complications are urethral fistulae and edema. Incomplete amputation of the foreskin can follow application of the plastic circumcision bell. These neonates should be referred to a surgeon or pediatrician quickly to increase the likelihood of a good outcome.

gauze or hemostat, taking care to go slightly beyond the incision line to minimize bleeding and provide a cosmetically pleasing result. If the foreskin will not retract, repeat the last two steps, only slightly deeper.

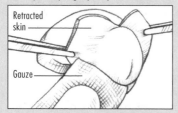

Place the cone over the glans and apply gentle pressure to the distal end or stem of the cone. At the same time, use the attached curved hemostat to ease the prepuce over the cone. The cone should sit between the glans and the prepuce against the corona. Suture the edges of the prepuce to the cone and release the hemostat.

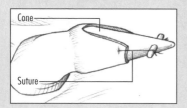

Insert the cone and the prepuce into the Yellen clamp, tighten slightly, verify placement (prepuce is even all around and the dorsal slit is fully visible inside the instrument), then tighten firmly. Position the scalpel at an angle slightly higher than horizontal. Press firmly against the cone and glide completely around the cone, being sure to penetrate all of the skin and mucosal layers. Remove all of the tissue within the instrument, as this may become a source of infection.

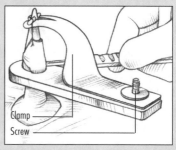

Immediately release the penis from the clamp and check for bleeding. Hemostasis may be enhanced by applying pressure, topical epinephrine, silver nitrate, or Gelfoam to the site of the bleeding. If this is ineffective, refer the patient immediately to a surgeon.

## Special considerations

■ A mohel usually brings his own equipment.

■ Always be sure to show the parents or caregivers the circumcision before discharge so they can ask any questions and you can teach them how to care for the area.

■ If the neonate's mother has human immunodeficiency virus (HIV) infection, circumcision should be delayed until the neonate's HIV status is known. The neonate whose mother has HIV infection has a higher-than-normal risk for infection.

■ Special care is needed in administering analgesia to neonates because of their increased skin permeability, susceptibility to apnea from opiates, and the prolonged pharmacologic half-lives of the drugs administered to them.

## Using a plastic bell

An alternative method of circumcision utilizes a plastic bell after making the dorsal slit. Using this method, the distal prepuce will become ischemic, then atrophic, eventually dropping off in 5 to 8 days. The prepuce will drop off with the plastic bell attached, leaving a clean, well-healed excision.

First, slide the plastic bell device between the foreskin and the glans penis; verify placement.

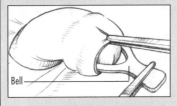

Excise the prepuce 1/8″ (3.2 mm) distal to the suture. Cut the suture to about 1/2″ (12 mm).

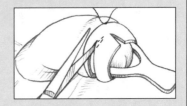

Find the bell indentation (at the coronal edge of the glans), and apply the suture lightly. After verifying the amount of skin to remove, and that the plastic bell can move freely on the glans penis, tighten the suture for 30 seconds before tying to promote hemostasis.

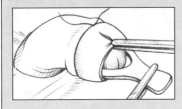

Holding the plastic bell in one hand, gently bend the stem portion with the other hand until it snaps.

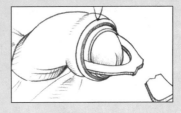

## Documentation

■ Note the time and date of the circumcision, procedure utilized, condition of the site, how the neonate tolerated the procedure, and any parent or caregiver teaching.

■ Document excessive bleeding or complications, the corrective actions taken, and the outcomes.

■ Note that options, along with potential adverse effects and complications, were discussed in detail. State that the parents or guardian desired circumcision.

# CLAVICLE IMMOBILIZATION

**CPT code**
23500 *Closed treatment of clavicle fracture without manipulation*

## Overview

A fractured clavicle is one of the most common skeletal injuries among all patients and the clavicle is the most commonly fractured bone in children. About 80% of fractures occur at the middle third of the clavicle, 15% occur at the distal site, and 5% occur proximally. The most common mechanisms of injury are a fall on an outstretched arm or hand and a direct blow or fall to the shoulder. Fracture can also result from high-energy direct blows sustained in motor vehicle accidents or contact sports, such as football, hockey, or wrestling. Clavicle fractures are classified according to location, degree of displacement, and involvement of articular surfaces or ligaments. (See *Classifying distal clavicular fractures,* page 106.)

Treatment includes immobilizing and stabilizing the fracture site to reduce pain and risk of additional injury, to maintain correct alignment during healing with minimal residual deformity or loss of function, to reduce the risk of nonunion, and to promote the patient's comfort.

Most middle third fractures can be managed appropriately by immobilization with a figure-eight bandage or sling.

## Indications

- To treat fractures of the middle third and medial third of the clavicle

## Contraindications

**ABSOLUTE**

- Fractures likely to require surgery, such as open fractures or fractures of the distal third of the clavicle with displacement
- Fractures in which neurovascular or respiratory compromise is suspected
- Fractures in which the shortening of the clavicle length is ½″ (1.3 cm) or more, which may increase risk for postoperative pain and dysfunction

## Preprocedure patient preparation

- Take a complete history and perform a physical examination. Include the mechanism of injury or degree of trauma, the onset and location of the pain, and the degree of movement or functioning after the injury.
- Reassure the patient that pain is usually greatly reduced after the fracture is immobilized. Explain that a "bump" may persist over the fracture site and won't impair function. Tell him when to expect full healing (4 to 6 weeks in adults, 3 to 4 weeks in children).

## Classifying distal clavicular fractures

Distal clavicular fractures may be minimally displaced (type I), displaced due to a fracture medial to the coracoclavicular ligaments (type II), or an articular surface fracture (type III).

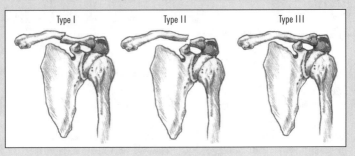

Type I    Type II    Type III

## Equipment

### For clavicle strap immobilization
Various commercial products are available

### For figure-eight immobilization
Bandage that's 6″ wide and 4′ to 6′ (1 to 2 m) long (length varies with size of the patient); may substitute stockinet filled with padding ◆ four to six large safety pins

### For sling-and-swathe immobilization
Sling (size based on size of patient) ◆ bandage (6″ wide and 4′ to 6′ long) ◆ two to three large safety pins

## Procedure
■ Explain the procedure to the patient, and address any questions or concerns he may have.

☑ OBTAIN
INFORMED CONSENT
■ Wash your hands.
■ Examine the clavicle for asymmetry and the ipsilateral shoulder for downward medial position. The proximal fragment of the clavicle will be positioned upward and posteriorly, causing tenting of the skin. The patient will frequently be splinting the affected side. Gentle palpation over the site will produce pain and crepitus.
■ Auscultate the lungs for symmetrical breath sounds. Verify the absence of underlying neurovascular injury. Evaluate pulses, skin temperature, and sensation and reflexes of the ipsilateral arm.
■ Obtain upright anteroposterior view X-rays to verify distal and middle third clavicle fractures. Also, note the appearance of the lungs and the position of the trachea. You may need a computed tomography scan to clearly visualize medial fractures. Anteroposteri-

or and lateral views of the thoracic spine may be indicated to rule out associated fracture of the first rib.

### For application of a clavicle strap

- Assist the patient to a comfortable seated position.
- Place the straps over his shoulders and under his arms.
- Standing behind and slightly above the patient, gently pull the straps toward the middle of his back, thus pulling both of his shoulders upward, laterally and backward.
- Maintain the position as you fasten the straps. (See *Clavicle strap immobilization,* pages 108 and 109.)
- Palpate the fracture for alignment and reevaluate neurovascular status.
- Repeat the X-ray to confirm alignment.

### For figure-eight immobilization

- Assist the patient to a comfortable seated position.
- Standing behind and slightly above the patient, hold one end of the long, wide bandage at the center of his back.
- Place the bandage over the top of one shoulder, bringing it down and under the axilla.
- Bring the bandage diagonally across his back, over the opposite shoulder, and under the axilla.
- With the bandage in place, gently tighten the ends until the shoulders are pulled slightly upward, laterally and backward.
- Pin the bandage in place.

- Palpate for alignment. Assess neurovascular status.
- Repeat the X-ray to confirm alignment.

### For sling-and-swathe immobilization

- Assist the patient to a comfortable seated position.
- Select a sling size appropriate to the patient's size, and place the sling on the ipsilateral arm.
- Wrap a 6″-bandage around the patient's torso and upper arm on the affected side, holding the arm against the chest wall to stabilize it. Fasten the bandage with safety pins.
- Palpate the fracture site for alignment. Assess neurovascular status.
- Repeat the X-ray to confirm alignment.

## Postprocedure patient teaching

- Remind the patient that he must wear the immobilizer constantly for 1 week. After that time, if he has no complications, he can remove it briefly for hygiene purposes. In any case, he must wear it until there's clinical evidence of union of the bone and until he can abduct the arm without pain.
- Tell a caregiver (such as a spouse or a parent) to frequently check the fit of the immobilizer or sling. If it feels too loose, it should be tightened. Instruct the patient to stand with his shoulders back in a "military position" while the caregiver tightens the immobilizer.
- Instruct the patient (or a re-

## Clavicle strap immobilization

To promote healing and comfort, you'll need to immobilize the patient's clavicle properly. Remember to use equipment that can be easily tightened and repositioned because the bandages and straps tend to loosen over time.

Clavicle immobilization is frequently achieved with tube stockinettes (shown in first illustration below) arranged in a figure-eight pattern (shown in second illustration below) and secured with safety pins. To increase patient comfort and compliance, pad the stockinette where it fits around the back of the neck and under the axillae.

Ready-made figure-eight clavicle immobilization straps use Velcro closures to permit a snug fit (as shown below). They can be adjusted to maintain proper positioning. Because the straps are thick, additional padding isn't usually necessary.

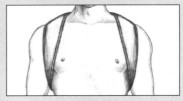

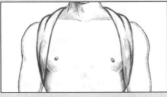

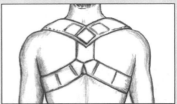

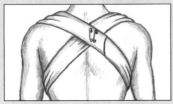

Whether you devise your own immobilization system or use a ready-made one, be sure the patient's shoulders are pulled upward and backward to allow the bones to knit in proper alignment, as shown (at top of next page) in this overhead view.

sponsible caregiver) to frequently check for swelling, color changes, or paresthesias of the hand and fingers. If any of these reactions occur, tell him to loosen the strap or sling until circulation and sensation are restored, and then to reapply it.
■ Ask the patient to frequently flex all his fingers, his wrist, and his elbow on the affected side to maintain flexibility and function.
■ Tell him not to raise the affected

arm above his shoulder for 6 weeks.
■ Promote his active participation in rehabilitation exercises, which should begin when the bone has fully healed. These exercises should include:
– the pendulum swing (Bend over from the waist. With the affected arm held down, gently swing it forward and backward in an arc, like a pendulum.)
– internal and external rotation (While lying down, use the unaf-

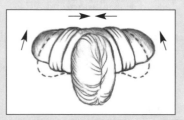

Some patients, particularly children or those with dementia, might be more compliant in a sling-and-swathe position. Immobilizing the arm on the affected side (as shown below) reminds the patient to limit movement. This position may also cause less discomfort.

The sling-and-swathe method (shown below) may also be more comfortable for a bedridden or chairbound patient because it doesn't require bulky strap connections along the middle of the patient's back.

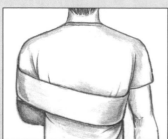

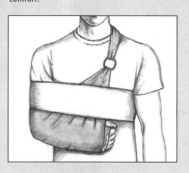

fected arm to gently pull the affected arm across the chest; then push it out laterally away from the affected side.)
—wall climbing. ("Walk" the fingers of the affected hand up a wall as far as they will comfortably go.)
■ Instruct him to use his unaffected hand to raise his affected arm forward in front of his chest.
■ If the patient is an athlete, urge him not to resume play until full range of motion (ROM) and strength are restored (usually

about 3 months). After that, special braces or splints aren't generally needed for play.
■ Urge him to contact you if he experiences persisting or worsening pain; numbness, tingling, or lack of sensation or decreasing function in the affected arm or hand; or any unusual swelling or coldness of the arm or hand.
■ Tell him to schedule a follow-up appointment in 1 week (sooner if he experiences problems).

## Complications

### ✳ COLLABORATION

■ *Nonunion, although rare, may occur with associated pain, deformity, and dysfunction; it requires referral to an orthopedist or a neurologist.*

■ *Malunion — with resultant clavicle deformity, compression of underlying structures, shortening of the clavicle, and impaired function — is also possible and requires referral to an orthopedist or a neurosurgeon.*

■ *Arthritis may result in fractures that involve articular surfaces; they require long-term management and referral to a rheumatologist.*

■ *Excess callus formation may put pressure on the brachial plexus or subclavian artery, causing thoracic outlet compression and paresthesia; these require referral to a neurologist or a neurosurgeon.*

## Special considerations

■ Some children may complain of discomfort and be uncooperative with the figure-eight or clavicle strap immobilizers. In this case, a simple sling or sling-and-swathe immobilizer may be better tolerated.

■ Include the patient's primary caregiver and support persons in the patient teaching.

■ Refer the patient to physical therapy for more intensive rehabilitation.

## Documentation

■ Review recent or pertinent documentation by other health team members; then initial their notes to signify that you're aware of their findings. This doesn't signify agreement with their comments or reduce your responsibility to conduct your own history and physical examination.

■ Before performing clavicle immobilization, document abnormal physical findings on the consent form and have the patient initial the comments and sign the form to signify acknowledgment of preprocedural abnormalities. In the chart, the preprocedural and postprocedural note must include an evaluation of function, ROM, and neurosensory testing (like two-point discrimination) along with a respiratory status evaluation. The differential diagnosis list or evaluation should indicate consideration of injury to the lung.

■ Record the mechanism of injury, any asymmetry or inability to raise the arm, the presence of pain, and radiologic verification of the fracture and postreduction alignment.

■ Record the patient's understanding of the instructions given after the procedure, particularly in the event of potential language barriers.

## *COLPOSCOPY AND CERVICAL BIOPSY*

### *CPT codes*

57452  *Colposcopy (separate procedure)*
57454  *Colposcopy with biopsy of cervix or endocervical curettage*
57500  *Biopsy, single or multiple, or local excision of lesion*

## Understanding how a colposcope works

The colposcope is a binocular microscope on a stand. It incorporates a light source, usually tungsten or halogen bulbs; some use a fiber-optic light source. The colposcope used in gynecologic examinations must be supplied with a green or blue filter that can be used to amplify findings. The filter absorbs red light reflected from blood vessels on the surface of the cervix, making them appear black against the surrounding tissue and enhancing their evaluation.

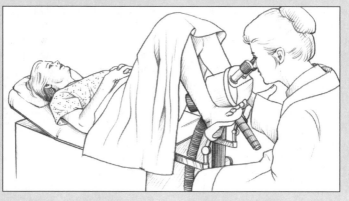

57505 *Endocervical curettage (separate procedure)*

## Overview

Colposcopy is an integral part of cervical cancer detection and treatment programs. Colposcopy more closely examines the cervix with the assistance of a special mounted microscope. It may be used to keep track of precancerous abnormalities and look for recurrent abnormalities after treatment. (See *Understanding how a colposcope works.*)

## Indications

■ To evaluate an abnormal Papanicolaou (Pap) smear result indicating cervical pathology

■ To treat a suspicious lesion visualized or palpated during pelvic examination
■ To rule out suspected human papilloma virus
■ To assess someone at high risk for dysplasia

## Contraindications
**RELATIVE**
■ Current menses, inflammation, or infection

## Preprocedure patient preparation

■ When scheduling a colposcopy, instruct the patient to avoid having intercourse or using vaginal medication, contraceptives, or douching for 48 hours before the examination.

■ Prepare the patient for the examination by describing the procedure. Sensations that may be experienced and should be discussed include stinging, which may accompany the application of acetic acid solution; a "pinch," which is how the biopsy of the cervix is experienced; and cramping that may accompany the endocervical curettage.

## Equipment

Colposcope ◆ gloves ◆ speculums ◆ biopsy forceps ◆ curettes ◆ endocervical speculum (optional) ◆ 3% to 5% acetic acid solution or normal saline solution ◆ Lugol's iodine solution ◆ Monsel's solution ◆ sponge forceps ◆ cotton-tipped and gynecologic applicator such as a Scopette ◆ sanitary napkins ◆ 4″ × 4″ sponges ◆ glass slide and preservative or vial with preservative

## Procedure

### For colposcopy

■ Explain the procedure to the patient, and address any questions or concerns she may have.

☑ OBTAIN
INFORMED CONSENT

■ Wash your hands.

■ After she has removed her undergarments, voided, and is appropriately draped, assist her to the lithotomy position, with her feet in the stirrups and her buttocks extended slightly beyond the edge of the table. Adjust the colpo-

scope's height to the examining table, chair, and yourself.

■ Put on gloves. Examine the external genitalia visually.

■ Using one gloved finger lubricated with water only, palpate the vaginal walls gently to detect subepithelial nodules or masses.

■ Also, ascertain the plane of the cervix so that insertion of the speculum will be atraumatic.

■ Insert a warm, clean, water-lubricated speculum of the appropriate size and open it to expose the cervix. (*Note:* To help the patient relax the pelvic musculature and ease the discomfort, encourage her to try to "push out" the speculum as you insert it.)

■ Obtain a Pap test specimen and cultures at this time, if needed.

■ Gently move the cervix with a cotton-tipped or gynecological applicator to clearly visualize the vaginal fornices.

■ Using a gynecologic applicator or a 4″ × 4″ sponge on a sponge stick, apply normal saline or acetic acid solution and clean the cervix of secretions. If acetic acid solution is used, it's necessary to wait several minutes before examining the cervix with the colposcope to allow aceto-whitening to fade.

■ Move the colposcope into position and focus to obtain the clearest cervical appearance. Examine the cervix under magnification. (See *Abnormal cervical findings*.)

■ Next, repeat the examination under blue or green light. This action makes abnormal surface blood vessels visible as black structures on the cervix.

■ After a complete and thorough

## Abnormal cervical findings

During the cervical examination, you're observing the appearance of the original squamous epithelium, the transformation zone (the area between the original squamous epithelium and columnar epithelium), and the columnar epithelium. Describe abnormal findings in detail, such as whether the lesion is flat, micropapillary, or microconvoluted. Iodine-negative epithelium results in a yellow color, as opposed to the normal iodine reaction, which is a dark mahogany color. The presence of atypical vessels in any lesion suggests more severe dysplasia. Leukoplakia is evidenced by white, thickened patches that can't be rubbed off and that sometimes show a tendency to fissure. Other abnormal findings that indicate the need for biopsy include:

■ Aceto-white epithelium (Note if it's mildly or intensely aceto-white.)

■ Punctuation with no blood vessel pattern and a pitted appearance

■ Mosaic with no blood vessel pattern and a geographic appearance

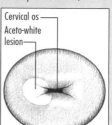

Cervical os
Aceto-white lesion

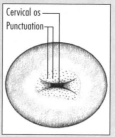

Cervical os
Punctuation

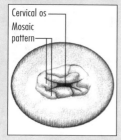

Cervical os
Mosaic pattern

examination, reapply 3% to 5% acetic acid solution to the cervix.

■ Allow at least 15 seconds for aceto-whitening to occur and reexamine the cervix with the colposcope without the light filter and then again with the light filter. If aceto-whitening fades during the examination, additional acetic acid solution can be applied without danger to the patient.

### For cervical biopsy

■ Repeat your examination for abnormal findings of the cervix.

■ Alternatively, some health care providers use Lugol's solution to paint the cervix for examination (Schiller's test). Lugol's is taken up

by normal, mature, glycogenated squamous epithelium, causing the tissue to attain a rich, mahogany color. Abnormal or neoplastic epithelium doesn't contain glycogen and won't stain, but looks a dirty yellow. Schiller's test is helpful in identifying the margins of lesions.

■ At this time, biopsy specimens of abnormal appearing cervical tissues are taken with the biopsy forceps. Always warn the patient before obtaining the biopsy that she'll feel a pinch. When identifying areas to biopsy, look for an area that will afford the pathologist with a border of normal and abnormal tissue, although it isn't

## Obtaining a cervical biopsy

Biopsy forceps are used to obtain a specimen of abnormal-appearing cervical tissues. The specimen should include the border of the lesion so the pathologist can compare normal and abnormal tissue.

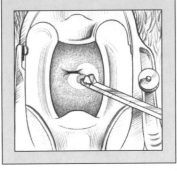

required. (See *Obtaining a cervical biopsy*.)

**CLINICAL TIP**
*Perform biopsies of abnormal areas of the posterior cervix before obtaining specimens from the anterior cervix. If anterior lesions are biopsied first, bleeding obscures the view of the posterior cervix and its lesions.*

■ Place the specimens immediately in preservative for transport to pathology.
■ Next, inform the patient that you'll be scraping cells from the canal of the cervix. Insert the curette ¾″ to 1¼″ (2 to 3 cm) into the cervical canal and scrape toward the external os. Repeat this procedure until you have scraped the canal two or three times in each quadrant. (For example, scrape the canal two or three times between the 9 o'clock and 12

o'clock quadrant, two or three times between the 12 o'clock and 3 o'clock quadrant, and so on.)
■ Place the endocervical specimen in preservative for transport to pathology.
■ Using an applicator, apply Monsel's solution to the biopsy areas to obtain hemostasis. Pressure may also be applied by a Scopette to control bleeding.
■ Remove the speculum, dispose of soiled equipment and supplies, and then assist the patient to a seated position. Instruct her that she may rest for a few minutes and then dress. Provide her with a sanitary napkin.

## Postprocedure patient teaching

■ Tell the patient that bleeding may continue like a light period for several days and that cramping may continue for the next few hours. Advise her that ibuprofen will relieve the cramps. Tell her to use sanitary napkins or panty liners for bleeding.
■ Explain to the patient that the Monsel's solution will drain out over the next day or so and will look like coffee grounds.
■ Tell the patient not to use tampons or vaginal preparations, to not douche unless instructed otherwise, and to abstain from intercourse for 1 week.
■ Instruct the patient to schedule follow-up in the facility when the results of the biopsies are received to discuss further therapy and a plan for her care.
■ Inform the patient to contact

you if she has heavier bleeding; a temperature higher than 100.4° F (38° C); a discharge with foul odor, burning, or itching; or other symptoms that cause concern.

■ Discuss lifestyle changes with the patient to reduce the risk of cervical cancer, including using condoms, stopping smoking, and avoiding exposure to sexually transmitted diseases by limiting the number of sexual partners.

## Complications

■ Excessive bleeding is treated with a second application of Monsel's solution.

■ Infection requires evaluation, testing, and treatment.

## Special considerations

■ Ideally, the time to perform the colposcopy in premenopausal women is at midcycle.

■ Refer to algorithms available for diagnostic decision making related to abnormal Pap smears and the performance of colposcopy (for example, at the National Testing Laboratories Web site, *www.cervicography.com/evaluating.html*).

■ There are a variety of colposcopy instruments available. Models with magnifications between 10× and 16× are practical for most diagnostic situations.

■ Graves metal bivalve speculums are preferred. Speculums with matte finishes may be used to overcome reflection problems.

■ The Kevorkian curette is used in a cervix with a wide os to obtain a specimen. The Novak curette is

more suitable for the narrow cervical os. A skin hook (optional) may be applied to the anterior cervical lip to stabilize the cervix if the curette doesn't slip easily into the os.

■ Cervicography is an adjunctive cervical screening procedure, intended to increase the sensitivity of the Pap smear in screening for cervical abnormalities. After a routine Pap Smear test is obtained, the cervix is swabbed with an acetic acid solution and the outside of the cervix is photographed with a special camera such as a cerviscope. The photos are then sent for evaluation by an expert. The slide is projected on a screen 10′ (3 m) or greater in width and observed at a distance of 3′ (1 m). This process approximates a colposcopic examination, and the information obtained can be used to allow the specialist to triage patients and see those with more severe dysplasia quickly. This isn't a substitute for colposcopy, but rather is performed as a prelude to colposcopy in areas where colposcopists aren't routinely available.

■ When performing cervicography, examine the cervix carefully and remove any hair, discharge, or other obstruction to visualization without rubbing or traumatizing tissue. Obstruction is the most common reason for a "technically defective" cervicography result.

## Documentation

■ Chart the indications for and the patient's response to the procedure. An efficient way to document colposcopic findings is by drawing the cervix with areas of aceto-whitened epithelium, abnormal vessels, mosaic, punctation, or leukoplakia drawn in and labeled as visualized. Areas biopsied should be marked by o'clock locations. It's important to draw lesions to scale to avoid misunderstanding about the size by professionals or laypersons who may review the chart in the future.

■ Classify the colposcopy as satisfactory (entire squamocolumnar junction visualized) or unsatisfactory (unable to inspect complete squamocolumnar junction).

■ Document patient teaching, instructions for follow-up care, and the need for further treatment or referral.

## CONDYLOMA ACUMINATUM TREATMENT

### CPT codes

56501 *Destruction of lesion(s), vulva; simple, any method*
56515 *Destruction of lesion(s), vulva; extensive, any method*

### Overview

Human papillomavirus (HPV) is a slow-growing deoxyribonucleic acid (DNA) virus that causes intradermal papilloma and is a sexually transmitted disease (STD). HPV infection creates the lesions commonly called genital warts. HPV may be external or internal.

External HPV lesions may be removed by self-applied medications (imiquimod [Aldara] or podofilox [Condylox]), 80% to 90% trichloroacetic acid (TCA), or 10% to 25% podophyllin. Cryotherapy with liquid nitrogen, vaporization with a carbon dioxide laser, electrodiathermy loop excision procedure, surgical excision, and interferon or 5-fluorouracil are methods used by physicians to treat internal lesions. The methods most commonly used by health care providers (TCA and podophyllin) are discussed here. Both of these methods are relatively inexpensive but can cause skin irritation. When choosing between them, remember that podophyllin and podofilox have a low systemic absorption rate, and TCA penetration is difficult to control. Health care providers who specialize in dermatology or STD clinics, or those who perform colposcopy, may use additional therapies.

The purpose of therapy is to remove genital warts and prevent progression of neoplasias. Because HPV is a virus and resides in human tissues even when dormant, it isn't possible to eradicate the infection, and recurrence of lesions is common.

### Indications

■ To treat external genital or vaginal condylomata
■ To remove symptomatic condylomata

## Contraindications

### RELATIVE
- Pregnancy (for podophyllin use)
- Internal HPV treatment
- Suspected malignancy

## Preprocedure patient preparation

- Teach the patient, and her partners if necessary, that although the first outbreak occurs after a 1- to 6-month incubation period, it isn't always symptomatic. Recurrent outbreaks can occur years later. Thus, diagnosing a patient with condyloma acuminata for the first time isn't "proof" of having intercourse with an infected person within the recent past.
- Warn the patient that the podophyllin or TCA may sting within minutes of application but usually resolves in about 5 minutes.

## Equipment

Cotton-tipped applicators ◆ 80% to 90% TCA or 10% to 25% podophyllin ◆ petroleum jelly ◆ light source ◆ gloves ◆ paper cup ◆ 3% to 5% acetic acid solution ◆ 4″ × 4″ gauze pads ◆ antiseptic such as povidone-iodine ◆ fenestrated drape ◆ tuberculin syringes ◆ interferon ◆ 27G or 30G needle

## Procedure

- Explain the procedure to the patient, and address any questions or concerns she may have.

✔ **OBTAIN INFORMED CONSENT**
- Wash your hands.
- After the patient has removed her undergarments and is appropriately draped, assist her to the lithotomy position, with her feet in the stirrups and her buttocks extended slightly beyond the edge of the table.
- Adjust the lamp so that it fully illuminates the genital area. Then fold back the corner of the drape to expose the perineum.
- Put on gloves. Warn the patient that you're about to touch her to avoid startling her.
- Using cotton-tipped applicators or gauze soaked with acetic acid solution, swab the area. Areas with HPV-DNA will turn white (called aceto-whitening).

### *For topical application*
- Apply a fenestrated drape, if desired, making sure all lesions are easily accessible.
- Using gloved fingers, coat the healthy skin adjacent to the lesions with petroleum jelly to protect it.
- Remove 0.5 ml of podophyllin from the container and place in a paper cup or open the TCA container. Dip a cotton-tipped applicator into the podophyllin or TCA.
- Apply the podophyllin or TCA to lesions, taking care to avoid touching the chemicals to healthy tissue. With TCA, the lesions will turn white.
- Dispose of each applicator after it touches tissue and use additional applicators until all lesions are treated.

### For lesion injection

■ Using 4″ × 4″ gauze pads and an antiseptic, such as povidone-iodine, clean the area in a circular motion from the site of the lesions outward.

■ Apply the fenestrated drape, ensuring that all lesions are easily accessible.

■ Using a separate tuberculin syringe with a 27G or 30G needle for each lesion, fill each syringe with the appropriate dose of interferon. A maximum of five lesions may be treated at each visit.

■ Insert the needle into the base of the lesion and form a wheal with the interferon. Repeat for each lesion.

■ Repeat the procedure twice weekly for 1 to 2 months for each lesion, depending on the response to treatment.

## Postprocedure patient teaching

■ Tell the patient to wash off the podophyllin in 2 to 4 hours.

■ Inform the patient that the area treated will be tender but should improve in a few hours. The tissues may be red, and leukorrhea may develop in females. These symptoms resolve in 2 to 3 days. The lesions will become smaller and finally disappear if therapy is successful.

■ Advise the patient to take warm water sitz baths to relieve perineal discomfort.

■ If the lesions are too sore to touch with a towel, tell the patient to use a hair dryer on low setting.

■ Tell the patient that over-the-counter (OTC) pain relievers (Tylenol or ibuprofen) may be used. Topical anesthetics may provide relief, but may also irritate.

■ Teach the signs and symptoms of podophyllin toxicity (nausea, vomiting, lethargy, coma, or paralysis), as indicated.

■ Instruct the patient to contact you if the symptoms aren't managed by sitz baths and OTC medications. Persistent tissue redness or leukorrhea may indicate infection.

■ Instruct the patient to use condoms to decrease the risk of transmitting the infection.

## Complications

■ The tissues may be red, swollen, and tender within a few hours after treatment with TCA or podophyllin. Sloughing of treated tissue may occur and referral to a gynecologist is indicated.

■ Anaphylactic reactions to podophyllin require emergency treatment.

## Special considerations

■ Use podophyllin and TCA on external HPV only. Use no more than 0.5 ml of podophyllin per treatment, and treat less than a 1.6-in$^2$ (10-cm$^2$) area per session.

■ Inject only five lesions per visit if using intralesional interferon.

🔹 COLLABORATION
*If there's no apparent improvement an alternative therapy, such as cryotherapy, may be needed, or refer the patient for surgical or electrocautery removal.*

## Documentation

- Document the onset, duration, symptoms, remedies tried, and outcomes.
- Describe the lesions and their number, size, location, and distribution.
- Note the differential diagnoses, which may include condyloma lata, molluscum contagiosum, carcinoma, and other STDs, such as syphilis, gonorrhea, and chlamydia.
- Record the type of treatment used, the number and approximate area of lesions treated, and protection of adjacent skin with petrolatum if topical agents are used.
- Report the patient's immediate reaction to therapy.
- Record the follow-up instructions and educational materials given, as appropriate, and the patient's understanding of the instructions and materials.

## CORNEAL ABRASION TREATMENT

### CPT codes

65205 *Removal of foreign body, external eye, conjunctival, superficial*
65210 *Removal of foreign body, external eye, conjunctival, embedded*
65220 *Removal of foreign body, external eye, conjunctival, corneal without slit lamp*
99070 *Eye tray: supplies and material provided by physician over and above what's usually included in office visit.*

## Overview

Corneal abrasion (injury to the covering of the cornea) treatment involves a thorough eye examination, irrigation, and daily follow-up evaluations until the abrasion heals completely or, if necessary, a referral.

The cornea has five layers: the epithelium (outer), Bowman's membrane, stroma (middle), Descemet's membrane, and endothelium (inner). An abrasion to the cornea can result from chemical or mechanical injury (trauma), typically a contact lens or other foreign body in the eye. Injury limited to the epithelium heals without scarring; if the injury extends to the Bowman's membrane, scar tissue may form. Signs and symptoms include pain, foreign body sensation, photophobia, tearing, blurred vision, and blepharospasm; the conjunctiva may also appear red from vascular response to the injury.

## Indications

- To treat known eye trauma, foreign body sensation, tearing, or unilateral pain on opening or closing of the eyelid
- To investigate photophobia or exposure to ultraviolet light (arc welding, tanning beds, excessive sunlight), or certain chemicals
- To alleviate continuing eye irritation in contact lens wearers
- To investigate unexplained crying, photosensitivity, unilateral tearing, and conjunctival inflammation in neonates and infants
- To treat mild chemical exposure

## Contraindications

**ABSOLUTE**

- Potential high-velocity injury such as metal fragments from heavy machinery
- Health care provider not familiar with treatment recommended by a poison control center
- Chemical exposure that's highly acidic, basic, or agent unknown
- Presence of eyelid, conjunctival, or corneal laceration
- Deeply imbedded foreign object
- Unsuccessful foreign body removal

**RELATIVE**

- Noncompliant patient

## Preprocedure patient preparation

- Perform a vision screening with a Snellen's chart.

## Equipment

Snellen's chart ◆ gloves ◆ tissues ◆ antibiotic ointment such as tobramycin (optional) ◆ eyelid retractors (optional) ◆ topical ophthalmic anesthetic (such as 0.5% proparacaine unless the patient is allergic to ester anesthetics) ◆ sterile fluorescein sodium strips ◆ sterile cotton-tipped applicators ◆ bright white light source (penlight) ◆ Wood's light or other source of cobalt-blue light ◆ 8- to 10-power magnification (magnifying glass, ophthalmoscope on the +20 to +40 diopter setting) ◆ isotonic irrigant (sterile normal saline or other ophthalmic irrigation solution, such as Dacriose) ◆ sterile eye patches and 1? paper tape (optional) ◆ cycloplegic drops for severe pain such as one drop of 1% cyclopentolate HCl (2% for heavily pigmented eyes) (optional)

## Procedure

- Explain the procedure to the patient, and address any questions or concerns he may have.

☑ **OBTAIN INFORMED CONSENT**

- Examine the patient's pupillary reflex, extraocular movements, anterior and posterior chambers, and fundi.
- Wash your hands, and put on gloves.
- Using a magnification source, inspect the eye and eyelid for erythema, drainage, and foreign bodies.
- Place the patient in the supine position with his head turned laterally to the affected side. Provide him with tissues to wipe drips.
- Open the affected eye, instill one to two drops of topical ophthalmic anesthetic, and wait for 1 to 2 minutes.
- Inspect the eye using the penlight, and compare it with the unaffected eye. The sclera should appear intact, the anterior chamber free from purulent material or blood, the iris and pupil symmetrical in size and shape, and the pupils equally reactive to light. If your examination reveals findings other than those listed above, refer the patient to an ophthalmologist.
- Evert the upper lid by placing a sterile cotton-tipped applicator on

the upper lid, grasping the eyelashes, and pulling the upper lid down and forward while pressing gently downward on the eyelid with the cotton-tipped applicator to expose the posterior surface of the upper lid. If available, use eyelid retractors to expose the conjunctiva.

- Examine the eye for signs of trauma, foreign bodies, infection, stye, or an inverted eyelash.

- Moisten a sterile fluorescein strip with one to two drops of sterile normal saline solution; you may also use the patient's own tears. Don't use too much solution because excessive fluorescein staining can occur which adheres to mucus, making it difficult to identify a defect.

- Retract the lower lid and touch the fluorescein strip to the conjunctiva.

- Instruct the patient to blink to distribute the stain.

- Use a Wood's light to examine the entire cornea and to identify areas of bright green concentrated fluorescence on the conjunctiva. The fluorescence indicates the location of the abrasion. (See *Fluorescein staining patterns,* page 122.) Note the size, shape, and location of the abrasion, if any.

- If you don't find a defect or if you note vertical streaking on the cornea, it's possible that a foreign body is embedded on the conjunctiva of the eyelid and you should then examine the entire conjunctiva.

**COLLABORATION**
*If you still can't find the cause of the patient's signs and symptoms, refer him to an ophthalmologist.*

- Gently rinse the eye with sterile normal saline solution to flush the fluorescein stain from the conjunctiva and to lessen further eye irritation.

- Administer cycloplegic drops for severe pain, if indicated. Instill antibiotic ointment for prophylaxis against infection. Administer the minimal effective amount of anesthetic because it could decrease the rate of healing, resulting in scarring.

- Cover the affected eye with a sterile eye patch to promote patient comfort. Have the patient close both eyes and firmly tape two eye patches (the first patch folded in half prevents the eye from opening) over the affected eye.

- Prescribe ophthalmic antibiotics for prophylaxis, such as tobramycin ointment or sulfacetamide ointment for 3 days.

## Postprocedure patient teaching

- Instruct the patient to schedule a return visit in 24 hours for reevaluation and for removal of the eye patch, if applicable.

- Tell the patient that it's crucial for you to monitor his progress every day until the eye is completely healed to catch complications such as infection at an early, treatable stage. Instruct him to contact you and return in 12 hours if symptoms persist.

- Tell him not to rub his eyes; doing so could disrupt new layers of epithelial granulation and delay healing.

## Fluorescein staining patterns

Abnormalities may be visible to the naked eye, such as the foreign body shown below. However, fluorescein staining may enhance physical findings. Fluorescein staining allows you to differentiate these diagnoses with the sharply demarcated circle or oval common in corneal abrasion.

Foreign bodies may become more visible with fluorescein staining.

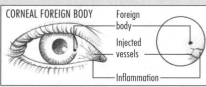

CORNEAL FOREIGN BODY
Foreign body
Injected vessels
Inflammation

Fluorescein staining permits the identification of the dendritic pattern of herpes simplex.

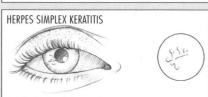

HERPES SIMPLEX KERATITIS

Here you can see the geographic appearance of keratitis sicca (dry eyes syndrome).

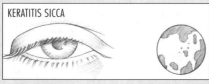

KERATITIS SICCA

Fluorescein staining enhances visibility of the band left by a chemical where it has been dragged across the eye's surface.

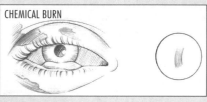

CHEMICAL BURN

Note the penetrating lines in this lateral view of corneal erosion.

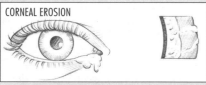

CORNEAL EROSION

Note the sharply demarcated circle or oval typical in cases of corneal abrasion.

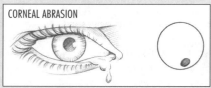

CORNEAL ABRASION

## How to administer eyedrops

Teach your patient how to administer his own eyedrops correctly. Have him follow these steps:

- Wash your hands thoroughly.
- Hold the medication bottle up to the light, and examine it. Don't use the medication if it's discolored or contains sediment. Instead, take it back to the pharmacy and have it examined. If the medication looks okay, warm it to room temperature by holding the bottle between your hands for 2 minutes.
- Moisten a cotton ball or a tissue with water, and clean any secretions from around your eyes. Use a fresh cotton ball or tissue for each eye.
- Stand or sit before a mirror or lie on your back, whichever is most comfortable for you. Squeeze the bulb of the eyedropper and slowly release it to fill the dropper with medication.
- Tilt your head slightly backward and toward the eye you're treating. Pull down your lower eyelid.

- Position the dropper over the conjunctival sac you've exposed between your lower lid and the white of your eye. Steady your hand by resting two fingers against your cheek or nose.
- Look up at the ceiling. Then squeeze the prescribed number of drops into the sac. Be careful not to touch the dropper to your eye, eyelashes, or finger. Wipe away excess medication with a clean tissue.
- Release the lower lid. Try to keep your eye open and not blink for at least 30 seconds. Apply gentle pressure to the corner of your eye at the bridge of your nose for 1 minute. This will prevent the medication from being absorbed through your tear duct.
- Repeat the procedure in the other eye, if ordered.
- Cap the bottle, and store it away from light and heat. If you're using more than one kind of drop, wait 5 minutes before you use the next one.

- To alleviate pain, the patient may take pain medicine, such as acetaminophen, or apply moist compresses if no eye patch was used. Inform him that the absence of pain doesn't guarantee complete resolution of the corneal injury.
- Tell the patient who isn't wearing an eye patch to rest his eye, especially if he's a child or has a history of amblyopia.
- Tell the patient to call you for signs and symptoms that persist or recur, acute changes in vision, and signs of infection (rapidly increasing redness, swelling, pain, and warmth; cloudy appearance of the eye; yellow, green, or brown drainage; or fever).
- Emphasize to the patient the importance of administering eyedrops as directed (See *How to administer eyedrops.*)

Encourage the patient to wear protective eyewear for high-risk occupational activities, such as arc welding and mixing chemicals.

## Complications

- Infection, scarring, corneal ulcers, permanent visual impairment, uveitis, and conjunctivitis are minimized by gentle handling and rapid treatment. However, these conditions may also be un-avoidable complications of the original injury. Early referral to an ophthalmologist is indicated when complications are suspected or if the patient has no relief within 12 hours of the initial visit.

## Special considerations

■ Cyclopentolate HCl may be re-peated in 5 minutes if needed (note that the drug's effects peak in about 45 minutes and have a duration of up to a day, so pupils may be unequal on follow-up ex-amination.)

■ Use individually packaged fluo-rescein sodium strips to avoid chemical preservatives or the in-creased infection risk associated with multiple-use vials.

✿ COLLABORATION
*Refer the patient immediately to an ophthalmologist for acute vi-sion loss, a herpes lesion, an intraoc-ular foreign body, blunt or sharp trauma to the eye, corneal infection, deterioration of vision or acute vi-sion loss, chemical burns (after im-mediate copious irrigation for 15 minutes with tap water from a shower or hose), a metallic foreign body, possible globe penetration (signs include hyphema, lens opacity, and pupil irregularity), noncompli-ance (for instance, a child who may need sedation), a foreign body that can't be irrigated out, an abrasion that isn't healing well within 24 hours or completely healed within 48 hours, or for signs of infection. Also refer the patient for dendritic, large, or centrally located defects found on fluorescein examination.*

*Inform the ophthalmologist if you've administered cycloplegic drops as di-lation may persist through the next day.*

■ The epithelium may become more fragile due to chronic hypox-ia associated with wearing hard contact lenses.

■ Look carefully for a foreign body in the cul-de-sac if you note a pattern of multiple vertical lines during conjunctival staining.

✿ COLLABORATION
*If you're unable to rule out the possibility of a penetrating ocular injury, apply a shield to the eye and refer the patient immediately to a nearby emergency department or ophthalmologist.*

■ Perform a Seidel's test if you sus-pect leakage of intraocular fluid. To do so, place a fluorescein strip directly over the site and look for a flow of green liquid.

■ Don't patch the eye in a patient with only a small peripheral defect (less than ¼″ [5 mm]), in children younger than age 5, or in cases of suspected infection.

■ Don't use topical corticosteroids; they may interfere with healing.

■ Use a slit lamp for eye examina-tion only if you're skilled in the technique.

## Documentation

■ Record a detailed case history before performing any procedures or treatments. Record the time, place, and type of injury as well as the presenting signs and symp-toms.

■ Note visual acuity in both eyes before the procedure.

■ Document the size and location of all abrasions. Illustrations can help, but be careful that the illustration doesn't magnify the size of the lesion. During subsequent examinations, document the degree of healing.

■ List any patient instructions and his understanding.

## CRUTCH WALKING AND CANE WALKING

**CPT code**
*No specific code has been assigned.*

## Overview

Ambulation aids, such as crutches and canes, remove full or partial weight from one or both legs, enabling the patient to support himself with his hands and arms. These aids protect injured legs from further injury and can help a patient with lower extremity weakness to walk.

To use ambulation aids successfully, the patient must have balance, stamina, control of his trunk, and upper-body strength. The patient's condition will determine the type of aid and the gait to use. Ambulation aids require the use of the abdominal and paraspinous muscles of the trunk, the muscles of the upper extremities, and those of the unaffected lower extremity. Canes are used for partial weight-bearing reduction. Crutches may be used for partial or full weight-bearing reduction.

The patient who can't use crutches may be able to use a walker.

Three types of crutches are commonly used. Standard aluminum or wooden crutches are used by the patient with a sprain, strain, or cast. They require stamina and upper-body strength. The paraplegic or other patient using the swing-through gait may use aluminum forearm crutches. These have a collar that fits around the forearm and a horizontal handgrip that provides support. Platform crutches are used by a patient with arthritis who has an upper-extremity deficit that prevents weight bearing through the wrist. They provide padded surfaces for the upper extremities.

## Indications

■ To aid ambulation in patients with sprains or strains, stress fractures, fractures of a lower extremity requiring partial or no weight-bearing, or neuromuscular deficits or injuries

## Contraindications

**RELATIVE**
■ Upper extremity injury or weakness
■ Balance abnormality

## Preprocedure patient preparation

■ Determine the appropriate ambulation aid for the patient based on his injury, upper-body strength, and neuromuscular deficit (if any).

# Equipment

Crutches with axillary pads, hand-grips, and rubber suction tips ◆ cane with handgrip and rubber suction tip (such as walking cane, quad cane, or platform crutch cane) ◆ walking belt (optional)

# Procedure

■ Explain the procedure to the patient, and address any questions or concerns he may have.

■ After choosing appropriate crutches for the patient, adjust their height with the patient standing or, if necessary, lying down.

■ To fit a patient for crutches, position each crutch so that it extends from a point 4″ to 6″ (10 to 15 cm) to the side and 4″ to 6″ in front of the patient's feet to 1½″ to 2″ (4 to 5 cm) below the axillae (about the width of two fingers). Adjust the handgrips so that the patient's elbows are flexed at a 15-degree angle when he's standing with the crutches in the resting position.

■ To fit a patient for a cane, have him hold the cane in the hand opposite the injured leg. The cane's length should be such that the patient's elbow is flexed at about 20 degrees with the rubber tip resting 3″ to 4″ (7.5 to 10 cm) lateral to the patient's shoe.

✴ **COLLABORATION**
*Consult with other health care providers (physical therapists or orthopedists) as needed to coordinate rehabilitation and teaching to optimize the patient's outcomes.*

■ If needed, place a walking belt around the patient's waist to help prevent falls. Tell him to position his crutches and to shift his weight from side to side. To facilitate learning and coordination, place the patient in front of a full-length mirror.

■ Describe the gait you'll teach and the reason for your choice. Demonstrate the gait as necessary. Tell the patient to perform a return demonstration.

# Postprocedure patient teaching

■ Provide the patient with a written copy of your instructions, as appropriate.

■ Teach the four-point gait to the patient who can bear weight on both legs. Although this is the safest gait, because three points are always in contact with the floor, it requires greater coordination than others because of its constant shifting of weight. Teach this sequence: right crutch, left foot, left crutch, right foot. Suggest counting to help develop rhythm, and make sure each short step is of equal length. If the patient gains proficiency at this gait, teach the faster two-point gait. This approach is used when weight bearing of a combination of extremities must be reduced (for example, in a patient with rheumatoid arthritis in both upper and lower extremities).

■ Teach the two-point gait to the patient with weak legs, but good coordination and arm strength. This is the most natural crutch-walking gait because it mimics walking, with alternating movement of the arms and legs. Instruct the patient to advance the right crutch and left foot simultaneously, followed by the left crutch and right foot. This approach only partially relieves weight bearing of legs.

■ Teach the three-point gait to the patient who can bear only partial or no weight on one leg. Instruct him to advance both crutches 6″ to 8″ (15 to 20 cm) along with the involved leg. Tell him to bring the uninvolved leg forward and to bear the bulk of his weight on the crutches. The patient may at this time place partial weight on the involved leg if allowed and pain-free. Stress the importance of taking steps of equal length and duration with no pauses. This approach completely eliminates weight-bearing of one extremity. The energy cost of this gait is twice as great as normal.

■ Teach the swing-to or swing-through gaits — the fastest ones — to the patient with complete paralysis of the hips and legs. Instruct him to advance both crutches simultaneously and to swing his legs parallel to (swing-to) or beyond (swing-through) the crutches. Caution him that this gait requires much energy.

■ If the patient will be using a cane, teach him to place it in the hand opposite the affected leg. Tell him to practice so that the cane and the heel of the injured leg strike the ground simultaneously.

■ Teach the patient who uses crutches to get up from a chair. Instruct him to hold both crutches in one hand, with the tips resting firmly on the floor. Then tell him to push up from the chair with his

free hand, supporting himself with the crutches.

■ Teach him to reverse this process to sit down. Tell him to support himself with the crutches in one hand and to lower himself with the other.

■ Teach the patient to ascend stairs using the three-point gait. Tell him to lead with his uninvolved leg and then follow with both crutches and the involved leg. To descend stairs, he should lead with the crutches and the involved leg and follow with the uninvolved leg.

## Complications

■ Atrophy of the hips and legs can occur if a patient who uses the swing-to or swing-through gait for a prolonged period neglects to perform appropriate therapeutic exercises routinely.

■ Brachial nerve palsy can develop in a patient who habitually leans on his crutches, causing prolonged pressure on the axillae. Instruct the patient to return to the clinic for reevaluation of gait and fitting if he feels tingling or numbness in the side of his chest, axillae, or upper arms.

## Special considerations

■ Encourage arm- and shoulder-strengthening exercises to prepare the patient for crutch walking. If possible, teach two techniques — one fast and one slow — so he can alternate between them to prevent excessive muscle fatigue and can adjust more easily to various walking conditions.

## Documentation

■ Before conducting patient teaching, document any abnormal physical findings and have the patient initial the documentation of pre-existing alterations in function or neurosensory findings.

■ Record the patient's level of understanding. Include barriers and use of an interpreter when indicated.

■ Describe the patient's condition and your assessment of his function, range of motion, and neurovascular status (paresthesia, pulses, pain, and pallor).

■ Record consultations (as indicated), preparation of the patient and equipment, and the gait trained.

■ Note any referrals, follow-up visits, and reasons the patient should contact you.

■ Record the type of gait the patient is to use, his ability to perform a return demonstration, his tolerance of the procedure, and anticipated duration of use.

■ Review recent or pertinent documentation by other health team members; then initial their notes to signify you're aware of their findings. This doesn't signify agreement with their comments or reduce your responsibility to conduct your own history and physical examination.

■ Record the quality and duration of the patient's ambulation (for instance, the patient can ambulate 30′ [9.1 m] without resting and can navigate a flight of stairs) and the use of proper technique independently, thus making the patient

safe for discharge per facility protocol.

# CRYOCAUTERY OF CERVIX

***CPT code***
57511   *Cryocautery of cervix, initial or repeat*

## Overview

Used to treat cervical intraepithelial neoplasia (CIN), cryocautery uses freezing temperatures to destroy the outermost layers of cervical cells. Temperatures of $-4°$ F ($-20°$ C) or lower for about 1 minute kill the infected or cancerous cervical cells. To perform the procedure, a probe that uses a refrigerant, such as nitrous oxide, to reach temperatures as low as $-103°$ F ($-75°$ C) is placed on the tissue and forms an ice ball (also called a cryolesion). Repeated cycles of freezing and thawing produce more tissue destruction than one freezing treatment that lasts an equal amount of time, provided that each freezing cycle produces the maximum effect. Smaller lesions may require only one treatment, but larger lesions may require multiple freeze cycles; persistent disease may require retreatment.

Three basic scenarios exist, only the first of which is an indication for cryocautery:

■ The lesion is covered by the 20- or 25-mm probe.

■ The lesion extends beyond the

probe, and the ice ball can only extend to the lesion periphery but not uniformly beyond 4 mm of the extent of the lesion.

- The lesion extends onto the vaginal fornices.

## Indications

- To remove CIN grade I or II lesion, precancerous cervical lesions, or carcinoma in situ

## Contraindications

### ABSOLUTE

- History of hypersensitivity or adverse reaction to cryotherapy
- Invasive cancer or dysplasia more than grade II
- Positive endocervical curettage
- Pregnancy
- Lack of correlation between a Papanicolaou test or colposcopic impression and biopsies
- Inability to see entire lesion or lesion greater than 2 cm in diameter
- Lesion extends beyond the reach of the probe
- Current sexually transmitted disease besides human papillomavirus
- Expected onset of menses within the next week

### RELATIVE

- Collagen disorders or immunoproliferative disorders
- Ulcerative colitis
- Glomerulonephritis
- High cryoglobulin levels (abnormal proteins that dissolve at body temperature but precipitate when cooled)
- History of endocarditis, syphilis, Epstein-Barr virus infection, high dose steroid use, cytomegalovirus infection, or chronic hepatitis B (because high-dose corticosteroid use can result in exaggerated tissue damage)

## Preprocedure patient preparation

- Tell the patient that cryosurgery will treat her cervical abnormality in the least-invasive effective manner, preventing progression or worsening of the abnormality.
- Tell the patient that mild cramping noted at the time of the procedure resolves within an hour in most cases.
- Have the patient premedicate with a nonsteroidal anti-inflammatory drug, such as ibuprofen, 1 hour before the procedure to decrease associated cramping and discomfort.

## Equipment

Cryogun with nitrous oxide tank and 20- and 25-mm flat and slightly conical cryoprobes ◆ warm water ◆ normal saline solution ◆ water-soluble lubricant ◆ timer or watch with a second hand ◆ vaginal speculum ◆ vaginal side-wall retractors or glove to place over the speculum ◆ drape

## Procedure

- Explain the procedure to the patient, and address any questions or concerns she may have.

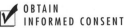
OBTAIN
INFORMED CONSENT

- Wash your hands.

■ After the patient has removed her undergarments and is appropriately draped, assist her to the lithotomy position, with her feet in the stirrups and her buttocks extended slightly beyond the edge of the table.

■ If the vaginal walls are at risk for contact with the cryoprobe (such as for an obese patient), use vaginal retractors. If one isn't available, you can cut the finger off a glove and snip the fingertip off as well. Slip this over the speculum before inserting it. When the speculum opens, the vaginal walls will be splinted.

■ Dip the speculum in warm water. Instruct the patient to take several deep breaths, and insert the speculum into the vagina. When it's in place, slowly open the blades to expose the lesion. Then lock the blades in place.

■ Select a cryoprobe tip that will cover the lesion plus ¼″ (5 mm) beyond the lesion's borders.

■ Select a flat or slightly conical tip. This will minimize the depth of freezing beyond diseased tissues. Dip the cryoprobe in warm water or normal saline solution and apply a thin layer of water-soluble lubricant to maintain good contact between the probe tip and the cervix.

■ Turn on the nitrous oxide tank and check the pressure. Insufficient pressure increases the time it takes the tissue to freeze.

■ Apply the cryoprobe and activate the freezing mechanism. Start timing the freeze, and tell the patient you've started the procedure. When adherence occurs (after 5 seconds), apply gentle outward traction to center the probe in the cervix. Your goal is to prevent the healthy tissue from being affected without tearing the cryoprobe free.

■ For benign cervicitis, freeze for one 3-minute period. For dysplastic CIN, freeze long enough to form an ice ball that extends at least 5 mm beyond the lesion (approximately 3 minutes). After freezing is stopped, allow the cryoprobe to defrost enough to fall away by itself. Most units automatically defrost the probe when freezing ceases. After the tissue thaws completely (5 to 10 minutes), repeat the process (called the freeze-thaw-refreeze cycle). Keep in mind that the timing isn't as important as formation of an adequate ice ball.

■ Between freeze cycles, place the tip in warm water to increase efficacy.

## Postprocedure patient teaching

■ Instruct the patient to return to the facility in 4 weeks for a postoperative examination, and tell her to follow up with a Pap test in 4 months; send her a reminder notice at that time.

■ Explain that a heavy, watery discharge for at least 3 weeks — occasionally up to 8 weeks — can be normal; the discharge may be blood-tinged for a few days but should change to darker red to brown and lessen over time. Suggest that she wear a sanitary pad and change it at least every 4 hours. After 3 weeks, she may douche with 1 tbs of vinegar in 1 cup of water or use a povidone-iodine vaginal suppository if odor becomes a problem.

■ Tell her that she can resume normal activities but must refrain from sexual intercourse and from putting anything in the vagina, including tampons, for 2 weeks.

■ Tell the patient to call you for severe cramping, bleeding, temperature above 100° F (37.8° C), or discharge that lasts longer than 3 weeks.

## Complications

■ Cramping and flushing commonly occur during the procedure but resolve spontaneously. The squamocolumnar junction may be deeper in the os after the procedure, making subsequent examinations more difficult.

■ Cervical stenosis may occur if a long tip is used.

■ Infertility, bleeding, menstrual irregularities for up to 3 months, and infection are rare, but are indications for referral to a gynecologist.

## Special considerations

■ To produce an adequate cryolesion, make sure the temperature at the periphery of the lesion and at ¼″ (5-mm) depth in the cervix reaches at least −4° F (−20° C) and is maintained for at least 1 minute. Adequate cryonecrosis at a depth of 5 mm requires a freeze-thaw-refreeze cycle of 5 minutes for each part of the cycle.

■ For larger lesions, consider using a 25-mm probe, which may produce better results than a 20-mm probe.

■ Be aware that many cryosurgical units have a defrost function that causes the cryoprobe to detach less than 15 seconds after freezing stops but the gas must remain on to activate this defrost function.

■ Keep in mind the following factors that increase freeze time: increased size of the ice ball needed, low tank pressure, increased vascularity, extra keratin covering on the cervix (remove or moisten the keratin to decrease freeze time), and poor physical contact between the cryoprobe and lesion. The type of system used also affects freeze time.

■ Most patients receive treatment in the facility setting and don't need an anesthetic.

## Documentation

■ Document a detailed description of the site pre- and postprocedure, a description of the procedure, the patient's reaction to the procedure, medications ordered, time frame for follow-up evaluation, and instructions given to the patient.

## *C*RYOTHERAPY FOR LESION REMOVAL

### CPT codes
*Note:* Precise code depends on lesion size.
17000 *Destruction by any method (including laser, with and without surgical curettement or local anesthesia) of all benign and premalignant lesions in any location, excluding cutaneous vascular proliferative lesions*

17003 *Destruction of multiple lesions*

17110 *Destruction by any method of less than 14 flat warts, molluscum contagiosum, or milia*

17260 *Destruction of less than 0.5-cm malignant lesion from trunk, arms, or legs*

17261 to 17266 *Destruction of malignant lesions from trunk, arms, or legs; varying lesion sizes*

17270 *Destruction of less than 0.5-cm malignant lesion from scalp, neck, hands, feet, or genitalia*

17271 to 17276 *Destruction of malignant lesions from scalp, neck, hands, feet, or genitalia; varying lesion sizes*

## Overview

Cryotherapy efficiently removes common skin lesions with minimal scar formation and pain. Pigment changes, which are more noticeable in darker skinned patients, are permanent. Cryotherapy uses freezing temperatures to destroy cells. Temperatures of 14° F ($-10°$ C) to $-4°$ F ($-20°$ C) destroy tissue; a temperature of $-58°$ F ($-50°$ C) destroys malignant cells. In the procedure, a blister forms at the dermal-epidermal junction, and the skin superficial to the blister is left essentially bloodless and without sensation. The time needed for freezing varies with the type of skin lesion and the freezing method used.

## Indications

■ To remove verruca vulgaris (common warts), verruca plantaris (plantar warts), actinic keratosis, condylomata acuminata, lentigines, molluscum contagiosum, papular nevi, sebaceous hyperplasia, seborrheic keratosis, and skin tags and polyps

## Contraindications

### ABSOLUTE

■ Sensitivity or adverse reaction to cryosurgery

■ Inability of the patient to accept the possibility of skin pigment changes

■ Areas with compromised circulation

■ Areas with a great deal of hair (cryotherapy destroys hair follicles)

■ Lesions that require pathologic evaluation

### RELATIVE

■ History of an exaggerated response

■ History of collagen disorders, ulcerative colitis, glomerulonephritis, or high cryoglobulin levels (abnormal proteins that dissolve at body temperature but precipitate when cooled)

■ Patients taking high-dose corticosteroids

## Preprocedure patient preparation

■ Inform the patient that wart removal will cause a blister to form. After the blister forms, he should remove the top layer of skin from the blister, apply a thin coat of antibiotic ointment, and then cover the area with an adhesive bandage. The top layer of skin from the blister may be removed by lightly rubbing the area with a washcloth or mild cloth, using soap and water. The patient shouldn't use his fingernails to remove the blister scab — he may get the wart virus under his nails.

## Equipment

Gloves ◆ tissue-freezing kit such as the Verruca Freeze unit, nitrous oxide cryotherapy unit, or liquid nitrogen in a foam cup ◆ cotton-tipped applicators ◆ water-soluble lubricating gel ◆ topical antibiotic such as triple antibiotic ointment ◆ dry 4″ × 4″ gauze pads ◆ tape

## Procedure

■ Explain the procedure to the patient, and address any questions or concerns he may have.

☑ OBTAIN
INFORMED CONSENT

■ Wash your hands, and put on gloves.
■ Place the patient in a comfortable position, with the lesion easily accessible.

### For verruca freeze

■ Choose the smallest size speculum that will cover the lesion and attach it to the cryogun.
■ Place the speculum firmly against the skin so no liquid can escape.
■ Depress the trigger gently until the speculum is filled approximately ⅛″ to ¼″ (3 to 6.5 mm). Hold the unit in place for 25 seconds to allow the fluid to evaporate before removing the speculum.

### For nitrous oxide

■ Use a cotton-tipped applicator to apply water-soluble lubricant to the lesion.
■ Choose the cryoprobe that best matches the size, shape, and depth of the lesion without being larger than the lesion. (See *Selecting the proper cryoprobe,* page 134.)
■ With the cryogun in your dominant hand, rest the cryoprobe against the lesion and press the trigger. The tip will form an ice ball that adheres to the skin in 5 to 10 seconds. (See *Guide to freezing lesions,* page 135.)

### For liquid nitrogen

■ Soak a cotton-tipped applicator in the liquid.
■ Apply the liquid to the lesion slowly to avoid splattering. The size of the cotton-tipped applicator and the amount of pressure affect how quickly and how deeply the area will freeze.
■ Alternatively, you may use a cryogun with a probe or spray-tipped nozzle to deliver the liquid nitrogen.
■ Stop freezing when you have an ice ball extending ⅛″ (2 mm) beyond the lesion's boundaries.
■ Apply a topical antibiotic.
■ Cover the area with dry gauze and tape.

## Postprocedure patient teaching

■ Inform the patient that immediate redness, swelling, and blisters

## Selecting the proper cryoprobe

Successfully freezing a lesion depends on selecting the appropriate cryoprobe tip. The shape of the tip determines the width of the freeze area. Applying pressure to the cryoprobe allows the probe to freeze at a greater depth.

The first two illustrations here show the use of appropriately shaped cryoprobes. The final illustration shows an inappropriate cryoprobe. In this example, the probe doesn't cover the lesion sufficiently.

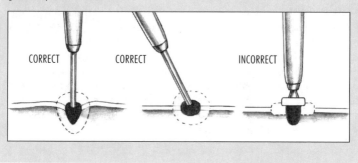

CORRECT    CORRECT    INCORRECT

are likely in the first 16 to 36 hours, but they decrease within 72 hours. Crusting occurs within 72 hours and resolves within 1 week.

■ Tell him to make an appointment in 3 to 4 weeks for evaluation and, possibly, retreatment.

■ Instruct the patient to keep the skin clean and dry. Explain the role of skin in defending the body against infection. Emphasize hygiene, sparing application of antibiotic ointment to the site, and the importance of keeping the site covered.

■ Tell the patient that his skin in that area may become lighter or the hair less plentiful but that only minimal scarring should occur. Advise him to wear sunscreen, particularly on that area.

■ If sensory nerves are affected, reassure the patient that recovery typically occurs within 2 months.

■ Urge the patient to notify you promptly if he experiences signs and symptoms of infection (increasing redness, swelling, pain, and warmth; cloudy yellow, green, or brown drainage; opening of wound; foul odor; a red streak from the site; or fever after 24 hours).

## Complications

■ Pigment changes and increased photosensitivity are permanent changes to the affected area.

■ Ischemia and infection are rare but require follow-up evaluation and treatment.

## Special considerations

■ Use caution when treating the palmar surface of the hand because cutaneous sensory nerves run superficially in the hands. If a nerve is affected, the patient usually recovers within 6 weeks. When freezing an area adjacent to a nerve, apply traction and advise the patient that temporary sensory loss may occur.

✿ COLLABORATION
*Refer the patient to a dermatologist for mucosal and periorbital cryosurgery because those require shorter freezing times and may produce excessive swelling that may be aesthetically and functionally disabling.*

■ Wart removal generally requires two freeze and thaw cycles, with the thaw time lasting 45 seconds.

## Documentation

■ Before performing cryotherapy, document any abnormal physical findings on the consent form. Have the patient initial the comments and sign the form to signify acknowledgment of preprocedural abnormalities. In the chart, the pre- and postprocedural notes must include an evaluation of potentially affected function, range of motion, and sensation.

■ When documenting consent, note that options and risks (particularly pigment changes and scarring) were discussed at length and that the patient wanted the procedure done.

■ Record indications for cryosurgery, freeze times, the time frame for follow-up evaluation, and any instructions given to the patient.

## Guide to freezing lesions

For cryotherapy to be successful, it's necessary to freeze different types of lesions for specific lengths of time. This table depicts the appropriate lengths of time needed to freeze a variety of skin lesions. If the freeze time noted yields insufficient coverage, allow the area to thaw and then refreeze. Subsequent refreezing yields deeper penetration of the cold.

| TYPE OF LESION | FREEZE TIME (IN SECONDS) |
|---|---|
| Actinic keratosis | 90 |
| Condyloma acuminata | 45 |
| Lentigines (freckles) | 10 to 15 |
| Molluscum contagiosum | 25 to 30 |
| Papular nevi | 30 to 45 |
| Sebaceous hyperplasia | 30 to 45 |
| Seborrheic keratosis | 30 |
| Skin tags and polyps | 30 to 45 |
| Verruca plantaris (plantar warts; after debridement) | 30 to 40 |

# *Culture of penis secretions*

***CPT codes***
87070 *Culture, bacterial, any source other than urine, blood, or stool, with isolation and presumptive identification of isolates*
87110 *Culture, chlamydia, any source*

## Overview

Proper collection and handling of a swab specimen of penile discharge will assist in the timely identification of the causative organism of a sexually transmitted disease, while preventing contamination from normal bacterial flora. After the specimen is collected, the swab should be placed in a sterile tube containing transport medium and should be immediately taken to the laboratory.

## Indications

■ To investigate the cause of urethral discharge, dysuria, or urinary frequency

## Contraindications

■ None known

## Preprocedure patient preparation

■ Explain to the patient the potential causes of his symptoms and that treatment with antibiotics may be indicated.
■ Inform the patient that there's some pain and discomfort associated with this procedure.

## Equipment

Gloves ◆ small sterile swab for obtaining urethral specimen ◆ culture tube with transport medium

## Procedure

■ Explain the procedure to the patient, and address any questions or concerns he may have.
■ Provide privacy and have the patient remove his garments from the waist down and sit upright on the side of a bed or stretcher.
■ Wash your hands, and put on gloves.
■ If there's visible urethral discharge on the tip of the penis, gently rotate sterile swab in a circular motion around the urethra, collecting a sufficient amount of discharge on the swab.
■ If there's no visible discharge, the sterile swab will need to be inserted into the urethra. Gently press open the meatus of the urethra with your nondominant hand. Then insert the swab into the urethra to approximately $\frac{3}{4}''$ (2 cm), and gently rotate. Be sure to complete a 360-degree rotation with the swab to obtain an appropriate sample. Gently withdraw the swab from the urethra.
■ Place the swab in a culture tube with transport medium, label it, and send it to the laboratory immediately.

## Postprocedure patient teaching

■ Inform the patient of the time it usually takes to receive the results, and assure him that he'll be notified of the results.
■ Instruct the patient to notify you if the following symptoms occur before or after culture results are obtained: increase in the amount of the discharge, change in the color of the discharge, or bleeding from the penis.

- Tell the patient that his sexual partners may also need to receive treatment, depending on the results of the culture.

## Complications
- None known

## Special considerations
- If there's no visible discharge, you may have the patient "milk" the penis for a few seconds to produce a discharge and avoid having to insert the swab into the urethra.

## Documentation
- Document the rationale for the procedure, and describe the discharge (amount, color, consistency) if visible.
- Record the date, time, and site of specimen collection and the patient's tolerance of the procedure.

## CYST EXCISION

### CPT codes
*Note:* Precise code depends on lesion size.
10060  *Incision and drainage of abscess (cutaneous or subcutaneous abscess or cyst); simple or single*
10061  *Incision and drainage of abscess (cutaneous or subcutaneous abscess or cyst); complicated or multiple*
11420 to 11426  *Excision, benign lesion; diameter 0.5 cm or less; except skin tag, scalp, neck, hands, feet, genitalia*

26160  *Excision of lesion of tendon sheath or capsule, hand or finger*

### Overview
A sebaceous or epidermal cyst consists of a small, mobile, superficial sac that contains sebum or keratin. It's commonly found on various areas of the body, such as the neck, back, scalp, and face. Its etiology is unknown. Cysts grow at varying rates, sometimes taking many years.

Cyst excision may be performed in two ways. In the first method, the cyst sac and its contents are removed simultaneously. In the second method, the cyst sac is removed only after expelling the contents. The site, size, and depth of the cyst all help determine which method is used.

After the cyst is removed, closure is done by suture or by secondary intention with iodoform packing. If the cyst sac can be easily identified and pulled through the incision, this method is preferred because it reduces the chance of recurrence.

### Indications
- To diminish the occurrence of scarring or infection

### Contraindications
**RELATIVE**
- Coagulopathies
- Anticoagulant therapy
- Anticipated complications or postsurgical scarring concerns
- Large cyst area

## Preprocedure patient preparation

■ Explain that healing from this procedure usually occurs in 10 to 14 days, depending on the surgical site, the size of the wound, complications that arise, and the presence of infection before the procedure.

## Equipment

1% or 2% lidocaine without epinephrine ◆ sterile 3-ml and 10-ml syringes ◆ 27G or 30G ½" needle ◆ 18G 1½" needle ◆ sterile #11 scalpel with handle ◆ sterile suture setup ◆ sterile curved hemostat ◆ sterile normal saline solution ◆ small sterile container with 10% formalin ◆ ¼" to 1" package iodoform gauze ◆ sterile 4" × 4" gauze pads ◆ sterile scissors ◆ tape ◆ antiseptic skin cleaner such as povidone-iodine ◆ sterile gloves ◆ sterile drape ◆ gloves

## Procedure

■ Explain the procedure to the patient, and address any questions or concerns that he may have.

☑ **OBTAIN INFORMED CONSENT**

■ Wash your hands.

■ Establish a sterile field and assemble the equipment.

■ Place the patient in the position that allows the best view of the surgical site.

■ Assess the surgical site for its size, consistency, redness, drainage, and tenderness.

■ Put on gloves.

■ Verify that the patient isn't allergic to iodine.

■ Clean the surrounding site with an antiseptic skin cleaner.

■ Remove and dispose of the gloves.

■ Put on sterile gloves.

■ Place the sterile drape appropriately over the cyst site.

■ Anesthetize the cyst perimeter with 1% or 2% lidocaine without epinephrine, using a 27G or 30G ½" needle and a 3-ml syringe, and inserting the needle at a 45-degree angle. Avoid direct injection into the cyst site.

■ Ask the patient if he notices any change in sensation. If he reports pain, indicating direct contact with the nerve, withdraw the needle 1 mm.

■ Aspirate to make sure there's no blood return. If there is, the needle is in a blood vessel. Withdraw the needle slightly and reinsert it in another area.

■ Inject 1 to 2 ml of lidocaine while partially withdrawing the needle. Then redirect the needle across the surface, advance it, and inject another 0.5 ml while withdrawing the needle. This method distributes the anesthetic uniformly, providing the optimal effect.

■ Massage the area gently. The maximum effect should occur in 5 to15 minutes.

■ Incise the cyst site lengthwise with a #11 scalpel to allow an easy extraction of the cyst sac and its contents.

■ Open the incised area with a curved hemostat, and pull the sac and its contents onto the skin.

■ Cut the elastic tissue of the sac around the outer edges until it's released. Removal of the entire sac reduces the likelihood of recurrence.

■ If the sac is already open after incision of the site, apply external pressure, using your fingers to remove its contents. This approach may also extrude the sac, depending on the site area. Never apply external pressure to a cyst on the face or mastoid.

■ Put the contents into the sterile container with formalin for pathology review.

■ Irrigate the wound site with sterile normal saline solution, using an 18G needle and 10-ml syringe.

■ Depending on the wound, use a suture or packing approach to close the wound.

■ If you're using a suture approach, close the wound with sutures at this time.

■ If you're using an iodoform packing approach (other than on a head site), pack the cavity site fully. Leave a small amount of packing outside the wound to facilitate easy removal. If the surgical site is on the head, suture the incision in two areas, loosely enough to facilitate drainage. Leave the ends of the sutures 2″ to 3″ (5 to 7.5 cm) long. Form a gauze roll with sterile 4″ × 4″ gauze pads, and place it on top of the incision. Secure it tightly to the incision by tying the ends of the sutures and forming a pressure dressing.

■ Apply a pressure dressing to the site with 4″ × 4″ gauze pads and tape.

■ Assess the need for over-the-counter or prescription-strength medications, depending on the patient's pain tolerance (using a pain scale) and degree of recovery.

## Postprocedure patient teaching

■ Advise the patient to apply cool compresses to the surgical site to help relieve pain and reduce swelling. Mild analgesics may also be necessary for the first few days after the procedure for pain control.

■ Inform the patient that his sutures can be removed in 7 to 10 days, depending on the size of the site and the appearance of complications.

■ Have the patient schedule a follow-up appointment in 48 hours to assess the site and wound status and then again in 7 to 10 days to have the sutures removed.

■ Instruct the patient to notify you promptly if he experiences increased pain after the first few days, fever, drainage with foul odor, a color change, increased site tenderness, bleeding, or a new opening in wound edges.

## Complications

■ Infection may be treated with local or systemic antibiotics and antiseptic soaks. It may also require consultation with a physician, a dermatologist, or an infectious disease specialist.

■ Scarring and keloids are minimized with gentle handling and the use of such techniques as undermining and layered suturing.

## Special considerations

- If using the iodoform gauze dressing, remove some of the gauze every 1 to 2 days until it's completely removed (approximately 10 to 14 days).

 **COLLABORATION**
*If the patient has a large cyst area or facial cysts in a highly visible area, if you anticipate complications, or if you have concerns about post-surgical scarring, consider referring the patient to a general surgeon or a plastic surgeon.*

## Documentation

- Before performing a cyst excision, document any abnormal physical findings on the consent form. Have the patient initial the comments and sign the form to signify acknowledgment of preprocedural abnormalities. In the chart, the preprocedural and postprocedural notes must include an evaluation of potentially affected function, range of motion, and sensation.
- Record when the informed consent was received and confirmed.
- Note whether you sent any specimens to the laboratory for analysis.
- Describe the surgical site before and after the procedure, the type of wound closure method used (suture or gauze packing), the patient's tolerance for the procedure, complications that arose, and any instructions given to the patient.

# CYST INJECTION, GANGLION

### CPT codes
20550  *Injection, tendon sheath, ligament, trigger point, or ganglion cyst*
20600  *Arthrocentesis, aspiration, or injection of a small joint, bursa, or ganglion cyst (leg, fingers, toes)*
20605  *Arthrocentesis, aspiration, or injection of an intermediate joint, bursa, or ganglion cyst (temporomandibular, acromioclavicular, wrist, elbow, ankle, olecranon bursa)*

## Overview

A ganglion cyst is a tumor that develops on or in a tendon sheath. The most common cause is chronic or recurrent inflammation from frequent strains or contusions at the site. Joints contain a thick, gel-like material. When this gel leaks from the joint into the weakened tendon sheath, it forms a cyst that not only is cosmetically unappealing but may also inhibit function and cause discomfort. Injection of an anesthetic, with or without a steroid, into the ganglion cyst provides pain relief and usually increases range of motion. However, these benefits may not be permanent.

## Indications

- To relieve discomfort and joint mobility interference caused by a ganglion cyst

## Contraindications

**ABSOLUTE**
- Cellulitis
- Infection

**RELATIVE**
- Coagulopathies

## Preprocedure patient preparation

- Advise the patient that he'll need to rest and elevate the affected joint for 24 hours after the procedure.

## Equipment

Antiseptic skin cleaner such as povidone-iodine ◆ sterile drape ◆ sterile gloves ◆ 3- and 10-ml syringes ◆ 18G 1½″ needle ◆ 22G or 25G 1½″ needle ◆ 1% lidocaine ◆ culture tube ◆ corticosteroid: short-acting (such as hydrocortisone), intermediate (such as methylprednisolone), or long-acting (such as dexamethasone) ◆ sterile 4″ × 4″ gauze pads ◆ tape

## Procedure

- Explain the procedure to the patient, and address any questions or concerns he may have.

☑ **OBTAIN INFORMED CONSENT**

- Wash your hands.
- Verify that the patient isn't allergic to iodine.
- Position the patient comfortably, with the cyst clearly exposed.
- Clean the site and surrounding area with povidone-iodine solution and gauze pads.
- Apply the sterile drape and put on sterile gloves.
- Use a 22G or 25G needle with the 3-ml syringe to draw up the appropriate dosages of 1% lidocaine and corticosteroid. Agitate gently.
- Using the 10-ml syringe with the 18G needle, insert the needle into the cyst and aspirate. If the aspirate appears cloudy, send the specimen for culture and sensitivity testing and continue the procedure; if the return is bloody, remove the needle, apply a dressing, and end the procedure.
- Unscrew the syringe and replace it with the second syringe that contains lidocaine and corticosteroid, and aspirate for blood. If no blood appears, inject the medications.
- Remove the needle and apply a pressure dressing.

## Postprocedure patient teaching

- Instruct the patient to leave the dressing on for 12 hours.
- Explain that some redness, oozing, swelling, and warmth are normal.
- Remind him to rest and elevate the joint for 24 hours.
- Recommend a nonnarcotic analgesic, such as acetaminophen or ibuprofen, for pain.
- Have the patient schedule a follow-up appointment in 1 week.
- Urge the patient to call you promptly if he experiences signs and symptoms of infection (rapid-

ly increasing redness, swelling, pain, and warmth; cloudy yellow, green, or brown drainage; opening of wound; foul odor; red streak from wound area; or fever).

## Complications

■ Recurrence is possible. Before giving a second injection, consider the effectiveness of the first one. Refer the patient to a surgeon if warranted.

■ Corticosteroid flare (increased pain after cyst injection) is rare but very painful. Manage the patient's pain with ice application and non-steroidal drug administration. If fever occurs or the condition doesn't resolve within 72 hours, corticosteroid flare is an unlikely cause of the symptoms.

■ Atrophy of subcutaneous tissue and depigmentation may occur. The risk increases with the number of injections and may be more of an issue for aesthetically conscious patients.

■ Adverse drug reactions generally require no action but are contra-indications for use of that drug in further treatments. To minimize the risk of adverse effects, use single-dose vials; many health care providers believe that adverse reactions result from preservatives in multi-dose vials.

■ Injection into a vein or artery can be avoided by aspirating to check for blood, before injecting the solution.

■ Infection is detected as early as possible through follow-up appointments and treated locally or systemically as indicated.

**COLLABORATION**

*Trauma to adjacent structures (such as bone, cartilage, and nerves) may require physical therapy or referral to an orthopedist or a surgeon; minimize the risk of this complication by limiting steroid injections to three per year.*

■ Tendon rupture is usually caused by multiple injections or overuse after injection. To minimize this risk, avoid injecting into tendons and against resistance.

## Special considerations

■ If the cyst recurs, consider excising it instead of administering a second injection.

## Documentation

■ Before performing this procedure, document any abnormal physical findings on the consent form. Have the patient initial the comments and sign the form to signify acknowledgment of preprocedural abnormalities. In the chart, the pre- and postprocedural notes must include an evaluation of potentially affected function, range of motion, and sensation.

■ Note whether a culture was sent to the laboratory.

■ Describe the site before and after the procedure, the type and amount of anesthetic used, the patient's reaction to the procedure, medications ordered, the time frame for follow-up evaluation, and any instructions given to the patient.

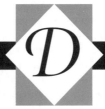

## DEFIBRILLATION

**CPT codes**
92950 *Cardiopulmonary resuscitation*
92960 *Cardioversion, elective, electrical conversion of arrhythmia; external*

## Overview

Always an emergency procedure, defibrillation delivers a controlled, untimed transcutaneous electrical charge to the myocardium, depolarizing the heart muscle in an attempt to get the sinoatrial node to resume its inherent rhythm. Its effectiveness depends on the amount of elapsed time from cardiac arrest to defibrillation. Because the patient requiring defibrillation is in a pulseless state, the rescuers should continue to perform cardiac compressions between attempts at defibrillation as well as maintain an airway.

Conditions that may contribute to lethal arrhythmias include hypoxia, severe acidosis, and electrolyte imbalance. If possible, the patient should receive treatment for the underlying cause while the resuscitation effort continues.

Defibrillation is the most important intervention for a patient in ventricular fibrillation or pulseless ventricular tachycardia; the patient's chances of survival decrease with any delay in defibrillation.

## Indications
■ To terminate ventricular fibrillation and pulseless ventricular tachycardia

## Contraindications
■ None known

## Preprocedure patient preparation
■ Make sure you're familiar with the conventional defibrillator or universal automated external defibrillator (AED) before using it.

## Equipment
Conventional defibrillator or universal AED with anterior-posterior or transverse paddles (manual or external automatic defibrillator) ◆

conductive medium pads or gel ◆ electrocardiogram (ECG) monitor with recorder ◆ I.V. line and solution ◆ oxygen administration and suction equipment ◆ oral or nasal airway or intubation equipment ◆ handheld resuscitation bag with 100% oxygen adapter and face mask ◆ emergency drugs, such as epinephrine, atropine, lidocaine, and vasopressors

## Procedure

■ Establish that the patient is unresponsive (by asking "Are you OK?" or gently shaking).
■ Call for help, and activate the emergency response system.
■ Open the airway, and assess for absence of spontaneous breathing.
■ Provide two slow, full ventilations.
■ Assess the patient for the absence of a carotid pulse (adult or child) or brachial pulse (infant).
■ Initiate cardiopulmonary resuscitation (CPR) until a monitor and defibrillator are available.
■ Expose the chest wall.
■ Apply the ECG monitor leads to the chest wall (avoiding paddle placement sites), or use "quick-look" paddles to determine cardiac rhythm. Quick-look paddles allow for single-lead interpretation of the cardiac rhythm.
■ Apply conductive pads to the chest wall, using transverse or anterior-posterior placement. If conductive pads aren't available, apply conductive gel to the paddles and place them in the transverse or anterior-posterior position. For anterolateral placement, place one

paddle to the right of the upper sternum, just below the right clavicle, and the other over the fifth or sixth intercostal space at the left anterior axillary line. For anteroposterior placement, place the anterior paddle directly over the heart at the precordium, to the left of the lower sternal border. Place the posterior paddle under the patient's body beneath the heart and immediately below the scapulae (but not under the vertebral column).

### For conventional defibrillator

■ Turn on the conventional defibrillator and monitor.
■ Charge the defibrillator for manual defibrillation to 200 joules, 300 joules, or 360 joules.

➤ **CLINICAL TIP**
*If you've successfully defibrillated a patient at 300 (or 360) joules and now need to defibrillate him again, start at the higher energy level; don't go back to 200 joules.*

■ Warn everyone to step back from the patient. Then quickly scan the area to make sure that everyone and all unnecessary equipment are clear of the patient and bed.
■ Make sure the rhythm is still ventricular fibrillation or pulseless ventricular tachycardia.
■ Activate the discharge buttons on the paddles of the manual defibrillator, and keep the paddles on the chest wall until the paddles discharge.
■ Assess the rhythm on the monitor, and check the patient for a pulse. If a shockable rhythm is present, follow the Assess-Charge-

Shock sequence as on previous page.

■ If defibrillation doesn't succeed, repeat three additional shocks at increasing energy levels in rapid succession, after making sure everyone and all nonessential equipment are clear of the patient and bed.

■ After three shocks, assess the patient's pulse.

■ If the three additional rapid shocks don't succeed, reinitiate CPR, provide manual ventilation, administer emergency drugs, and continue to defibrillate according to advanced cardiac life support (ACLS) protocol while transporting the patient to an acute care facility.

### For universal AED

■ Turn on the AED.

■ Attach the AED electrode pads to the patient's bare, dry chest.

■ Analyze the rhythm — stop CPR during this to avoid interference.

■ Some AED models begin charging as soon as they recognize a shockable rhythm. Make sure everyone and all nonessential equipment are clear of the patient and bed.

■ Discharge the shock by pressing the appropriate button on the AED.

■ After three shocks or after any "No Shock Indicated" message, check the patient's pulse. If there's no pulse, perform CPR for 1 minute. Repeat cycles of three shocks and 1 minute of CPR until the "No Shock Indicated" message is displayed on the screen. Trans-

port the patient to an acute care facility.

### For both types of defibrillation

■ If defibrillation succeeds, assess the patient's vital signs, peripheral pulses, level of consciousness, and respiratory effort. Administer emergency cardiac medications, oxygen or ventilation, and I.V. fluids according to ACLS recommendations and continue cardiac monitoring while transporting the patient to an acute care facility.

■ Obtain a postdefibrillation ECG rhythm strip or 12-lead ECG.

## Postprocedure patient teaching

■ After successful defibrillation, explain to the patient or family that the patient will be admitted to an acute care facility or a critical care unit.

■ Explain to the patient that he may feel muscle soreness for a few days after defibrillation.

■ Address the patient's and family's other educational needs after the initial crisis has passed.

## Complications

■ Chest wall injury or burns may occur. The patient may require pain management, surgical intervention, rib stabilization, or treatment to prevent infection.

## Special considerations

■ As needed, treat hypoxia, hypothermia, and acidosis because these underlying conditions may inhibit the success of defibrillation.

- Select correct energy levels sequentially from 200 to 360 joules according to ACLS protocol for external defibrillation in adults. Use 2 joules/kg for children.
- Maintain about 25 p.s.i. on each paddle during defibrillation.
- Avoid defibrillating directly over a pacemaker or an implanted cardioverter-defibrillator generator because defibrillating over the device may interfere with its functioning.
- If the patient has on a transdermal nitroglycerin patch, remove it before defibrillating. Because of the aluminum backing on the patch, the electric current may cause arcing that can result in damage to the paddles and burns to the patient.

## Documentation

- Document the patient's rhythm (asystole) before defibrillation, the time of each defibrillation, the energy levels used, the results of each defibrillation, and all other resuscitation measures used.
- Document the final outcome of the resuscitative effort and the disposition of the patient.

# *DEPO-PROVERA INJECTIONS*

### *CPT code*
90782  *Therapeutic or diagnostic injection (specify material injected); subcutaneous or intramuscular*

## Overview

Depo-Provera is a 150-mg injection of medroxyprogesterone acetate given every 3 months for contraception. The injection prevents follicular maturation and ovulation as well as thinning of the endometrium. It's more than 99% effective in the prevention of pregnancy when used as directed.

## Indications

- To prevent pregnancy

## Contraindications

### ABSOLUTE

- Active thrombophlebitis, or current or past history of thromboembolic disorders, or cerebral vascular disease
- Known hypersensitivity to Depo-Provera (medroxyprogesterone acetone or any of its other ingredients)
- Known or suspected malignancy of the breast
- Known or suspected pregnancy
- Liver dysfunction or disease
- Undiagnosed vaginal bleeding

**RELATIVE**

- Cervical intraepithelial neoplasia
- Desire for pregnancy within 1 year (consider methods with faster return to fertility)
- Diabetes mellitus
- Gallbladder disease
- History of depression
- Migraine headaches
- Uncontrolled hypertension

## Preprocedure patient preparation

- Discuss birth control options with the patient, including the benefits, risks, efficacy rate, and adverse effects of each, to help her select the option that's best for her.
- A current complete physical examination including cervical cytology is recommended but not required prior to initiating Depo-Provera.
- Patients should be counseled about potential adverse effects, particularly changes in bleeding patterns, weight gain, and mood changes.

◢ **CLINICAL TIP**
*Adequate counseling about probable adverse effects has been shown to increase continuation rates of Depo-Provera use.*

- Advise patients that return to fertility may occur as soon as the next injection is due but may take as long as 18 months.

## Equipment

Depo-Provera 1 ml vial or prefilled syringe ◆ needle ($\frac{1}{3}$″), 21G to 23G) ◆ alcohol pad ◆ gloves

### *Equipment preparation*

- Depo-Provera should be stored at room temperature and shaken vigorously just before use.

## Procedure

- Review the patient's history and physical examination. Confirm that she's an appropriate candidate for Depo-Provera.
- Explain the procedure to the patient, and address any questions or concerns she may have.
- Wash your hands.
- Obtain the patient's blood pressure measurement.
- Put on gloves.
- Prepare the prefilled syringe or draw the medication from the vial into a syringe.
- Wipe the area to be injected with the alcohol pad.
- Inject the medication I.M. deep in the gluteus or deltoid muscle.
- Remove the syringe and dispose of properly.
- Don't massage the injection site.

## Postprocedure patient teaching

- Tell the patient that injections should be repeated every 3 months (11 to 13 weeks). Receiving the injections as scheduled is crucial to the effectiveness of the medication. Give the patient the date she should return for the next injection, or schedule her an appointment.
- Inform her that Depo-Provera doesn't provide protection from sexually transmitted diseases. Con-

doms should be used in addition to the injection for the patient at risk for infection.

■ Encourage a low-fat, calcium-rich diet, weight-bearing exercise, and avoidance of smoking because long-term use of Depo-Provera may reduce bone mineral density.

■ Advise the patient to contact you if she develops sharp chest pain, coughing up of blood, sudden shortness of breath, sudden severe headache or vomiting, dizziness or fainting, problems with vision or speech, weakness, numbness in an extremity, severe pain or swelling in the calf, unusually heavy vaginal bleeding, severe pain or tenderness in the lower abdomen, or persistent pain, pus, or bleeding at the injection site.

## Complications

■ Common adverse reactions include menstrual irregularities (bleeding or amenorrhea, or both), weight changes, headache, nervousness, abdominal pain or discomfort, dizziness, and asthenia (weakness or fatigue).

■ Occasional adverse reactions include decreased libido or anorgasmy, backache, leg cramps, depression, nausea, insomnia, leukorrhea, acne, vaginitis, pelvic pain, breast pain, no hair growth or alopecia, bloating, rash, edema, hot flashes, and arthralgia.

## Special considerations

■ The initial Depo-Provera injection should be administered:

– during the first 5 days of a normal menstrual period
– within the first 5 days postpartum if not breast-feeding
– at 6 weeks postpartum if exclusively breast-feeding.

If it has been more than 13 weeks since a previous injection was given, determine whether the patient is pregnant prior to administering another injection.

## Documentation

■ In the patient's chart, record her desire for contraception with Depo-Provera, counseling provided about risks and benefits, the dose and lot number of medication along with the site of injection, and the date her next injection is due.

## DIAPHRAGM FITTING

**CPT code**
57170  *Diaphragm or cervical cap fitting with instructions*

## Overview

The diaphragm is a barrier contraception method that mechanically blocks sperm from entering the cervix. It consists of a soft latex rubber dome that's supported by a round metal spring on the outside. A diaphragm is available in various sizes and must be fitted to the individual. When used with spermicidal jelly, its effectiveness ranges from 80% to 93% for new users and increases to 97% for long-term users.

## Indications

- To prevent pregnancy

## Contraindications

**ABSOLUTE**

- History of toxic shock syndrome or repeated urinary tract infections (UTIs)
- Vaginal stenosis
- Pelvic abnormalities
- Allergy to spermicidal jellies or latex
- Less than 6 weeks postpartum
- Personal factors that interfere with insertion and removal of the diaphragm

**RELATIVE**

- Uterine prolapse or retroversion
- Large cystocele or rectocele

## Preprocedure patient teaching

- Discuss birth control options with the patient, including the benefits, risks, efficacy rate, and adverse effects of each, to help her select the method that's right for her.
- Explain the insertion and removal procedures necessary for diaphragm use.
- Tell the patient that minimal discomfort during the procedure typically resolves by the end of the procedure.

## Equipment

Diaphragm fitting rings or set of fitting diaphragms ♦ water-soluble lubricant ♦ diaphragm introducer (optional) ♦ gloves

## Procedure

- Explain the procedure to the patient, and address any questions or concerns she may have.
- Check the patient's history for allergies, especially to latex.
- Instruct the patient to undress below the waist, and assist her into the dorsal lithotomy position.
- Wash your hands, and put on gloves.
- Insert your index and middle fingers into the vagina as if performing a pelvic examination.
- Measure from the symphysis bone to the posterior of the cervix by touching the posterior fornix with your middle finger and raising your hand until the index finger touches the pubic arch.
- Use your thumb tip of the inserted hand to mark where the pubic bone touches the middle finger.
- While maintaining your thumb position, withdraw your hand from the patient.
- Place one end of the diaphragm rim or fitting ring on the tip of the middle finger with the opposite side lying just in front of the thumb. This action will give you the approximate diameter of the diaphragm. Diaphragms are manufactured in sizes of 60 to 90 mm, with the average being 75 to

## Proper diaphragm measurement

To determine the correct size of the diaphragm, extend and hold together your index and middle fingers and insert them into the patient's vagina. With the middle finger touching the posterior fornix, raise your hand until your index finger touches the pubic arch. Press your thumb against your hand directly under the pubic bone.

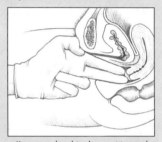

Keep your hand in that position and smoothly withdraw it. The correctly sized diaphragm is the one that fits with one end of the diaphragm rim on the tip of the middle finger and the opposite side of the rim lying just in front of the thumb tip.

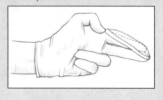

diaphragm ring, feeling for gaps. Several insertions and removals of diaphragms may be required until the proper size is found.

■ To remove the diaphragm, insert your index finger under the symphysis pubis and hook the diaphragm under the proximal rim. Gently pull the diaphragm down and out. Or, slide one finger under the rim until the suction is released.

■ Teach the patient how to insert and remove the diaphragm. Then leave the patient with the diaphragm in place so that she can practice inserting and removing it in private. Have her leave it in when she has finished.

▶ CLINICAL TIP
*To ease insertion, advise the patient to try inserting the diaphragm while squatting, laying on her back with both knees bent, or standing and putting one foot on a stool.*

■ Examine the patient to see whether she inserted the diaphragm correctly. With the diaphragm inserted, have the patient squat and move around to ensure proper fit.

■ Demonstrate how to properly clean the diaphragm with warm, soapy water.

80 mm. (See *Proper diaphragm measurement.*)

■ Select the appropriate-sized diaphragm, and lubricate the rim or dome. (See *Inserting the diaphragm.*)

■ Check the diaphragm to ensure that it fits snugly against the vaginal walls. Follow the edges of the

## Postprocedure patient teaching

■ Emphasize that the patient is to call you if she experiences symptoms of toxic shock syndrome, including fever greater than 101° F (38.3° C), nausea, vomiting, diarrhea, sore throat, body aches, a

## Inserting the diaphragm

Instruct the patient as you insert the diaphragm, identifying structures and associated feelings to prepare her for inserting it herself. Lubricate the rim or dome of the fitting ring or diaphragm to lessen the discomfort of insertion.

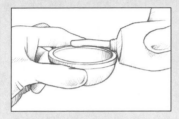

Hold the vulva open with your other hand. Fold the diaphragm in half with one hand by pressing the opposite sides together.

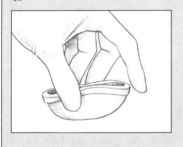

Slide the folded diaphragm into the vagina and toward the posterior cervicovaginal fornix.

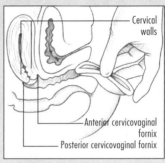

It should fit from below the symphysis and cover the cervix. The proximal rim should fit behind the pubic arch with minimal pressure. Note that the cervix is palpable behind the diaphragm. The cervix feels like a "nose."

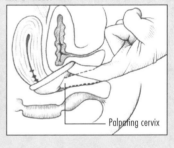

rash, or feeling dizzy, faint, or weak.

■ If the patient is new to diaphragm use and misses a menstrual cycle, she should consider a pregnancy test; contraceptive failure is more common in new users.

■ Instruct the patient to return for follow-up for any complications or concerns. Proper fit should be veri-fied annually, after weight change of more than 15 lb (6.8 kg), after giving birth, after pelvic surgery or an abortion, or for such symptoms as dyspareunia, cramping, and bladder or rectal pain. Diaphragms are replaced every 2 years even if they still fit well.

■ Emphasize to the patient the importance of using the dia-

phragm with spermicidal jelly
every time she has intercourse. Explain that she should apply about
a teaspoon of spermicidal jelly
(such as nonoxynol-9) to the concave surface as well as a thin layer
around the rim. Instruct her to
avoid oil-based products because
they'll cause the diaphragm to deteriorate.

■ Teach her to insert one rim behind the pubic bone and the opposite rim behind the cervix and
to confirm placement by feeling
the cervix behind the dome.

■ Tell her that for subsequent intercourse, she should leave the diaphragm in place and insert more
spermicidal jelly into the vagina;
she shouldn't douche.

■ Tell her to leave the diaphragm
in place at least 6 hours after the
last session of intercourse (but less
than 24 hours).

■ Instruct the patient to wash the
diaphragm with mild soap and dry
it after each use and to inspect it at
least once a month for holes and
wear of the latex.

■ Emphasize that diaphragms
don't prevent sexually transmitted
diseases.

## Complications

■ Pregnancy resulting from not
using spermicidal jelly or from improperly placing the diaphragm
(the result of poor technique or
body changes, such as weight gain
or loss of more than 15 lb [6.8 kg]
and surgery).

■ Recurrent UTIs, discomfort,
and ulceration from an improper
fit are indications for removal.

## Special considerations

■ Although you shouldn't use
spermicidal jelly for the demonstration, explain to the patient that
she'll use it whenever she uses the
diaphragm.

■ You can obtain diaphragm fitting rings free from such companies as Ortho Pharmaceuticals in
sizes that increase in 5-mm increments.

■ Several types of diaphragms exist:
– The arching spring is the most
common in the United States and
has a firm rim, needs no introducer, and is helpful to patients who
have less pelvic support, cystocele,
rectocele, or a retroverted uterus.
It tends to be easier to insert.
– The coil spring has a flexible rim
and needs no introducer but requires good internal support and
the cervix in the midplane or anterior position.
– The flat spring has flat-plane
flexibility and may need an introducer. It's recommended for smaller women, those with a narrow
pelvic shelf, and women who have
never been pregnant.

■ A diaphragm introducer may be
used to insert the diaphragm.

## Documentation

■ Document details of the procedure, including the patient's reaction to the procedure, ability to demonstrate proper technique, time frame for follow-up evaluation, and instructions given to the patient.

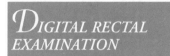

# $\mathcal{D}$IGITAL RECTAL EXAMINATION

**CPT code**
*No specific code has been assigned.*

## Overview

A digital rectal examination may be performed for screening and diagnostic purposes (such as to assess rectal sphincter tone), to check for abnormalities (such as a tumor), and to assess other body structures (such as the prostate gland in the male or the posterior part of the uterus in the female). It's also part of the physical examination for patients age 40 and older.

## Indications

■ To assess external rectal sphincter tone, check for hemorrhoids, and determine the presence of any mass or irregularity of the rectal wall
■ To assess the prostate gland in males or posterior uterus in females
■ To relieve fecal impaction
■ To obtain stool sample for guaiac test

## Contraindications

■ None known

## Preprocedure patient preparation

■ Explain to the patient the importance of and need for the examination.

## Equipment

Gloves ◆ water-soluble lubricant ◆ guaiac test kit (optional)

## Procedure

■ Explain the procedure to the patient, and address any questions or concerns he may have.

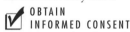
■ Wash your hands, and put on gloves.
■ Providing privacy, have the patient undress from the waist down. Assist the pediatric or geriatric patient into the left lateral Sims' position. When performing the procedure for a pelvic gynecologic examination, assist the patient into the lithotomy position. For male patients, have the patient stand at the side of the bed and lean over the table. Drape appropriately.
■ Spread the patient's buttocks with your nondominant hand to expose the anus and surrounding tissue, checking for fissures, lesions, scars, inflammation, discharge, rectal prolapse, and external hemorrhoids.

■ Apply a water-soluble lubricant to the gloved index finger of your dominant hand. Warn the patient that he may feel some pressure, and ask him to bear down to relax the sphincter. As relaxation occurs, gently insert your finger into the rectum, toward the umbilicus. Palpate as much of the rectal wall as possible by rotating your finger clockwise and then counterclockwise.

■ Remove your finger from the rectum, and inspect the glove for stool, blood, and mucus. Test any fecal matter adhering to the glove for occult blood using a guaiac test, if appropriate.

## Postprocedure patient teaching

■ Review your findings with the patient.

■ Instruct the patient to notify you for any bleeding, pain, diarrhea, or other symptoms that weren't present before or were aggravated by the examination.

■ Tell the patient that a warm tub bath may help to relieve any mild discomfort he experiences after the examination.

## Complications

■ Iatrogenic perforation, pain, or incontinence may result from the examination and require further evaluation.

## Special considerations

■ Rectal sphincter muscle tone can be assessed as you insert and remove your finger through the anus.

■ The prostate gland should feel smooth, rubbery, and about the size of a walnut. Note any tenderness, nodules, or enlargement.

## Documentation

■ Record your examination findings, including any tenderness, pain and, if present, the location of nodules, masses, or other lesions.

■ Record the patient's tolerance of the procedure.

# $\mathcal{D}$ISLOCATION REDUCTION

***CPT codes***
23650   *Closed treatment of shoulder dislocation, with manipulation*
24600   *Closed treatment of elbow dislocation*
26700   *Closed treatment of metacarpophalangeal dislocation, single, with manipulation*
26770   *Closed treatment of interphalangeal joint dislocation, single, with manipulation*
27550   *Closed treatment of knee dislocation*

## Overview

Dislocation is the partial or complete displacement of one bone from another. It can occur spontaneously due to structural defect, traumatic injury, or joint disease. A dislocated joint is reduced when normal position is returned. Reduction decreases pain, helps prevent structural defects and lost or decreased use of the joint, and facilitates healing.

## Indications

■ To alleviate pain and promote healing of a dislocated shoulder, elbow, finger, patella, or toe

## Contraindications

**ABSOLUTE**
■ Fracture of the joint
■ Separation of the acromioclavicular joint
■ Fracture of the joint capsule
■ Abnormal neurovascular status of the extremity
■ Dislocation of the hip or knee

## Preprocedure patient preparation

■ Take a complete history, and perform a physical examination.
■ Obtain radiographic confirmation to rule out fractures and to determine the direction of dislocation. If a fracture is found, immobilize the joint and refer the patient to an orthopedic specialist.

## Equipment

Cleaning solution, such as povidone-iodine or alcohol ◆ lidocaine without epinephrine ◆ 5-ml syringe with 25G needle

## Procedure

■ Explain the procedure to the patient, and address any questions or concerns he may have.

✔ **OBTAIN INFORMED CONSENT**
■ Wash your hands.
■ If necessary, use an assistant to help stabilize the patient. (For a pediatric patient, the parents usually provide the best assistance and can help calm the child.)
■ As needed, use an oral narcotic or a muscle relaxant, or both. Have naloxone (Narcan) available, and monitor the patient's vital signs and airway patency during and after the procedure for signs of overdose.

### *Finger or toe reduction*

■ Use a digital nerve block. Clean the digit with povidone-iodine or alcohol. Infiltrate lidocaine (without epinephrine) using a 25G needle for field anesthesia.
■ Grasp and stabilize the proximal segment in one hand.
■ With your other hand, grasp and apply firm and steady longitudinal traction to the distal segment in the direction of angulation.
■ Slowly move the distal segment in the opposite direction of the angulation while continuing to apply steady traction and pressure to the dorsal side.
■ Continue moving the distal segment toward the neutral position until reduction occurs.
■ Check joint stability.
■ Apply an aluminum finger splint with tape to maintain the joint in a functional position; you

can tape a stable joint to the adjacent finger.

■ As needed, obtain an X-ray to confirm positioning of the joint.

### Shoulder reduction
*Manual reduction*
■ With the patient supine, grasp and support his upper arm above the elbow with both hands and support the forearm under your own arm against your body. Make sure the arm is adducted, externally rotated, and flexed.

■ Apply firm, steady, distracting axial traction to the arm, pulling it distally. ("Distracting" in this context means to pull away from the skeletal attachment.)

■ While maintaining traction, slowly ease the arm into the shoulder until reduction occurs. You may also need to provide some internal or external rotation or slight pressure directed anteriorly from beneath the upper arm.

■ As needed, ask an assistant to apply countertraction to stabilize the patient. Do this by wrapping a bed sheet around the patient's upper torso and having the assistant apply countertraction from the side opposite the affected shoulder.

■ Obtain anteroposterior and axillary lateral X-rays to confirm reduction.

■ Apply a sling and swathe to prevent shoulder external rotation and abduction.

*Passive reduction (Stinson's method)*
■ Use this method for patients with recurrent dislocations. Place the patient in a prone position on the examination table with the in-

volved extremity hanging off the table toward the floor.

■ Place a folded towel under the shoulder.

■ Apply steady traction to the distal extremity, either manually or with a 10- to 15-lb (4.5- to 7-kg) weight attached to the patient's wrist. Allow weights to pull on the arm for 15 to 20 minutes. Reduction should occur spontaneously. If it doesn't, immobilize the extremity and call an orthopedic specialist. You may need to provide some rotation or flexion of the extremity.

### Patella reduction
■ Place the patient in the supine position. Apply steady manual pressure to the lateral aspect of the patella with one hand while slowly extending the knee with the other hand until reduction occurs.

■ Rule out patella fracture or rupture of the patellar or quadriceps tendon.

■ Apply a knee immobilizer to prevent knee flexion.

### Radial head subluxation in children (nursemaid's elbow)
■ Rule out elbow, shoulder, and clavicle fracture or dislocation.

■ Seat the child in the parent's lap. Explain to the parent that the child may experience brief pain with the procedure but then should experience immediate relief of symptoms after reduction occurs.

■ Grasp the patient's wrist and distal forearm in one hand, and support the elbow with the opposite hand, with the thumb over the radial head.

■ Supinate the forearm, rotating the hand palm up.

■ Flex the elbow until you feel a snap over the radial head, indicating that the orbicular ligament has reduced. The child shouldn't require a sling or immobilization.

## Postprocedure patient teaching

■ Explain that the joint will probably swell for 24 to 48 hours after the injury and that keeping the joint elevated and applying ice for 20 minutes intermittently should minimize pain and swelling.

■ Promote use of an anti-inflammatory medication, which will help decrease pain and swelling.

■ Tell the patient with a patella or shoulder dislocation — especially those younger than age 30 — that the risk of recurrence is high. After reduction, refer him to an orthopedic surgeon for evaluation within 1 week. Rest the joint until evaluated by the surgeon.

■ Tell the patient to call or return at once if he experiences redislocation, loss of normal sensation of the limb (numbness and tingling), or increased pain.

## Complications

✣ COLLABORATION
*Malposition or failure to maintain reduction, vascular compromise, and neurologic compromise require collaboration with or referral to an orthopedic specialist.*

■ Narcotic overdose can be reversed with naloxone. Monitor the patient for several hours, and repeat naloxone administration as needed.

## Special considerations

✣ COLLABORATION
*Don't attempt reduction of a large joint or a joint with a concurrent fracture if acute vascular or neurologic compromise threatens the limb. Refer the patient immediately to an orthopedic specialist, or send him to the emergency department for reduction. Dislocations of the elbow, hip, knee (femorotibial), and ankle also require an emergency referral unless acute neurovascular compromise exists.*

## Documentation

■ Review recent or pertinent documentation by other health team members; then initial their notes to signify that you're aware of their findings. This doesn't signify agreement with their comments or reduce your responsibility to conduct your own history and physical examination.

■ Before performing this procedure, document abnormal physical findings on the consent form. Have the patient initial the comments and sign the form to signify acknowledgment of preprocedural abnormalities. In the chart, the preprocedural and postprocedural note must include an evaluation of function, range of motion, and such neurosensory testing as two-point discrimination.

■ Record indications and details of the procedure, the patient's reaction to it, medications ordered, the time frame for follow-up evaluation, and any instructions given to the patient.

# DOPPLER ULTRASONOGRAPHY

## CPT code
93922 *Noninvasive physiologic studies of upper or lower extremity arteries, single-level, bilateral (includes ankle and brachial indices, Doppler waveform analysis, volume plethysmography, and transcutaneous oxygen tension measurement)*

## Overview
Doppler ultrasound consists of an audio unit, a volume control, and a transducer that detects the movement of red blood cells. It's useful in critical care settings in which vasopressors that constrict peripheral circulation are in use. It's also used when a patient has had trauma to a limb that could impede or divert blood flow.

## Indications
■ To determine arterial blood flow when blood flow may be compromised (for instance, in a cool, edematous, pale, cyanotic, or apparently pulseless extremity)

■ To determine placement for an arterial insertion or puncture

## Contraindications
**ABSOLUTE**
■ Use over an open or draining lesion

## Preprocedure patient preparation
■ Tell the patient that he'll feel no pain but that the gel may feel cold. Explain that he may hear loud noises but that this is normal.

## Equipment
Doppler ultrasound ◆ ultrasound transmission gel (not water-soluble lubricant) ◆ marking pen ◆ soft cloth and antiseptic solution or soapy water

## Procedure
■ Explain the procedure to the patient, and address any questions or concerns he may have.
■ Wash your hands.
■ Position the patient comfortably with the affected area accessible.
■ Apply a small amount of coupling or transmission gel to the ultrasound probe.
■ Position the probe on the skin directly over the selected artery.
■ Set the volume control to the lowest setting. If your model doesn't have a speaker, plug in the earphones and slowly raise the volume.

■ To obtain the best signal, tilt the probe at a 45-degree angle from the artery, making sure that you apply gel between the skin and the probe.

■ Slowly move the probe in a circular motion to locate the center of the artery and the Doppler signal — a hissing noise at the heartbeat. Don't move the probe rapidly because this will distort the signal.

■ After you've assessed the pulse, clean the probe with a soft cloth soaked in antiseptic solution or soapy water. Don't immerse the probe or bump it against a hard surface.

■ Wipe the gel from the patient's skin, and mark the selected artery with the marking pen.

### Postprocedure patient teaching

■ Provide further teaching based on the test results, diagnosis, and prognosis.

### Complications
■ None known

### Special considerations

■ Be aware that failure to position the transducer properly can interfere with results.

■ If the patient has a threat to vascular integrity, such as recent orthopedic surgery or an indwelling central venous catheter above the affected site, frequently check pulses for any changes in circulation.

■ If you don't hear any noise when you turn the Doppler ultrasound on, replace the battery.

■ To avoid a loud static noise, turn the volume all the way down and hold the probe against the skin before turning the Doppler ultrasound on.

### Documentation

■ Document the indication for the procedure, the site of evaluation, whether you found a pulse, a description of the pulse (full and bounding, thready, irregular), and all patient instructions given.

## $\mathcal{E}$AR PIERCING

**CPT code**
69090  *Ear piercing*

### Overview

Ear piercing is a voluntary procedure (typically for cosmetic reasons) that's requested by patients
of all ages. The procedure involves
inserting a needle or piercer
through the earlobe, then inserting
a hypoallergenic earring in the
hole. Informed consent may be
necessary before the procedure.

### Indications

■ To perform an elective ear
piercing

### Contraindications

**RELATIVE**
■ Immunocompromised patient
■ Predisposed to keloid formation
■ Coagulopathy
■ Skin disorder at the site

### Preprocedure patient preparation

■ Tell the patient that minimal
and temporary pain is anticipated
with this procedure and that an ice
pack will be applied to the earlobes before the piercing.

### Equipment

Commercial ear-piercing tool ◆
topical antiseptic skin cleaner such
as alcohol swabs ◆ surgical marking pen ◆ ice pack ◆ gloves ◆ sterile earrings (use 14-karat gold or
surgical steel posts)

### Procedure

■ Explain the procedure to the patient, and address any questions or
concerns she may have.

☑ **OBTAIN INFORMED CONSENT**

■ Assess external ear for shape,
symmetry, defects, or other ear
puncture sites.
■ Position the patient either sitting in high Fowler's position or
lying on her side.
■ Wash your hands, and put on
gloves.

■ Ask the patient to point to the area where she wants the piercing to take place. Mark the site anteriorly with a surgical marking pen. Have the patient verify placement selection.

■ Apply an ice pack to the front and back of the earlobe for 2 minutes.

■ Clean the piercing site with a topical antiseptic cleanser such as alcohol.

■ Position the earlobe between the front and rear portions of the piercing tool, with the nose of the device over the placement box. (See *Piercing the earlobe.*)

▶ **CLINICAL TIP**
*When piercing a young child's ears, one piercer can stand on each side of the child to perform the piercing of both ears simultaneously.*

■ Clean around the earring and new puncture site with an alcohol swab.

■ Repeat procedure to the opposite earlobe, if desired.

## Postprocedure patient teaching

■ Tell the patient that cool compresses may be applied to the earlobes for comfort as necessary. Tell her to contact you if any colored discharge, swelling, redness, or ongoing pain is noted.

■ Teach the patient to clean the new piercing site daily with soap and water or alcohol.

■ Teach the patient to turn her earrings (keeping them in her ear) two to four times daily for the first few weeks.

■ Tell the patient to call you if the

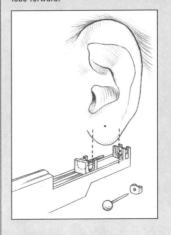

## Piercing the earlobe

After marking the site and inserting the earring post and back into the ear-piercing tool, insert the earlobe and depress the handle. To release the earring back, stop applying pressure and ease the earlobe forward.

earlobe becomes tender, red, and crusty.

## Complications

■ Infection may occur at the puncture site if appropriate postprocedure care isn't initiated and maintained.

■ Keloid formation is reduced by minimizing trauma during insertion, but keloids may be permanent.

■ Ear deformity due to the earring pulling through the earlobe can be avoided by inserting the earring more than $\frac{1}{4}''$ (0.6 cm) from the edge of the lobe.

■ Auricular hematoma is treated

with pressure and drainage as needed.

■ Nickel dermatitis is avoided by using solid gold or surgical steel earrings.

■ The risk of an embedded earring post or backing is minimized by turning the earring in the hole several times daily.

## Special considerations

■ For the first ear piercing, mark the site at the center of each earlobe. For second piercings, the existing earring must be removed and the second mark should be placed approximately ⅜″ (1 cm) up from the first hole along the natural line of the earlobe.

■ Earrings must remain in place for 6 weeks before being removed or replaced with different earrings so that complete healing and epithelialization of the earlobe sinus tract can occur.

## Documentation

■ Document if informed consent was received, if necessary.

■ Record the pre- and postprocedure assessment of ear.

■ Document procedure, method of puncture, and location.

■ Note the patient's understanding of instructions, such as site care, pain control, and to contact you with signs of infection.

# ECHOCARDIOGRAPHY

**CPT codes**
93307  *Echocardiography, transthoracic; complete*
93308  *Echocardiography, transthoracic; follow-up or limited study*

## Overview

Echocardiography is a noninvasive test that shows the size, shape, and motion of cardiac structures. It's useful for evaluating patients with chest pain, enlarged cardiac silhouettes on X-ray films, electrocardiographic changes unrelated to coronary artery disease, and abnormal heart sounds on auscultation.

In this test, a transducer directs ultrahigh-frequency sound waves toward cardiac structures, which reflect these waves. The echoes are converted to images that are displayed on a monitor and recorded on a strip chart or videotape. Results are correlated with clinical history, physical examination, and findings from additional tests. An electrocardiogram (ECG) is done simultaneously to time events in the cardiac cycle.

The techniques most commonly used in echocardiography are M-mode (motion-mode), for recording the motion and dimensions of intracardiac structures, and two-dimensional (cross-sectional), for recording lateral motion and providing the correct spatial relationship between cardiac structures. (See *M-mode echocardiograms.*)

## M-mode echocardiograms

In the normal motion-mode echocardiogram of the mitral valve shown below (top illustration), valve movement appears as a characteristic lopsided M-shaped tracing. The anterior and posterior mitral valve leaflets separate (D) in early diastole, quickly reach maximum separation (E), then close during rapid ventricular filling (E-F).

Leaflet separation varies during mid-diastole, and the valve opens widely again (A) following atrial contraction. The valve starts to close with atrial relaxation (A-B) and is completely closed during the start of ventricular systole (C). The steepness of the E-F slope indirectly shows the speed of ventricular filling, which is normally rapid.

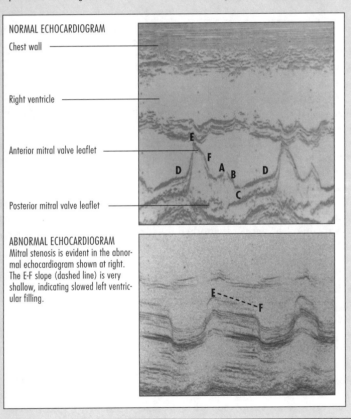

NORMAL ECHOCARDIOGRAM

Chest wall

Right ventricle

Anterior mitral valve leaflet

Posterior mitral valve leaflet

ABNORMAL ECHOCARDIOGRAM
Mitral stenosis is evident in the abnormal echocardiogram shown at right. The E-F slope (dashed line) is very shallow, indicating slowed left ventricular filling.

## Indications

■ To diagnose and evaluate valvular abnormalities

■ To measure the size of the heart's chambers

■ To evaluate chambers and valves in congenital heart disorders

■ To aid diagnosis of hypertrophic and related cardiomyopathies
■ To detect atrial tumors
■ To evaluate cardiac function or wall motion after myocardial infarction
■ To detect pericardial effusion

## Contraindications

■ None known

## Preprocedure patient preparation

■ Explain to the patient that this test is used to evaluate the size, shape, and motion of various cardiac structures.
■ Inform him that he needn't restrict food or fluids before the test.
■ Inform the patient that the procedure is painless. Discomfort may arise from cold gel that's placed on his chest and on the transducer wand.
■ Explain to the patient that other procedures (ECG and phonocardiography) will be performed simultaneously.
■ Explain to the patient that during the procedure, he may be asked to reposition or inhale a gas with a slightly sweet odor (amyl nitrite) while changes in heart function are recorded; describe the possible adverse effects of amyl nitrite (dizziness, flushing, and tachycardia), but assure the patient that such symptoms quickly subside.

## Equipment

Echocardiography ultrasound machine ◆ ultrasound transmission gel (not water-soluble lubricant) ◆ soft cloth and antiseptic solution or soapy water ◆ equipment to perform an ECG

## Procedure

■ Explain the procedure to the patient, and address any questions or concerns he may have.

☑ **OBTAIN INFORMED CONSENT**

■ Providing privacy, have the patient disrobe from the waist up and lie supine on the bed.
■ Wash your hands.
■ Place electrodes on the chest and begin an ECG. (See "Electrocardiography," page 165.)
■ Dim the lighting in the room for better monitor viewing. The echocardiography ultrasound machine should be positioned next to the bed.
■ Apply transmission gel to the third or fourth intercostal space to the left of the sternum, and place the transducer directly over it.
■ Systematically angle the transducer to direct ultrasonic waves at specific parts of the patient's heart.
■ Record significant findings on a strip chart recorder (M-mode echocardiography) or on a videotape recorder (two-dimensional echocardiography).
■ For a different view of the heart, place the transducer beneath the xiphoid process or directly above the sternum.
■ For a left lateral view, assist the

patient to reposition on his left side.

■ To record the heart function under various conditions, ask the patient to inhale and exhale slowly, to hold his breath, or to inhale amyl nitrite.

■ Remove the transmission gel from the patient's skin and from the transducer wand. Clean the transducer wand with a soft cloth soaked in antiseptic solution or soapy water. Don't immerse the wand or bump it against a hard surface.

## Postprocedure patient teaching

■ Tell the patient that results won't be readily available. The study must be fully analyzed before disclosing the results to the patient. Inform the patient that further care will be based upon the results of the echocardiogram and diagnosis as appropriate.

## Complications

■ None known

## Special considerations

■ Incorrect transducer placement and excessive patient movement may interfere with the echocardiogram.

■ Poor imaging is possible if the patient has a thick chest, chest wall abnormalities, or chronic obstructive pulmonary disease.

■ Test results may be invalidated if the patient has an arrhythmia during the procedure.

## Documentation

■ Document the indication for the procedure, any medications or positions used during the procedure, the patient's tolerance of the procedure, and the quality of the imaging obtained.

## *E*LECTRO-CARDIOGRAPHY

*CPT codes*
93000 *Electrocardiogram (ECG), routine ECG with at least 12 leads; with interpretation and report*
93005 *ECG, routine ECG with at least 12 leads; tracing only, without interpretation and report*

## Overview

The most commonly used test for evaluating cardiac status, the electrocardiogram (ECG) is a graphic recording of the electrical current generated by the heart. This current radiates from the heart in all directions and, on reaching the skin, is measured by electrodes connected to an amplifier and a strip chart recorder. The standard resting ECG uses 10 electrodes to measure the electrical potential from 12 different leads: the standard limb leads (I, II, III), the augmented limb leads ($aV_F$, $aV_L$, $aV_R$), and the precordial or chest leads ($V_1$ through $V_6$).

ECG tracings normally consist of three identifiable waveforms: the P wave, the QRS complex, and the T wave. The P wave depicts atrial depolarization, the QRS complex reflects ventricular depolarization, and the T wave indicates ventricular repolarization. The manner in which these waveforms appear, their relationship to one another, and changes in their configuration allow identification of a patient's underlying cardiac status.

## Indications

■ To help identify primary conduction abnormalities, cardiac arrhythmias, cardiac hypertrophy, pericarditis, electrolyte imbalances, myocardial ischemia, and the site and extent of myocardial infarction (MI)
■ To monitor recovery from MI
■ To evaluate the effectiveness of cardiac medication
■ To observe pacemaker performance
■ To determine the effectiveness of thrombolytic therapy and the resolution of ST-segment depression or elevation and T-wave changes
■ To establish a baseline for a patient who is starting an exercise program, at risk for cardiac problems, or in need of surgery

## Contraindications

■ None known

## Preprocedure patient preparation

■ Explain to the patient that this test evaluates the heart's function by recording its electrical activity and that it doesn't require any special preparation.
■ Reassure the patient that the test won't hurt and that he won't get an electric shock. Tell him it will take from 3 to 10 minutes to perform.
■ Inform the patient that he'll have electrodes attached to his arms, legs, and chest and that the gel or paste may feel cold.
■ Tell the patient to lie quietly and relax and to breathe normally during the procedure.
■ Advise the patient not to talk during the test because the movement of his chest and diaphragm may distort the ECG tracing.

## Equipment

Drape ◆ ECG machine ◆ pregelled disposable electrodes or electrodes and paste or gel ◆ alcohol pads ◆ ECG paper ◆ clippers (optional)

### Equipment preparation

■ Place the ECG machine close to the patient.
■ Plug the power cord into the wall outlet, or confirm that the battery is charged.
■ Keep the patient away from electrical fixtures and power cords to minimize electrical interference.

## Procedure

■ Explain the procedure to the patient, and address any questions or concerns he may have.
■ Provide privacy, and have the patient lie supine in the center of the bed or examination table with his arms relaxed at his sides. You

can elevate the head of the bed to make the patient more comfortable.

■ Wash your hands.

■ Drape the patient so that you expose his arms, legs, and chest.

■ If the bed or examination table is too narrow for the patient to relax or the patient is trembling and is nonresponsive to common measures such as a blanket for warmth, ask him to place his hands under his buttocks to reduce muscle tension, which can interfere with the ECG tracing.

■ Select flat, fleshy surfaces to place the extremity electrodes. Avoid muscular and bony areas. If the patient has an amputated limb, choose a site on the stump.

■ If you need to place an electrode on a hairy area, clip the patient's hair. Remove the clipped hair; wipe the area with alcohol, and allow it to dry.

■ Apply electrodes to the medial aspects of the wrists and ankles and to the appropriate locations on the chest. Drape the female patient's chest to provide privacy. (See *Positioning chest electrodes*.)

   ➤ **CLINICAL TIP**
*If you're using pregelled disposable electrodes, peel off the contact paper and apply them directly to the prepared sites. If you're using paste or gel, apply it first and then promptly secure the electrodes. Never substitute the recommended paste or gel with another conductive medium because it may impair the quality of the transmission of electrical impulses. Position the electrodes with the lead connection pointing superiorly.*

■ For female patients, place the electrodes beneath the breast tis-

## Positioning chest electrodes

To ensure accurate test results, position the chest electrodes as follows:

■ Place $V_1$ at the fourth intercostal space and right sternal border.

■ Place $V_2$ at the fourth intercostal space and left sternal border.

■ Place $V_3$ midway between $V_2$ and $V_4$.

■ Place $V_4$ at the fifth intercostal space and left midclavicular line.

■ Place $V_5$ at the fifth intercostal space and left anterior axillary line.

■ Place $V_6$ at the fifth intercostal space and left midaxillary line.

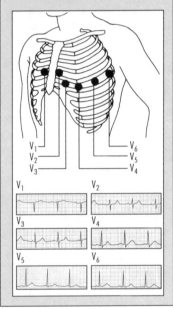

sue. In a large-breasted woman, displace breast tissue laterally.

■ Connect the limb leadwires to the electrodes as follows:

– RA to the right arm

– RL to the right leg

– LA to the left arm

– LL to the left leg.

■ Then connect the chest leadwires. Make sure you connect the leadwires properly.

■ Make sure the paper speed selector is set to the standard 25 mm/second and that the machine is set to full voltage.

■ Enter requested information into the machine — typically, the patient's name, identification number, current medications, and your name.

■ Ask the patient to relax, lie still, breathe normally, and not talk while you record the ECG.

■ Press the AUTO or RECORD button, and observe the quality of the tracing. The machine will record all 12 leads automatically, recording 3 consecutive leads simultaneously. Most machines have a display screen so you can preview waveforms before they are recorded on paper.

■ If the ECG machine display screen reads "check leads" or "lead XX off," make sure the lead connections are secure and attempt to record again.

■ If the waveform extends beyond the paper during recording, reduce the settings to one-half of the standard and note this on the ECG tracing (it will affect the interpretation).

■ Make sure all leads are represented on the tracing. If not, determine which lead has become loose, reattach it, and restart the tracing.

■ When the machine has finished recording, remove the cables from the patient and reposition the patient's gown or clothes. If the patient is to have serial ECGs, you may want to leave the electrodes in

place to ensure that the next ECG is performed with the same lead placement as the first. If not, remove the electrodes, clean the skin with alcohol pads, disconnect the electrodes from the leadwires, and dispose of or clean the electrodes.

## Postprocedure patient teaching

■ Tell the patient that you'll interpret the 12-lead ECG for abnormalities or changes and direct the patient's care appropriately.

## Complications

■ None known

## Special considerations

■ Provide a quiet, private area to obtain the ECG.

■ If the patient has sweaty, oily, or scaly skin, rub the electrode sites with a dry gauze pad or alcohol before applying the electrodes.

■ If the patient's respirations interfere with the quality of the recording, ask him to hold his breath briefly while you record the ECG.

■ If the patient has a pacemaker, you can perform the ECG with or without a magnet. A magnet may be placed over the pacemaker to deactivate it, thereby allowing the underlying heart rhythm to be assessed. If a magnet isn't used, the ECG will evaluate the function of the pacemaker as well.

## Documentation

- Document the indications for performing the ECG.
- Note the patient's name, age, and gender and the date on the ECG tracing.
- Include a copy of the ECG with any documentation.
- Document an interpretation of the ECG, including relevant normal and abnormal results.
- List any medications the patient is currently taking, especially those that can affect the heart.
- Note any management or treatment initiated or changed based on the results of the ECG.

# $\mathcal{E}$MERGENCY DELIVERY

### CPT codes
59409 *Vaginal delivery only (with or without forceps or episiotomy)*
59410 *Vaginal delivery only (with or without forceps or episiotomy) plus postpartum care*

## Overview

Emergency delivery, the unplanned birth of a neonate outside of a health care facility, may occur when labor progresses very quickly or when circumstances prevent the patient from entering a facility. Whether assisting at an emergency delivery or instructing the person who is, your objectives include establishing a clean, safe, private birth area; promoting a controlled delivery; preventing injury, infection, and hemorrhage; and ensuring the safety of the neonate.

## Indications

- To perform a delivery outside of a hospital or birthing center

## Contraindications

- None known

## Preprocedure patient preparation

- As you perform each step, calmly explain what you're doing to the patient. If a support person is present, encourage him to help the patient focus on her breathing. Initially, she'll need to take small panting breaths. As the baby emerges, she'll need to breathe quickly four times, exhaling as if she's blowing out a candle, then take a deep breath as she bears down.
- Have someone call for emergency medical service.

## Equipment

Boiling water ◆ unopened newspaper or large, clean cloth (such as a tablecloth, towel, or curtain) ◆ bath towel, blanket, or coat (to cushion and support the patient's buttocks) ◆ gloves ◆ at least two small, clean cloths ◆ clean, sharp object for cutting (such as a pair of scissors, new razor blade, knife, or nail file) ◆ ligating material (such as string, yarn, ribbon, or new shoelaces) ◆ clean blanket or towel (to cover the neonate) ◆ boiling water

***Equipment preparation***
■ Boil the ligating and cutting materials for at least 5 minutes, if possible.

## Procedure

■ Offer support and reassurance to help relieve the patient's anxiety. Encourage the patient to pant during contractions to promote a controlled delivery. To the extent possible, provide privacy, wash your hands, and put on gloves.
■ Position the patient comfortably on a bed, a couch, or the ground. Open the newspaper or the large, clean cloth and place it under the patient's buttocks to provide a clean delivery area. Elevate the buttocks slightly with the bath towel, blanket, or coat to provide additional room for delivery.
■ Check for signs of imminent delivery, such as bulging perineum, an increase in bloody show, urgency to push, and crowning of the presenting part.
■ As the fetal head reaches and begins to pass the perineum, instruct the patient to pant or blow through the contractions because bearing down forcefully could cause extensive maternal lacerations. Place one hand gently on the perineum to cover the fetal head, control birth speed, and prevent sudden expulsion.
■ Avoid forcibly restraining fetal descent because undue pressure can cause cephalohematoma or scalp lacerations, head trauma, and

vagal stimulation. Undue pressure may also compress the umbilical cord, which may cause fetal bradycardia, circulatory depression, and hypoxia.
■ As the fetal head emerges, immediately break the amniotic sac if it's intact. Support the head as it emerges. Instruct the patient to continue blowing and panting.
■ Locate the umbilical cord. Insert one or two fingers along the back of the emergent head to be sure the cord isn't wrapped around the neck. If the cord is wrapped loosely around the neck, slip it over the head to prevent strangulation during delivery. If it's wrapped tightly around the neck, ligate the cord in two places. Then carefully cut between the ligatures, using a clean, sharp object or, if possible, a sterile one.
■ Carefully support the head with both hands as it rotates to one side (external rotation). Gently wipe mucus and amniotic fluid from the nose and mouth in a downward motion with a clean, small cloth to prevent aspiration.
■ Instruct the patient to bear down with the next contraction to aid delivery of the shoulders. Position your hands on either side of the neonate's head, and support the neck. Exert gentle downward pressure to deliver the upper shoulder. Then exert gentle upward pressure to deliver the lower shoulder. Don't force the shoulder — this could damage the neonate's spinal cord. Instead, wait for the patient to bear down again. (See *Delivering the neonate's shoulders.*)

**➤ CLINICAL TIP**
*Remember that amniotic fluid and vernix are slippery, so take care to support the neonate's body securely after freeing the shoulders. Cup one hand around the head, and grasp the buttocks or feet as they emerge.*

■ Keep the neonate in a slightly head-down position to encourage mucus to drain from the respiratory tract. Wipe excess mucus from his face. If the neonate doesn't breathe spontaneously, gently pat the soles of his feet or stroke his back. Never suspend a neonate by his feet.

■ Note the time of delivery.

■ Dry and cover the neonate quickly with the blanket or towel. Ensure that his head is well covered to minimize exposure and heat loss.

■ Cradle the neonate at the level of the maternal uterus until the umbilical cord stops pulsating. This prevents the neonatal blood from flowing to or from the placenta and leading to hypovolemia or hypervolemia, respectively. Hypovolemia can lead to circulatory collapse and neonatal death; hypervolemia can cause hyperbilirubinemia.

■ Place the neonate on the mother's abdomen in a slightly head-down position. Encourage the mother to start breast-feeding right away if she wants to and if the neonate is pink in color and breathing without difficulty. Skin-to-skin contact will warm the neonate. Cover the patient and neonate with a warm blanket, but

## Delivering the neonate's shoulders

Depending on the neonate's size, delivering the shoulders may be rapid or slow. You should deliver the shoulders with the contraction following the one that frees the head. Tell the patient to breathe quickly four times, exhaling as if she's blowing out a candle, then to push hard.

Place a hand on either side of the neonate's head for support. As the contraction begins, gently guide the neonate's head downward to deliver the upper shoulder, as shown.

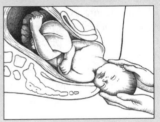

Then, at the next contraction, guide the neonate's head upward to help deliver the lower shoulder, as shown.

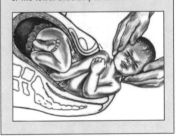

leave the patient's legs uncovered so you can deliver the placenta.

■ Ligate the umbilical cord at two points, 1″ to 2″ (2.5 to 5 cm) apart. Place the first ligature 4″ to 6″ (10 to 15 cm) from the neonate. Ligation prevents autotransfusion, which may cause he-molysis and hyperbilirubinemia.

▪ Cut the umbilical cord between the two ligatures, using sterile equipment if available.

▪ Watch for signs of placental sep-aration, such as a slight gush of dark blood from the vagina, cord lengthening, and a firm uterine fundus rising within the abdomi-nal area. Usually, the placenta sep-arates from the uterus within 5 minutes after delivery (though it may take as long as 30 minutes). When you see these signs, encour-age the patient to bear down to ex-pel the placenta. As she does, ap-ply gentle downward pressure on her abdomen to aid placental de-livery. Never tug on the umbilical cord to initiate or aid placental de-livery because this may invert the uterus or sever the cord from the placenta.

▪ Examine the expelled placenta for intactness. Retained placental fragments may cause hemorrhage or lead to intrauterine infection.

▪ Place the cord and the placenta inside the towel or blanket cover-ing the neonate to provide extra warmth and also to ensure that the cord and placenta will be trans-ported to the hospital for closer examination.

▪ Palpate the maternal uterus to make sure it's firm. Gently mas-sage the atonic uterus to encourage contraction and prevent hemor-rhage. Encourage breast-feeding, if appropriate, to stimulate uterine contraction.

▪ Check the patient for excessive bleeding from perineal lacerations. Apply a perineal pad, if available, and instruct the patient to press her thighs together. Provide com-fort and reassurance, and offer flu-ids, if available. Await the arrival of an emergency medical service, or arrange transportation to the hospital for the patient and neonate. Make sure that the pa-tient and neonate are warm and dry while they await transport.

## Postprocedure patient teaching

▪ Provide information to the pa-tient and her support person as ap-propriate.

## Complications

▪ The risk of intrauterine infec-tion may increase if an object is in-troduced into the vagina to facili-tate delivery. This may also cause injury to the cervix, uterus, fetus, cord, or placenta and should never be done.

▪ Never try to delay the birth or tell the patient to wait because fe-tal distress may occur. Also, don't deny that the birth is about to take place.

▪ Never try to deliver a neonate whose foot, arm, or shoulder ap-pears first. The neonate and the mother could die in this situation. Instead, make every effort to get the patient to a health care pro-vider with expertise in obstetrics or to a hospital.

## Special considerations

▪ Maintain a warm environment and close all doors and windows to prevent heat loss from the neonate.

■ In a breech presentation, make every effort to transport the patient to a nearby hospital. If the patient begins to deliver, carefully support the fetal buttocks with both hands. Gently lift the body to deliver the posterior shoulder. Then lower the neonate slightly to deliver the anterior shoulder. Flexion of the head usually follows. Never apply traction to the neonate's body because his head may lodge in the cervix. Allow the neonate to rotate and emerge spontaneously.

■ If the umbilical cord emerges first, elevate the presenting part throughout delivery to prevent occluding the cord and causing fetal hypoxia. This obstetric emergency usually necessitates a cesarean section. If the cord is protruding from the vagina, place a saline-soaked, sterile gauze over it to prevent it from drying out.

■ If the neonate fails to breathe spontaneously after birth, vigorously dry him to stimulate breathing. If he still isn't breathing, begin to breathe for him. Place your open mouth over his nose and mouth. Using air collected in your cheeks, deliver four short puffs. Next, check the umbilical cord for pulsation. If you find no pulse, begin cardiopulmonary resuscitation (CPR). Place your index and middle fingers over the lower third of the neonate's sternum. The other hand supports the back with the fingers encircling the torso. Administer a breath of air; then use your fingers gently but firmly to pump the heart, making sure the chest wall returns to its relaxed position between compressions.

Pump five times for each breath of air delivered, for a rate of 100 beats/minute. Continue performing CPR until the neonate breathes and his heart beats.

■ Some patients prefer to squat or sit at the edge of a chair, letting gravity aid the delivery. If that's the case, be prepared to catch the neonate so he won't hit the floor.

■ Some neonates emerge quickly and all neonates are very slippery at birth, so cup one hand around the head and grasp the buttocks or feet as they emerge.

## Documentation

■ Give the medical care team the following information, if possible: the time of delivery; the presentation and position of the fetus; any delivery complications (such as the cord wrapped around the neonate's neck); the color, character, and amount of amniotic fluid; and the patient's blood type and Rh factor, if known.

■ Note the time of placental expulsion, the placental appearance and intactness, the amount of postpartum bleeding, the status of uterine firmness (tone) and contractions, and the patient's response.

■ Document the sex of the neonate, his estimated Apgar score, and any resuscitative measures used.

■ Record whether the patient began breast-feeding the neonate.

■ Identify and quantify any fluids given to the patient.

# EPISTAXIS CONTROL

### CPT codes
30901  *Control nasal hemorrhage, anterior, simple (limited cautery or packing), any method*
30903  *Control nasal hemorrhage, anterior, complex (extensive cautery or packing), any method*
30905  *Control nasal hemorrhage, posterior, with posterior nasal packs or cautery, initial*
30906  *Control nasal hemorrhage, posterior, with posterior nasal packs or cautery, subsequent*

## Overview

Epistaxis is spontaneous, typically self-limited bleeding from the nasal cavity or nasopharynx. One in 10 persons experiences at least one significant episode in his lifetime. However, recurrent or persistent episodes may signal an underlying disorder.

There are two main types of nosebleeds. The first type is anterior epistaxis, in which moderate, continuous bleeding typically occurs in one nostril. Almost all cases of nosebleeds in children and adults are of this type. The blood typically has a venous source, although elderly people are more prone to arterial bleeding because of vascular and mucosal atrophy. Episodes typically last from a few minutes to half an hour. The second type is posterior epistaxis, which occurs in about 10% of nosebleeds and in which bleeding is heavier and the blood may run from both nostrils if the patient is leaning forward. The blood may also flow into the pharynx, causing profound nausea and possibly coffee-ground emesis. Bleeding is brisk and intermittent, and the source of blood is typically arterial. This type of epistaxis occurs most commonly in elderly people. It can be difficult to treat because the rupture is usually slightly superior or inferior to the posterior tip of the inferior turbinate.

There are several causes of epistaxis, including trauma, such as direct trauma to the nose or nosepicking, which is a primary cause of disruption to nasal mucosa. Other causes include allergies, hypertension, a dry environment where excessive heat may dry and crack the nasal mucosa, and infections, especially upper respiratory tract infections and influenza. A spontaneous rupture of a blood vessel (typical in children and elderly people, usually in the anterior septum) and cocaine use (which induces vasospasm and can lead to tissue necrosis) can also trigger epistaxis. If an X-ray of the patient's sinuses appears opaque and he has a sinus infection that doesn't respond to conservative therapy, then epistaxis may indicate the presence of a neoplasm.

## Indications

■ To control nasal hemorrhage that isn't controlled by applying pressure to the nostril for 5 to 10 minutes

## Contraindications

**RELATIVE**

- Nasal trauma that might involve internal structure injury
- Coagulopathy
- Potential cerebrospinal fluid leak

## Preprocedure patient preparation

- If possible, obtain a detailed history, including frequency and duration of nosebleeds, associated trauma or history, and coagulopathies.

## Equipment

### *For anterior and posterior packing*

Gowns ◆ protective eyewear ◆ masks ◆ sterile gloves ◆ nasal speculum ◆ directed illumination source (such as headlamp or strong flashlight) or fiber-optic nasal endoscope ◆ sterile tray or sterile towels ◆ sterile cotton-tipped applicators ◆ local anesthetic spray (topical 4% lidocaine) or vial of local anesthetic solution (such as 2% lidocaine or 1% to 2% lidocaine with epinephrine 1:100,000) ◆ sterile cotton balls or cotton pledgets ◆ silver nitrate sticks ◆ small-tip topical nasal vasoconstrictor (such as 1.5% to 2% phenylephrine or 4% cocaine) ◆ oxidized regenerated cellulose (such as Gelfoam, Avitene, Surgicel, or thrombin) ◆ petroleum gauze strip ◆ sterile normal saline solution (1-g container and 60-ml syringe with luer-lock tip, or 5-ml bullets for moistening nasal tampons) ◆ antibiotic ointment ◆ equipment for measuring vital signs ◆ equipment for drawing blood

### *For anterior packing*

Two packages 1½″ petroleum strip gauze (3″ to 4″ [1 to 1.5 m]) ◆ two nasal tampons ◆ petroleum jelly

### *For posterior packing*

Two #14 or #16 French catheters with 30-cc balloon or two single- or double-chamber nasal balloon catheters ◆ Kelly clamps or bayonet forceps ◆ 4″ × 4″ gauze ◆ suture material

### *Equipment preparation*

- Wash your hands.
- Assemble all equipment. Make sure the headlamp or flashlight works.
- Create a sterile field. (Use the sterile towels or the sterile tray). Using aseptic technique, place all sterile equipment on the sterile field. Thoroughly lubricate the anterior or posterior packing with antibiotic ointment.

## Procedure

- Explain the procedure to the patient, and address any questions or concerns he may have.
- Put on protective equipment, including a gown, gloves, protective eyewear, and a mask.
- Check vital signs and observe for hypotension with postural changes. Also monitor airway patency.
- To prevent blood from going down the nasopharynx and to reduce venous pressure, position the

patient sitting up and leaning forward.

■ To inspect the nasal cavity, use a nasal speculum and an external light source or a fiber-optic nasal endoscope. To remove collected blood and help visualize the bleeding vessel, use cotton-tipped applicators and wick away the blood. Consider applying a topical vasoconstrictor such as phenylephrine to slow bleeding and aid visualization.

■ If bleeding is located anteriorly, apply continuous external pinching pressure with the thumb and forefinger to the anterior nasal septum for 15 minutes without stopping.

■ If blood still hasn't clotted, insert a cotton pledget of vasoconstricting nasal drops or epinephrine into the nasal passage. Apply pressure for an additional 10 minutes.

■ Remove the pledget to observe for rebleeding.

■ If these measures fail, anesthetize the mucous membrane with a cotton pledget of 4% lidocaine.

■ If you can see the bleeding site and it's accessible, apply a silver nitrate stick to the site and any prominent vessels.

■ If bleeding recurs after a short time, repeat the previous two steps immediately and then pack the nasal passage with a petroleum gauze strip or oxidized regenerated cellulose for 24 hours.

### For anterior nasal packing

■ Apply topical vasoconstricting agents to control bleeding, or use chemical cautery with silver nitrate sticks. To enhance the vasoconstrictor's action, apply continuous external pinching pressure with the thumb and forefinger to the anterior nasal septum for 15 minutes without stopping.

■ If bleeding persists, insert an absorbable hemostatic nasal pack directly on the bleeding site. The pack swells to form an artificial clot. If these methods fail, insert anterior nasal packing. Even if only one side is bleeding, both sides may require packing to control bleeding. (See *Types of nasal packing*.)

■ While the anterior pack is in place, instruct the patient or parent to use cotton-tipped applicators to apply petroleum jelly to the patient's lips and nostrils to prevent drying and cracking. Recheck the patient's vital signs after 5 to 10 minutes.

■ Alternatively, nasal balloon catheters may be used to control epistaxis (See *Nasal balloon catheters*, page 178.)

### For posterior nasal packing

■ Wash your hands, and put on sterile gloves.

■ Roll 4″ × 4″ gauze and tie with suture material, leaving ends long enough to tie to the catheters.

■ If the bleeding source is in the posterior nasal cavity, lubricate the soft catheters to ease insertion. Instruct the patient to open his mouth and to breathe normally through his mouth during catheter insertion to minimize gagging as the catheters pass through the nostril.

■ Advance one or two soft catheters into the patient's nostrils. As

# Types of nasal packing

Your patient's nosebleed may be controlled with anterior or posterior nasal packing.

## ANTERIOR NASAL PACKING

You may treat an anterior nosebleed by packing the anterior nasal cavity with a 3' to 4' (1 to 1.5-m) strip of antibiotic-impregnated petroleum gauze or with a nasal tampon.

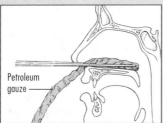

Petroleum gauze

A nasal tampon is made of tightly compressed absorbent material with or without a central breathing tube. Insert a lubricated tampon along the floor of the nose (shown above) and, with the patient's head tilted backward, instill 5 to 10 ml of antibiotic or normal saline solution. The tampon expands as a result, stopping the bleeding. Instruct the patient to moisten the tampon periodically.

In a child or a patient with blood dyscrasia, you may fashion an absorbable pack by moistening a gauzelike, regenerated cellulose material with a vasoconstrictor. Applied to a visible bleeding point, this substance will swell to form a clot. The packing is absorbable and doesn't need removal.

## POSTERIOR NASAL PACKING

Posterior packing consists of a gauze roll shaped and secured by three sutures (one suture at each end and one in the middle). To insert the packing, advance a soft catheter or catheters into the patient's nostrils. When the catheter tips appear in the nasopharynx, grasp them with a Kelly clamp or bayonet forceps and pull them forward through the mouth. Secure the two end sutures on the nasal packing to the catheter tip, and draw the catheters back through the nostrils. This step brings the packing into place with the end sutures hanging

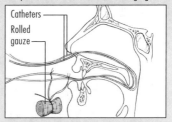

Catheters

Rolled gauze

from the patient's nostril. (The middle suture emerges from the patient's mouth to free the packing, when needed.) You may weight the nose sutures with a clamp. Then pull the packing securely into place behind the soft palate and against the posterior end of the septum (nasal choana).

After you examine the patient's throat (to ensure that the uvula hasn't been forced under the packing), insert anterior packing and secure the whole apparatus by tying the posterior packing sutures around rolled gauze or a dental roll at the nostrils (shown below).

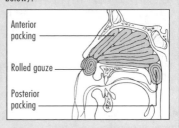

Anterior packing

Rolled gauze

Posterior packing

they appear in the nasopharynx, grasp them with a clamp and pull them out through the mouth. Tie the two end sutures to the catheter, and gently pull the catheter back out from the nose until the rolled gauze passes the uvula and is snug against the nasal passage.

## Nasal balloon catheters

To control epistaxis, you may use a balloon catheter instead of nasal packing. Self-retaining and disposable, the catheter may have a single balloon or a double balloon to apply pressure to bleeding nasal tissues.

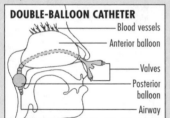

**SINGLE-BALLOON CATHETER**

- Blood vessels
- Balloon
- Valve
- Collapsible bulb

When inserted and inflated, the single-balloon catheter (shown above) used for anterior bleeding compresses the blood vessels while a soft, collapsible external bulb prevents the catheter from dislodging posteriorly.

**DOUBLE-BALLOON CATHETER**

- Blood vessels
- Anterior balloon
- Valves
- Posterior balloon
- Airway

The double-balloon catheter is used for simultaneous anterior and posterior nasal packing. It compresses the posterior vessels serving the nose and the posterior bleeding vessels; the anterior balloon compresses bleeding intranasal vessels. This catheter contains a central airway for breathing comfort.

### INSERTION

To insert a single- or double-balloon catheter, prepare the patient as you would for nasal packing. Be sure to discuss the procedure thoroughly to alleviate the patient's anxiety and promote his cooperation.

Explain that the catheter tip will be lubricated with an antibiotic or a water-soluble lubricant to ease passage and to prevent infection. The tip of the single-balloon catheter will be inserted in the nostrils until it reaches the posterior pharynx. Then the balloon will be inflated with normal saline solution, pulled gently into the posterior nasopharynx, and secured at the nostrils with the collapsible bulb. With a double-balloon catheter, the posterior balloon is inflated with normal saline solution; then the anterior balloon is inflated.

### ROUTINE CARE

To prevent damage to nasal tissue, order the balloon deflated for 10 minutes every 24 hours. If bleeding recurs or remains uncontrolled, reinflate the balloon immediately.

### RECOGNIZING COMPLICATIONS

The patient may report difficulty breathing, swallowing, or eating, and the nasal mucosa may sustain damage from pressure. Balloon deflation may dislodge clots and nasal debris into the oropharynx, which could prompt coughing, gagging, or vomiting. If these occur, remove the catheter. Under these circumstances, arterial ligation, cryotherapy, or arterial embolization should be considered.

- Help the patient assume a comfortable position with his head elevated 45 to 90 degrees.
- Assess him for airway obstruction or any respiratory changes.

## Postprocedure patient teaching

- Instruct the patient to contact you for recurrent bleeding within 1 hour or for a second episode within 1 week.

■ Tell the patient to schedule an appointment for removal of the nasal packing, usually in 2 to 5 days. After an anterior pack is removed, instruct the patient to avoid rubbing or picking his nose, inserting any object into his nose, and blowing his nose forcefully for 48 hours.

■ Tell the patient to expect reduced smell and taste ability. Make sure he has a working smoke detector at home.

■ Advise him to eat soft foods because his eating and swallowing abilities will be impaired. Instruct him to drink fluids often or to use artificial saliva solution or spray to cope with dry mouth.

■ Teach him measures to prevent nosebleeds, and instruct him to seek medical help if these measures fail to stop bleeding.

■ Suggest rubbing a lubricant (such as A&D ointment or bacitracin) over the nasal septum twice a day for 3 to 5 days to promote healing and hydration. Suggest using a humidifier or pot of water on the radiator to increase humidity in the home, especially in sleeping areas and during the winter.

■ If the patient is a child, tell the parents to keep their child's fingernails trimmed.

■ Provide the patient with written information on epistaxis management.

## Complications

■ Blood loss and infection are treated on a case-by-case basis.

■ Hypoxemia is treated with oxygen by mask and is monitored closely.

■ Airway obstruction is relieved by adjusting or removing the packing.

■ Pressure necrosis risk is minimized by not pulling the packing too tight and removing it as soon as possible.

■ Hypotension is treated with fluid replacement, rest and, if needed, blood transfusion.

## Special considerations

**COLLABORATION**
*Refer the patient to an otolaryngologist or emergency medical facility for massive bleeding, persistent and continuous epistaxis, an inaccessible or poorly visualized bleeding site, or posterior epistaxis.*

■ Patients with posterior packing may be hospitalized for monitoring.

■ After the packing is in place, compile assessment data carefully to help detect the underlying cause of nosebleeds. Mechanical factors include a deviated septum, injury, and a foreign body. Environmental factors include drying and erosion of the nasal mucosa. Other possible causes are upper respiratory tract infection, anticoagulant or salicylate therapy, blood dyscrasia, cardiovascular or hepatic disorders, tumors of the nasal cavity or paranasal sinuses, chronic nephritis, and familial hemorrhagic telangiectasia.

■ If significant blood loss occurs or if the underlying cause remains unknown, order a complete blood count and coagulation profile as soon as possible. As indicated, order an arterial blood gas analysis to detect any pulmonary complications, and arterial oxygen saturation monitoring to assess for hypoxemia. If necessary, administer supplemental humidified oxygen with a face mask. Prescribe antibiotics, decongestants, and analgesics without aspirin or ibuprofen, as indicated.

■ If needed, obtain hemoglobin and hematocrit studies (if the patient has a history of significant bleeding); type and crossmatch (if the patient may need a transfusion); prothrombin time, partial thromboplastin time, and international normalized ratio (if the patient tends to bleed easily from external stimuli); or sinus X-rays (if you suspect a neoplasm).

## Documentation

■ Record a detailed history, including frequency and duration of nosebleeds, associated trauma or history, and coagulopathies.

■ Document any measures taken for hemostasis as well as outcomes. Record the type of packing and when it should be removed. Note the patient's vital signs, any laboratory studies performed, and the results. Record any complications and subsequent measures taken.

■ Record patient instructions and verification of comprehension.

## *EXTERNAL FETAL MONITORING*

### CPT codes

59050 *Fetal monitoring during labor by consulting physician (i.e.,*
*non-attending physician) with written report (separate procedure); supervision and interpretation*
59051 *Fetal monitoring during labor by consulting physician (i.e., non-attending physician) with written report (separate procedure); interpretation only*

## Overview

An indirect, noninvasive procedure, external fetal monitoring uses two devices strapped to the patient's abdomen to evaluate fetal well-being during labor. The use of the external fetal monitor has a number of drawbacks. (See *Drawbacks of external fetal monitoring.*)

One device used for fetal monitoring, an ultrasound transducer, transmits high-frequency sound waves through soft body tissues to the fetal heart. The waves rebound from the heart, and the transducer relays them to a monitor. Another device used for fetal monitoring, a pressure-sensitive tocotransducer, responds to the pressure exerted by uterine contractions and simultaneously records their duration and frequency. (See *Applying external fetal monitoring devices*, page 182.) The monitoring apparatus traces fetal heart rate and uterine contraction data onto the same printout paper.

## Indications

■ To monitor fetal status in high-risk pregnancy
■ To monitor fetal status in oxytocin-induced labor
■ To monitor fetal status during

antepartal nonstress and contraction stress test

■ To monitor fetal status after rupture of membranes

## Contraindications

■ None known

## Preprocedure patient preparation

■ Inform the patient and her support person that "external fetal monitoring" is the term used for measuring the fetal heart rate as it reacts to her uterine contractions during labor. The fetal heart rate and the pattern of the patient's contractions are displayed as a graph on the monitor. This helps determine how the fetus is handling the stress of labor.

■ Inform the patient and her support person that the monitor may make noise if the pen set tracer moves above or below the printed paper. Reassure them that this doesn't indicate fetal distress. As appropriate, explain other aspects of the monitor to help reduce maternal anxiety about fetal well-being.

■ Explain to the patient and her support person how to time and anticipate contractions with the monitor. Inform them that the distance from one dark vertical line to the next on the printout grid represents 1 minute. The support person can use this information to prepare the patient for the onset of a contraction and to guide and slow her breathing as the contraction subsides.

### Drawbacks of external fetal monitoring

Use of external fetal monitoring may be uncomfortable for a woman in labor. To avoid dislodging the transducers, she must restrict her movement, changing position as little as possible. Remaining still is also necessary to keep from creating static noise — anything that brushes the surface of the transducer or even the patient's own bowel sounds can interfere with obtaining a clear recording of the fetal heart rate or uterine activity.

The need for a supine position may interfere with placental blood flow, increasing the risk of supine hypotensive syndrome (caused by the weight of the uterus and its contents on the maternal inferior vena cava).

The transducers and straps need frequent adjustments because they can cause redness around the patient's abdomen and easily slip out of place.

■ Advise the patient and her support person that external fetal monitoring may be done for about 20 minutes at the start of labor, then for a few minutes each hour. The monitor may be left on for continuous monitoring as well. The monitor allows you to see signs of fetal distress early and take steps to help the fetus.

■ Explain to the patient that the external fetal monitors are held in place by straps around her abdomen. A pressure gauge measures the pressure of the contractions, and an ultrasonic device detects fetal heart rate. Explain to her that there's no pain associated with the monitors and that she's free to change positions; however, movement can temporarily interfere with monitoring information.

## Applying external fetal monitoring devices

To ensure clear tracings that define fetal status and labor progress, be sure to precisely position external monitoring devices, such as an ultrasound transducer and a tocotransducer.

### FETAL HEART MONITOR

Palpate the uterus to locate the fetus's back. If possible, place the ultrasound transducer over this site where the fetal heartbeat sounds the loudest. Then tighten the belt. Use the fetal heart tracing on the monitor strip to confirm the transducer's position.

### LABOR MONITOR

A tocotransducer records uterine motion during contractions. Place the tocotransducer over the uterine fundus where it contracts, either midline or slightly to one side. Place your hand on the fundus and palpate a contraction to verify proper placement. Secure the tocotransducer's belt; then adjust the pen set so that the baseline values read between 5 and 15 mm Hg on the monitor strip.

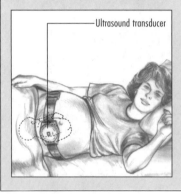

Ultrasound transducer

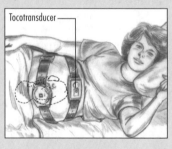

Tocotransducer

■ Advise the patient that you're able to disconnect the monitor temporarily to allow her to walk around or go to the bathroom.

## Equipment

Electronic fetal monitor ◆ ultrasound transducer and cable ◆ tocotransducer and cable ◆ conduction gel ◆ transducer straps ◆ damp cloth ◆ printout paper

### Equipment preparation

■ Because fetal monitor features and complexity vary, review the operator's manual before proceeding. If the monitor has two paper speeds, select the slower speed

(typically 3 cm/minute) to ensure an easy-to-read tracing. At higher speeds (for example, 1 cm/minute), the printed tracings are difficult to decipher and interpret accurately. Many facilities now have the monitors preset to a certain setting to produce standardized test results.

■ Plug the tocotransducer cable into the uterine activity jack and the ultrasound transducer cable into the phono-ultrasound jack. After the straps are placed around the patient's abdomen, attach them to the tocotransducer and the ultrasound transducer.

■ Label the printout paper with the patient's identification number or birth date and name, the date, maternal vital signs and position, the paper speed, and the number of the strip paper to maintain accurate, consecutive monitoring records.

## Procedure

■ Explain the procedure to the patient, and address any questions or concerns she may have.

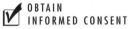 **OBTAIN INFORMED CONSENT**

■ Wash your hands, and provide privacy.

### *Beginning the procedure*

■ Assist the patient to the semi-Fowler or left-lateral position with her abdomen exposed. Don't let her lie supine because pressure from the gravid uterus on the maternal inferior vena cava may cause maternal hypotension and decreased uterine perfusion and may induce fetal hypoxia.

■ Palpate the patient's abdomen to locate the fundus — the area of greatest muscle density in the uterus. Then, using transducer straps, secure the tocotransducer over the fundus.

■ Adjust the pen set tracer controls so that the baseline values read between 5 and 15 mm Hg on the monitor strip. This prevents triggering the alarm that indicates the tracer has dropped below the paper's margins. The proper setting varies among tocotransducers.

■ Apply conduction gel to the ultrasound transducer crystals to promote an airtight seal and optimal sound-wave transmission.

■ Use Leopold's maneuvers to palpate the fetal back, through which fetal heart tones resound most audibly.

■ Start the monitor. Then apply the ultrasound transducer directly over the site having the strongest heart tones.

■ Activate the control that begins the printout. On the printout paper, note any coughing, position changes, drug administration, vaginal examinations, and blood pressure readings that may affect interpretation of the tracings.

### *Monitoring the patient*

■ Observe the tracings to identify the frequency and duration of uterine contractions, but palpate the uterus to determine intensity of contractions.

■ Mentally note the baseline fetal heart rate (FHR) — the rate between contractions — to compare with suspicious-looking deviations. FHR normally ranges from 110 to 160 beats/minute.

■ Assess periodic accelerations or decelerations from the baseline FHR. Compare the FHR patterns with those of the uterine contractions. Note the time relationship between the onset of an FHR deceleration and the onset of a uterine contraction, the time relationship of the lowest level of an FHR deceleration to the peak of a uterine contraction, and the range of FHR deceleration. These data help distinguish fetal distress from benign head compression. (See *Reading a fetal monitor strip,* page 184.)

■ Move the tocotransducer and the ultrasound transducer to accommodate changes in maternal

## Reading a fetal monitor strip

Presented in two parallel recordings, the fetal monitor strip records the fetal heart rate (FHR) in beats/minute in the top recording and uterine activity (UA) in mm Hg in the bottom recording. You can obtain information on fetal status and labor progress by reading the strips horizontally and vertically.

Reading horizontally on the FHR or the UA strip, each small block represents 10 seconds. Six consecutive small blocks, separated by a dark vertical line, represent 1 minute.

Reading vertically on the FHR strip, each block represents an amplitude of 10 beats/minute. Reading vertically on the UA strip, each block represents 5 mm Hg of pressure.

Assess the baseline FHR — the "resting" heart rate — between uterine contractions when fetal movement diminishes. This baseline FHR (normal range: 110 to 160 beats/minute) pattern serves as a reference for subsequent FHR tracings produced during contractions.

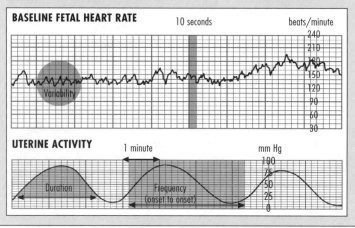

or fetal position. Readjust both transducers every hour, and assess the patient's skin for reddened areas caused by the strap pressure. Document skin condition.

■ Clean the ultrasound transducer periodically with a damp cloth to remove dried conduction gel, which can interfere with ultrasound transmission. Apply fresh gel as necessary. After using the ultrasound transducer, place the cover over it.

## Postprocedure patient teaching

■ Advise the patient as appropriate based on the results of the monitoring.

## Complications
■ None known

## Special considerations
■ If the monitor fails to record uterine activity, palpate for con-

tractions. Check for equipment problems as the manufacturer directs, and readjust the tocotransducer.

■ If the patient reports discomfort in the position that provides the clearest signal, try to obtain a satisfactory 5- to 10-minute tracing with the patient in this position before assisting her to a more comfortable position. As the patient progresses through labor and abdominal pressure increases, the pen set tracer may exceed the alarm boundaries.

■ Monitoring devices, such as phonotransducers and abdominal electrocardiogram transducers, are available. However, facilities use these devices less frequently than they use the ultrasound transducer.

■ The Association of Women's Health, Obstetric, and Neonatal Nurses maintains that intermittent auscultation of the fetal heart with a 1:1 nurse-patient ratio is equivalent to continuous external fetal monitoring. For low-risk patients, the suggested auscultation frequency is 30-minute intervals in active first-stage labor and 15-minute intervals in second stage labor. For high-risk patients, the suggested auscultation frequency is 15-minute intervals in active first-stage labor and 5-minute intervals in second-stage labor.

## Documentation

■ Make sure you've numbered each monitor strip in sequence and labeled each printout sheet with the patient's identification number or birth date and name, the date, the time, maternal vital signs and position, the paper speed, and the number of the strip paper.

■ Record the time of any vaginal examinations, membrane rupture, drug administration, and maternal or fetal movements.

■ Record maternal vital signs and the intensity of uterine contractions.

■ Document each time that you moved or readjusted the tocotransducer and ultrasound transducer, and summarize this information in your notes.

# *E*YE IRRIGATION

### CPT codes
65205 *Removal of foreign body, external eye, conjunctival, superficial*
68399 *Unlisted procedure, conjunctiva*

## Overview

The goal of eye irrigation is to flush and eliminate irritants to the eye itself, its cavity, and surrounding tissue. This may include foreign bodies, chemicals, or bodily secretions. The type of irritant (if known) should be identified before irrigation. Some irritants (such as alkali chemicals) are highly damaging to the eye, and patients should be referred for emergency or specialist care.

In an emergency, tap water may serve as an irrigant. The amount of solution needed to irrigate an eye depends on the contaminant. Secretions require a moderate volume; major chemical burns require a copious amount. Usually, an I.V. bottle or a bag of normal saline solution (with I.V. tubing attached) supplies enough solution for continuous irrigation of a chemical burn. (See *Three devices for eye irrigation*.)

## Indications

- To remove a chemical irritant or foreign particles and prevent further damage to the eye

## Contraindications

**RELATIVE**
- Noncompliant patient
- Possibility of orbital fracture
- Suspected globe penetration or rupture injury

## Preprocedure patient preparation

- Ask the patient what the eye irritant is, when symptoms started, and about any relief measures he may have attempted.
- Tell the patient that discomfort should be minimal. Notable relief should be identified after the procedure or within a few hours.
- If the patient has a chemical burn, ease his anxiety by explaining that irrigation prevents further damage.

## Equipment

Gloves ◆ towels ◆ eyelid retractor ◆ cotton balls or 4″ × 4″ gauze pads ◆ ophthalmoscope ◆ magnifying glass ◆ protective eyewear ◆ reservoir basin

### *Optional*

Litmus paper ◆ proparacaine hydrochloride topical anesthetic ◆ prepackaged, commercially prepared sterile irrigation solution ◆ fluorescent stain ◆ prepackaged eye irrigation kit ◆ eye patch ◆ tape

### *For moderate-volume irrigation*

Sterile ophthalmic irrigant ◆ cotton-tipped applicators ◆ 20-ml sterile syringe

### *For copious irrigation*

1 or more 1,000-ml bottles or bags of normal saline solution ◆ standard I.V. infusion set without needle ◆ I.V. pole

### *Equipment preparation*

- All solutions should be at body temperature: 98.6° F (37° C). Read the label on the sterile ophthalmic irrigant. Double-check its sterility, strength, and expiration date.

### *For moderate-volume irrigation*

- Remove the cap from the irrigant container, and place the container within easy reach. (Be sure to keep the tip of the container sterile.)

### *For copious irrigation*

- Use aseptic technique to set up the I.V. tubing and the bag or bottle of normal saline solution. Hang the container on an I.V. pole, fill the I.V. tubing with the solution, and adjust the drip regulator valve to ensure an adequate but not forceful flow. Place all other equipment within easy reach.

## Three devices for eye irrigation

Depending on the type and extent of injury, a patient's eye may need to be irrigated using different devices.

**SQUEEZE BOTTLE**
For moderate-volume irrigation — to remove eye secretions, for example — apply sterile ophthalmic irrigant to the eye directly from the squeeze bottle container. Direct the stream at the inner canthus, and position the patient so that the stream washes across the cornea and exits at the outer canthus.

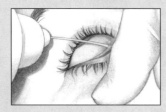

**I.V. TUBE**
For copious irrigation — to treat chemical burns, for example — set up an I.V. bag and tubing without a needle. Use the procedure described above for moderate irrigation to flush the eye for at least 15 minutes.

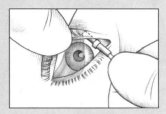

**MORGAN LENS**
Connected to irrigation tubing, a Morgan lens permits continuous lavage and also delivers medication to the eye. Use an adapter to connect the lens to the I.V. tubing and the solution container. Begin the irrigation at the prescribed flow rate. To insert the device, ask the patient to look down as you insert the lens under the upper eyelid. Then tell him to look up as you retract and release the lower eyelid over the lens.

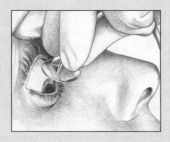

■ Ensure that there's adequate lighting for an ophthalmic examination.

## Procedure

■ Explain the procedure to the patient, and address any questions or concerns he may have.

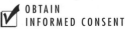
OBTAIN
INFORMED CONSENT

■ Wash your hands, and put on gloves and protective eyewear.
■ Inspect the eyelids. Assess external and then internal structures with the magnifying glass and the ophthalmoscope.
■ Assist the patient into a supine position. Turn his head slightly toward the affected side to prevent solution flowing over his nose and into the other eye.
■ Place a towel under the patient's

head and let him hold another towel against his affected side to catch excess solution.

■ If the patient has identified the irritant as a chemical, place a piece of litmus paper in the inner canthus area. This will identify whether it's an alkali- or acid-based chemical.

■ Using the thumb and index finger of your nondominant hand, separate the patient's eyelids.

■ If indicated, instill proparacaine hydrochloride eyedrops as a comfort measure. Use them only once because repeated use retards healing. Wait a few minutes for maximal anesthetic effect.

■ To irrigate the conjunctival cul-de-sac, continue holding the eyelids apart with your thumb and index finger.

■ To irrigate the upper eyelid (the superior fornix), use an eyelid retractor. Steady the hand holding the retractor by resting it on the patient's forehead. The retractor prevents the eyelid from closing involuntarily when solution touches the cornea and conjunctiva.

■ Position the reservoir basin close to the side of the patient's head to catch used irrigant.

### For moderate-volume irrigation

■ With your nondominant hand, place your thumb along the lower eyelid and pull down. Place your index finger on the upper eyelid, and separate the upper and lower eyelids.

■ Holding the bottle of sterile ophthalmic irrigant or a sterile 20-ml syringe filled with sterile normal saline about 1″ (2.5 cm) from the eye, direct a constant, gentle stream at the inner canthus so that the solution flows across the cornea to the outer canthus.

■ Evert the lower eyelid and then the upper eyelid to inspect the eye cavity and eye structures for retained foreign particles. Flush the entire area of the cavity and eye structures.

■ Remove any foreign particles by gently touching the conjunctiva with sterile, wet cotton-tipped applicators. Don't touch the cornea.

■ Resume irrigating the eye until it's clean of all visible foreign particles.

### For copious irrigation

■ Hold the control valve on the I.V. tubing about 1″ (2.5 cm) above the eye, and direct a constant, gentle stream of normal saline solution at the inner canthus so that the solution flows across the cornea to the outer canthus.

■ Ask the patient to rotate his eye periodically while you continue the irrigation. This action may dislodge foreign particles.

■ Evert the lower eyelid and then the upper eyelid to inspect for retained foreign particles. (This inspection is especially important when the patient has caustic lime in his eye.)

■ At this time, you may place the sterile I.V. tubing tip under the eyelid to hold it in place as irrigation continues.

■ After eye irrigation, gently dry the eyelids with cotton balls or sterile gauze pads, wiping from the inner to the outer canthus. Use a new cotton ball or pad for each wipe. This reduces the patient's need to rub his eye.

■ Reassess external and internal eye structures with the magnifying glass and ophthalmoscope.

■ If corneal abrasion is suspected, apply fluorescent stain and evaluate for color changes.

■ When you are finished, place an eye patch over the eye, secure it with tape, and tell the patient to keep it in place for 24 hours.

■ Remove and discard your gloves and protective eyewear.

■ Wash your hands to avoid burning, residual chemical contaminants.

## Postprocedure patient teaching

■ Instruct the patient to keep the eye patch in place for 24 hours. If further irritation, pain, or discomfort is noted, tell the patient to contact you for further evaluation. Generally, no antibiotics or further medications are necessary for this procedure.

■ Instruct the patient to call if any increased or ongoing discomfort is noted or if any change in vision, eye pain or sensation, or eye drainage is noted. Tell the patient to avoid rubbing his eyes. Reinforce good hand-washing practices. Tell the patient that applying clean, cool compresses to the affected eye may help alleviate any postprocedure discomfort.

## Complications

■ Trauma or infection may be caused secondary to the original injury or procedure and must be evaluated and treated on a case-by-case basis.

## Special considerations

■ If symptoms continue, vision changes are noticed, or irritation is seen on the ophthalmoscopic examination, a fluorescent stain examination should be completed.

**✦ COLLABORATION**
*If any suspicious findings are noted during the procedure or assessment, refer the patient to an ophthalmologist for evaluation.*

■ Immediate irrigation with normal saline solution is the single best initial treatment for chemical burns to the eye and reduces the ultimate physical damage to the eye.

■ For chemical burns, irrigate each eye for at least 15 minutes with normal saline solution to dilute and wash away the harsh chemical. (After irrigating any chemical, note the time, date, and chemical for your own reference in case you develop contact dermatitis.)

**✦ COLLABORATION**
*Most acid burns with mild to moderate stromal haze will get better with time. Alkaline burns may initially look far better than how they will appear at day 2 or 3. Therefore, it's important to refer the patient to a facility or an ophthalmologic practice immediately after irrigating the eye.*

■ When irrigating both eyes, have the patient tilt his head toward the side being irrigated to avoid cross-contamination.

■ Proparacaine hydrochloride ophthalmic anesthetic should be stored tightly closed in its original container and refrigerated. Don't use discolored solution.

## Documentation

- Record the results of the preprocedure and postprocedure external and internal ophthalmoscopic examinations. Note any abnormal color, drainage, assessment of vision changes, and pain or discomfort before and after irrigation.
- Document whether ophthalmic anesthetic was used and how much.
- Note the type of irritant seen, removed, or irrigated. If litmus paper was used, document the findings.
- Record the type of irrigating procedure used.
- List what patient instructions were given and the patient's understanding of those instructions.
- Note the duration of irrigation, the type and amount of solution, and characteristics of the drainage. Record your assessment of the patient's eye before and after irrigation. Also note his response to the procedure.

## EYE PROPHYLAXIS (CREDÉ'S TREATMENT)

### CPT code
*No specific code has been assigned.*

## Overview

Named for its developer, Credé's treatment prevents damage and blindness from conjunctivitis due to *Neisseria gonorrhoeae,* which is transmitted to the neonate during birth from the infected mother. This procedure is also used to treat chlamydial conjunctivitis transmitted during birth.

Required by law in the United States, Credé's treatment consists of instilling 1% silver nitrate solution into the neonate's eyes. Most states permit alternative treatment with 1% tetracycline ointment or 0.5% erythromycin ophthalmic ointment. By this method, the neonate may avoid chemical irritation from silver nitrate yet benefit from the antimicrobial effects of broad-spectrum antibiotics.

The solution or ointment is instilled in the conjunctival sac (from the eye's inner canthus to its outer canthus). The treatment, which may cause conjunctival swelling, may also disturb the typically quiet but alert neonate at birth. Therefore, although silver nitrate treatment is usually given at delivery, it can be delayed for up to 1 hour to allow initial parent-child bonding.

## Indications

- To prevent *N. gonorrhoeae* infection in all neonates

## Contraindications

- None known

## Preprocedure patient preparation

- If the patient and her support person are present for the procedure, explain that state law mandates Credé's treatment. Forewarn them that the neonate may cry and that the treatment may irritate his eyes. Reassure them that these are temporary effects.

## Equipment

Silver nitrate ampule or ophthalmic antibiotic ointment ◆ sterile needle or pin supplied by silver nitrate manufacturer (as needed) ◆ gloves

### Equipment preparation

■ Puncture one end of the wax silver nitrate ampule with the needle or pin. If you're administering ophthalmic antibiotic ointment (such as tetracycline or erythromycin), remove the cap from the ointment container. A single-dose ointment tube should be used to prevent contamination and spread of infection.

## Procedure

■ Explain the procedure to the parents, and address any questions or concerns they may have.
■ Wash your hands, and put on gloves.
■ To ensure comfort and effectiveness, shield the neonate's eyes from direct light, tilt his head slightly to the side of the intended treatment, and instill the medication. (See *How to instill medication for Credé's treatment.*)
■ Close and manipulate the eyelids to spread the medication over the eye.

## How to instill medication for Credé's treatment

Using your nondominant hand, gently raise the neonate's upper eyelid with your index finger and pull down the lower eyelid with your thumb. Using your dominant hand, apply the ophthalmic antibiotic ointment, such as tetracycline or erythromycin, in a line along the lower conjunctival sac (as shown). Repeat the procedure for the other eye.

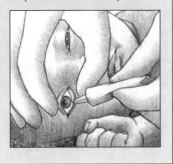

## Postprocedure patient teaching

■ If chemical conjunctivitis occurs or if the skin around the neonate's eyes discolors, reassure the patient that these temporary effects will subside within a few days.

## Complications

■ Chemical conjunctivitis may cause redness, swelling, and drainage, especially after silver nitrate instillation.

## Special considerations

■ Instill another drop if the silver nitrate solution touches only the eyelid or eyelid margins to ensure complete prophylaxis.

## Documentation

- If you perform Credé's treatment in the delivery room, record the treatment on the delivery room form.
- If you perform the treatment in the nursery, document it in your notes.

## EYE TRAUMA STABILIZATION

### CPT code
*No specific code has been assigned.*

## Overview

Eye trauma stabilization procedures are dependent on the type of injury, such as chemical burns and blunt and sharp trauma. Eye trauma is a major cause of monocular blindness, visual impairment, and disfiguring disability. There is little statistical data on the incidence, type, severity, and etiology of eye trauma. A 1993 study by the National Center for Health Statistics, Centers for Disease Control and Prevention, found that males sustained more ocular injuries in all diagnostic categories and were more likely to be injured by a foreign body during a fight, a sporting event, or a motor vehicle accident. The sports most commonly associated with ocular injuries were basketball (with another player coming in contact with the eye), racquetball, ice hockey, and squash. Ocular injuries in women are more often the result of assaults and falls. Severe injuries include chemical and thermal burns of the globe, lacerations and open wounds of the globe, avulsions and severe burns of the periorbital tissues and eyelids, and extensive orbital fractures. Penetrating injuries in the past had the worst prognosis until the advent of current microsurgical techniques. A patient presenting with ocular trauma commonly will have sustained other trauma, typically to the head and neck. In the event of potentially life-threatening trauma, evaluation and treatment of the eye are delayed until the patient is stabilized.

Chemical burns to the eye are most likely to occur in the occupational setting or as a result of accidents. (See *Chemical burns: Sources, presentation, and effects.*) Radiation injury of the eye commonly occurs secondary to prolonged exposure to bright sunlight or blinding snow, sun lamps, tanning booths, and welders' arcs.

## Indications

- To prevent further trauma to the eye while transporting or preparing for eye surgery
- To minimize duration of exposure to a chemical irritant
- To prevent or minimize risk of permanent visual loss or cosmetic disfigurement
- To alleviate ocular pain

# Chemical burns: Sources, presentation, and effects

| TYPE | SOURCE | PRESENTATION | EFFECTS |
|------|--------|--------------|---------|
| **ACIDS** | | | |
| Acetic acid | Vinegar and household cleaners | ■ Decreased visual acuity<br>■ Corneal erosion<br>■ Conjunctiva inflamed<br>■ Necrosis of cornea and conjunctiva | ■ Penetration limited<br>■ Damage immediate and limited to area of contact<br>■ Posterior of eye rarely injured<br>■ Delayed damage possible<br>■ Necrosis of cornea and conjunctiva; outcome related to concentration and duration of exposure |
| Hydrochloric acid | Household cleaners | | |
| Sodium hydrochlorite | Bleach | | |
| Sulfuric acid | Toilet cleaners and battery acid | | |
| Hydrofluoric acid | Etching and gasoline production | | |
| **ALKALI** | | | |
| Magnesium hydroxide | Fireworks | ■ Painless vision loss<br>■ Few symptoms initially<br>■ Conjunctival chemosis<br>■ Corneal erosion<br>■ Whitened or blanched appearance of cornea, sclera, or conjunctiva due to necrosis<br>■ Degree of opacification of cornea and ischemia of limbus indicative of the degree of damage and prognosis | ■ Exposure more serious than acid exposure<br>■ Damage proportionate to pH, concentration, and time elapsed before lavage is initiated<br>■ Can penetrate deeply and continue penetration for hours to days<br>■ Potential outcomes: blindness; glaucoma; chronic inflammation of iris and ciliary body (iridocyclitis) and globe, lens, and iris; scarring; lid deformity; cataract formation |
| Calcium hydroxide | Lime, plaster, mortar, and cement | | |
| Potassium hydroxide | Drain cleaners | | |
| Sodium hydroxide | Drain cleaners, lye, and automobile air bags | | |

## Contraindications

■ None known

## Preprocedure patient preparation

■ Obtain a detailed history about the trauma to the eye.

■ Inform the patient that further evaluation and education will be performed after the crisis is resolved.

## Equipment

Equipment will depend on the nature of the injury.

Eye lavage basin ◆ gloves ◆ sterile saline solution, lactated Ringer's solution, or sterile water ◆ Morgan or Medi-flow irrigation lens (optional) ◆ I.V. tubing ◆ standard Snellen chart or near-vision card ◆ large metal or plastic eye shield or paper or Styrofoam drinking cup ◆ 4″ × 4″ gauze bandage and tape ◆ ophthalmic anesthetic agent (such as pontocaine) and antibiotic (such as gentamicin) ◆ sterile pH strips ◆ eye patches

## Procedure

■ Explain the procedure to the patient, and address any questions or concerns he may have.

☑ **OBTAIN INFORMED CONSENT**

■ Wash your hands and put on gloves.

### Stabilization for eye trauma: Chemical burns

➤ **CLINICAL TIP**
*Irrigation of lens is contraindicated if a deep corneal injury, penetrating foreign body, orbital fracture, or rupture of the globe is suspected.*

■ Position the eye lavage basin close to the side of the patient's head.

■ Begin immediate eye lavage using an I.V. bag, tubing, and copious amount of sterile normal saline, lactated Ringer's solution, or sterile water, directing flow from inner to outer canthus and under the lid.

■ Identify the chemical causing the injury. If the chemical is unknown, use a pH strip to determine presence of acid or alkali.

■ If the chemical is a known alkali, irrigate continuously without stopping to check the pH until the patient reaches the emergency department. Otherwise, irrigate continuously for 15 to 20 minutes and then check the pH. Place a pH strip in the conjunctival sac of the lower lid. Don't touch the cornea. Continue lavage until the pH reaches at least 7. (The normal pH of tears is 7.3 to 7.7.)

■ Instill ophthalmic anesthetic and place the Morgan or Medi-flow lens to facilitate irrigation and examination, if necessary.

■ If the chemical is hydrofluoric acid, mix five 10-ml vials of 10% calcium gluconate in 1,000 ml of sterile water and flush the eye continuously until the patient reaches the emergency department.

■ Assess visual acuity with the Snellen chart or near-vision card.

### Stabilization for eye trauma: Blunt or sharp injury

■ First, rule out life-threatening trauma.

■ Perform a neurologic examination to rule out possible accompanying head or cervical spine injuries. Stabilize these injuries first.

## Protective eye covering

Provide a protective cover for the eye during transport to the emergency department. To do this, make padding by wrapping gauze loosely around your hand several times to form a "donut" with a central opening diameter large enough to avoid any pressure on the globe. Secure with an over and under wrap of gauze to form a firm edge.

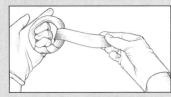

Apply the "donut" over the orbit of the eye, avoiding contact with the globe.

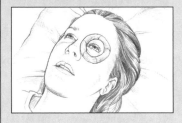

Lay an eye shield (or Styrofoam cup) on top of the donut.

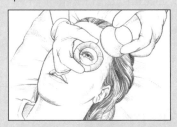

Apply an eye patch to the unaffected eye to prevent consensual movement of and further trauma to the affected eye. Secure the eye patch and the eye shield by wrapping 4" gauze around the head several times.

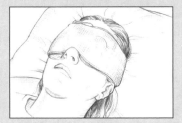

- In a conscious, stable patient, first test visual acuity with the Snellen chart or near-vision card.
- Perform an eye examination, taking special note of critical signs and symptoms. If rupture of the globe is suspected or present, defer the rest of the examination.
- If retinal tears or detachment is suspected, place the patient in the supine position, if possible.
- Don't attempt to remove any penetrating foreign body.
- If the eyelid is lacerated and the globe is injured, apply cool saline compress using 4" × 4" gauze, tape, and a protective shield.
- Provide protective cover for the eye during transport to the emergency department. (See *Protective eye covering*.)
- If the eyelid is avulsed, locate lid fragments and place on sterile saline gauze and in a sterile container. Transport the container with the patient.

## Postprocedure patient teaching

- Generally, patient instruction is dependent on the type of trauma.
- Instruct the patient to not remove the eye patch.
- Tell the patient to keep his head still during transport.
- Make sure the patient doesn't bend or lift his head.

## Complications

 COLLABORATION

*Eye trauma necrosis, blindness, glaucoma, adhesions, cataracts, deformity, and infection can result but are minimized by emergency evaluation and treatment by an ophthalmologist.*

## Special considerations

- If life-threatening trauma, head injury, or cervical spine injury is present, stabilization of these injuries takes priority. In the event of potential chemical injury, lavage of the eye takes priority, even before the nature of the chemical is determined.
- Don't attempt to open the eyelid of a severely traumatized eye if the patient is uncooperative.
- Fluorescein staining is contraindicated if injury to the globe is suspected.
- Pain and tearing from a corneal abrasion or chemical exposure may result in an inaccurate visual acuity assessment. If the patient is unable to read the eye chart, assess for his ability to see finger movement or to discriminate light.

- Avoid pressure on the globe in case of blunt or penetrating injury to reduce the risk of globe rupture and loss of vision.
- With corneal lacerations, less interference is better. Assess the injury, arrange for immediate referral and evaluation, and then shield the eye gently for protection while the patient is in transit.
- Immediate irrigation is the single best initial treatment for chemical burns to the eye and reduces the ultimate physical damage to the eye.
- Most acid burns with mild to moderate stromal haze will get better with time. Alkaline burns may initially look far better than they will appear at day 2 or 3. Therefore, it's important to refer the patient as soon as the eye is irrigated.
- Don't deny that the current level of visual acuity may be permanent or make promises. Although vision may improve significantly, it's best to foster conservative expectations because the outcome is unknown.

## Documentation

- Document patient history along with a detailed description of the event, including the object causing trauma, the direction and force of the blow, and the type of foreign body or chemical involved.
- Note whether the patient was using protective gear or safety goggles at the time of the accident.
- Record pretrauma visual acuity and function; other visual symptoms, such as flashes, floaters,

pain, and diplopia; and previous ocular disease.

■ List current medications, allergies (especially to local anesthetics or PABA sunscreen lotions), and the use of over-the-counter preparations.

■ Document current visual acuity, symptoms, and physical findings.

■ Note pupil size and reactivity, extraocular movements, symmetry of facial and orbital bones, tissue integrity (lids and globe), color, swelling, presence of a foreign body, and neurologic examination findings if head injury also occurred.

■ Record any informed consents obtained. Document the patient's level of understanding.

■ List treatments or stabilization procedures initiated, and document patient response to treatments.

■ Note patient disposition (referrals or transport to the emergency department) and status when discharged from immediate care.

## *E*YEBROW *LACERATION REPAIR*

### *CPT codes*
12011 *Simple repair of superficial wounds of face, ears, eyelids, nose, lips, and/or mucous membranes: 2.5 cm or less*
12013 to 12018 *Wounds 2.5 cm or greater*

## Overview

Eyebrow lacerations may be caused by facial trauma, typically from sports or contact activities. Because of the strong bone structure beneath the eyebrow, these lacerations are rare, but when occurring, they commonly require medical attention and repair.

Depending on the wound, three options are available for repairing eyebrow lacerations: application of Steri-Strips, a topical skin adhesive, or sutures.

## Indications
### *Application of Steri-Strips or a topical skin adhesive*
■ To repair eyebrow lacerations that are in relatively nonmoving areas with minimal tension and good laceration edge approximation

### *Application of sutures*
■ To repair eyebrow lacerations that are under tension or have poor laceration edges

## Contraindications
### ABSOLUTE
■ Underlying facial bone fracture

## Preprocedure patient preparation

■ Determine the history of the injury, associated symptoms, and interventions the patient has used. Assess any associated injuries such as cervical trauma.

■ Assess the patient's tetanus immunization status, and provide tetanus prophylaxis as warranted.

## Equipment

Sterile gloves ◆ antiseptic solution such as povidone-iodine ◆ sterile normal saline solution ◆ 60-ml syringe with a large-bore (18G to 20G) cannula tip ◆ sterile 4″ × 4″ gauze pads ◆ #15 scalpel blade

### Steri-Strips
Steri-Strips ◆ forceps ◆ tincture of benzoin (optional)

### Topical skin adhesive
Topical skin adhesive (such as 2-octyl cyanoacrylate [Dermabond])

### Sutures
Equipment for administering local anesthesia ◆ equipment for suturing, including 5.0 nonabsorbable suture material ◆ topical antibiotic ointment

## Procedure

■ Explain the procedure to the patient, and address any questions or concerns he may have.

☑ **OBTAIN INFORMED CONSENT**

■ Wash your hands and put on gloves.
■ Irrigate the laceration with normal saline solution and the 60-ml syringe, being careful not to get the saline into the patient's eyes.
■ If necessary, remove dead tissue with the #15 scalpel blade, leaving clean edges on the laceration.
■ Cleanse the area around the laceration with povidone-iodine and

gauze. Avoid getting the povidone-iodine directly into the wound — it may be toxic to the tissue. Allow it to dry.

### Steri-Strips
■ To apply Steri-Strips, no anesthesia is needed. Grasp one end of the Steri-Strip with the forceps, and place it on one side of the laceration. Using your other hand to approximate the laceration edges, gently pull the Steri-Strip across and place on the other side of the laceration for a good fit.

◢ **CLINICAL TIP**
*For better adhesion, apply tincture of benzoin along either side of the laceration and allow it to become tacky before placing Steri-Strips.*

■ Continue to apply Steri-Strips until adequate wound closure is achieved.
■ Leave the site open to air.

### Topical skin adhesive
■ To apply the topical skin adhesive, no anesthesia is required. Approximate the laceration edges with one hand while painting the laceration with the topical skin adhesive (according to manufacturer instruction) with the other. Apply just enough adhesive to hold the edges of the laceration together.
■ The adhesive usually takes less than 1 minute to cure, at which point it becomes a strong and flexible bond.
■ Leave the site open to air.

### Sutures
■ Administer local anesthesia. (See

"Anesthesia: Topical, local, and digital nerve block," page 20.)

■ Suture the laceration using simple interrupted suturing and 5.0 nonabsorbable suture material. (See "Suturing of simple lacerations," page 459.) Be sure to approximate the edges of the laceration precisely for the best cosmetic result.

▶ CLINICAL TIP
*If the eyebrow hairs obliterate the view of the laceration, apply a small amount of topical antibiotic ointment to the brow and part the hairs as necessary. Never shave the eyebrow; the hairs may grow back irregularly or not at all.*

■ Apply a topical antibiotic ointment.

## Postprocedure patient teaching

■ Teach the patient signs of infection, such as redness, swelling, yellow or green drainage, foul odor, or increase in temperature, and have him notify your office if he experiences any of these.

■ Inform the patient with Steri-Strips or topical skin adhesive that the laceration should heal in approximately 7 to 10 days.

■ If the Steri-Strips become loose or dislodged, ask the patient to return to the office to have them replaced. Have the patient return to the office in 7 days for Steri-Strip removal.

■ The topical skin adhesive requires no removal; it disappears naturally. The patient may get the area wet (such as from a shower); however, the area should not be soaked. Have the patient return to the office in 7 days for reevaluation.

■ The patient requiring sutures should return to the office in 3 to 5 days for suture removal. If necessary, Steri-Strips or paper tape may be applied to the healing laceration to enhance approximation of the edges.

## Complications

■ Infection may occur with eyebrow laceration, requiring antibiotic therapy.

✦ COLLABORATION
*Scarring or cosmetically undesirable results may require consultation with a plastic surgeon.*

## Special considerations

■ Choose the best wound closure method for the type of laceration your patient presents with. For lacerations with minimal tension and good wound approximation or for patients who are afraid of needles, Steri-Strips or a topical skin adhesive are best. However, wounds that are under tension or have poor edge approximation will necessitate suturing.

■ Great care should be taken to precisely approximate the laceration edges for the best cosmetic results despite the method used for closure.

## Documentation

■ Document pre- and postprocedure visual function.

■ Thoroughly document the location, size, depth, and mechanism of the eyebrow laceration, using illustrations as necessary.

■ Document the method of wound closure used and a description of the procedure.

■ If suturing was required, record the type of analgesia and anesthetic used, the type and number of sutures placed, and the patient's tolerance of the procedure.

■ Document the patient's scheduled follow-up visit and discharge instructions given.

# Eyelid eversion

**CPT code**
*No specific code has been assigned. Eyelid eversion is usually performed with another procedure.*

## Overview

Eyelid eversion is a technique for manipulating the upper eyelid to allow inspection of the lid and conjunctiva for a foreign body, lesions, or swelling. Careful inspection of the eye must be performed when the patient complains of a foreign body sensation, excessive tearing, blurred vision, light sensitivity, or a history of a known foreign body hitting the eye. The foreign body sensation originates from the superficial layer of the cornea and, if left untreated, can lead to a variety of visual disturbances.

## Indications
■ To remove a known foreign body
■ To treat eye trauma
■ To evaluate unexplained eye irritation

## Contraindications
■ Uncooperative or combative patient
■ Penetrating eye injury
■ Eyelid laceration

## Preprocedure patient preparation
■ Inform the patient that he may experience some discomfort during the procedure.

## Equipment
Cotton-tipped applicator ◆ gloves ◆ magnification (such as a slit lamp [optional])

## Procedure
■ Explain the procedure to the patient, and address any questions or concerns he may have.
■ Ask the patient to lie supine to ensure comfort and to facilitate the examination.
■ Wash your hands, and put on gloves.
■ Instruct the patient to look downward.
■ Tell him to try to relax the eye.
■ Without putting pressure on the eyeball, place a cotton-tipped ap-

plicator along the upper edge of the eyelid. (See *Eyelid eversion.*)

■ Examine the under surface of the lid under magnification such as a slit lamp, if necessary. If a foreign body is identified, gently remove it with a dampened cotton-tipped applicator.

■ To release the eyelid, have the patient look up while gently pulling the eyelashes outward.

## Postprocedure patient teaching

■ Tell the patient that he'll experience minimal discomfort from the procedure. Follow-up may be required.

## Complications

■ Trauma (minimized by gentle handling)
■ Infection (minimized by using standard precautions)

## Special considerations

■ None

## Documentation

■ Document eyelid eversion as part of the eye examination.
■ Record findings on examination and how the foreign body was removed, if applicable.
■ Note any and all instructions, medications prescribed, and expected follow-up.

### Eyelid eversion

To evert the eyelid, place a cotton-tipped applicator along the upper edge of the eyelid approximately ¹⁄₃″ (0.8 cm) above the lid margin. Grasp the upper eyelashes with the thumb and forefinger.

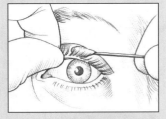

Pull the upper lid down and forward. Press gently downward on the eyelid (but not pressing against the globe) with the cotton-tipped applicator while lifting the eyelashes up. This will evert the eyelid for inspection. Stabilize the everted eyelid with the thumb against the superior orbital ridge.

To release the eyelid, have the patient look up while gently pulling eyelashes outward.

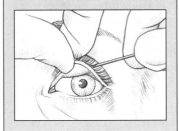

## FEEDING TUBE INSERTION AND REMOVAL

**CPT code**
91100  *Intestinal feeding tube passage, positioning, and monitoring*

### Overview

A feeding tube is inserted nasally or orally into the stomach or duodenum to give nourishment to patients refusing or unable to eat. The feeding tube also permits supplemental feedings in patients with high nutritional requirements, such as those who are unconscious or have extensive burns. The preferred route is nasal, but the oral route may be used for patients with such conditions as deviated septums or head or nose injuries.

Feeding tubes differ somewhat from standard nasogastric tubes. Made of silicone, rubber, or polyurethane, feeding tubes have smaller diameters and greater flexibility. This reduces oropharyngeal irritation, necrosis from pressure on the tracheoesophageal wall, distal esophageal irritation, and discomfort from swallowing. To facilitate passage, some feeding tubes are weighted with tungsten while others need a guide wire to keep them from curling in the back of the throat. These small-bore tubes usually have radiopaque markings and a water-activated coating, which provides a lubricated surface.

### Indications

- To permit feeding of patients at high risk for aspiration with gastric feeding or who otherwise can't tolerate it
- To permit short-term nutrient replacement

### Contraindications

**ABSOLUTE**
- Absence of bowel sounds
- Possible intestinal obstruction
- Intractable vomiting
- Upper GI bleeding

## Preprocedure patient preparation

■ Explain to the patient and significant others why the patient needs a feeding tube and how long it's expected to be in place. Explain that the tube must move into the intestine by gravity. Therefore, small amounts of tubing will be advanced periodically for about 6 to 12 hours if the patient is ambulatory, or 12 to 24 hours if the patient is on bed rest. An X-ray will then be taken to verify the location of the tube.

■ Show the patient the feeding tube to promote cooperation through helping him better understand the procedure.

## Equipment

### For insertion

Feeding tube (#6 to #18 French, with or without guide wire) ◆ linen-saver pad ◆ gloves ◆ hypoallergenic tape ◆ water-soluble lubricant ◆ skin preparation (such as tincture of benzoin) ◆ facial tissues ◆ penlight ◆ small cup of water with a straw or ice chips ◆ emesis basin ◆ 60-ml syringe ◆ stethoscope

### For removal

Linen-saver pad ◆ tube clamp

### Equipment preparation

■ Have the proper size of tube available (usually the smallest-bore tube that will allow free passage of the liquid feeding formula). Read the instructions on the tubing package carefully because tube characteristics vary according to the manufacturer. (For example, some tubes have marks at the appropriate lengths for gastric, duodenal, and jejunal insertion.)

■ Examine the tube to make sure it's free from defects, such as cracks or rough or sharp edges.

■ Next, place the tube in water and run water through it. This checks for patency, activates the coating, and facilitates removal of the guide.

## Procedure

■ Explain the procedure to the patient, and address any questions or concerns he may have.

■ Provide privacy.

■ Wash your hands, and put on gloves.

■ Assist the patient into semi-Fowler's or high Fowler's position. Place a linen-saver pad across the patient's chest to protect him from spills.

■ Determine the tube length needed to reach the stomach by first extending the distal end of the tube from the tip of the patient's nose to his earlobe. Coil this portion of the tube around your fingers so the end stays curved until you insert it. Then extend the uncoiled portion from the earlobe to the xiphoid process. Use a small piece of hypoallergenic tape to mark the total length of the two portions.

### Inserting the tube nasally

■ Using the penlight, assess nasal patency. Inspect nasal passages for a deviated septum, polyps, or other obstructions. Occlude one nostril, then the other, to determine which has the better airflow. Assess the patient's history of nasal injury or surgery.

■ Lubricate the curved tip of the tube (and the feeding tube guide, if appropriate) with a small amount of water-soluble lubricant to ease insertion and prevent tissue injury.

■ Ask the patient to hold the emesis basin and facial tissues in case he needs them.

■ Insert the curved, lubricated tip into the more patent nostril, and direct it along the nasal passage toward the ear on the same side. When it passes the nasopharyngeal junction, turn the tube 180 degrees to aim it downward into the esophagus. Instruct the patient to lower his chin to his chest to close the trachea. Then give him a small cup of water with a straw or ice chips. Direct him to sip the water or suck on the ice and swallow frequently. This will ease the tube's passage. Advance the tube as he swallows.

### Inserting the tube orally

■ Have the patient lower his chin to close his trachea, and ask him to open his mouth.

■ Place the tip of the tube at the back of the patient's tongue, give water, and instruct the patient to swallow. Remind him to avoid clamping his teeth down on the tube. Advance the tube as he swallows.

### Positioning the tube

■ Keep passing the tube until the tape marking the appropriate length reaches the patient's nostril (for nasal insertion) or lips (for oral insertion).

■ To check tube placement, attach the syringe filled with 10 cc of air to the end of the tube. Gently inject the air into the tube as you auscultate the patient's abdomen with the stethoscope about 3″ (7.5 cm) below the sternum. Listen for a whooshing sound, which signals that the tube has reached its target in the stomach. You may also pull back on the syringe to remove the air and to verify stomach contents. If the tube remains coiled in the esophagus, you'll feel resistance when you inject the air or the patient may belch. If you can't hear verification of placement, the tube may be in the esophagus. You'll need to advance the tube or reinsert it before proceeding.

■ After confirming proper tube placement, remove the tape marking the tube length.

■ Tape the tube to the patient's nose.

■ Verify tube placement in the stomach by X-ray as needed; then remove the guide wire.

■ To advance the tube to the duodenum, especially a tungsten-weighted tube, position the patient on his right side. This lets gravity assist tube passage through the pylorus. Write orders for the tube to be advanced 2″ to 3″ (5 to 7.5 cm) hourly for a total of about 8″ (20 cm) until X-ray studies confirm duodenal placement. (An X-ray must confirm placement before feeding begins because duodenal feeding can cause nausea and vomiting if accidentally delivered to the stomach.)

■ Apply a skin preparation to the patient's cheek before securing the tube with tape. This helps the tube adhere to the skin and also prevents irritation.

■ Tape the tube securely to the patient's cheek to avoid excessive pressure on his nostrils, as needed.

### Removing the tube

■ Protect the patient's chest with a linen-saver pad.

■ Flush the tube with air, clamp or pinch it to prevent fluid aspiration during withdrawal, and withdraw it gently but quickly. Place it on the linen-saver pad.

■ Promptly wrap the used tube in the pad and discard it.

■ Assist the patient to cleanse his nostril or rinse his mouth as needed.

## Postprocedure patient teaching

■ Advise the patient that there will be some discomfort with the tube. (Minimize such discomfort by secondarily fastening the tube after it's positioned in the duodenum to keep it from pulling as the patient moves. To do this, place tape around the tube; then place a safety pin through the tape and pin this to the patient's clothing. Emphasize that he'll need to unpin the tube before changing clothing.)

■ Detail the goals that the patient must achieve before the tube can be removed (such as a positive gag reflex or cessation of food pocketing as he eats), and outline how he can actively participate in achieving them, as indicated.

■ Teach the patient and caregivers how to use and care for a feeding tube if the patient will go home with the feeding tube in place. Teach them how to obtain equipment, insert and remove the tube, prepare and store feeding formula, and solve problems with tube position and patency.

■ Instruct the patient or caregiver to contact you immediately if the tube moves or if the patient experiences abdominal pain or cramping or difficulty breathing.

■ Teach the patient or caregiver to retape the tube at least daily and as needed. Alternate taping the tube toward the inner and outer side of the nose to avoid constant pressure on the same nasal area. Inspect the skin for redness and breakdown.

■ Teach the patient or caregiver how to perform nasal hygiene using cotton-tipped applicators and water-soluble lubricant to remove crusted secretions.

■ Advise the patient or caregiver to brush the patient's teeth, gums, and tongue with mouthwash or a mild saltwater solution at least twice daily.

## Complications

■ Pulmonary aspiration is a life-threatening complication. Reduce the risk of pulmonary aspiration by ensuring tube placement well below the pyloric sphincter.

■ Skin erosion at the nostril, sinusitis, esophagitis, esophagotracheal fistula, gastric ulceration, and pulmonary and oral infection are associated with prolonged intubation.

## Special considerations

■ Write orders to flush the feeding tube every 8 hours with up to 60 ml of normal saline solution or water to maintain patency.
■ If the patient can't swallow the feeding tube, use a guide wire to aid insertion.
■ Always compare the potential risks and benefits for the patient. For instance, supplementing nutrition through tube feeding may not improve or prolong the life of a patient with end-stage dementia, but it's likely to cause significant discomfort and distress.
■ Precise feeding-tube placement is especially important because small-bore feeding tubes may slide into the trachea without causing immediate signs or symptoms of respiratory distress, such as coughing, choking, gasping, or cyanosis. However, the patient will usually cough if the tube enters the larynx. To be sure that the tube clears the larynx, ask the patient to speak. If he can't, the tube is in the larynx. Withdraw the tube at once and reinsert.
■ If the feeding tube needs to be repositioned after the guide wire has been removed, fluoroscopic guidance is required.
■ If your patient will use a feeding tube at home, write for home care services. Include the anticipated start and end date of services, the number and duration of skilled nursing visits, and as-needed visits

for problems related to the tube. Note the amount and frequency of feedings, any durable medical equipment and supplies needed, frequency of such laboratory studies as electrolytes and creatinine, and daily or weekly weighing of the patient.

## Documentation

■ Record the date, time, tube type and size, insertion site, area of placement, and confirmation of proper placement.
■ For tube removal, record the date and time and the patient's tolerance of the procedure.

# *F*ETAL HEART RATE MONITORING

***CPT code***
*No specific code has been assigned.*

## Overview

A major clue to fetal well-being during gestation and labor, the fetal heart rate (FHR) may be assessed by auscultating with a fetoscope or a Doppler ultrasound stethoscope placed on the maternal abdomen. This ultrasound device emits low-energy, high-frequency sound waves that rebound from the fetal heart to a transducer, which transmits the impulses to a monitor strip for recording.

Because FHR normally ranges from 110 to 160 beats/minute, auscultation yields only an average rate at best. However, because auscultation can detect gross (but often late) fetal distress signs (tachycardia and bradycardia), the technique remains useful in an uncomplicated, low-risk pregnancy. In a high-risk pregnancy, indirect external or direct internal electronic fetal monitoring gives more accurate information on fetal status. However, internal fetal monitoring may be performed only if the membranes are ruptured.

## Indications

■ To screen for fetal well-being or fetal distress

## Contraindications

■ None known

## Preprocedure patient preparation

■ If using a Doppler stethoscope, tell the patient that the lubricant will feel cold and wet.
■ Advise the patient that you may reposition the listening instrument frequently to hear the loudest fetal heart tones. (See *Finding fetal heart tones*.)

## Equipment

Fetoscope or Doppler stethoscope ◆ water-soluble lubricant (for ultrasound instrument) ◆ watch with second hand ◆ drape

## Procedure

■ Explain the procedure to the pa-

### Finding fetal heart tones

When explaining the procedure to the patient, advise her that you may reposition the listening instrument frequently to hear the loudest fetal heart tones. If you're unable to detect the fetus with the fetoscope, use a Doppler stethoscope to locate the heartbeat first and then place the fetoscope in the same spot. It's a good idea to develop a systematic approach to locating fetal heart tones so that you don't miss or unnecessarily repeat areas.

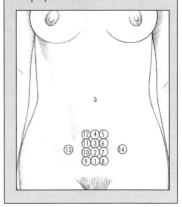

tient, and address any questions or concerns she may have.
■ Wash your hands, and provide privacy.
■ Assist the patient to a supine position, and drape her appropriately to minimize exposure. If you're using a Doppler stethoscope, apply the water-soluble lubricant to the patient's abdomen. (See *Instruments for hearing fetal heart tones,* page 208.) This gel or paste creates an airtight seal between the skin and the instrument and promotes optimal ultrasound wave conduction and reception.

## Instruments for hearing fetal heart tones

The fetoscope and the Doppler stethoscope are basic instruments for auscultating fetal heart tones and assessing fetal heart rate.

### FETOSCOPE
This instrument can be used to help determine gestational age. If you can hear fetal heart tones (FHTs) with a fetoscope between 18 and 20 weeks' gestation, it can either confirm or lend support to the estimated due date. The FHTs are best heard when the tubing of the fetoscope is no longer than 10″ (25.4 cm). The fetoscope must be placed with the metal against your forehead. Metal against bone facilitates the conduction of sound. Use of a fetoscope later in pregnancy may not require the use of your forehead, because the uterus is thinner. When listening for early FHTs with the fetoscope, you may need to turn off air conditioners and have the patient empty her bladder.

### DOPPLER STETHOSCOPE
This instrument can detect fetal heartbeats as early as the 10th gestational week. Useful throughout labor, the Doppler stethoscope has greater sensitivity than the fetoscope.

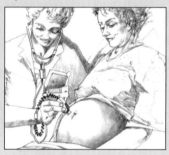

### *Calculating FHR during gestation*

■ To assess FHR in a fetus age 20 weeks or older, place the earpieces in your ears and position the bell of the fetoscope or Doppler stethoscope on the abdominal midline above the pubic hairline of the patient.

■ After 20 weeks' gestation, when you can palpate fetal position, use Leopold's maneuvers to locate the back of the fetal thorax. Then position the listening instrument over the fetal back. (See *Performing Leopold's maneuvers,* pages 210 and 211.) Because the presentation and position of the fetus may change, most health care providers don't perform Leopold's maneuvers until 32 to 34 weeks' gestation.

■ Using a Doppler stethoscope, place the earpieces in your ears and press the bell gently on the patient's abdomen. Start listening at the midline, midway between the umbilicus and the symphysis pubis. If using a fetoscope, place the earpieces in your ears with the fetoscope positioned centrally on your forehead. Gently press the bell about ½″ (1.3 cm) into the patient's abdomen. Remove your hands from the fetoscope to avoid extraneous noise.

■ Move the bell of either instrument slightly from side to side, as necessary, to locate the loudest heart tones. After locating these tones, palpate the maternal pulse.

■ While monitoring the maternal pulse rate (to avoid confusing maternal heart tones with fetal heart tones), count the fetal heartbeats for at least 15 seconds. If the maternal radial pulse and FHR are the same, try to locate the fetal thorax by using Leopold's maneuvers; then reassess FHR. Usually, the fetal heart beats faster than the maternal heart does. Record FHR.

***Counting FHR during labor***

■ Position the fetoscope or Doppler stethoscope on the abdomen — midway between the umbilicus and symphysis pubis for cephalic presentation or at the umbilicus or above for breech presentation. Locate the loudest heartbeats and simultaneously palpate the maternal pulse to ensure that you're monitoring fetal rather than maternal pulse.

■ Monitor maternal pulse rate and count fetal heartbeats for 60 seconds during the relaxation period between contractions to determine baseline FHR. In a low-risk labor, assess FHR every 60 minutes during the latent phase, every 30 minutes during the active phase, and every 15 minutes during the second stage of labor. In a high-risk labor, assess FHR every 30 minutes during the latent phase, every 15 minutes during the active phase, and every 5 minutes during the second stage of labor.

■ Auscultate FHR during a contraction and for 30 seconds after the contraction to identify fetal response to the contraction.

■ Notify the collaborating physician immediately if you observe marked changes in FHR from baseline values (especially during or immediately after a contraction, when signs of fetal distress typically occur). If fetal distress develops, begin indirect or direct electronic fetal monitoring.

■ Repeat the procedure as indicated.

■ Also auscultate before administration of medications, before ambulation, and before artificial rupture of membranes.

■ Auscultate after rupture of membranes, after any changes in the characteristics of the contractions, after vaginal examinations, and after administration of medications.

## Postprocedure patient teaching

■ Tell the patient that the fetal heart rate will be assessed periodically to evaluate the status of the fetus.

## Complications

■ None known

## Special considerations

■ Allow the patient and her support person to listen to the fetal heart if they wish. This helps to make the fetus a greater reality for them. Record their participation.

■ Auscultating FHR is a noninva-

## Performing Leopold's maneuvers

You can determine fetal position, presentation, and attitude by performing Leopold's maneuvers. Ask the patient to empty her bladder, assist her to a supine position, and expose her abdomen. Then perform the four maneuvers in order.

### FIRST MANEUVER
Warm your hands and face the patient. Place your hands on the patient's abdomen to determine fetal position in the uterine fundus. Curl your fingers around the fundus. With the fetus in vertex position, the buttocks feel irregularly shaped and firm. With the fetus in breech position, the head feels hard, round, and movable.

### SECOND MANEUVER
Move your hands down the sides of the abdomen, and apply gentle pressure. If the fetus lies in vertex position, you'll feel a smooth, hard surface on one side — the fetal back. Opposite, you'll feel lumps and knobs — the knees, hands, feet, and elbows. If the fetus lies in breech position, you may not feel the back at all.

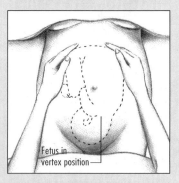

Fetus in vertex position

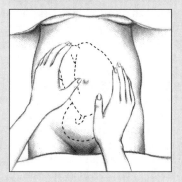

sive method that screens for fetal distress while leaving the patient mobile and unencumbered. However, this method may not be adequate and an external or internal monitor may become necessary as labor progresses.

■ If you're auscultating FHR with a Doppler stethoscope, be aware that obesity and hydramnios can interfere with sound-wave transmission, making accurate results more difficult to obtain. For continuous FHR monitoring, apply the ultrasound transducer (also called a tocotransducer) to the pa-

tient's abdomen. The monitor will provide a printed record of FHR.
■ The tocotransducer may also be applied to monitor the contractile pattern.

## Documentation
■ Record both FHR and maternal pulse rate on the flowchart.
■ Document each auscultation and indications for monitoring.
■ Note the patient's and her support person's participation in counting FHR during labor.

## THIRD MANEUVER

Spread apart the thumb and fingers of one hand. Place them just above the patient's symphysis pubis. Bring your fingers together. If the fetus lies in vertex position and hasn't descended, you'll feel the head. If the fetus lies in vertex position and has descended, you'll feel a less distinct mass.

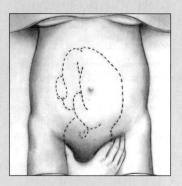

## FOURTH MANEUVER

Use this maneuver in late pregnancy. The purpose of the fourth maneuver is to determine flexion or extension of the fetal head and neck. Place your hands on both sides of the lower abdomen. Apply gentle pressure with your fingers as you slide your hands downward, toward the symphysis pubis. If the head presents, one hand's descent will be stopped by the cephalic prominence. The other hand will be unobstructed.

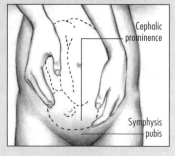

# *F*ISHHOOK REMOVAL

## CPT codes

10120 *Removal of subcutaneous foreign body, simple*
10121 *Incisional removal of foreign body, complex*
20520 *Incision and removal of foreign body in muscle, simple*

## Overview

Most fishhook injuries are minor and can be treated at the scene or in a facility. However, all fishhook injuries require an evaluation of the location, type of hook, and surrounding tissues before attempting removal. (See *Types of fishhooks,* page 212.) There are four basic techniques for fishhook removal: the "retrograde" and the "string and yank" techniques for barbless and superficial injuries; the "needle cover" technique for large, superficially imbedded hooks; and the "advance and cut" technique, which leads to the best results, for all multiple-barbed

## Types of fishhooks

Although there are many types of fishhooks available, most have one or more barbs, as shown below.

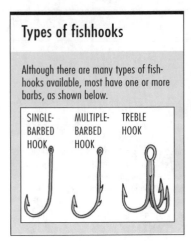

SINGLE-BARBED HOOK

MULTIPLE-BARBED HOOK

TREBLE HOOK

hooks and deeply imbedded hooks.

## Indications

■ To remove a fishhook embedded in the subcutaneous tissue

## Contraindications

**ABSOLUTE**

■ Fishhooks that have penetrated the orbit or whose location are such that attempting removal may result in eye injury (refer these patients immediately to an ophthalmologist)

## Preprocedure patient preparation

■ Determine the type of fishhook involved in the injury.
■ Assess the neurologic and vascular status proximal and distal to the site of the injury.
■ Assess the depth of the wound and which method of extraction

will be used. (At times, more than one method may be attempted before extraction is successful; prepare your equipment for the worst-case scenario.)
■ If there's more than one hook, as with a treble hook, the other hooks should be covered or removed with a wire cutter to prevent further injury to the patient and the health care provider.
■ If a lure is attached to the hook, remove the lure with a wire cutter.
■ Determine the amount and method of anesthesia needed.

## Equipment

Normal saline solution ◆ larger syringe, such as a 20- to 60-ml syringe ◆ antiseptic solution, such as povidone-iodine or hexachlorophene ◆ sterile 4″ × 4″ gauze pads and tape ◆ gloves and protective eyewear ◆ topical antibiotic ointment ◆ equipment to provide local anesthesia or digital nerve block ◆ 2′ (0.6-m) length of fishing line or size 0 silk suture or thread (for the "string-yank" technique) ◆ 18 G or larger needle (for the "needle cover" technique) ◆ hemostat and wire cutter (for the "advance and cut" technique)

## Procedure

■ Explain the procedure to the patient, and address any questions or concerns he may have.
■ Wash your hands, and put on gloves and protective eyewear.
■ Irrigate the wound with normal saline using a 20- to 60-ml syringe without a needle.

- Cleanse the wound using gauze pads and antiseptic solution.

### Retrograde technique

- This technique generally requires no local anesthetic.
- Apply slight downward pressure to the shaft of the hook. This maneuver will disengage the barb from the skin.
- Gently back the hook out along the path it entered.
- If any resistance occurs, consider an alternative method.
- Explore the wound for dirt and foreign material (such as bait), and irrigate with saline
- Apply a topical antibiotic ointment and a simple dressing with gauze and tape.
- If the patient hasn't had a tetanus booster in the past 5 years, give tetanus toxoid.

### String-yank technique

- This technique generally requires no local anesthetic.
- Stabilize the involved skin against a flat surface, such as a table or countertop.
- Loop a string, such as 2′ (0.6 m) of fishing line or size 0 silk suture or thread, around the midpoint of the bend of the hook.
- Secure the free end by wrapping it once around your index finger and grasping it between the thumb and index finger.
- Depress the shank of the hook against the skin and maintain pressure, ensuring that the shaft remains parallel to the skin.
- With the string parallel to the shaft and continuous downward pressure applied to the shaft with

the opposing hand, give a quick firm yank on the string.

- Explore the wound for dirt and foreign material (such as bait), and irrigate with saline.
- Apply a topical antibiotic ointment and a simple dressing with gauze and tape.
- If the patient hasn't had a tetanus booster in the past 5 years, give tetanus toxoid.

### Needle cover technique

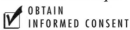 **OBTAIN INFORMED CONSENT**

- Administer a local anesthetic. (See "Anesthesia: Topical, local, and digital nerve block," page 20.)
- Introduce an 18G needle (or larger depending upon the size of the hook) along the entrance wound, parallel to the shank of the hook. The bevel must be pointed toward the inside curve of the hook, allowing the lumen to engage the barb.
- Advance the needle until you reach the barb; then pull back on the hook to engage the barb into the lumen of the needle.
- The hook and needle are then removed together.
- Explore the wound for dirt and foreign material (such as bait), and irrigate with saline.
- Apply a topical antibiotic ointment and a simple dressing of gauze and tape.
- If the patient hasn't had a tetanus booster in the past 5 years, give tetanus toxoid.

### *Advance and cut technique*

> ◤ CLINICAL TIP
> *Although this method does create additional trauma, it's almost always successful and is the preferred method for removing multibarbed or deeply embedded fishhooks.*

☑ OBTAIN
INFORMED CONSENT

■ Administer a local anesthetic over the point of the hook or, if necessary, administer a digital nerve block. (See "Anesthesia: Topical, local, and digital nerve block," page 20.)

■ For a single-barbed hook, use a hemostat to grasp the shaft of the hook and advance the point upward, using a rotating motion of the wrist.

■ Pass the hook up and through the skin until the barb is exposed.

■ Cut off the barb using a wire cutter; then back the hook out through the original entrance wound.

■ For multibarbed hooks, use the same technique of advancing the needle forward, but when the barbs are exposed remove the eye of the hook, grasp the hook at the barbed end, and pull it through the exit wound you just created.

■ Explore the wound for dirt and foreign material (such as bait), and irrigate with saline.

■ Apply a topical antibiotic ointment and a simple dressing of gauze and tape.

■ If the patient hasn't had a tetanus booster in the past 5 years, give tetanus toxoid.

## Postprocedure patient teaching

■ Inform the patient that he should be seen for follow-up in 2 to 3 days to ensure proper healing and to be assessed for infection.

■ Advise the patient on appropriate pain medications as necessary.

■ Instruct the patient that he should keep the wound elevated as much as possible. The wound dressing should be changed at least twice daily and a moist healing environment ensured.

## Complications

■ Damage to nerves, blood vessels, and tendons may occur and require further evaluation and management.

■ Infection may occur and require topical or systemic antibiotic therapy.

## Special considerations

> ✱ COLLABORATION
> *Fishhooks may involve deeper structures, such as bones, tendons, vessels, and nerves; injuries that have compromised neurologic or vascular status should be approached with caution, and the patient may need referral to a health care provider with expertise in this area.*

■ Routine antibiotic prophylaxis isn't warranted but should be considered for immunocompromised patients; in deeper wounds involving tendons, bones, and cartilage; in wounds that occurred more than 8 hours prior to removal; or in patients with a history of poor wound healing (such as in a patient with diabetes mellitus or peripheral vascular disease).

## Documentation

■ Record the type of hook involved, the time and circumstances of the injury, justification for the chosen procedure, and a brief description of the procedure.

■ Document neurovascular checks to the area pre- and postprocedure.

■ Document the medications administered, including dosage and time of administration.

■ Document patient teaching done for wound care, dressing changes, and follow-up care.

## $F$OOT CARE

### CPT codes

11055  *Paring or cutting of benign hyperkeratotic lesion (corn or callus), single lesion*
11056  *As above, for 2 to 4 lesions*
11057  *As above, for more than 4 lesions*
11719  *Trimming of nondystrophic nails, any number*

### Overview

The goal of foot care is to improve comfort of the feet. Nails, skin, and circulation must be assessed for abnormalities, such as corns, calluses, and plantar warts. Identification and monitoring of these abnormalities reduces the risk of infection and complications of untreated conditions.

Corns are caused by pressure from bony prominences against a shoe, the ground, or another bony prominence. A corn may be hard or soft, but either type requires smoothing and flattening of hyperkeratotic tissue to reduce pressure and pain. After it has been reduced, the corn has a white core and should be evaluated for a possible sinus tract. If this is present, treatment with an antibiotic (such as triple antibiotic cream or ointment) may be necessary. Padded and correctly fitted shoes are essential to reduce pressure.

Calluses are caused by excessive friction and pressure, typically on the plantar aspect of the foot. Calluses (diffuse hyperkeratotic tissue) may also be smoothed and flattened with a sanding tool, a pumice stone, or a file to reduce pressure and pain. The underlying tissue is pink, making it easier to identify adequate reduction of hyperkeratotic tissue. Padding is essential to reduce friction. Arch support or other orthotics may be necessary to restore balance to gait.

Plantar warts, caused by a common wart virus, are very painful. Located on the metatarsal head or heel of the foot, they differ from corns or calluses in that they have a soft, central core and are surrounded by a firm hyperkeratotic ring. Multiple tiny black spots on the surface represent coagulated blood. A plantar wart is usually painful when squeezed. This helps distinguish a plantar wart from a callus, which is generally not painful when squeezed. Reduction of hyperkeratotic tissue reduces pain. Surgical removal may lead to deep, painful scarring. Avoid acidic removal preparations, especially in the diabetic patient.

## Indications

- To prevent foot and wound complications, especially in patients with diabetes or peripheral vascular disease
- To relieve pressure, pain, or discomfort caused by corns, calluses, or plantar warts
- To achieve cosmetic improvements

## Contraindications

### ABSOLUTE

- Open wounds on feet
- Infected, ingrown toenails
- Injured, ecchymotic feet, toes, or nails
- Severe fungal infections
- Numbness or tingling

### RELATIVE

- Use of warfarin (Coumadin) or aspirin
- Previous surgery

## Preprocedure patient preparation

- Inform the patient that he should experience immediate relief from pressure and pain after the procedure.
- Teach him how corns, calluses, bunions, and hammer toes develop, and review ways to prevent their formation.

## Equipment

Foot-soaking basin with disposable liner ◆ bath thermometer ◆ warm water not to exceed 105° F (40.6° C) ◆ mild liquid soap (may use commercial foot bath preparation with antibacterial properties) ◆ towel ◆ paper towels ◆ comfortable chair ◆ gloves ◆ impervious gown ◆ mask (high-efficiency particulate air [HEPA] filter) ◆ protective eyewear ◆ toenail clippers ◆ nail file ◆ manicure stick ◆ sanding tool with grinder ◆ assorted corn and callus pads ◆ moleskin ◆ lambs' wool ◆ massage oil or lotion ◆ assessment tool ◆ topical antibiotic, such as bactroban, neosporin, or polysporin ◆ adhesive bandage ◆ #17 scalpel

## Procedure

- Assemble all equipment in the room. Seat the patient in a comfortable chair. Before beginning the procedure, decide how you will sit (on a cushion placed on the floor or on a low stool in front of the patient).
- Take a brief history per the assessment tool. (See *Foot assessment and care*.) Specifically ask questions regarding use of warfarin or aspirin, diabetic status, peripheral vascular disease, foot or leg pain, and previous foot or leg surgery.
- Verify that the patient isn't allergic to iodine (an ingredient in many commercial foot baths).
- Explain the procedure to the patient, and address any questions or concerns he may have.

☑ OBTAIN INFORMED CONSENT

- Place a towel on the floor under the patient's feet and chair, and wash your hands.
- Fill a lined basin with warm

# Foot assessment and care

**Name:** Robert Messer      **Physician:** K. Diehl
**Age:** 72    **Male/Female:** Male     **Initial Visit:** 6/29/02
**Date:** 6/29/02      **Subsequent Visit:** _____

**Medical History:** __ Amputation __Arthritis __HTN __Diabetes ✗ Foot/Leg Pain
         ✗ PVD/CAD/CVI __Smoker __Stroke __Previous Surgery __Other

**Medications:** _____

**Vascular Status:** Pulses (DP) + R + L    Pulses (PT) + R + L    Temperature W R W L
Color DR R DR L    Edema +/ R +/ L
(+) Present   (D) Diminished   (−) Absent   (N) Normal   (W) Warm   (C) Cool   (DR) Dependent Rubor
           (EP) Elevation Pallor   (1+ - 4+) Edema

**Nails:** Excess Length ✗ R ✗ L   Thick ✗ R ✗ L   Discolored __R __L   Ingrown __R ✗ L
Debris __R __L   Incurvated __R __L   Thick Cuticles __R __L   Capillary Refill __R __L

**Skin:** Calluses __R __L   Corns ✗ R ✗ L   Dry __R __L   Fat Padding __R __L
Fissures __R __L   Maceration __R __L   Moist __R __L   Ulcer(s) __R __L

**Deformities:** Bunions __R __L   Crossover Toes __R __L   Hammer Toes __R __L
Flat Foot __R __L   Plantar Wart __R __L

**Sensation:** ✗ R   Comments Decreased _____
          ✗ L   Comments Decreased _____

**Nursing Interventions:** ✗Hygiene   __Clip, 5 or less   ✗ Clip, 5 or more   __Grind, 5 or less
__Grind, 5 or more   ✗ Buff Corns   __Buff Callus   __Apply Lotion   __Instruction

**Recommendations:** ✗ Daily Hygiene   ✗ Daily Foot Inspection   __Footwear   __Nail Care
__Skin Care Stockings (compression)   __Other

**Referral(s):** _____

**Label Feet Below:**    C-Callus   **CN**-Corn   E-Edema   M-Maceration   P-Pain   R-Redness
                **W**-Warmth   **U**-Ulcer(s)   **PW**-Plantar Wart

R                L   R                L

**Signature:** Paula Smith, CRNP
   ✓   Check if narrative is written on reverse side.

water (not to exceed 105° F [40.6° C]) and antibacterial soap or foot bath preparation.

- Tell the patient to soak his feet for 10 minutes.
- Adjust room lighting as needed.
- Put on an impervious gown, protective eyewear, and gloves. Remove the patient's feet from the bath. Using a paper towel, pat the feet dry. Using a second paper towel, dry between the toes.
- Examine the feet. Use feet maps to record findings, including any abnormalities.
- Clip the patient's toenails, taking small clips across the entire nail border. Follow the shape or contour of the top of the toe. Don't cut deeply into the corners. Run a thumb over the nail and the top of the toe to be sure the nail is short enough. Avoid clipping any skin surfaces. Cut thickened, discolored, or unhealthy nails last to prevent transmission of possible infection to healthy nails.
- File rough edges with a nail file.
- Use a manicure stick to remove debris around and under the nails.
- Check between the toes for nail clippings; remove them with a paper towel.
- Use the sanding tool and grinder to flatten and smooth any corns or calluses. Don't exceed the #2 setting on the sanding tool. (*Note:* You and the patient must wear masks and the room must be properly ventilated when grinding and sanding is taking place. Instead of using a sanding tool, you may use a #17 scalpel blade.) Slowly and gently sand the surface of the corn or callus. Avoid abrading the surrounding healthy skin.

Apply light pressure while sanding across the entire corn or callus, until the area feels soft and flexible. Don't sand below the level of healthy tissue. Stop if the tissue feels warm or if the patient reports feeling "heat."

- Pare corns with a #17 scalpel. Remove the corn core carefully, avoiding damage to healthy skin. Apply topical antibiotic and an adhesive bandage.
- Pad bony areas with moleskin, corn pads, or lambs' wool.
- Massage the foot, using a light oil (such as almond or baby oil) or a massage lotion without alcohol. Begin with a gentle thumb massage at the Achilles tendon, and circle the malleolus. Hold the foot in the left hand, and massage the dorsum with the heel of the right palm. Change hands. Massage the outer aspect of the foot between the thumb and fingers. Massage each toe. Knead the ball of the foot down through the arch, using the flat surface of the fist. Use thumbs and small circles to massage the heel. Reknead the arch.
- Assist the patient with his socks and shoes.
- With gloves still on, empty the water basin and discard the liner. Discard the paper towels and manicure stick.
- Clean equipment per facility policy.
- Remove gloves, eyewear, and gown. Dispose of them according to facility policy. Wash your hands. Place the towel in the hamper.
- Assist the patient to the waiting area.

## Postprocedure patient teaching

■ Review proper foot care with the patient. Instruct him to:
– wash his feet daily with lukewarm water and a mild soap and dry them well, especially between the toes.
– trim his toenails straight across, using an emery board to shape the nails even with the toes and to smooth rough edges.
– keep skin supple with a moisturizing lotion or light oil (but tell him not to apply lotion or oil between the toes).
– change socks daily and wear proper-fitting shoes that are free from cracks, pebbles, nails, or anything that can hurt the feet.
■ Demonstrate the proper way to inspect shoes. (See *Footwear inspection.*)
■ Caution him not to walk barefoot, indoors or outdoors.
■ Teach him to check his feet daily for blisters, cuts, sores, and other abnormalities.
■ Urge him to notify you immediately if he experiences signs or symptoms that persist, worsen, or cause anxiety, such as tingling, numbness, open lesions, dark toes, skin maceration with heavy odor, cracks between toes and on heels (especially if bleeding), drainage, or pain in toenails, heels, metatarsal pads, or other areas of the foot.
■ Schedule a follow-up appointment as needed for calluses. Instruct the patient to return to the office in 1 week for a follow-up for corns.

---

## Footwear inspection

Many foot problems arise from shoes that fit improperly. You can help the patient avoid unnecessary foot problems by instructing him in proper footwear inspection.

**PROPER FIT**
Shoes should extend ½" (1.3 cm) beyond the longest toe. They should also be wide enough to ensure no unnecessary pressure on any part of the foot.

**QUALITY AND TYPE OF SHOE**
Shoes should be firm and well constructed and shouldn't cause feet to perspire.

**SHOE INTERIOR**
Inspect the inside of the shoes for tears in the lining or insole; pebbles, nails, or other debris; cracks; holes; or odor indicating moisture. Hold the shoe firmly by the toe, and tap the heel on the floor. This will loosen any debris that may have adhered to the shoe lining.

---

■ Recommend foot care every 4 to 6 weeks as indicated.

## Complications
■ None known

## Special considerations
✦ COLLABORATION
*Refer the patient to a podiatrist for treatment of secondary infections, split toenails, or separating nails. Nail removal may be indicated.*
■ As a person ages, the toenails become more yellow and grow slower as the nail plate thickens.

Nails may also thicken and develop transverse ridges.
- Nails appear pink in whites and may have a bluish hue in dark-skinned people.

## Documentation

- In the chart, the preprocedural and postprocedural note must include an evaluation of potentially affected function, range of motion, and neurosensory testing such as two-point discrimination.
- Record a brief history, with attention to medication, pain in feet or legs, diabetic status, and peripheral vascular disease.
- Note all abnormal findings on the assessment sheet.
- Describe the type of care provided (for example, hygiene, padding, or massage with oil), instructions given to the patient as well as his understanding of them, and his ability to perform return demonstrations of foot and shoe inspections.
- Describe referrals, if any, and their purpose.

---

# FOREIGN BODY REMOVAL FROM THE EAR

### CPT codes
69200 *Removal of foreign body from external auditory canal without general anesthesia*
69210 *Removal of impacted cerumen (one or both ears)*

## Overview

Removal of foreign bodies from the ear involves manually removing an object from the ear. Cerumen is the most common material requiring removal in most adults. However, other objects also become lodged in the external ear, such as parts of toys, beans, peas, nuts, coins, cotton-tipped applicators, and insects. It's important to get a firm grip on the foreign body so as to avoid pushing it deeper into the ear canal.

## Indications

- To remove a foreign body in the outer two-thirds of the external ear canal

## Contraindications

### ABSOLUTE
- Visibility obscured due to trauma
- Tympanic membrane perforation or infection suspected
- Object likely to swell with moisture (such as a pea or a bean)

### RELATIVE
- Noncompliant patient
- Object not easily accessible or visible

## Preprocedure patient preparation

- Obtain a detailed history from the patient, including the type of object in the ear and how it became lodged in the ear.
- Explain that there may be some

discomfort with the removal procedure.

## Equipment

Otoscope ◆ ear speculum ◆ gloves ◆ ear curette, loop, or hook (plastic or wire) curette with soft tubing ◆ alligator forceps ◆ small magnet ◆ alcohol or peroxide ◆ cotton-tipped applicator ◆ protective cover or towel ◆ viscous lidocaine, topical anesthetics, or mineral oil (optional) ◆ otic antibiotic or corticosteroid such as Cortisporin (optional) ◆ adjustable light such as a gooseneck lamp

## Procedure

■ Explain the procedure to the patient, and address any questions or concerns he may have.
■ Wash your hands, and put on gloves.
■ Position the light source to shine on the ear. Inspect the external ear for signs of infection or injury. Refer patients with trauma to the ear canal to an ear, nose, and throat (ENT) specialist or the emergency department.
■ Drape the patient with a protective cover or towel.
■ Using the otoscope, inspect the external ear canal for edema and erythema, and determine the presence and type of foreign body. Determine the appropriate extraction tool. For vegetation and fabric, use alligator forceps. For smooth objects, such as beads, popcorn kernels, or nuts, use the loop. Harder objects such as batteries may be retrieved with a 1-mm right-angle hook. Metal items may be re-trieved with a small magnet. Insects need to be immobilized or killed before removal is attempted; instill viscous lidocaine, mineral oil, or topical anesthetic into the ear canal, and allow 5 minutes for these agents to work.
■ Grasping the pinna of the ear, straighten the external ear canal by pulling the ear up and back (on an adult) or down and back (on a child).
■ Hold the patient's head in place with your nondominant hand. Rest your dominant hand on the patient's head to steady it and to move with the patient if he moves suddenly.
■ Insert the ear speculum; then introduce the retrieval instrument through the speculum. Grasp the object firmly with the forceps, or place the loop or hook behind the object. Withdraw the instrument and speculum with a slow, steady motion.
■ If these steps are ineffective, try flushing out the object. However, if the object may swell (such as might occur with an organic foreign body), don't instill fluid into the ear canal. If removal is successful but small particles or debris remain, irrigate the ear.
■ Inspect the external ear canal for patency after extraction; repeat the procedure as needed until the canal is clear.
■ Dry the external ear canal to remove any blood and swab with an alcohol- or peroxide-saturated cotton-tipped applicator to reduce the risk of otitis externa.
■ Instill a topical antibiotic or corticosteroid (such as Cortisporin) to

control external edema, erythema, and infection.

## Postprocedure patient teaching

■ Tell the patient not to clean the external ear with a cotton-tipped applicator and not to place any small object into the ear canal.

## Complications

✻ **COLLABORATION**
*Risk of tympanic membrane rupture and laceration of the external ear canal are minimized with gentle handling but may be unavoidable. Depending on the extent of injury, consider consulting with your collaborating physician or an ENT specialist.*

■ Middle ear effusion is more common with ear irrigation if the tympanic membrane is perforated. This infection and otitis externa may be treated with local antibiotics such as chloramphenicol.

## Special considerations

■ If the object is a live insect, try placing the patient in a dark room and shining a penlight into the ear canal. Many times the insect will move toward the light, easing extraction.

■ Don't push the foreign body toward the tympanic membrane during extraction; doing so could cause injury.

■ Stop trying to extract the object if the patient experiences pain, severe vertigo, or nausea.

■ Battery parts can leak acid. Avoid irrigation, which would spread caustic material throughout the canal.

■ Patients, particularly small children, may require sedation before attempting removal.

✻ **COLLABORATION**
*Refer the patient to the collaborating physician or otolaryngologist if the extraction effort wasn't successful or if the patient has a perforated tympanic membrane, myringotomy tubes, or chronic otitis media.*

■ If the patient has impacted earwax, consider instilling carbamide peroxide or mineral oil three times a day for 3 to 5 days to soften it before attempting removal.

## Documentation

■ Document which ear was affected, and identify the suspected foreign body, if possible.

■ Note the date and time of extraction, including the instruments used for manual extraction and whether irrigation was necessary.

■ Record your assessment of the appearance of the ear canal, noting any signs of infection and any change in hearing ability both before and after the procedure. Note how the patient tolerated the procedure and any concerns he had, particularly related to his hearing acuity.

■ Document patient teaching and include that the patient was instructed to notify you for any signs or symptoms of infection, such as increasing pain, drainage, swelling, or fever.

# FOREIGN BODY REMOVAL FROM THE EYE

### CPT codes
65205 *Removal of foreign body, external eye, conjunctival, superficial*
65210 *Removal of foreign body, external eye, conjunctival, embedded*
65220 *Removal of foreign body, external eye, corneal without slit lamp*
65222 *Removal of foreign body, external eye, corneal with slit lamp*
99070 *Eye tray: supplies and materials provided over and above what is usually included in office visit*

## Overview

Foreign body removal of the eye involves removing foreign matter through irrigation or dislodgement without causing further injury. A patient who complains of eye pain, burning, and the feeling that he has something in his eye may have a foreign body in the eye — typically dust, dirt, or a particle of metal, plastic, or wood. If the patient also displays photophobia and a tearing eye, he may have a corneal abrasion. People who take part in such activities as digging, drilling, hammering, welding, and woodworking without appropriate eye protection are at increased risk for eye injury.

The health care provider should evaluate the patient complaining of eye pain for one or more foreign bodies in the eye because some types of injuries can scatter fragments across the cornea. The foreign body typically lodges underneath the upper eyelid or in the superior temporal cul-de-sac, where the upper lid attaches to the eyeball; foreign bodies can also lodge in the inferior cul-de-sac below the lower lid.

## Indications

■ To treat foreign body sensation, photophobia, tearing, or unilateral pain on opening or closing the eyelid
■ To remove extraocular foreign bodies

## Contraindications
### ABSOLUTE
■ High-velocity injury
■ Hyphema
■ Lens opacity
■ Pupil irregularity
■ Penetrating object or injury

### RELATIVE
■ Metallic object

## Preprocedure patient preparation

■ Have the patient remove contact lenses before beginning the procedure.
■ Inform the patient that the ophthalmic anesthetic may cause a burning sensation until it takes effect.

## Equipment

Short-acting ophthalmic anesthetic solution (0.5% proparacaine) ◆ vision-screening device such as a Snellen chart ◆ gloves ◆ cotton-tipped applicators or eyelid retractor ◆ ophthalmoscope ◆ sterile fluorescein stain strips ◆ sterile saline solution ◆ ophthalmic antibiotic solution or ointment, such as gentamicin, tobramycin, and ciprofloxacin ◆ eye patches or eye shield and adhesive tape (if indicated) ◆ binocular loupe or slit lamp (if available) ◆ small-gauge needle (may be attached to a syringe for stability) (optional) ◆ 3-ml syringe ◆ small burr drill (if you're skilled in this procedure)

## Procedure

■ Explain the procedure to the patient, and address any questions or concerns he may have.

✓ OBTAIN
INFORMED CONSENT

■ Inspect the eye and lid for erythema, drainage, and hemorrhage. If you suspect intraocular perforation or open globe injuries, refer the patient to an ophthalmologist at once.

■ Perform a vision screening using a Snellen chart.

■ Examine the pupillary reflex, extraocular movements, anterior and posterior chambers, and fundi.

■ Wash your hands and put on gloves.

■ Open the affected eye, and instill one or two drops of short-acting ophthalmic anesthetic.

■ While the patient looks down, evert the upper lid by placing a cotton-tipped applicator on the upper lid, grasping the eyelashes, and pulling the upper lid down and forward while pressing gently downward on the eyelid with the cotton-tipped applicator to expose the inner surface of the upper lid;

you can also use an eyelid retractor to expose the conjunctiva.

■ Examine the entire cornea, including the cul-de-sac, with an ophthalmoscope, slit lamp, or binocular loupe to locate and determine the depth of a foreign body.

■ Locate the foreign body, assess whether or not it's embedded, and determine the best technique of removal.

■ If the foreign body is lying on the surface, use an oblique stream of sterile saline solution to flush the eye or use a saline-moistened, cotton-tipped applicator in a gentle rolling motion to gently attempt to remove the foreign body without causing embedding or scratching of the conjunctiva.

■ If you can't remove the object with the applicator, gently attempt to dislodge the object with a small-gauge needle attached to a syringe for stability. (See *Extraction with a needle*.)

■ Gently irrigate the eye with sterile saline solution to clean the area.

■ Stain the conjunctiva with fluorescein to assess for corneal abrasion.

■ Apply ophthalmic antibiotic solution or ointment.

■ Cover the affected eye to promote patient comfort and protect the eye. Have the patient close both eyes, and tightly tape two eye patches or an eye shield over the affected eye.

## Postprocedure patient teaching

■ Tell the patient to schedule a return office visit within 24 hours for reevaluation of the eye and restaining of the cornea as indicated.

■ Instruct the patient that the eye patch shouldn't be removed and to avoid any rubbing of the eye.

■ Encourage the patient to wear protective eyewear for high-risk occupational and recreational activities, such as arc welding, mixing chemicals, and lighting fireworks.

## Complications

■ Corneal ulcer or abrasion, intraocular foreign body, uveitis, or conjunctivitis (viral or bacterial) may resolve with time and antibiotics, such as gentamicin, tobramycin, or ciprofloxacin. If any of these conditions don't resolve, refer the patient to an ophthalmologist.

## Special considerations

■ If the patient complains of increased pain during the procedure, stop at once.

■ If the patient has a metallic object in his eye — especially from a high-velocity injury — an X-ray should be taken or a computed tomography scan of the orbit should be performed to make sure no object penetrated the eye itself. The patient shouldn't undergo magnetic resonance imaging if there is a metal object in the eye, although this type of scan may be indicated for a nonmetallic foreign body as well.

■ Use an ophthalmic magnet to remove metallic foreign bodies.

■ Use a syringe or small burr drill

### Extraction with a needle

If other methods are unsuccessful, you may gently attempt to dislodge the object with a small-gauge needle attached to a syringe for stability. Under magnification, approach the object from the side rather than from the front to avoid scratching the cornea.

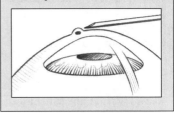

to remove rust rings only if you are skilled in the procedure.

**COLLABORATION**
*Signs of intraocular perforation include softness of the orbit on gentle palpation, any change in pupillary size or reaction, abnormality of the anterior chamber, and leakage of fluid from the chamber. If any of these signs is present, cover the eye with a patch and protective shielding, instruct the patient to rest the eye and elevate his head, and refer him to an ophthalmologist. Call to ensure that the patient will be seen immediately.*
*Refer the patient to an ophthalmologist if there's a metallic injury with rust rings that can't be removed, a corneal ulceration that won't heal, signs of uveitis, or vision loss.*

■ Don't apply a topical corticosteroid or pain medication because they may mask changes or interfere with healing.

## Documentation

- Document the indications for the procedure and any visual or cosmetic defects. Note that you have discussed with the patient at length the potential for vision loss due to unavoidable scarring, particularly when a corneal foreign body encroaches on the visual axis.
- Record the type, number, and location of foreign bodies. Note the removal procedure used.
- List any patient instructions and the patient's understanding of them.
- Record whether the patient was referred to an opthalmologist.

# *FOREIGN BODY REMOVAL FROM THE NOSE*

### *CPT code*
30300  *Removal of foreign body, intranasal; office-type procedure*

## Overview

The primary goal of foreign body removal from the nose is to remove the object without trauma to the nasal cavity and without aspiration of the object. For extremely anxious or noncompliant patients, sedation may help the health care provider perform a safe and effective removal.

Children and mentally incapacitated patients are among the high-risk groups for placing foreign bodies in the nose (and ears). Small toy parts and beans are among the most common intruders, but a wide variety of objects have been reported. Children may inform parents that they have inserted objects into their noses. However, sometimes the history isn't as clear, and the child may present with a purulent nasal discharge from the obstructed nostril. A visual examination may reveal the object, or it may show a grossly inflamed area with purulent discharge. After the diagnosis is made, every attempt should be made to remove the foreign body noninvasively and with direct visualization of the object.

Noninvasive steps should be taken first to reduce the incidence of trauma to the patient or the nose. Noninvasive methods include blowing the nose forcefully, mouth-to-mouth technique, and bag-valve mask positive pressure. Invasive methods include the hooked probe (bayonet or alligator forceps), suction, and the balloon technique with indwelling urinary or Fogarty catheters.

## Indications

- To remove a known foreign body from the nose

## Contraindications
**RELATIVE**
- Combative or uncooperative patients
- Large amount of swelling around the object

✿ COLLABORATION
*Patients with edema around the object that inhibits removal may require general anesthesia and refer-*

*ral to an ear, nose, and throat (ENT) specialist.*

## Preprocedure patient preparation

■ Explain that there will be some discomfort and that aspiration deeper into the nasal cavity or posterior nasopharynx is possible.

## Equipment

Phenylephrine spray ◆ topical lidocaine epinephrine solution ◆ suction machine ◆ #3 or #5 curved suction catheter ◆ indwelling urinary or #4 Fogarty catheter ◆ alligator forceps ◆ bayonet forceps ◆ bright portable light source ◆ gloves ◆ drape or towel ◆ suction tips ◆ nasal speculum ◆ bag-valve mask (optional)

## Procedure

■ Explain the procedure to the patient and his parents, and address any questions or concerns they may have.

☑ OBTAIN
INFORMED CONSENT

■ Place the patient in a supine position. This allows for increased patient comfort and facilitates the procedure for the health care provider.
■ Stress the importance of the patient remaining completely still for the procedure.
■ Wash your hands, put on gloves, and drape the patient to protect clothing.
■ Using a nasal speculum and a bright light source, inspect the nare and try to visualize the object.

Extending the head may aid visualization.
■ Suction any pus or debris that may occlude visualization of the object.
■ Administer phenylephrine and lidocaine into affected nostril to reduce intranasal inflammation and to provide topical anesthesia. Sedate if necessary.

◢ CLINICAL TIP
*Some children may need to be physically restrained to perform the procedure. If difficulty continues, stop and refer the patient to an ENT specialist due to the risk of forcing the object farther inside.*

### For noninvasive procedures

■ If the patient is cooperative and able, tell him to forcefully blow his nose while occluding the unaffected nostril. This should help dislodge the object.
■ Another noninvasive technique is the mouth-to-mouth technique. Instruct the parent to blow a sharp breath into the child's mouth while occluding the opposite nostril. The positive pressure from behind the object should help dislodge it. This technique allows for parental involvement, which may help to calm the child and is especially useful with infants.
■ The bag-valve mask works similarly to the mouth-to-mouth technique, providing a positive pressure force behind the object. Again, the unaffected nare is occluded while delivering positive pressure into the mouth of the patient using a bag-valve mask.

### For invasive procedures

■ If noninvasive methods are unsuccessful and you're able to visualize the object, choose an extraction tool based on the type of object. Use alligator forceps to withdraw soft objects, such as paper, cotton, and cloth. Harder objects can be removed with bayonet forceps.

■ Insert the chosen tool gently into the nose, with the patient lying completely still. If you meet resistance or the patient is combative, refer the patient to an ENT specialist.

■ Open the clamps as you approach the object. Grasp the object and withdraw slowly.

■ Use a suction catheter for smooth, round objects that are difficult to grasp with the above tools. Place the suction catheter gently against the object, and then turn on the suction while removing the catheter. Be careful not to push the object further into the nasal passage.

■ An indwelling urinary or Fogarty (balloon technique) catheter can also be used. Pass the catheter carefully past the object, inflate the balloon with approximately 1 cc of air, and withdraw slowly, pulling the object out of the nose.

## Postprocedure patient teaching

■ Although the risk of infection is small, instruct the patient and parents to observe for signs and symptoms, including increased pain within 24 hours of the procedure, increased temperature, yellow or green drainage from nose, and foul odor. If any of these symptoms appears, the patient should return to the office as soon as possible. Otherwise, he should follow up with you 1 to 2 days after the procedure. Following removal of nasal foreign bodies, the patient should irrigate with saline two to three times a day for 2 to 3 days.

■ Educate parents about the significant risk of aspiration of these objects in small children, especially those under age 5. Also educate parents about objects, such as marbles and beads, often found lodged in the nose and ears. Advise them that young children shouldn't be allowed to play with small objects.

## Complications

■ Trauma to mucous membranes increases the possibility of postprocedure bleeding or infection and may require application of a topical hemostatic agent.

✦ COLLABORATION
*Injury to nasal passages can be life-threatening. To prevent this, refer combative patients to an ENT specialist.*

*Aspiration or deeper progression of the object resulting in the inability to remove the object requires referral to an acute care facility or an ENT specialist.*

## Special considerations

■ The nasal mucosa may be premedicated with 0.5% phenylephrine (Neo-Synephrine) and aerosolized lidocaine or tetracaine to reduce any mucosal edema and to provide local anesthesia. However, some health care providers prefer using nebulized epinephrine instead. Parents can hold the nebulizer mask close to the child's face. The inhaled medication helps reduce nasal inflammation and makes removing the object easier. Children generally tolerate this better than nasal inhalers, and removal with instruments may be avoided.

■ Patients with edema around the object that inhibits removal may require general anesthesia and referral to an ENT specialist.

■ Usually instillation of lidocaine into the nose provides sufficient anesthesia. However, with the combative child, it may be necessary to administer I.V. sedation.

■ In all procedures, placing any instrument into the nasal canal should be done with a steady hand resting on the patient's head in case of sudden movement, which can be an involuntary response to pain.

■ After the foreign body is removed, inspect the nasal cavity again for additional foreign bodies or bleeding.

■ Any bleeding can be stopped by inserting cotton into the nostril temporarily.

■ Some health care providers recommend always using a topical anesthetic (for comfort) and a vasoconstrictive agent (to decrease edema in surrounding tissues) before attempting to remove a nasal foreign body.

■ It's important to rule out a foreign body as the source of any unilateral nasal discharge.

➤ **CLINICAL TIP**
*Always use care when performing these procedures. Aspiration of foreign bodies has resulted in death in some children younger than age 5.*

## Documentation

■ Document the patient's condition on arrival, history and duration of symptoms, any behavioral changes, and whether the object was visualized.

■ Note the actual procedure, instruments used (if any), technique, and how the patient tolerated it.

■ List all medications given to the patient and whether any restraints were used.

■ Document any instructions given to patient and parents postprocedure, including preventive measures to avoid a recurrence.

*F*OREIGN BODY
REMOVAL FROM
THE THROAT

**CPT code**
42809  *Removal of foreign body, pharynx*

## Overview

Peanuts in children and chicken or fish bones in adults are some of the most common objects that become lodged in the throat. However, foreign bodies in the throat occur most commonly in infants and children younger than age 4. The patient may complain of a sensation of having something stuck in the throat, pain, dysphagia, drooling, coughing, or gagging. More serious complications such as respiratory compromise require immediate emergency management. Evaluation for and removal of a foreign body from the throat is necessary for a patient presenting with the above-mentioned symptoms.

## Indications

- To evaluate and remove a foreign body from the throat in the patient who presents with a feeling of something stuck in the throat, pain, dysphagia, drooling, coughing, or gagging

## Contraindications

**ABSOLUTE**
- Epiglottiditis

**RELATIVE**
- Acute throat inflammation or infection

## Preprocedure patient preparation

- Obtain a detailed history from the patient to determine what may have been aspirated. The patient is often able to identify on which side the object may be.
- Perform a thorough examination of the head and neck.

## Equipment

Gloves ◆ protective eyewear ◆ topical anesthetic, such as 2% to 4% lidocaine spray or 14% benzocaine spray ◆ bright light source (such as a headlight) ◆ bayonet forceps ◆ laryngeal mirrors (No. 4 and No.

5 or size appropriate for patient) ◆ 4″ × 4″ gauze pads

## Procedure

- If the patient shows signs of respiratory distress or can't cough or talk, proceed directly to emergency management. (See "Obstructed airway management," page 336.)
- Explain the procedure to the patient, and address any questions or concerns he may have.
- Wash your hands and put on gloves and protective eyewear.
- Assist the patient to a comfortable position, sitting up and leaning slightly forward. For children, a supine position may be more effective; a mummy restraint may be necessary for infants. (See "Child restraint techniques," page 95.)
- Ask the patient to open his mouth wide. Using a bright light source, examine the mouth. If the aspirated object is visible, consider using topical anesthetic spray; then use bayonet forceps to gently remove it.

➤ **CLINICAL TIP**
*Don't force an object out of the throat because this could cause laceration or perforation of surrounding tissue. If the object is unremovable with forceps, endoscopy or bronchoscopy may be necessary.*

- If no object is visible at the back of the mouth, spray the back of the mouth with topical anesthetic spray. This will prevent the gag reflex from being stimulated.
- Extend the tongue by grasping it firmly with gauze pads.
- Using the largest laryngeal mirror size that will fit comfortably in

the patient's mouth and directing your light source appropriately, examine the throat. With the laryngeal mirror, lift the uvula out of the way and gently move the mirror to assess for any foreign objects, masses, or nodules in the larynx, hypopharynx, or oropharynx. Avoid touching surrounding structures (such as the posterior wall of the throat) with the mirror to prevent gag reflex stimulation.

■ Remove any visible objects with the bayonet forceps. If you can't remove the object or if you don't see an object, refer the patient to an otolaryngologist or an acute care facility for further management, which may include endoscopy or bronchoscopy.

■ Gently release the patient's tongue.

## Postprocedure patient teaching

■ Instruct the patient not to eat or take anything by mouth until the local anesthetic has worn off.

■ Discuss the treatment plan and further consultations that may be necessary.

■ Teach the patient to drink cool liquids or to eat ice cream or popsicles for topical pain relief.

## Complications

■ Vomiting may occur due to inadequate anesthetic application.

## Special considerations

■ Consider X-rays to aid in diagnosis and treatment.

## Documentation

■ Record the patient's history and physical examination findings, the indications for the procedure, the method of removal or throat examination necessary, and the object removed. Document the anesthetic used, if necessary, and the patient's tolerance of the procedure.

■ Chart any referrals that were necessary.

# *F*RENOTOMY

***CPT code***
41010 *Incision of lingual frenulum (frenotomy)*

## Overview

Frenotomy is performed to repair the condition called ankyloglossia, also known as "tongue-tie." In ankyloglossia, the lingual frenulum (the band of tissue that connects the tongue to the floor of the mouth) is too short and tight, restricting the movement of the tongue up and down and from side to side. Infants with this condition are unable to touch the roof of their mouth with their tongue (the tip of the tongue may have a heart-shaped appearance when this is attempted) or protrude the tongue past the lower teeth or gum line. (See *Viewing ankyloglossia,* page 232.) The effects of ankyloglossia, while controversial, include poor breast-feeding and impaired speech development.

## Viewing ankyloglossia

The illustration below shows how the tongue is attached to the floor of the mouth by the lingual frenulum in this infant with ankyloglossia. Because the lingual frenulum extends almost to the gum line, the tongue's movement is restricted.

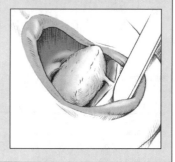

Although most cases of ankyloglossia may resolve spontaneously with the natural stretching of the lingual frenulum, intervention may be necessary for an infant with poor weight gain or a failure to thrive due to impaired breastfeeding — the tongue is unable to extend to allow for proper latchon — or if there's impaired swallowing or impaired speech development. Frenotomy may be performed at any age, although it's typically done on infants or children.

## Indications

■ To release the tongue with restricted movement due to ankyloglossia

## Contraindications

### ABSOLUTE
■ Bleeding disorders
■ Severe ankyloglossia (extremely impaired movement of the tongue), which requires referral to a surgeon for repair requiring general anesthesia

## Preprocedure patient preparation

■ Explain the risks of the procedure to the parents, including bleeding or infection.
■ Inform the parents that there's usually minimal pain from the procedure — it has been likened to getting one's ears pierced. Also inform them it takes only minutes and that the infant will need to be restrained.

## Equipment

Gloves ◆ cotton-tipped applicators ◆ topical 20% benzocaine ◆ tongue retractor (4″ × 4″ gauze pads or wooden tongue depressor with a slit in the end to grasp the tongue) ◆ hemostat ◆ sterile iris scissors ◆ 1% lidocaine with epinephrine

## Procedure

■ Explain the procedure to the parents, and address any questions or concerns they may have.

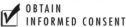
OBTAIN
INFORMED CONSENT
■ Wash your hands, and put on gloves.

- Position the patient comfortably. The parents or an assistant may hold the patient, stabilizing the head and providing easy access to the mouth.
- Apply topical 20% benzocaine to the lingual frenulum using a cotton-tipped applicator.
- Retract the tongue. To extend the tongue, an assistant may hold it using sterile $4'' \times 4''$ gauze pads or use the wooden tongue blade with a slit in the end.
- Determine the area to be "clipped." Apply the hemostat to that area, clamping down on the tissue. Leave it in place for a few seconds and then remove.
- Use the iris scissors to snip the tissue demarcated by the hemostat.
- If bleeding occurs, saturate a cotton-tipped applicator with 1% lidocaine with epinephrine and apply to the site until bleeding stops.

## Postprocedure patient teaching

- Instruct the breast-feeding mother that she may feed the infant immediately after the procedure.
- For pain relief, inform the parents that they may administer children's acetaminophen.
- Teach the parents signs and symptoms of infection, such as redness, edema, yellow or green drainage, or a foul odor at the site. They should notify your office immediately if any of these signs or symptoms arise.
- Instruct the parents that the patient should return to the office in 2 weeks for a follow-up check.

## Complications

- Infection may require treatment with systemic antibiotic therapy.
- Bleeding or damage to the surrounding tissue may occur, requiring further evaluation and management.

## Special considerations

- Many cases of ankyloglossia are brought to the attention of the health care provider by the parents. Signs and symptoms that may lead to the discovery of ankyloglossia include a clicking noise when breast-feeding, poor latching ability, impaired weight gain, inability of the tongue to protrude, and a mother with frequent mastitis and sore nipples.

## Documentation

- Record the indications for the procedure, any medications administered during the procedure, the patient's tolerance of the procedure, and any complications that occurred.
- Document patient teaching and instructions given.

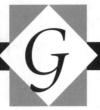

## GASTROSTOMY FEEDING BUTTON CARE

**CPT code**
*No specific code has been assigned.*

### Overview

A gastrostomy feeding button serves as an alternative feeding device for an ambulatory patient receiving long-term enteral feedings. It can be used to replace a gastrostomy tube if necessary; the Food and Drug Administration has approved the feeding button for 6-month implantation.

The feeding button has a mushroom dome at one end and two wing tabs and a flexible safety plug at the other. When inserted into an established stoma, the button lies almost flush with the skin, with only the top of the safety plug visible. The button can usually be inserted into a stoma in less than 15 minutes.

In addition to its cosmetic appeal, the device is easily maintained, reduces skin irritation and

breakdown, and is less likely than an ordinary feeding tube to become dislodged or migrate. A one-way, antireflux valve mounted just inside the mushroom dome prevents accidental leakage of gastric contents. The device usually requires replacement after 3 to 4 months, typically because the antireflux valve wears out.

### Indications

■ To replace a dislodged gastrostomy feeding button, clear an obstruction, or care for red, irritated skin around the gastrostomy site

### Contraindications

■ Stoma not adequately visible

### Preprocedure patient preparation

■ Show the patient or caregiver the dislodged gastrostomy feeding button. Demonstrate how to reinsert the feeding button because they may do this at home if the feeding button becomes dislodged again.

## Equipment

Gastrostomy feeding button of the correct size (all three sizes, if the correct one isn't known) ♦ obturator ♦ water-soluble lubricant ♦ gloves ♦ antiseptic solution such as povidone-iodine ♦ water ♦ hydrogen peroxide ♦ 10-ml syringe ♦ cotton-tipped applicators ♦ 4″ × 4″ gauze pads

## Procedure

■ Explain the procedure to the patient or his caregiver, and address any questions or concerns he may have.
■ Wash your hands, and put on gloves.
■ Ask the patient to lie in a supine position, and provide a pillow to raise his head slightly.
■ Reinsert the feeding button. If the patient saved the button, it may be reused. (See *How to reinsert a gastrostomy feeding button,* page 236.)
■ If the button is obstructed, flush with 10 ml of water in a 10-ml syringe to dislodge formula or food particles. Then clean the inside of the feeding catheter with a cotton-tipped applicator to preserve patency. Snap the safety plug in place to keep the lumen clean and prevent leakage if the antireflux valve fails.
■ When the skin around the stoma is red or irritated, gently clean with gauze pads and a solution of 50% water, 50% hydrogen peroxide. Then wipe the area with povidone-iodine solution. Allow to air-dry.

## Postprocedure patient teaching

■ Make sure the patient can insert and care for the gastrostomy feeding button as above. Offer written instructions, and answer his questions on obtaining replacement supplies.
■ Instruct the patient to clean the peristomial site once daily with mild soap and water or povidone-iodine solution and let the skin air-dry for 20 minutes to avoid skin irritation. Also, instruct him to clean the site whenever spillage of feeding solution or medication occurs.

## Complications

■ Infection at the site may occur necessitating treatment with antibiotics.

## Special considerations

■ Slowing tube feedings or changing the feeding solution may help the patient with diarrhea.
■ Ranitidine may be prescribed for a patient with indigestion. Smaller feedings given more frequently may also provide relief.

## Documentation

■ Note the indications for the procedure. Record the appearance of the stoma and surrounding skin. Document care necessitated by the gastrostomy feeding button.
■ Document all instructions given to the patient and statements that

# How to reinsert a gastrostomy feeding button

If your patient's feeding button pops out (with coughing, for instance), you or he will need to reinsert the device. Here are some steps to follow.

### PREPARE THE EQUIPMENT
Collect the feeding button, an obturator, and water-soluble lubricant. If the button will be reinserted, wash it with soap and water and rinse it thoroughly.

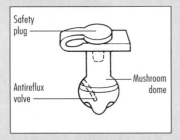

### INSERT THE BUTTON
■ Check the depth of the patient's stoma to make sure you have a feeding button of the correct size. Then clean around the stoma.
■ Lubricate the obturator with a water-soluble lubricant and distend the button several times to ensure the patency of the antireflux valve within the button.
■ Lubricate the mushroom dome and the stoma. Gently push the button through the stoma into the stomach.

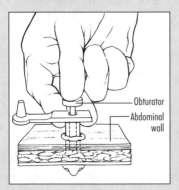

■ Remove the obturator by gently rotating it as you withdraw it, to keep the antireflux valve from adhering to it. If the valve sticks nonetheless, gently push the obturator back into the button until the valve closes.
■ After removing the obturator, make sure the valve is closed. Then close the flexible safety plug, which should be relatively flush with the skin surface.

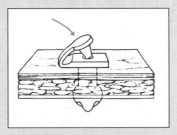

■ If you need to administer a feeding right away, open the safety plug and attach the feeding adapter and feeding tube. Then deliver the feeding.

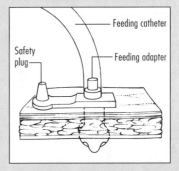

indicate his understanding of them.

## GRAM STAIN, WET MOUNT, AND POTASSIUM HYDROXIDE

**CPT codes**
87205  *Smear, primary source, with interpretation; routine stain for bacteria, fungi, or cell types*
87210  *Smear, primary source, with interpretation; wet mount with saline, india ink, or KOH prep*
87220  *Tissue examination for fungi*

## Overview

Specimen collection involves obtaining a fluid sample from the vagina for testing. As a procedure in gynecology, a Gram stain is used to assist in the diagnosis of sexually transmitted diseases (STDs), particularly *Neisseria gonorrhoeae.* The Gram stain enhances detection of bacteria and polymorphonuclear (PMN) leukocytes. A thin smear of cervical secretions is dried and then Gram-stained. Under oil emersion microscopy (100×), gram-negative *N. gonorrhoeae* can be visualized as pink diplococci within PMN cells of the specimen.

The wet mount is another technique used to assist in the diagnosis of vaginal disorders. Specimens of vaginal secretions are taken from several sites on the vaginal walls and fornices with a clean applicator. The specimen is then mixed with normal saline or 10% to 20% potassium hydroxide (KOH) on a glass slide. The slide is viewed microscopically at 10× and 40×, and any of the following may be identified: *Candida albicans* (and other *Candida* species), *Trichomonas vaginalis,* and the clue cells of bacterial vaginosis. The presence of candidiasis and trichomoniasis may be confirmed by wet mount. Diagnosis of bacterial vaginosis is further confirmed by a vaginal pH of more than 4.7 measured by litmus tape and a fishy odor (caused by release of amines) when KOH is mixed with the vaginal secretions.

## Indications

- To identify suspected STD
- To assess vaginal discharge, itching, burning, or irritation

## Contraindications

- Current menses
- Recent intercourse, douching, or intravaginal medication

## Preprocedure patient preparation

- Obtain the gynecologic history from the patient, including the onset and a description of her present symptoms.

## Equipment

Gloves ◆ cotton-tipped applicators ◆ glass slide ◆ coverslips ◆ dropper bottle of normal saline ◆ dropper bottle of 10% to 20% KOH ◆ small test tubes (optional) ◆ microscope ◆ vaginal speculum ◆ litmus paper ◆ drape

## Procedure

■ Explain the procedure to the patient, and address any questions or concerns she may have.

■ Have the patient disrobe from the waist down and put on a gown or drape and assist her into the lithotomy position.

■ Wash your hands, and put on gloves.

■ Examine the external genitalia and mons, and insert a warmed speculum that has been moistened with water.

■ Visualize the cervix, and collect a Papanicolaou (Pap) specimen if appropriate.

■ Collect the specimen for Gram stain from the cervical os using a cotton-tipped applicator. Roll a thin specimen of the secretions onto a glass slide, and set aside to air-dry before Gram-staining.

■ Discard the applicator.

■ Collect a specimen for the wet mount from several areas along the vaginal walls and fornices with another cotton-tipped applicator.

■ Touch the applicator to a sample of litmus paper, and note the pH.

■ Option 1 (slide):
– Set this applicator on a glass slide while you complete the speculum examination.

■ Option 2 (test tube):
– Place the applicator in a glass test tube with 0.5 to 1.0 ml of normal saline. Repeat this step, placing the second applicator in 0.5 to 1.0 ml KOH.

■ Remove the speculum.

■ Perform a bimanual examination, and evaluate carefully for tenderness in the uterus or adnexa.

■ Remove soiled gloves, and wash your hands; explain your findings to the patient, and assist her to a seated position.

■ Instruct her to dress while you complete the laboratory studies.

■ Put on a clean pair of gloves. Take the applicator you placed on the clean slide or the test tube to the area where the microscope is located.

■ Option 1:
– Apply a thin sample of discharge directly to a glass slide from the cotton-tipped applicator.
– Allow a drop of normal saline to fall on the specimen and use the wooden applicator end to mix.

■ Option 2:
– Gently agitate the cotton-tipped applicator in the normal saline. Transfer a drop of the saline solution to a glass slide.
– Cover the slide with a coverslip.

■ Prepare the KOH slide similarly, noting any existence of an amine odor (fishy) or whiff.

■ Alternatively, use two slides, placing both the normal saline and KOH specimens on the opposite ends of a single slide. Standardize your technique by always placing normal saline at one end of the slide and KOH at the other end of the slide.

■ Place a slide under the microscope. Allow the other to air-dry.

■ Examine the normal saline slide first under 10× and again at 40×. Examine the KOH slide the same way. Examine at least 5 different microscopic fields. (See *Identifying microscopic findings*.)

■ Retrieve the first slide that air-dried. Apply Gram stain, and see if it adheres to the specimen. If it "stains" the sample, the result is gram-positive. If it doesn't adhere to the sample, it's gram-negative.

■ Correlate laboratory findings with clinical information, and diagnose the cause of the complaint. (See *Differential diagnosis of vaginal discharge,* page 240.)

## Postprocedure patient teaching

■ Tell the patient that the appropriate therapy for the identified vaginal malady will generally resolve the abnormal discharge and that no complications are common with this procedure.

■ Instruct the patient to complete the course of drug therapy and schedule a follow-up appointment after drug therapy is completed. As appropriate, teach the patient how to administer vaginal medication.

■ Review proper use of condoms as indicated.

■ Advise the patient to contact you if symptoms aren't resolved by completion of the medication, if symptoms escalate or don't improve, or if additional symptoms develop.

■ Warn the patient that vaginal preparations suspended in petrolatum will weaken latex condoms and diaphragms. Advise her to ab-

## Identifying microscopic findings

To identify microscopic findings, first examine the specimen with saline. Potential findings are trichomonads, leukocytes, and clue cells.

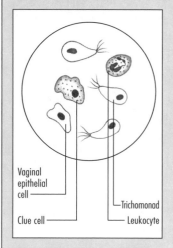

Vaginal epithelial cell

Clue cell

Trichomonad

Leukocyte

Next, examine the specimen with potassium hydroxide. Potential findings are pseudohyphae, spores, and leukocytes.

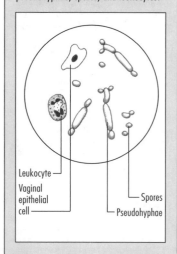

Leukocyte

Vaginal epithelial cell

Spores

Pseudohyphae

## Differential diagnosis of vaginal discharge

Although individual presentations vary, there are some common findings that help differentiate the cause of vaginal discharge. To review these findings, check below.

| DISORDER AND CAUSATIVE ORGANISM | CHARACTERISTICS OF DISCHARGE | VULVO-VAGINAL FINDINGS | DIAGNOSTIC TESTS |
|---|---|---|---|
| **CANDIDAL VAGINITIS** <br> *Candida albicans, C. glabrata, C. tropicalis* | Mild more than profuse; thin more than thick; white, curdlike discharge; adherent to vaginal walls | Possible erythema, excoriation, edema | ■ pH 4.0 to 4.7 <br> ■ KOH: positive for hyphae or spores <br> ■ Saline: white blood cells (WBCs) <br> ■ Gram stain: positive for budding *Candida* |
| **TRICHOMONAL VAGINITIS** <br> *Trichomonas vaginalis* | Yellow to gray to green, odorous discharge; varying consistency; may have bubbles | Possible erythema and edema; may have "strawberry" patches | ■ pH greater than 6.0 <br> ■ KOH: amine odor <br> ■ Saline: motile trichomonads, elevated WBCs, decreased lactobacilli present on Papanicolaou test |
| **BACTERIAL VAGINOSIS** <br> Polybacterial *Mobiluncus, Bacteroides, Peptococcus, Peptostreptococcus, Eubacterium, Fusobacterium, Mycoplasma hominis* | White to gray or yellow to green, thin, homogenous, malodorous discharge; adherent to walls and at introitus; may have erythema | Discharge at introitus; may have erythema | ■ pH 5.5 to 7.0 <br> ■ KOH: amine odor <br> ■ Saline: increased parabasal cells, decreased lactobacilli, clue cells <br> ■ Gram stain: *G. vaginalis, Mobiluncus* |
| **CYTOLYTIC VAGINITIS** <br> None; exfoliative vaginitis and greater turnover of squamous epithelial cells secondary to over-production of lactobacilli; may occur from self-treatment of a vaginal infection. | Thick, white discharge | Within normal limits; may see thick vaginal discharge | ■ pH 4.0 to 4.5 <br> ■ Saline: increased epithelial cells, increased lactobacilli, elevated or decreased WBCs <br> ■ Gram stain: lactobacilli, gram-positive rods |

stain from intercourse while treatment for vaginal infection continues.

■ Review with the patient behaviors to control vaginal infections, such as wearing cotton underwear; avoiding tight-fitting jeans, nylons, and slacks; wiping from front to back after going to the bathroom; using mild soap; and avoiding douching.

■ Discuss the presence and characteristics of natural vaginal lubrication. Advise the patient against excessive treatment of simple vaginal discharge (one unaccompanied by itching, irritation, or malodor) with over-the-counter (OTC) preparations to prevent cytolytic vaginitis.

## Complications

■ None known

## Special considerations

■ With the availability of OTC vaginal medications, the patient may come for diagnosis after self-treating. Cytolytic vaginitis is a reaction that occurs from treatment or overtreatment of vaginal infections. An overgrowth of lactobacilli produces excess acid that results in cytolysis of epithelial cells. The discharge of cytolytic vaginitis contains no pathogens. Treatment is alkaline douche (1 tsp baking soda in 1 pint of warm water) once or twice as necessary.

■ Consider postponing specimen collection until the next day if the patient has douched, used intravaginal medication, or had intercourse within the previous 24 hours.

■ Consider testing all patients with vaginal complaints, especially if the symptoms don't resolve with treatment.

■ The specimen for Gram stain may be sent out for analysis, at which time the laboratory technician will also review the slide for diplococci.

## Documentation

■ Record subjective data, such as complaints, symptoms, duration, exacerbating or ameliorating factors, remedies tried, and effects of remedies.

■ Document findings of external genitalia and pelvic examinations and wet mount, normal saline, and KOH slides. Documentation of wet mount is in the form of what's present on the slide (for example, normal saline: no hyphae, positive for motile trichomonads, no clue cells; KOH: positive for whiff).

■ List the prescribed treatment for diagnosed vaginal malady and follow-up care as appropriate.

■ Document any patient teaching and the patient's understanding.

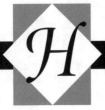

## HAIR-THREAD TOURNIQUET REMOVAL

**CPT code**
10120 *Removal of subcutaneous foreign body, simple*

## Overview

Hair-thread tourniquet syndrome is a condition that involves infants and young children. It generally involves a hair (80% of the time) that becomes wrapped around an appendage, such as a toe, finger, or genital part. Examples of other offending agents are strings or fibers from a mitten or garment. Although the mechanism is not completely understood, generally, the hair becomes wrapped around the appendage, causing constriction and subsequent lymphedema. As the appendage continues to swell, the hair cuts through the skin and underlying structures (the urethra in cases involving the penis). If this condition isn't recognized and treated, the hair eventually causes strangulation and necrosis of the involved ap-

pendage. Recognition of this condition is crucial but commonly elusive because the tourniquet may be difficult to visualize.

## Indications

- To remove a hair or fiber wrapped around an appendage

## Contraindications

**RELATIVE**
- While removal of the hair is always imperative, the health care provider must determine who's most qualified to perform the procedure. When necrosis of the distal portion of the appendage is possible or if the penile urethra has been compromised, further consultation and management may be necessary.

## Preprocedure patient preparation

- When a patient presents with a swollen finger, toe, penis, or clitoris, begin by identifying the cause. Inspect the appendage carefully for a circumferential constriction or laceration. If this is found, hair-thread tourniquet syndrome is the most likely cause.

■ Because this condition affects infants and young children, discuss with the parents how this occurred and how you plan to proceed. Offer them the option of a surgical consultation.

## Equipment

Gloves ◆ equipment for local anesthesia or a digital nerve block ◆ normal saline solution ◆ 30- to 60-ml syringe ◆ 4″ × 4″ gauze pads ◆ hexachlorophene solution ◆ skin hook ◆ small forceps without teeth ◆ #11 scalpel blade or small iris scissors ◆ device for magnification, such as a magnifying lense or otoscope ◆ topical antibiotic ointment ◆ a depilatory such as Nair (optional)

## Procedure

■ Explain the procedure to the patient and parents, and address any questions or concerns they may have.

■ Wash your hands, and put on gloves.

■ Administer the appropriate local or digital nerve block. (See "Anesthesia: topical, local, and digital nerve block," page 20.)

■ Clean the area using hexachlorophene solution. Avoid using povidone-iodine solution because it will reduce visibility of the site.

■ Irrigate the area with normal saline solution, using a 30- to 60-ml syringe. Thoroughly dry the area with 4″ × 4″ gauze pads.

■ Using magnification, attempt to see and identify the hair, fiber, or other offending agent. The degree of swelling and ability to identify the hair or fiber dictates your approach to treatment.

■ If an end of the hair or fiber can be grasped with forceps, use small forceps without teeth to unwind it.

■ If the hair can be seen but can't be unwound, use a skin hook to get under the hair. Then use a #11 scalpel blade or iris scissors to cut the hair and remove it. Have an assistant hold the wound edges apart if necessary.

**▲▶ CLINICAL TIP**
*In most cases, the hair or fiber is wrapped around several times. Make sure you remove the entire tourniquet. It's also important not to amputate apparently dead tissue during the initial presentation. Even tissue that appears badly damaged can revitalize, especially in infants and young children.*

**✿ COLLABORATION**
*If the wound is very deep and a hair or fiber can't be identified, refer the patient for surgical exploration (a dorsal slit allows deeper exploration).*

■ An alternative method, using a depilatory, such as Nair, can be attempted if the tourniquet is a hair. Once the hair is identified, the depilatory is applied to the site. Several minutes later, the hair becomes fragile and may be picked out with small forceps. This technique is best for superficial tourniquets but won't work on fibers.

■ After the tourniquet has been removed, apply a topical antibiotic ointment such as Polysporin. Leave the site uncovered to allow air circulation.

## Postprocedure patient teaching

- Advise the parents that the swelling will decrease slowly and the color should return to normal over time.
- Instruct the parents that the child should be seen in 24 hours. Any increase in swelling or further cyanosis should alert you to a retained hair or fiber necessitating reexploration or surgical consultation.

## Complications

- Irreversible tissue necrosis requires surgical consultation because amputation may be necessary.
- A deep tourniquet or damage to underlying structures, such as nerves, tendons, blood vessels, or the urethra, necessitates a surgical and, possibly, urological consultation.
- Infection at the site may necessitate treatment with topical or systemic antibiotics.

## Special considerations

- Close monitoring may be needed if you suspect any damage to underlying structures. In case of penile involvement, be sure to observe the child urinating to check for a ureteral cutaneous fistula.
- The earliest recorded case of hair-thread tourniquet syndrome

was in 1832, involving a 4-week-old infant with a hair wrapped around the penis. It was later found to be an intentional act by a disgruntled nanny. Nonaccidental trauma (NAT) is always a consideration in pediatric injury and should be considered in the case of hair-thread tourniquet syndrome, although this is an unusual presentation of NAT.

- Because follow-up care in these cases is so important, be sure to call the parents if they fail to return for a scheduled follow-up visit.

## Documentation

- Record the condition of the appendage at the time the patient presented, the steps taken in determining the cause of the swelling, and the technique used to remove the tourniquet.
- Document any postprocedure instructions given and the scheduled follow-up appointments.

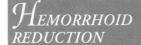

## *Hemorrhoid Reduction*

**CPT code**
*No specific code has been assigned.*

## Overview

Hemorrhoids are varicosities in the superior or inferior hemorrhoidal venous plexus. Dilation and enlargement of the superior plexus produce internal hemorrhoids; dilation and enlargement of the inferior plexus produce external hemorrhoids that may protrude from the rectum. (See *Types of hemorrhoids.*)

Hemorrhoids occur in both sexes and probably result from increased venous pressure in the hemorrhoidal plexus. Although hemorrhoids may be asymptomatic, they characteristically cause painless, intermittent bleeding, which occurs on defecation. Bright red blood appears on the stool or on the toilet paper because of injury to the fragile mucosa covering the hemorrhoid. Such first-degree hemorrhoids may itch. When second-degree hemorrhoids prolapse, they're usually painless and spontaneously return to the anal canal after defecation. Third-degree hemorrhoids cause constant discomfort and prolapse in response to any increase in intra-abdominal pressure. They must be manually reduced because they don't spontaneously return to the anal canal.

## Indications

■ To temporarily relieve painful and bleeding external hemorrhoids

## Contraindications

■ Severe pain

## Preprocedure patient preparation

■ Explain to the patient that manual reduction is only a temporary solution to hemorrhoids and that they will most likely recur. How-

### Types of hemorrhoids

Covered by mucosa, internal hemorrhoids bulge into the rectal lumen and may prolapse during defecation. Covered by skin, external hemorrhoids protrude from the rectum and are more likely to thrombose than internal hemorrhoids. The illustrations below show frontal and cross-sectional views.

INTERNAL HEMORRHOIDS

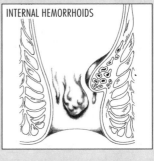

EXTERNAL HEMORRHOIDS

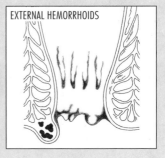

ever, manual reduction may provide relief until further treatment can be done.

■ Evaluate the hemorrhoid for degree and type. Differentiate it from an anal fissure, which can produce similar symptoms.

## Equipment

Gloves ◆ water-soluble lubricant ◆ drape or sheet

## Procedure

- Explain the procedure to the patient, and address any questions or concerns he may have.
- Provide privacy and ask the patient to disrobe from the waist down.
- Wash your hands, and put on gloves.
- Assist the patient to lie on his left side, flexing either the right knee or both knees toward his chest. Drape the patient to provide privacy.
- Apply a small amount of lubricant to the fingers of your dominant hand.

> **CLINICAL TIP**
> *Use only a small amount of lubricant because too much lubricant can cause the hemorrhoid to easily slip back out after reduction.*

- Gently guide the hemorrhoid back through the anal sphincter using your thumb and index finger.
- Wipe away any excess lubricant from the site before assisting the patient back to a sitting position.

## Postprocedure patient teaching

- Encourage the patient to stay off his feet for several hours following the procedure.
- For comfort, instruct the patient to use sitz baths or warm water soaks as necessary. To relieve constipation, thereby preventing hemorrhoids from becoming more severe, encourage the patient to increase his fluid intake and to eat a high-fiber diet (including foods such as raw vegetables and fruits and whole grain cereals) or to take a fiber supplement.
- Instruct the patient to use a hydrocortisone suppository (available over the counter) if the hemorrhoids are inflamed.

## Complications

- Reducing hemorrhoids offers only a temporary solution; hemorrhoids recur after manual reduction. For recurring hemorrhoids that are symptomatic, refer the patient to a colorectal surgeon.

## Special considerations

> **COLLABORATION**
> *Hemorrhoidectomy, the most effective treatment, is necessary for patients with severe bleeding, intolerable pain and pruritus, and a large prolapse. For a patient with internal hemorrhoids, banding — or ligation — or infrared coagulation therapy may be performed. These procedures require referral to a colorectal surgeon.*

- When evaluating the patient's symptoms, don't confuse hemorrhoids with an anal fissure, which can produce anal tags and similar symptoms.
- When the patient is experiencing severe pain and bleeding, do what is necessary to relieve his symptoms. The patient should always return to the facility for fur-

ther investigation of rectal bleeding (such as by anoscopy or sigmoidoscopy) after the symptoms are less intense.

## Documentation

▪ Record the indications for the procedure, the patient's toleration of the procedure, and the plans made for follow-up evaluation or referral.
▪ Document all instructions given to the patient and his understanding of them.

## *H*EMORRHOID, TREATMENT OF THROMBOSED

### CPT codes
46083 *Incision of thrombosed hemorrhoid, external*
46320 *Enucleation or excision of external thrombosed hemorrhoid*

## Overview

Thrombosis of external hemorrhoids produces sudden rectal pain and a subcutaneous, large, firm lump that the patient can feel. Management depends on timing and the severity of the patient's symptoms. If it has only been 1 to 2 days since the patient's symptoms developed, or if it has been longer than 2 days and the symptoms remain severe, the thrombosed hemorrhoids may be treated. However, if the patient's symptoms have been present for longer

than 2 days or are lessening in severity, treatment isn't necessary except to provide measures to ease pain, combat swelling and congestion, and regulate bowel habits.

Before incising the hemorrhoids, be certain that they're external and not internal hemorrhoids that have prolapsed. Internal thrombosed hemorrhoids should never be incised.

## Indications

▪ To remove the clot of thrombosed hemorrhoids that have been present for fewer than 2 days or that produce severe symptoms

## Contraindications

**ABSOLUTE**
▪ Blood dyscrasia (acute leukemia, aplastic anemia, or hemophilia)
▪ GI carcinoma
▪ Prolapsed internal hemorrhoids
▪ Rectal prolapse
▪ First trimester of pregnancy
▪ Thrombosed hemorrhoids present for longer than 2 days with less severe symptoms

## Preprocedure patient preparation

▪ Tell the patient that injection of the anesthetic will be painful because the area is already tender. However, once the anesthetic takes effect, pain will be minimal.

## Equipment

Gloves ◆ antiseptic solution such as povidone-iodine ◆ equipment to provide local anesthesia, including lidocaine with epinephrine ◆ #11 scalpel ◆ iris scissors ◆ forceps ◆ equipment for suturing, including 3-0 chromic suture material ◆ 4″ × 4″ gauze pads ◆ tape

## Procedure

■ Explain the procedure to the patient and address any questions or concerns he may have.

☑ **OBTAIN INFORMED CONSENT**

■ Wash your hands, and put on gloves.

■ Assist the patient to lie on his left side, flexing either his right knee or both knees toward his chest. Drape patient to provide privacy.

■ Wash the anal area with an antiseptic solution, such as povidone-iodine, and gauze pads and allow to dry.

■ Administer local anesthesia to the site. (See "Anesthesia: topical, local, and digital nerve block," page 20.)

■ Incise the thrombosed hemorrhoid using the #11 scalpel or iris scissors to make an opening just large enough to remove the clot. The clot may pop out spontaneously or you may need to use forceps to remove it.

■ Gently explore the hemorrhoid to make sure all clots have been removed.

■ Bleeding is usually minimal. If suturing is necessary, as with larger incisions, use chromic suture material to close the incision. (See "Suturing of simple lacerations," page 459.)

■ Apply a dressing with 4″ × 4″ gauze pads and tape to cover the site.

## Postprocedure patient teaching

■ Prescribe pain medication for the patient, and give instructions for use.

■ Tell the patient to stay off his feet for several hours following the procedure. He may remove the dressing when he has his first bowel movement after the procedure. If there's still drainage, tell the patient (male or female) that sanitary napkins may be used to prevent soiling clothing.

■ Tell the patient to take sitz baths or warm soaks 3 to 4 times per day, starting after his first bowel movement or 12 hours after the procedure.

■ If the patient required suturing, tell him that his sutures are absorbable and won't need to be removed. However, if his symptoms worsen or he experiences signs or symptoms of infection, such as swelling, yellow or green drainage, foul odor, or increase in temperature, he'll need to return to the facility for evaluation.

■ To relieve constipation, thereby preventing hemorrhoids from becoming more severe, encourage the patient to increase his fluid intake and to eat a high-fiber diet (raw vegetables and fruits and whole grain cereals) or take a fiber supplement.

## Complications

- Infection may require treatment with antibiotics. Bleeding and further pain may also occur.
- Thrombosed hemorrhoids may recur, requiring multiple treatments or hemorrhoidectomy.

## Special considerations

- When the patient is experiencing severe pain and bleeding, do what's necessary to relieve his symptoms. However, the patient should always return to the facility for further investigation (such as by anoscopy or sigmoidoscopy) of rectal bleeding after his symptoms are less intense.
- Not all thrombosed hemorrhoids require treatment. If it has been longer than 2 days since the patient's symptoms developed, it may be best to allow healing to occur naturally.

## Documentation

- Document the type and location of the hemorrhoids.
- Record the indications for the procedure, medications given during the procedure, and the patient's toleration of the procedure.
- If suturing was required, document the type of suture material used, the number of sutures placed, and the location of the sutures.
- Record all patient instructions given and the patient's understanding of them.

# *H*OLTER MONITORING

### *CPT codes*
*93230 Electrocardiograph (ECG) monitoring for 24 hours by continuous original ECG waveform recording with device producing a full miniaturized printout; includes recording, microprocessor-based analysis with report, and physician review and interpretation*
*93231 ECG monitoring for 24 hours by continuous original ECG waveform recording, includes hookup, recording, and disconnection*
*93232 ECG monitoring for 24 hours by continuous original ECG waveform recording, includes microprocessor-based analysis with report*
*93236 ECG monitoring for 24 hours by continuous computerized monitoring and noncontinuous recording, monitoring, and real-time data analysis with report*

## Overview

Holter monitoring, also called continuous ECG monitoring, allows measurement of cardiac activity over a period of time without confining a patient to a facility. Holter monitoring records variations in ECG waveforms during normal activity. During monitoring, the patient needs to maintain a log of activities and associated symptoms he may experience.

## Indications

- To determine the status of a patient recuperating from an acute myocardial infarction
- To assess pacemaker functioning after implantation
- To evaluate cardiac signs and symptoms, such as angina or unexplained fainting
- To evaluate the frequency and type of cardiac arrhythmias
- To assess the effectiveness of antiarrhythmic drug therapy
- To determine the relationship between cardiac events, the patient's activities, and associated symptoms (such as chest pain, light-headedness, syncope or presyncope, and palpitations)

## Contraindications

**ABSOLUTE**

- Hypertensive crisis that requires immediate intervention

## Preprocedure patient preparation

- Explain that the patient will have 24 hours of cardiac activity monitored before the monitor is removed. Tell him that he'll feel no pain from the procedure but that the tape and monitor may cause mild discomfort.
- Tell the patient that he'll need to wear a small microprocessor for 24 hours after activation of the monitor. Tell him not to remove the microprocessor unless told to do so. Explain that he'll have a carrying case with strap to carry the 2-lb monitor.
- Tell the patient he'll need to maintain an activity logbook during the 24-hour monitoring period. He should record the time, activities he performs, and any symptoms (such as headache, dizziness, light-headedness, palpitations, or chest pain) that may occur. Explain the importance of maintaining his usual routine, including working, eating, sleeping, using the bathroom, driving, and taking his medication. He should be sure to record the time medications are taken.

- Suggest wearing a watch to make it easier to keep an accurate log.
- Encourage the patient to wear loose-fitting clothes with tops that open in the front.
- Tell the patient that he can sponge bathe, but he shouldn't get the equipment wet.
- Tell the patient to take the usual steps for medical emergencies (such as taking nitroglycerin and going to the emergency department for chest pain).
- Inform the patient to avoid power lines with high voltage areas, metal detectors, electric blankets, and magnetic force fields because these could affect the monitoring and recording.
- Tell the patient to call your facility if any problems or questions arise.

## Equipment

Holter unit with new battery ◆ cable wires ◆ disposable pregelled electrodes ◆ carrying case with strap ◆ 4″ × 4″ gauze pad or alcohol pad ◆ logbook or diary ◆ clippers (optional)

## Procedure

- Explain the procedure to the patient and address any questions or concerns he may have.
- As applicable, ask the patient if he has any allergies to adhesive tape, electrode gel, or alcohol.
- Place the equipment into the carrying case, and connect the neck strap.
- As appropriate, tell the patient that you need to clip the hairs on his chest so that you can place the electrodes properly. After clipping, wash the areas with soap and water to remove body oils.
- If the patient's skin is extremely oily, scaly, or diaphoretic, rub the electrode site with a dry 4" × 4" gauze pad or alcohol pad before applying the electrode.
- Connect the wires to the electrodes and to the monitor.
- Apply each electrode to the patient's chest by removing the paper backing, securing the edges of the electrode, and then pressing the center to ensure proper contact. (See *Placing electrodes for Holter monitoring.*)
- Place the strap over the patient's neck and position the unit comfortably. Make sure there isn't too much slack or pull on the cables because artifact may occur.

### Postprocedure patient teaching

- Tell the patient he'll need a follow-up appointment to review results 48 to 72 hours after removal of the monitor.
- Show the patient how to reattach loosened electrodes by de-

---

### Placing electrodes for Holter monitoring

This illustration shows you one method that is used to place electrodes with a 5-lead system. Make sure you place the electrodes over bone, not intercostal spaces. The two negative electrodes are placed on the manubrium. Positive electrodes are placed on the $V_1$ and $V_5$ positions. A ground electrode is placed at the lower right rib margin. Refer to your facility's policy or manufacturer instructions for preferred electrode placement.

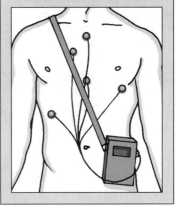

---

pressing the center, and tell him to return to the facility if an electrode becomes fully dislodged.

### Complications

- None known

### Special considerations

- If the patient can't return to the facility immediately after the monitoring period, show him how to remove the equipment and store the monitor and log.
- If the patient is wearing a patient-activated Holter monitor, tell

him that he can wear the monitor for up to 7 days. Tell him how to initiate the recording manually when symptoms occur.

## Documentation

- Document the indications for monitoring.
- Note the date and time the monitor was applied.
- Record the patient's medication regimen before monitoring.
- Include the patient's event log in documentation.
- Document postprocedure results and actions taken.

---

## HOME APNEA MONITORING

**CPT code**
*No specific code has been assigned.*

## Overview

Home apnea monitoring allows for detection of apneic breathing episodes and bradycardia. An alarm will sound when these events occur, alerting parents or caregivers. Home apnea monitoring requires that parents or caregivers be prepared to operate the equipment safely, correctly, and confidently.

## Indications

- To monitor infants who have experienced one or more episodes of prolonged apnea (cessation of breathing for at least 20 seconds or a briefer episode of apnea associated with bradycardia, cyanosis, or pallor) that isn't associated with a reversible etiology
- To monitor infants with continued apneic spells requiring prolonged, electronic, cardiorespiratory monitoring in the hospital who might otherwise be considered for home discharge
- To monitor infants who have a history of bronchopulmonary dysplasia or intraventricular hemorrhage
- To monitor infants who have a family history of siblings with sudden infant death syndrome (SIDS)

## Contraindications

- None known

## Preprocedure patient preparation

- Explain to parents or caregivers how monitoring equipment is used to detect episodes of apnea and bradycardia. Reiterate to parents that monitoring can't guarantee against SIDS.
- Instruct parents or caregivers on additional methods to decrease the risk of SIDS such as placing the infant on his back while sleeping.
- Emphasize to parents or caregivers the normal care and development of the infant.
- Have the parents or caregivers prepare their home and family for the equipment. Store the monitor on a sturdy, flat surface, and post emergency telephone numbers of the health care provider, equipment supplier, and ambulance in an accessible area.

## Equipment

Home monitoring equipment available through local home nursing care or medical supplies resource

➤ **CLINICAL TIP**

*Most authorities recommend monitoring both cardiac and respiratory function. Many different monitors are available. It's the health care provider's responsibility to prescribe equipment with demonstrated reliability. Some monitors also record oximetry, which may be helpful in distinguishing a true apneic spell from a false-positive alarm.*

## Procedure

■ Explain the procedure to the parents or caregivers, and address any questions or concerns they have.

■ Perform a thorough evaluation to identify and treat reversible causes of apnea.

■ If necessary, arrange for the setup of equipment through a local home nursing care or medical supplies resource.

■ Teach the parents and other caregivers how to operate the monitor, such as how to turn the unit on and how to attach the electrodes or band. Advise them to make sure the respiration indicator goes on each time the infant breathes. If it doesn't, describe troubleshooting techniques such as moving the electrodes slightly.

➤ **CLINICAL TIP**

*A representative from the monitor equipment company is usually available to review procedures with parents and other caregivers.*

■ Show the parents or caregivers how to respond to the apnea and bradycardia alarm. Direct them to check the color of the infant's oral tissues. If the tissues appear bluish and the infant isn't breathing, tell them to call loudly and touch him — gently at first, then move urgently as needed but not to shake the infant. If he doesn't respond, urge them to begin cardiopulmonary resuscitation (CPR).

■ Also, advise the parents or caregivers to keep the operator's manual attached to or beside the monitor and to consult it as needed. Explain that problems such as an activated loose-lead alarm may indicate a dirty electrode, a loose electrode patch, a loose belt, or a disconnected or malfunctioning wire monitor.

■ Develop, with the family, a care plan that includes periodic (at least monthly) physical, historical, developmental, and laboratory reassessment. Emphasize the need for continued monitoring or other interventions. Information from the monitor (frequency of alarms) should be downloaded periodically and reviewed by the health care provider.

■ Discontinue home monitoring when the infant is 12 months old or after the infant has been free from symptomatic apnea or apnea requiring intervention for at least three months.

## Performing infant CPR

Although the objective of cardiopulmonary resuscitation (CPR) in an infant is the same as for a child and an adult, the techniques for an infant vary. If bystanders are present, first tell someone to call emergency medical services. If you're alone, perform resuscitation measures for 1 minute; then call for help. You may move an uninjured infant close to a telephone if necessary.

### CLEAR THE AIRWAY

■ To remove an airway obstruction, place the infant facedown on your forearm, with his head lower than his trunk. Support your forearm on your thigh.
■ Use the heel of your free hand to deliver five blows between the infant's shoulder blades (as shown below). Back blows are safer than abdominal thrusts in infants because of the size of the infant's liver, the close proximity of vital organs, and the poor abdominal muscle tone.

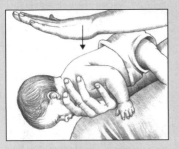

■ If the airway remains obstructed, sandwich the infant between your hands and forearms and flip him over onto his back.
■ Keeping the infant's head lower than his trunk, give five midsternal chest thrusts, using your middle and ring fingers only (as shown above right), to raise intrathoracic pressure enough to force a cough that will

expel the obstruction. Remember to hold the infant's head firmly to avoid injury.

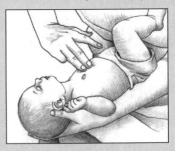

■ Repeat this sequence until the obstruction is dislodged or the infant loses consciousness.
*Caution:* Don't do a blind finger-sweep to discover or remove an obstruction. In an infant, this maneuver may push the object back into the airway and cause further obstruction. Only place your fingers in the infant's mouth to remove an object you can see.

### RESTORE CONSCIOUSNESS

■ If the infant loses consciousness, position him to open the airway. Deliver two breaths as described below.
■ If he doesn't regain consciousness, reposition his head and try breathing for him again. If this attempt fails, repeat the procedure for removing a foreign object.

## Postprocedure patient teaching

■ Teach parents how to perform infant CPR or provide them with a resource for appropriate instruction. (See *Performing infant CPR.*)

Teach other family members, such as older siblings, grandparents, and baby-sitters or other caregivers, how to use the monitor safely and perform CPR.
■ Instruct the parents and other caregivers in observation tech-

■ When the foreign object is removed, assess respirations and pulse. Continue revival efforts as needed.

### PROVIDE VENTILATION
■ Take a breath, and tightly seal your mouth over the infant's nose and mouth (as shown below).

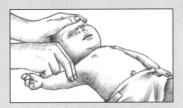

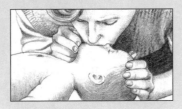

■ Deliver a gentle puff of air because an infant's lungs hold less air than an adult's. If the infant's chest rises and falls, the amount of air is probably adequate.

■ Continue rescue breathing with one breath every 3 seconds (20 breaths/minute) if you can detect a pulse.

### RESTORE HEARTBEAT AND CIRCULATION
■ Assess the infant's pulse by palpating the brachial artery located inside the upper arm between the elbow and shoulder (as shown above right). If you find a pulse, continue rescue breathing but don't initiate heart compressions.

■ Begin heart compressions if you find no pulse. To locate the infant's heart, draw an imaginary line between the infant's nipples. Place three fingers directly below — and perpendicular to — the nipple line. Then, lift up your index finger so that the middle and ring fingers lie one finger's width below the nipple line (as shown below). Use these two fingers to depress the sternum here $\frac{1}{3}$ to $\frac{1}{2}$ the depth of the chest at least 100 compressions/minute.

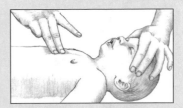

■ Supply one breath after every five compressions. Maintain this ratio whether you're the helper or the lone rescuer. This ratio allows for about 100 compressions and 20 breaths per minute for an infant.

niques, including techniques for observing the infant's color and breathing patterns and distinguishing between false and true apnea alarms.

■ Instruct the parents or caregivers to notify local service authorities, such as police, ambulance service, telephone company, and electric company, that their infant uses an apnea monitor so that alternative power can be supplied if a failure occurs.

## Complications

- False alarms may be triggered by loose or incorrect placement of the electrodes, improperly set sensitivity to respiratory activity, or movement by the infant.

## Special considerations

**COLLABORATION**

*If consultative resources and expertise aren't locally available, consider referral to a specialized infant evaluation center.*

- Respiratory or cardiorespiratory monitoring at home may be considered for infants born prematurely or with other conditions that necessitate at-home use of oxygen therapy or medications or infants who are at increased risk for SIDS. There's no reliable test to identify specific infants at risk for SIDS. Although SIDS is more common in premature infants, no clear relationship exists between SIDS and apnea. Home apnea monitoring is a controversial and unproven method for preventing SIDS.
- The need for home apnea monitoring can be a source of significant anxiety for parents. This may predispose a parent to hypervigilance, decreased nurturance, and possible abuse. The use of home electronic monitoring equipment when it isn't indicated should be avoided.
- Prolonged apnea can be a symptom of many disorders, including infection, seizures, airway abnormalities, hypoglycemia or other metabolic problems, anemia, gas-troesophageal reflux, impaired regulation of breathing during sleeping and feeding, and abuse. Diagnosis and treatment of these disorders may prevent the need for ongoing home monitoring.
- Because the infant with prolonged apnea requiring home monitoring has such a significant psychological impact on parents and siblings, the entire family should be evaluated and supported. Psychosocial and respite care should be available.

## Documentation

- Document the indications for home apnea monitoring.
- Record care and treatment plan, including the criteria for termination of monitoring.
- Document teaching to parents or caregivers regarding infant CPR, use of the equipment, and observation techniques.
- Document follow-up examinations, including historical and laboratory data and monitor downloads and the psychosocial status of the parents and family.

# *H*PV-DNA TESTING OF THE CERVIX

### *CPT code*

87621 *Infectious agent detection by nucleic acid (deoxyribonucleic acid [DNA] or ribonucleic acid [RNA]); papillomavirus, human, amplified probe technique*

## Overview

Human papillomavirus (HPV) is a widespread, sexually transmitted infection. Low-risk types of genital HPV can cause condyloma (genital warts). High-risk HPV types are present in almost all cervical carcinomas and precancerous lesions. HPV-DNA testing is used to detect the presence of HPV and differentiates between low- and high-risk types. Some studies have shown that the presence of HPV can be used to predict development of cervical carcinoma and that the type of HPV correlates with the risk of lesion progression. The only available HPV-DNA test is the Hybrid Capture HPV-DNA Assay.

## Indications

■ To investigate abnormal Papanicolaou (Pap) test results

## Contraindications

■ None known

## Preprocedure patient preparation

■ Explain why and how the procedure will be performed. Review the equipment used, applicable pelvic anatomy, and associated discomforts (cramping and bleeding).
■ Review the patient history and cervical cytology and biopsy results.

## Equipment

Cervical sampler containing a cervical brush and a tube with specimen transport medium ◆ vaginal speculum ◆ gloves ◆ light source ◆ drape

### Equipment preparation

■ Warm and lubricate the speculum with warm water.
■ Store cervical samplers at room temperature, and be sure to use them before the expiration date marked on the package.

## Procedure

■ Explain the procedure to the patient, and address any questions or concerns she may have.
■ Ensure that the patient has emptied her bladder.
■ Wash your hands.
■ Place the patient in the dorsal lithotomy position with her legs draped.
■ Adjust the light source so it's focused on the patient's external genitalia.
■ Put on gloves.
■ Visualize the cervix using the speculum, and observe for any abnormalities, including lesions and inflammation.
■ Gently insert the cervical brush into the endocervical canal. A few bristles should still be visible outside the cervix.
■ Rotate the cervical brush three full turns.
■ Remove the cervical brush, and insert it to the bottom of the transport tube.

- Snap off the shaft of the cervical brush at the score line, then cap the tube securely.
- Ensure that any bleeding occurring during endocervical sampling has stopped.
- Remove the speculum.
- Specimens may be stored at room temperature for up to 2 weeks.

➤ **CLINICAL TIP**
*When performing a Pap test and HPV-DNA testing at the same visit, conduct the Pap test first. When performing a colposcopy and HPV-DNA testing at the same visit, collect the HPV sample before acetic acid or other solution is applied.*

## Postprocedure patient teaching

- Tell the patient that she may experience bright red or brownish vaginal spotting after the procedure.
- Remind the patient that HPV-DNA testing doesn't diagnose cancer.
- Stress the importance of appropriate follow-up care.

## Complications

- Patients may experience mild cramping and bleeding during sample collection. Hemostasis of significant bleeding can be achieved by applying pressure or by using silver nitrate or Monsel's solution.

## Special considerations

- The specific Pap test abnormality for which HPV-DNA testing is indicated is controversial. HPV-DNA testing appears to be most useful in patients with atypical squamous cells of undetermined significance to determine the best management strategy for follow-up of this result.
- HPV-DNA testing should never be used in lieu of clinically warranted colposcopy.
- An HPV assay can be performed on cervical specimens rinsed in Cytyc PreservCyt Solution (the ThinPrep Pap test). Many laboratories offer reflex testing for HPV-DNA when specific abnormalities (of the health care provider's choosing) are identified on a Thin-Prep Pap test.

## Documentation

- Record the findings of the speculum examination, particularly noting abnormalities of the cervix such as difficulty entering the endocervical canal.
- Document that HPV-DNA testing was sent, including date, time collected, and which laboratory received the specimen.
- Document instructions given to the patient for follow-up care and her understanding of these.

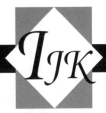

## INCONTINENCE EVALUATION, URINARY

### CPT codes
51725 *Simple cystometrogram (CMG)*
51736 *Simple uroflowmetry (UFR), such as stopwatch flow rate or mechanical flowmeter*
51795 *Voiding pressure studies (VP); bladder voiding pressure, any technique*

### Overview

Incontinence is an uncontrollable passage of urine resulting from either bladder abnormality or neurologic disorder. Incontinence is a common urologic sign that may be transient or permanent and may involve large volumes of urine or scant dribbling.

Incontinence is classified as stress, overflow, urge, or total incontinence. Stress incontinence refers to intermittent leakage resulting from a sudden physical strain, such as a cough, sneeze, or quick movement. Overflow incontinence is a dribble resulting from urine retention, which fills the bladder and prevents it from contracting with sufficient force to expel a urinary stream. Urge incontinence refers to the inability to suppress a sudden urge to urinate. Total incontinence is continuous leakage resulting from the bladder's inability to retain any urine.

If the patient's urinary incontinence developed within the last 2 weeks, causes of acute urinary incontinence should be ruled out, such as urinary tract infection, an adverse effect from medication, or vaginal infection, and appropriate treatment should be prescribed. For persistent urinary incontinence (present longer than 2 weeks), diagnostic evaluation includes assessment of lower urinary tract function through the stress maneuver, normal voiding, postvoid residual determination, bladder filling, repeat stress maneuver, and bladder emptying.

### Indications

■ To evaluate persistent urinary incontinence when the cause is unknown

## Contraindications

### ABSOLUTE

- Acute urinary incontinence
- An uncooperative patient
- A patient who can't be catheterized for urine

## Preprocedure patient preparation

- Obtain a complete history and physical examination and determine if the patient meets the indications for urine flow studies.
- Inform the patient that samples of urine obtained from the procedure will be sent for urinalysis and urine culture.
- Explain the entire procedure to the patient and discuss why it's necessary and how it will be performed (in a series of steps). Review the anatomy of the lower urinary tract.
- Tell the patient that he may feel pressure during the procedure but that the entire procedure should take only about 15 minutes.

## Equipment

Drape ◆ gloves ◆ antiseptic solution such as povidone-iodine ◆ sterile 4″ × 4″ gauze pads ◆ sterile catheter tray and 14 French straight catheter ◆ 50-ml syringe without needle ◆ 1 L of sterile water ◆ urine receptacle (bedpan or measuring "hat" for females or urinal for males) ◆ commode ◆ absorbent pads ◆ disposable 32-oz graduated cylinder

## Procedure

- Explain each step of the procedure to the patient as you perform it, and address any questions or concerns he may have.

☑ **OBTAIN INFORMED CONSENT**

- Wash your hands, and put on gloves.
- Obtain baseline vital signs.
- Provide privacy, and ask the patient to disrobe from the waist down and lie in a supine position on the examination table. Drape the patient appropriately.

### For a stress maneuver test

- Perform a stress maneuver test when the patient's bladder feels full; it can be done first or after the cystometry.
- Place the absorbent pad over the urethral area. Ask the patient to cough forcefully three times. Leakage of urine during the coughing confirms stress incontinence; prolonged leakage of urine that occurs after the coughing doesn't indicate stress incontinence.

➤ **CLINICAL TIP**
*If no urinary leakage occurs with coughing when the patient is in a supine position, repeat the procedure with the patient standing.*

### For a normal voiding test

- Clean the urethral area with povidone-iodine solution and gauze pads.
- Providing privacy, ask the patient to void into a measuring container (measuring "hat" or graduated urinal) over a commode. Determine the approximate urine flow rate by dividing the amount

of urine voided by the time required to void. The normal urine flow rate is 15 to 20 ml/second. Hesitancy, straining, or intermittent urine stream while voiding may indicate an obstruction.

### For a postvoid residual determination test

■ Assist a female patient to the supine position over a fractured bedpan and a male patient to the supine position with a urinal positioned to catch leakage.
■ Within 5 to 10 minutes after the patient has voided, perform a sterile straight catheterization using a 14 French catheter and the catheter kit. Measure residual urine volume. The bladder normally retains approximately 50 ml of urine; greater than 100 ml after voiding indicates an obstruction or contractility problem.

⮕ CLINICAL TIP
*Inability to insert the catheter may be caused by bladder obstruction.*

■ Send the collected urine specimen for urinalysis and urine culture.

### For a bladder filling test

■ After all urine is drained from the bladder, leave the catheter in place.
■ Remove the plunger of the 50-ml syringe, and attach the syringe to the end of the catheter to act as a funnel. Position the syringe approximately 15 cm above the urethra.
■ Gradually fill the bladder by allowing 50 ml at a time of room temperature sterile water to flow

in by gravity (keeping track of how much water you instill).
■ Continue to fill until the patient expresses feeling an urge to void. After that point, fill by only 25 ml increments until the patient feels unable to hold any more urine; however, don't exceed filling 500 ml of water into the bladder. Then remove the catheter. Feelings of urgency to urinate at a low bladder volume (less than 300 ml) may indicate urge incontinence.

### Repeat stress maneuver test

■ Ask the patient to forcefully cough three times while in a supine position and then three times when standing to recheck for stress incontinence or to perform this test if the patient's bladder wasn't full for the first stress maneuver.

### For a bladder emptying test

■ Ask the patient to void into a measuring container, and measure the amount of urine. Subtract this from the amount of water instilled. The result is the amount of postvoid residual urine left in the bladder. Compare this value with the result from the postvoid residual determination step.

## Postprocedure patient teaching

■ Provide teaching and further treatment based on the results of your clinical findings and test results.
■ Teach the patient signs and symptoms of a urinary tract infection (increased urinary frequency, burning, pain, or further inconti-

## Correcting incontinence with bladder retraining

The incontinent patient typically feels frustrated, embarrassed and, sometimes, hopeless. Fortunately, however, his problem can often be corrected by bladder retraining — a program that aims to establish a regular voiding pattern. Here are some guidelines for establishing such a program:

■ Before you start the program, assess the patient's intake pattern, voiding pattern, and behavior (for example, restlessness or talkativeness) before each voiding episode.

■ Encourage the patient to use the toilet 30 minutes before he's usually incontinent. If this isn't successful, readjust the schedule. Once he can stay dry for 2 hours, increase the time between voidings by 30 minutes each day until he achieves a 3- to 4-hour voiding schedule.

■ When your patient voids, make sure that the sequence of conditioning stimuli is always the same.

■ Ensure that the patient has privacy while voiding — any inhibiting stimuli should be avoided.

■ Keep a record of continence and incontinence for 5 days — this may reinforce your patient's efforts to remain continent.

**CLUES TO SUCCESS**

Remember, a positive attitude for you and your patient is crucial to his successful bladder retraining. Here are some additional tips that may help your patient succeed:

■ Make sure the patient is close to a bathroom or portable toilet. Leave a light on at night.

■ If your patient needs assistance getting out of his bed or chair, promptly answer his call for help.

■ Encourage him to wear his accustomed clothing, as an indication that you're confident he can remain continent. Acceptable alternatives to diapers include condoms for the male patient and incontinence pads or panties for the female patient.

■ Encourage him to drink 2,000 to 2,500 ml of fluid each day. Less fluid doesn't prevent incontinence but does promote bladder infection. Limiting his fluid intake after 5 p.m., however, will help him remain continent during the night.

■ Reassure your patient that any episodes of incontinence don't signal a failure of the program. Encourage him to maintain a persistent, tolerant attitude.

nence), and tell him to notify your facility if these symptoms occur.

## Complications

■ Urinary tract infection is rare after these procedures, but make sure the patient is aware of the signs and symptoms of infection.

## Special considerations

■ Have the patient keep a daily bladder log for 1 week to obtain more information about the amount of fluids consumed and voided and the frequency of incontinence.

■ Begin management of incontinence by implementing a bladder retraining program. (See *Correcting incontinence with bladder retraining*.)

■ To help prevent stress incontinence, teach the patient exercises to strengthen the pelvic floor muscles.

## Documentation

- Record findings from the history and physical examination.
- Document the patient's tolerance of the procedures, complaints of discomfort, the amount of sterile water instilled (if applicable), a description of the urine voided, and any samples sent for laboratory testing.
- Record instructions given to the patient and statements indicating understanding of them.

# *I*NGROWN TOENAIL CARE

### *CPT codes*
11730 *Avulsion of nail plate, partial or complete, simple; single*
11732 *Avulsion of each additional nail plate*
11750 *Excision of nail and nail matrix, partial or complete*

## Overview

An ingrown toenail is a common condition that can cause a great deal of disability and discomfort for the patient. It occurs when the proper fit of the toenail into the lateral nail groove is altered. The great toe is generally the only one affected, and the problem may occur on either the medial or lateral aspect of the toe. Causes include:
- improperly fitting shoes
- toenails cut at an inappropriate angle (rounded rather than flat)

- accumulation of debris under the nail
- congenital malformation of the great toenail (an autosomal dominant trait)
- curling or deformity of the nail caused by trauma or excessive length.

A splinter or small piece of the great toenail invades the sulcus and subcutaneous tissue, resulting in inflammation of the surrounding area. This leads to callous formation, edema, and perforation into the nail groove as a result of rubbing. The nail edge becomes imbedded in the lateral skin fold, causing pain, erythema and, ultimately, infection. Either partial or total removal of the toenail is commonly indicated at this point.

The three stages of this disorder must be understood to develop a sound treatment plan:
- Stage I is characterized by tenderness on palpation and when wearing shoes, erythema, and slight swelling at the site (paronychia).
- Stage II is associated with erythema, tenderness with associated suppuration, and a small collection of pus.
- Stage III is characterized by all of the above signs and symptoms, plus hypertrophy of the nail wall and granulation tissue formation.

Each stage requires a different approach to care. Stage I warrants conservative management with toenail elevation and wicking. Stage II may require partial toenail removal in the facility (as described in this procedure). Stage III should be referred to a health care provider with expertise in this area for more aggressive treatment under appropriate sedation or anesthesia.

## Indications

■ To treat ingrown toenail, medial or lateral aspect (onychocryptosis); chronic, recurrent inflammation of the nail fold (paronychia); or deformed or curved nail (onychogryposis)

## Contraindications

**ABSOLUTE**

■ Coagulopathies likely to inhibit hemostasis
■ Allergy to local anesthetics
■ Use of phenol solution in pregnancy

**RELATIVE**

■ Diabetes mellitus (may refer to a health care provider with expertise in this area)
■ Peripheral vascular disease
■ Immunocompromised status
■ Peripheral neuropathy

## Preprocedure patient preparation

■ Obtain a detailed history, and conduct a physical examination.
■ Position the patient comfortably on the examination table.

## Equipment

### Conservative management (stage I)

Splinter forceps or disposable tweezers ◆ nail file ◆ cotton for packing (3 mm × 2.5 mm) ◆ tincture of iodine or 60% alcohol solution (optional) ◆ scissors ◆ gloves ◆ antiseptic, germicidal solution such as povidone-iodine ◆ a basin for soaking the foot ◆ dressing material and tape ◆ antibiotic ointment

### Partial toenail removal (stage II)

Equipment above plus: narrow periosteal elevator (nail elevator) ◆ english nail splitter or sterile scissors with straight blades ◆ phenol solution (88%) or 60% alcohol solution (optional) ◆ sterile drapes ◆ two sterile straight hemostats ◆ local anesthetic such as lidocaine without epinephrine ◆ rubber band or Penrose drain ◆ 5-ml syringe with 1" 27G or 25G needle ◆ alcohol pads

## Procedure

■ Explain the procedure to the patient, and address any questions or concerns he may have.
■ Verify that the patient isn't allergic to latex and iodine.
■ Soak the affected foot in an antiseptic, germicidal solution.
■ Wash your hands.

### For conservative management

■ Have the patient lie comfortably with knees flexed and feet flat on the examination table. Put on gloves.
■ Thin the middle-third of the nail on the affected side by filing the upper surface until you can see the nail matrix.
■ Using scissors, cut cotton to proper length. Stretch and roll the

cotton to form a wick. (See *Using conservative management.*)

■ Optional: Soak cotton in a 60% alcohol or tincture of iodine solution to prevent infection.

■ Lift the nail edge using forceps, and gently push the wick firmly under the distal portion of the affected lateral nail groove.

■ Apply antibiotic ointment to the infected cuticle edge.

■ Tape the cotton wick to prevent displacement (tape the lateral edge between the first and second toes to prevent irritation; tape the medial edge to the medial aspect of the toe to prevent rubbing from shoes).

■ Cover with a dressing.

### *For partial toenail removal*

☑ **OBTAIN INFORMED CONSENT**

■ Put on gloves, and drape the foot with a sterile drape.

■ Administer a digital block to the affected toe. (See "Anesthesia: topical, local, and digital nerve block," page 20.) Massage the area gently. The maximum effect should occur in 5 to 15 minutes.

➤ **CLINICAL TIP**
*Always ensure that the local anesthetic doesn't contain epinephrine; failure to do so can lead to vasoconstriction and tissue hypoxia.*

■ When adequate anesthesia is attained (usually in 5 to 15 minutes), wrap a rubber band or Penrose drain securely around the proximal toe as a tourniquet (optional).

■ Remove the affected portion of the nail. (See *Removing part of a nail*, page 266.)

## Using conservative management

An ingrown toenail in stage I usually requires conservative management. Using forceps, lift the nail away from the inflamed soft tissue. Gently push a cotton wick under the nail and leave in place for 1 week; replace as indicated. This allows the edema and inflammation to resolve and the nail to grow out in a normal manner.

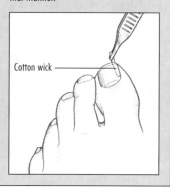

Cotton wick

■ Examine the nail bed and remove any debris.

■ Remove the tourniquet, if used. Never leave the tourniquet in place for more than 10 minutes.

■ Apply antibiotic ointment to the nail bed, and then cover with a sterile dressing. Cut to proper size with scissors.

■ Optional: Use phenol to cauterize the matrix where the nail was removed.

## Postprocedure patient teaching

■ Inform the patient that serosanguineous drainage should be minimal within 24 hours and that pain

## Removing part of a nail

Partial nail removal (partial avulsion) is indicated for more advanced cases of paronychia.

Administer a digital block proximal to the toenail on the outer edge of the toe, inserting the needle toward the plantar surface on the affected side.

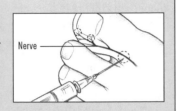

Nerve

Use a gauze pad to separate the toes. Loosen and lift the affected nail edge, using the periosteal elevator or hemostat. Introduce and advance the elevator, applying upward pressure against the nail (freeing the nail sulcus and eponychium from the nail plate) and away from the nail bed to minimize bleeding and injury.

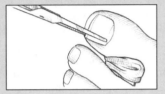

Using the nail splitter or sterile scissors, wedge off a 2- to 3-mm section of the affected nail. Then use the nail elevator to free the wedge from the nail bed. Grasp the nail wedge with a hemostat. In one steady, continuous movement, pull the wedge out while simultaneously twisting toward the affected side of the toe.

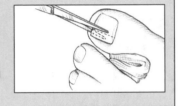

should be well controlled with nonnarcotic analgesia and foot elevation. Explain that sterile exudate may be present for up to 4 weeks, that the toe should be fully healed in 4 to 6 weeks, and that complete nail regrowth takes 8 to 12 months in an adult.

■ Instruct the patient to rest the affected foot and elevate it for 24 hours.

■ Advise him to change the dressing in 24 hours and to observe for signs of infection (redness, swelling, pain, and purulent drainage).

■ Instruct him to begin ambulation with open-toed shoes or sandals after 24 hours and to wear

only this type of shoe for 2 weeks. Have him avoid tight or poorly fitting footwear at all times.

■ Teach him proper wound care. Tell him to soak the toe in warm water for 20 minutes twice daily for 4 days, to dry the toe and apply a thin layer of antibiotic ointment to the toe's affected edge, to reapply nail packing (if used) after each soaking, and to keep a bandage on the toe until it heals.

■ Advise the patient to take acetaminophen or ibuprofen as directed for pain.

■ Instruct him to avoid running or strenuous activity for 2 weeks.

■ Urge him to notify you promptly if he experiences chills, fever higher than 100° F (37.8° C), pus, foul-smelling odor, increased warmth or red streaks, bleeding after the first 48 hours, pain unrelieved by acetaminophen or ibuprofen, or a return of symptoms as the nail regrows.

■ Encourage him to schedule a follow-up appointment in 1 week for evaluation of the wound, including a neurosensory evaluation.

## Complications

■ Infection is treated with antimicrobial soaks and antibiotics.

■ Excessive bleeding may be cauterized with handheld cautery or silver nitrate sticks. Refer the patient to a physician or an acute care center if you can't control the bleeding.

■ Nail regrowth with paronychia is treated with a repeat procedure.

## Special considerations

■ Many patients don't realize how long it takes to clear paronychia. They may stop treatment when results aren't evident in 1 or 2 months. Before initiating treatment and with each visit, reinforce that the nail takes 1 year to regrow.

## Documentation

■ Before performing this procedure, document any abnormal physical findings on the consent form. Have the patient initial the comments and sign the form to signify acknowledgment of preprocedural abnormalities. In the chart, the preprocedural and postprocedural note must include an evaluation of potentially affected function, range of motion, and sensation.

■ In documenting the patient's consent to the procedure, note that you discussed treatment options, duration of treatment, and the significant risk for recurrence of infection.

■ If applicable, indicate the type, amount, and placement of local anesthesia administered; the needle gauge used; and the patient's reaction to the injection.

■ Record the time of tourniquet placement and removal.

■ Describe the wound appearance (including amount of bleeding) after the procedure.

■ Note discharge instructions explained to the patient and family.

# Inguinal Hernia Reduction

### CPT code
*No specific code has been assigned.*

## Overview

In inguinal hernia, the large or small intestine, omentum, or bladder protrudes into the inguinal canal. An inguinal hernia may be indirect or direct. An indirect inguinal hernia, the more common form, results from weakness in the fascial margin of the internal inguinal ring. In an indirect hernia, abdominal viscera protrudes from the abdomen through the inguinal ring and follows the spermatic cord (in males) or round ligament (in females); they emerge at the external ring and extend down the inguinal canal, commonly into the scrotum or labia. An indirect inguinal hernia may develop at any age, is three times more common in males, and is especially prevalent in infants younger than age 1.

A direct hernia results from weakness in the fascial floor of the inguinal canal. Instead of entering the canal through the internal ring, the hernia passes through the posterior inguinal wall, protrudes directly through the transverse fascia of the canal (in an area known as Hesselbach's triangle), and comes out at the external ring.

In males, during the 7th month of gestation, the testicle normally descends into the scrotum, preceded by the peritoneal sac. If the sac closes improperly, it leaves an opening through which the intestine can slip. In either sex, a hernia can result from weak abdominal muscles (caused by congenital malformation, trauma, or aging) or increased intra-abdominal pressure (caused by heavy lifting, pregnancy, obesity, or straining).

An inguinal hernia may be reduced if it can be manipulated back into place with relative ease. An incarcerated inguinal hernia can't be reduced because adhesions have formed, obstructing the intestinal flow. A strangulated hernia occurs when part of the herniated intestine becomes twisted or edematous, seriously interfering with normal blood flow and peristalsis and, possibly, leading to intestinal obstruction and necrosis. An incarcerated hernia can become strangulated, requiring surgery for repair. A strangulated hernia necessitates immediate surgery.

## Indications
- To temporarily push herniated contents back into place to avoid incarceration or strangulation
- To relieve the sharp, steady pain caused by herniation

## Contraindications
**ABSOLUTE**
- Strangulated hernia (patient appears ill and has severe pain, an irreducible mass in the groin, and diminished bowel sounds)

## Preprocedure patient preparation
- Assess the herniated area. A large hernia appears as an obvious swelling or lump in the inguinal area; with a small hernia, the affected area may simply appear full. Palpation of the inguinal area while the patient is performing Valsalva's maneuver confirms the diagnosis.

## Equipment
Gloves ◆ narcotic analgesic or muscle relaxant (optional)

## Procedure
- Explain the procedure to the patient, and address any questions or concerns he may have.

- Wash your hands.
- Assist the patient to the Trendelenburg position. Have him bend his knees slightly to decrease abdominal muscle tension.
- Encourage the patient to relax, and allow 30 minutes for passive reduction to occur. In passive reduction, the herniated contents slip back into place by gravity.

▶ CLINICAL TIP
*Consider administering a narcotic analgesic or muscle relaxant to aid passive reduction. Monitor the patient closely if either of these is administered.*

- If passive reduction fails, attempt active reduction. Put on gloves, and encourage the patient to remain relaxed. With your dominant hand, gently guide the herniated contents back through the external ring. Use your nondominant hand to aid in compressing and guiding the herniated contents.
- If the patient is an infant or child, surgical repair is necessary following passive or active reduction. An adult patient should consider elective surgical repair following passive or active reduction.

## Postprocedure patient teaching

- Warn the patient against lifting heavy objects or straining during bowel movements.
- Instruct the patient to drink plenty of fluids to maintain hydration and prevent constipation.
- If surgery might be hazardous (such as in an elderly or debilitated patient) or while awaiting an elective repair, the patient may wear a truss to keep the abdominal contents from protruding into the hernial sac. Tell him to bathe daily and apply liberal amounts of cornstarch or baby powder to prevent skin irritation. Warn against applying the truss over clothing.
- Teach the patient the signs and symptoms of intestinal obstruction, such as anorexia, vomiting, and pain and tenderness in the groin. If these symptoms occur, tell the patient to notify your facility or go to the emergency department immediately.

## Complications

- Intestinal obstruction or strangulation can occur after passive or active reduction if the hernia reprotrudes, in which case, surgical repair is immediately necessary.

## Special considerations

- Surgical repair consists of either herniorrhaphy or hernioplasty. In herniorrhaphy, the contents of the hernial sac are replaced into the abdominal cavity and the opening is closed. In hernioplasty, the weakened area is reinforced with steel mesh, fascia, or wire.
- If bowel obstruction is suspected, X-rays and a white blood cell count (which may be elevated) are required.

## Documentation

- Record the patient's medical history and physical examination findings. Document the indica-

tions for the procedure, medications administered, and the patient's toleration of the procedure.
■ Document any further treatment plans such as surgery.
■ Document instructions given to the patient and teaching.

# INJECTION, INTRADERMAL

### CPT code
90799 *Unlisted therapeutic, prophylactic, or diagnostic injection*

## Overview

Intradermal injections are administered in small volumes (usually 0.5 ml or less) into the outer layers of the skin. They're used primarily for diagnostic purposes because little systemic absorption takes place.

The ventral forearm is the most commonly used site for intradermal injection because of its easy accessibility and lack of hair. In extensive allergy testing, the outer aspect of the upper arms may be used as well as the area of the back located between the scapulae. (See *Intradermal injection sites.*)

## Indications

■ To administer agents requiring little systemic absorption; this type of injection is used primarily to produce a local effect, such as in allergy or tuberculin testing

## Contraindications

■ Dependent on agent being injected

## Preprocedure patient preparation

■ Tell the patient he'll feel a prick when the needle is inserted in the skin, but that discomfort will be minimal after the injection.
■ Show him where you'll be giving the injection.

## Equipment

Tuberculin syringe with a 26G or 27G ½″ to ⅜″ needle ♦ medication to be injected ♦ gloves ♦ alcohol pads

### Equipment preparation
■ Verify the medication order on the patient's record. Note whether the patient has any allergies.
■ Inspect the medication to make sure it isn't abnormally discolored or cloudy and doesn't contain precipitates.
■ Check the medication against the patient's record, and read the label again as you draw up the medication for injection.

## Procedure

■ Explain the procedure to the patient and address any questions or concerns he may have.
■ Wash your hands, and put on gloves.
■ Instruct the patient to sit up and to extend his arm and support it

on a flat surface, with the ventral forearm exposed.

■ With an alcohol pad, clean the surface of the ventral forearm about two or three fingers' width distal to the antecubital space. Make sure the test site you have chosen is free from hair or blemishes. Allow the skin to dry completely before administering the injection.

■ While holding the patient's forearm in your hand, stretch the skin taut with your thumb.

■ With your free hand, hold the needle at a 10- to 15-degree angle to the patient's arm, with its bevel up.

■ Insert the needle about ⅛″ (0.3 cm) below the epidermis at sites 2″ (5 cm) apart. Stop when the needle's bevel tip is under the skin, and inject the antigen slowly. You should feel some resistance as you do this, and a wheal should form as you inject the antigen. (See *Giving an intradermal injection,* page 272.)

**CLINICAL TIP**
*If no wheal forms, you have injected the antigen too deeply; withdraw the needle, and administer another test dose at least 2″ from the first site.*

■ Withdraw the needle at the same angle at which it was inserted. Don't rub the site. This could irritate the underlying tissue, which may affect test results.

■ Circle each test site with a marking pen, and label each site according to the recall antigen given. Instruct the patient to refrain from washing off the circles until the test is completed.

## Intradermal injection sites

The most common intradermal injection site is the ventral forearm. Other sites (indicated by dotted areas) include the upper chest, upper arm, and shoulder blades. Skin in these areas is usually lightly pigmented, thinly keratinized, and relatively hairless, facilitating detection of adverse reactions.

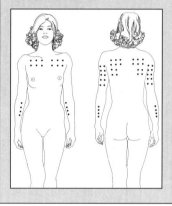

■ Dispose of needles and syringes according to your facility's policy.

■ Remove and discard your gloves, and wash your hands.

## Postprocedure patient teaching

■ Instruct the patient to return to the facility in 24 to 48 hours to assess his response to the skin testing.

## Complications

■ In patients who are hypersensitive to the test antigens, a severe anaphylactic response can result. This requires immediate epineph-

## Giving an intradermal injection

Secure the forearm. Insert the needle at a 10- to 15-degree angle so that it just punctures the skin's surface. The antigen should raise a small wheal as it's injected.

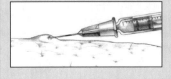

rine injection and other emergency resuscitation procedures.

## Special considerations

■ Be especially alert for signs and symptoms of an anaphylactic response after giving a test dose of penicillin or tetanus antitoxin.

## Documentation

■ Record the type and amount of medication given, the time it was given, and the injection site.
■ Note skin reactions and other adverse reactions.

# *Injection, intramuscular*

## CPT codes
90782 *Therapeutic, prophylactic, or diagnostic injection (specify material); subcutaneous or intramuscular*

90788 *Intramuscular injection of antibiotic (specify)*

## Overview

I.M. injections deposit medication deep into muscle tissue. This route of administration provides rapid systemic action and absorption of relatively large doses (up to 5 ml in appropriate sites). Because muscle tissue has few sensory nerves, I.M. injection allows less painful administration of irritating drugs.

The site for an I.M. injection must be chosen carefully, taking into account the patient's general physical status and the purpose of the injection. I.M. injections require sterile technique to maintain the integrity of muscle tissue.

## Indications

■ To administer medications requiring rapid systemic action or absorption of relatively large doses (up to 5 ml) as indicated
■ To administer medications for patients who can't take medication orally, when I.V. administration is inappropriate, or for drugs that are altered by digestive juices

## Contraindications
### ABSOLUTE
■ Not to be given at inflamed, edematous, or irritated sites, or at sites that contain moles, birthmarks, scar tissue, or other lesions

### RELATIVE
■ Impaired coagulation mechanisms, occlusive peripheral vascu-

lar disease, edema, and shock; after thrombolytic therapy; and during an acute myocardial infarction because these conditions impair peripheral absorption

■ Oral or I.V. routes are preferred for administration of drugs that are poorly absorbed by muscle tissue, such as phenytoin, digoxin, chlordiazepoxide, and diazepam

## Preprocedure patient preparation

■ Tell the patient he'll feel a prick when the needle is inserted in the skin, but that discomfort will be minimal after the injection. (This is dependent on the agent being injected. Some agents, such as tetanus toxoid, can cause soreness at the site for several days after the injection.)

■ Show him where you'll be giving the injection.

■ If the patient has experienced pain or emotional trauma from repeated injections, consider numbing the area before cleaning it by holding ice on it for several seconds. If you must inject more than 5 ml of solution, divide the solution and inject it at two separate sites.

■ Always encourage the patient to relax the muscle you'll be injecting because injections into tense muscles are more painful than usual and may bleed more readily.

## Equipment

Medication as indicated ◆ diluent or filter needle, if needed ◆ 3- or 5-ml syringe ◆ 20G to 25G 1″ to

3″ needle ◆ gloves ◆ alcohol pads ◆ gauze pad, 1″ tape, and ice (optional)

### *Equipment preparation*

■ Verify the medication order on the patient's record. Note whether the patient has any allergies.

■ Inspect the medication to make sure it isn't abnormally discolored or cloudy and doesn't contain precipitates.

■ The prescribed medication must be sterile.

■ Determine appropriate needle length. Needle length depends on the injection site, the patient's size, and the amount of subcutaneous fat covering the muscle. A larger needle gauge accommodates viscous solutions and suspensions.

■ Check the medication against the patient's record, and read the label again as you draw up the medication for injection.

■ Wipe the stopper of the vial with alcohol, and draw the prescribed amount of medication into the syringe.

## Procedure

■ Explain the procedure to the patient, and address any questions or concerns he may have.

■ Wash your hands, and select an appropriate injection site. The gluteal muscles (gluteus medius and minimus and the upper outer corner of the gluteus maximus) are most commonly used for healthy adults, although the deltoid muscle may be used for a small-volume injection (2 ml or less). Remember to rotate injection sites for patients who require repeated injections.

**◢▶ CLINICAL TIP**
*For infants and children, the vastus lateralis muscle of the thigh is used most commonly because it's usually better developed and contains no large nerves or blood vessels, minimizing the risk of serious injury. The rectus femoris muscle may also be used in infants but is usually contraindicated in adults.*

■ Position and drape the patient appropriately, making sure the site is well exposed and that lighting is adequate.

■ Loosen the protective needle sheath, but don't remove it.

■ After selecting the injection site, gently tap it to stimulate the nerve endings and minimize pain when the needle is inserted. (See *Locating I.M. injection sites.*) Clean the skin at the site with an alcohol pad. Move the pad outward in a circular motion to a circumference of about 2″ (5 cm) from the injection site, and allow the skin to dry. Keep the alcohol pad for later use.

■ Put on gloves. With the thumb and index finger of your nondominant hand, gently stretch the skin of the injection site taut.

■ While you hold the syringe in your dominant hand, remove the needle sheath by slipping it between the free fingers of your nondominant hand and then drawing back the syringe.

■ Position the syringe at a 90-degree angle to the skin surface with the needle a couple of inches from the skin. Tell the patient that he'll feel a prick as you insert the needle. Then quickly and firmly

thrust the needle through the skin and subcutaneous tissue, deep into the muscle.

■ Support the syringe with your nondominant hand, if desired. Pull back slightly on the plunger with your dominant hand to aspirate for blood. If no blood appears, slowly inject the medication into the muscle. A slow, steady injection rate allows the muscle to distend gradually and accept the medication under minimal pressure. You should feel little or no resistance against the force of the injection.

■ If blood appears in the syringe on aspiration, the needle is in a blood vessel. If this occurs, stop the injection, withdraw the needle, prepare another injection with new equipment, and inject another site. Don't inject the bloody solution.

■ After the injection, gently but quickly remove the needle at a 90-degree angle.

■ Using a gloved hand, cover the injection site immediately with the used alcohol pad, apply gentle pressure and, unless contraindicated, massage the relaxed muscle to help distribute the drug.

■ Remove the alcohol pad, and inspect the injection site for signs of active bleeding or bruising. If bleeding continues, apply pressure to the site; if bruising occurs, you may apply ice.

■ Watch for adverse reactions at the site for 10 to 30 minutes after the injection.

**◢▶ CLINICAL TIP**
*An elderly patient is likely to experience bleeding or oozing from*

# Locating I.M. injection sites

## DELTOID
Find the lower edge of the acromial process and the point on the lateral arm in line with the axilla. Insert the needle 1″ to 2″ (2.5 to 5 cm) below the acromial process, usually two or three fingers' width, at a 90-degree angle or angled slightly toward the process. Typical injection: 0.5 ml (range: 0.5 to 2.0 ml).

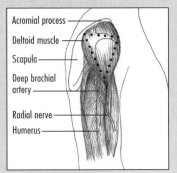

Acromial process
Deltoid muscle
Scapula
Deep brachial artery
Radial nerve
Humerus

## DORSOGLUTEAL
Inject above and outside a line drawn from the posterior superior iliac spine to the greater trochanter of the femur. Or, divide the buttock into quadrants and inject in the upper outer quadrant, about 2″ to 3″ (5 to 7.5 cm) below the iliac crest. Insert the needle at a 90-degree angle. Typical injection: 1 to 4 ml (range: 1 to 5 ml).

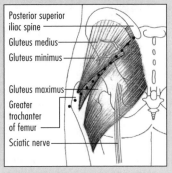

Posterior superior iliac spine
Gluteus medius
Gluteus minimus
Gluteus maximus
Greater trochanter of femur
Sciatic nerve

## VENTROGLUTEAL
Locate the greater trochanter of the femur with the heel of your hand. Then spread your index and middle fingers from the anterior superior iliac spine to as far along the iliac crest as you can reach. Insert the needle between the two fingers at a 90-degree angle to the muscle. (Remove your fingers before inserting the needle.) Typical injection: 1 to 4 ml (range: 1 to 5 ml).

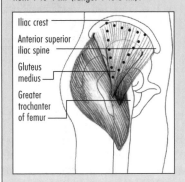

Iliac crest
Anterior superior iliac spine
Gluteus medius
Greater trochanter of femur

## VASTUS LATERALIS
Use the lateral muscle of the quadriceps group, from a hands' width below the greater trochanter to a hands' width above the knee. Insert the needle into the middle third of the muscle parallel to the surface on which the patient is lying. You may have to bunch the muscle before insertion. Typical injection: 1 to 4 ml (range: adults, 1 to 5 ml; infants, 1 to 3 ml).

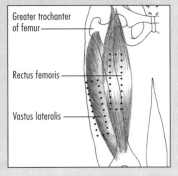

Greater trochanter of femur
Rectus femoris
Vastus lateralis

*the site after the injection because of decreased tissue elasticity. In this case, apply a small pressure bandage.*

■ Discard all equipment according to standard precautions and your facility's policy. Don't recap needles; dispose of them in an appropriate sharps container to avoid needle-stick injuries.

## Postprocedure patient teaching

■ Tell the patient he may apply ice to the site if soreness is present, as indicated. Also tell him adverse effects of the medication administered, as appropriate.

■ Teach the patient to monitor the injection site for signs and symptoms of local infection (such as redness, swelling, and yellow or green drainage), which can occur any time the skin is punctured. He should notify your facility if any of these occur.

## Complications

■ Accidental injection of concentrated or irritating medications into subcutaneous tissue or other areas where they can't be fully absorbed can cause sterile abscesses to develop. These abscesses result from the body's natural immune response in which phagocytes attempt to remove the foreign matter.

■ Failure to rotate sites in patients who require repeated injections can lead to deposits of unabsorbed medications. These deposits can reduce the desired pharmacologic

effect and may lead to abscess formation or tissue fibrosis.

## Special considerations

■ To slow their absorption, some drugs for I.M. administration are dissolved in oil or other special solutions. Mix these preparations well before drawing them into the syringe.

■ The gluteal muscles can be used as the injection site in a toddler only after he has been walking for about 1 year.

■ Never inject into sensitive muscles, especially those that twitch or tremble when you assess site landmarks and tissue depth. Injections into these trigger areas may cause sharp or referred pain such as the pain caused by nerve trauma.

■ Keep a rotation record that lists all available injection sites, divided into various body areas, for patients who require repeated injections. Rotate from a site in the first area to a site in each of the other areas. Then return to a site in the first area that is at least 1″ (2.5 cm) away from the previous injection site in that area.

■ I.M. injections can damage local muscle cells, causing elevation of serum enzyme levels (creatine kinase [CK]) that can be confused with the elevation resulting from cardiac muscle damage such as in myocardial infarction. To distinguish between skeletal and cardiac muscle damage, diagnostic tests for suspected myocardial infarction must identify the isoenzyme of CK specific to cardiac muscle (CK-MB) and include tests to determine lactate dehydrogenase and aspartate aminotransferase levels. If it's important to measure these enzyme levels, consider switching to I.V. administration and adjust dosages accordingly.

■ Dosage adjustments are usually necessary when changing from the I.M. route to the oral route.

■ Because elderly patients have decreased muscle mass, I.M. medications can be absorbed more quickly than expected.

## Documentation

■ Chart the drug administered, dose, date, time, route of administration, and injection site.

■ Note the patient's tolerance of the injection and the injection's effects, including any adverse effects.

# INJECTION, SUBCUTANEOUS

## CPT code

90782 *Therapeutic, prophylactic, or diagnostic injection (specify material); subcutaneous or intramuscular*

## Overview

When injected into the adipose (fatty) tissue beneath the skin, a drug moves into the bloodstream more rapidly than if given by mouth. Subcutaneous (S.C.) injection allows slower, more sustained drug administration than I.M. injection; it also causes minimal tissue trauma and carries little risk of striking large blood vessels and nerves.

Absorbed mainly through the capillaries, drugs recommended for S.C. injection include nonirritating aqueous solutions and suspensions contained in 0.5 to 2 ml of fluid. Heparin and insulin, for example, are usually administered S.C. (Some patients with diabetes, however, may benefit from an insulin infusion pump.)

Drugs and solutions for S.C. injection are injected through a relatively short needle, using a meticulous sterile technique. The most common S.C. injection sites are the outer aspect of the upper arm, anterior thigh, loose tissue of the lower abdomen, upper hips, buttocks, and upper back. (See *Locating subcutaneous injection sites,* page 278.)

## Indications

■ To administer an injection allowing for slower, more sustained drug administration than I.M. injection, as indicated

## Contraindications

### ABSOLUTE

■ Sites that are inflamed, edematous, scarred, or covered by a mole, birthmark, or other lesion

### RELATIVE

■ Impaired coagulation mechanisms

## Locating subcutaneous injection sites

Subcutaneous (S.C.) injection sites (as indicated by the dotted areas shown below) include the fat pads on the abdomen, upper hips, upper back, and lateral upper arms and thighs. For S.C. injections administered repeatedly, such as insulin, rotate sites. Choose one injection site in one area, move to a corresponding injection site in the next area, and so on.

When returning to an area, choose a new site in that area. Preferred injection sites for insulin are the arms, abdomen, thighs, and buttocks. The preferred injection site for heparin is the lower abdominal fat pad just below the umbilicus.

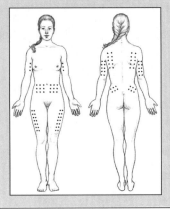

## Preprocedure patient preparation

■ Tell the patient he'll feel a prick when the needle is inserted in the skin, but that discomfort will be minimal after the injection.
■ Show him where you'll be giving the injection.

## Equipment

Medication for injection ◆ 25G to 27G ⅝″ to ½″ needle ◆ gloves ◆ 1- or 3-ml syringe ◆ alcohol pads ◆ antiseptic cleaning agent, filter needle, and insulin syringe (optional)

### Equipment preparation

■ Verify the medication order on the patient's record. Note whether the patient has any allergies.
■ Inspect the medication to make sure it isn't abnormally discolored or cloudy and doesn't contain precipitates.
■ Check the medication against the patient's record, and read the label again as you draw up the medication for injection.

## Procedure

■ Explain the procedure to the patient, and address any questions or concerns he may have.
■ Select an appropriate injection site. Rotate sites according to a schedule for repeated injections, using different areas of the body unless contraindicated. (Heparin, for example, should be injected only in the abdomen if possible.)
■ Wash your hands, and put on gloves.
■ Position the patient, and expose the injection site.
■ Clean the injection site with an alcohol pad, beginning at the center of the site and moving outward in a circular motion. Allow the skin to dry before injecting the drug to avoid a stinging sensation

from introducing alcohol into subcutaneous tissues.

■ Loosen the protective needle sheath.

■ With your nondominant hand, grasp the skin around the injection site firmly to elevate the subcutaneous tissue, forming a 1″ (2.5-cm) fat fold.

■ Holding the syringe in your dominant hand, insert the loosened needle sheath between the fourth and fifth fingers of your nondominant hand while still pinching the skin around the injection site. Pull back the syringe with your dominant hand to uncover the needle by grasping the syringe like a pencil. Don't touch the needle.

■ Position the needle with the bevel up.

■ Tell the patient he'll feel a needle prick.

■ Insert the needle quickly in one motion at a 45- or 90-degree angle. (See *Technique for subcutaneous injections.*) Release the patient's skin to avoid injecting the drug into compressed tissue and irritating nerve fibers.

■ Pull back the plunger slightly to check for blood return. If none appears, begin injecting the drug slowly. If blood appears on aspiration, withdraw the needle, prepare another syringe, and repeat the procedure.

**CLINICAL TIP**
*Don't aspirate for blood return when giving insulin or heparin. It isn't necessary with insulin and may cause a hematoma with heparin.*

■ After injection, remove the nee-

## Technique for subcutaneous injections

Before giving the injection, elevate the subcutaneous tissue at the site by grasping it firmly.

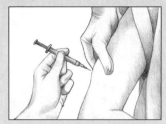

Insert the needle at a 45- or 90-degree angle to the skin surface, depending on needle length and the amount of subcutaneous tissue at the site. Some medications, such as heparin, should always be injected at a 90-degree angle.

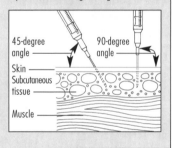

45-degree angle

90-degree angle

Skin
Subcutaneous tissue

Muscle

dle gently but quickly at the same angle used for insertion.

■ Cover the site with an alcohol pad, and massage the site gently (unless contraindicated, as with heparin and insulin) to distribute the drug and facilitate absorption.

■ Remove the alcohol pad, and check the injection site for bleeding and bruising.

■ Dispose of injection equipment according to your facility's policy.

To avoid needle-stick injuries, don't resheath the needle.

## Postprocedure patient teaching

■ Tell the patient the adverse effects of the medication administered, as appropriate.
■ Teach the patient to monitor the injection site for signs and symptoms of local infection (such as redness, swelling, and yellow or green drainage), which can occur any time the skin is punctured. He should notify your facility if any of these occur.

## Complications

■ Concentrated or irritating solutions may cause sterile abscesses to form. Repeated injections in the same site can cause lipodystrophy. A natural immune response, lipodystrophy can be minimized by rotating injection sites.

## Special considerations

■ When using prefilled syringes, adjust the angle and depth of insertion according to needle length.

## Documentation

■ Record the time and date of the injection, medication and dose administered, injection site and route, and patient's reaction.

# INJECTION, Z-TRACK

## CPT code
90782 *Therapeutic, prophylactic, or diagnostic injection (specify material); subcutaneous or intramuscular*

## Overview

The Z-track method of I.M. injection prevents leakage, or tracking, into the subcutaneous tissue. Lateral displacement of the skin during the injection helps to seal the drug in the muscle.

This procedure requires careful attention to technique because leakage into subcutaneous tissue can cause patient discomfort and may permanently stain some tissues.

## Indications

■ To administer drugs that irritate and discolor subcutaneous tissue — primarily iron preparations such as iron dextran

## Contraindications

ABSOLUTE
■ Not to be given at inflamed, edematous, or irritated sites or at sites that contain moles, birthmarks, scar tissue, or other lesions

RELATIVE
■ Impaired coagulation mechanisms, occlusive peripheral vascular disease, edema, and shock; after thrombolytic therapy; and during an acute myocardial infarction be-

cause these conditions impair peripheral absorption

## Preprocedure patient preparation

- Tell the patient he'll feel a prick when the needle is inserted in the skin, but that discomfort will be minimal after the injection. (This is dependent on the agent being injected.)
- Show him where you'll be giving the injection.
- If the patient has experienced pain or emotional trauma from repeated injections, consider numbing the area before cleaning it by holding ice on it for several seconds. If you must inject more than 5 ml of solution, divide the solution and inject it at two separate sites.
- Always encourage the patient to relax the muscle you'll be injecting because injections into tense muscles are more painful than usual and may bleed more readily.

## Equipment

Medication as indicated ♦ patient's medication record and chart ♦ two 20G 1¼″ to 2″ needles ♦ 3- or 5-ml syringe ♦ gloves ♦ alcohol pads

### Equipment preparation

- Verify the medication order on the patient's record. Note whether the patient has any allergies.
- Inspect the medication to make sure it isn't abnormally discolored or cloudy and doesn't contain precipitates.

- The prescribed medication must be sterile.
- Determine appropriate needle length. Needle length depends on the injection site, the patient's size, and the amount of subcutaneous fat covering the muscle. A larger needle gauge accommodates viscous solutions and suspensions. Make sure the needle you're using is long enough to reach the muscle.
- Attach one needle to the syringe, and draw up the medication to be administered. Then draw 0.2 to 0.5 cc of air (depending on your facility's policy) into the syringe. Remove the first needle and attach the second to prevent tracking the medication through the subcutaneous tissue as the needle is inserted.
- Check the medication against the patient's record, and read the label again as you draw up the medication for injection.

## Procedure

- Explain the procedure to the patient, and address any questions or concerns he may have.
- Wash your hands.
- Place the patient in the lateral position, exposing the gluteal muscle to be used as the injection site.
- Clean an area on the upper outer quadrant of the patient's buttock with an alcohol pad.
- Put on gloves. Then displace the skin laterally by pulling it away from the injection site. (See *Displacing the skin for Z-track injection,* page 282.)

## Displacing the skin for Z-track injection

By blocking the needle pathway after an injection, the Z-track technique allows I.M. injection while minimizing the risk of subcutaneous irritation and staining from such drugs as iron dextran. The illustrations here show how to perform a Z-track injection.

Before the procedure begins, the skin, subcutaneous fat, and muscle lie in their normal positions.

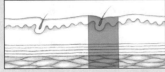

To begin, place your finger on the skin surface, and pull the skin and subcutaneous layers out of alignment with the underlying muscle. You should move the skin about ½" (1 cm).

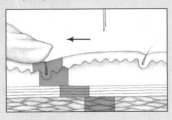

Insert the needle at a 90-degree angle at the site where you initially placed your finger. Inject the drug and withdraw the needle.

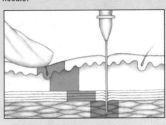

Finally, remove your finger from the skin surface, allowing the layers to return to their normal positions. The needle track (shown by the dotted line) is now broken at the junction of each tissue layer, trapping the drug in the muscle.

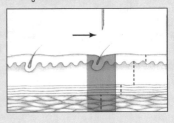

■ Insert the needle into the muscle at a 90-degree angle.

■ Aspirate for blood return; if none appears, inject the drug slowly, followed by the air. Injecting air after the drug helps clear the needle and prevents tracking the medication through subcutaneous tissue as the needle is withdrawn.

■ Wait 10 seconds before withdrawing the needle to ensure dispersion of the medication.

■ Withdraw the needle slowly. Then release the displaced skin and subcutaneous tissue to seal the needle track. Don't massage the injection site or allow the patient to wear a tight-fitting garment over the site because it could force the medication into subcutaneous tissue.

■ Discard the needles and syringe in an appropriate sharps container. Avoid needle-stick injuries by not recapping needles.

■ Remove and discard your gloves.

## Postprocedure patient teaching

■ Encourage the patient to walk or move about in bed to facilitate absorption of the drug from the injection site.

■ Tell the patient the adverse effects of the medication administered, as appropriate.

■ Teach the patient to monitor the injection site for signs and symptoms of local infection (such as redness, swelling, and yellow or green drainage), which can occur any time the skin is punctured. He should notify your facility if any of these occur.

## Complications

■ Discomfort and tissue irritation may result from drug leakage into subcutaneous tissue.

■ Failure to rotate sites in patients who require repeated injections can interfere with the absorption of medication. Unabsorbed medications may build up in deposits. These deposits can reduce the desired pharmacologic effect and may lead to abscess formation or tissue necrosis.

## Special considerations

■ Never inject more than 5 ml of solution into a single site using the Z-track method. Alternate gluteal sites for repeat injections.

## Documentation

■ Record the medication, dosage, date, time, and site of injection on the patient's medication record. Include the patient's response to the injected drug.

# INSECT BITE CARE

***CPT code***
*No specific code has been assigned.*

## Overview

Individuals react differently to the bites of insects or arachnids, depending on the immunologic status of the individual and what organism is involved. Immunologically sensitive patients have more widespread or severe reactions than patients who are immunologically tolerant and may demonstrate no reaction at all. Medically important spiders in the United States include the brown recluse and black widow spiders. These spiders cause life-threatening systemic venom reactions. Other spiders can cause pain and limited local necrosis of the skin.

## Indications

■ To treat reactions that are allergic in nature or severe such as bites from known medically important spiders (Minor reactions usually require no treatment.)

## Contraindications

**ABSOLUTE**

■ Allergy to any medication to be used for treatment

## Preprocedure patient preparation

■ Obtain a detailed history from the patient regarding the offending insect, when the bite occurred, and any immediate reactions that occurred.

## Equipment

Topical calamine lotion ◆ oral antihistamine ◆ ice packs ◆ tongue blade or scalpel ◆ epinephrine hydrochloride 1:1000 in aqueous solution ◆ tuberculin syringe with 27G ½″ needle ◆ tetanus toxoid ◆ elastic bandage

## Procedure

■ Explain the procedure to the patient, and address any questions or concerns he may have.
■ Wash your hands.

### General care

> **CLINICAL TIP**
> *Application of meat tenderizer containing papain hasn't been proven to be helpful or valuable for the management of itching and swelling caused by insect bites.*

■ Elevate the affected site or limb.
■ Apply topical calamine lotion to relieve itching.
■ Administer oral antihistamines as necessary.

### For bee or wasp stings

■ Remove the stinger containing venom if still present. This may be done by gently scraping the skin with a horizontal motion using a tongue blade or other such object.

Try not to crush the stinger; this will release more venom.
■ After the stinger is removed, apply ice to the area.
■ Have the patient elevate the affected area to reduce the reaction. Administer antihistamines as necessary to decrease itching and swelling.
■ Treat anaphylactic reactions immediately with epinephrine hydrochloride 1:1000 in aqueous solution. Repeat treatment every 20 to 30 minutes if necessary. Additionally, injectable corticosteroids, oxygen, bronchodilators, and I.V. fluids may be necessary. (See "Anaphylaxis management," page 17.)

### For ant or spider bites

■ Most minor spider and ant bites require no treatment. Significant pain or itching may be treated with the application of ice packs, topical steroids, and antihistamines.
■ The female black widow spider is 1 to 1.5 cm long, shiny black, and has a red hourglass on the ventral abdomen. Because a black widow spider bite can be fatal if treatment isn't started immediately, transfer the patient directly to an acute care facility for treatment with tetanus toxoid and antiserum for the black widow spider. The male black widow spider doesn't bite.
■ The brown recluse spider is 1 cm long, brown, and has a dark, violin-shaped spot on the dorsal surface. A bite of the brown recluse spider causes pain and itching that increase in intensity. The toxin causes skin necrosis and a

hemolytic reaction that leads to severe and potentially life-threatening hemolysis. Central necrosis develops with surrounding white skin and a red halo peripherally. Gravity causes the venom to spread to dependent areas. Initial treatment consists of first aid measures, including rest, ice, compression, and elevation. These measures decrease the activity of the necrotoxin. The patient should then be transferred to an acute care facility for further treatment and close monitoring.

### For mosquito bites

- For severe reactions, apply ice to the site and administer topical corticosteroids or antihistamines as necessary for significant itching or swelling.

## Postprocedure patient teaching

- Teach the patient to apply cool compresses or an ice pack as necessary for local pain relief.
- Tell the patient to watch the site for signs of infection (redness, drainage, increased temperature, or foul odor from the site) and to call your facility if these symptoms arise. Treatment with a topical or systemic antibiotic may be necessary.
- Teach the patient avoidance strategies when going outdoors, such as not using hair sprays or perfumes, covering the skin with long sleeves and pants, using nets and screens, and using insect repellents such as deet.

### For bee or wasp stings

- Instruct the patient to watch for signs of systemic toxicity or allergic reaction (tachycardia; sweating; generalized edema, especially around the mouth, face, or tongue; nausea and vomiting; diarrhea; shortness of breath; generalized pruritus; or collapse). He should go directly to an emergency department if any of these symptoms occur.
- Because most fatal reactions to bee or wasp stings occur within the first hour or two after exposure, instruct patients with known anaphylactic reactions in self-administering epinephrine injections (such as EpiPen, BD Auto-Injector, and Ana-kit) to enable immediate intervention. These kits are available by prescription and should be carried at all times when exposure is possible.

## Complications

- Anaphylactic reactions are possible with bee or wasp stings and must be treated immediately. Once stabilized, the patient may need to be transferred to an acute care facility.
- A severe reaction to a black widow or brown recluse spider bite requires immediate treatment at an acute care facility.

## Special considerations

- Multiple bee or wasp stings can cause vomiting, diarrhea, hypotension, dyspnea, edema, and collapse. Rhabdomyolysis and intravascular hemorrhage can cause renal failure. Death has been known to occur following a significant number of stings at the same time because of the toxic dose of the venom. The number of stings needed for a toxic dose is approximately 8.6 stings per pound of body weight. A healthy adult would need to be stung over 1,000 times for death to occur. However, any patient stung multiple times should see their health care provider or go to the emergency department.

■ Black widow spiders are found in all 48 contiguous states. Patient awareness is essential.

■ Brown recluse spiders hide in undisturbed areas, such as cracks, crevices, dark storage areas, and closet corners. The spider may bite when disturbed and may not be seen at the time of the bite.

## Documentation

■ In case of bee or wasp stings, record the procedure used to remove stinger, the patient's reaction to the sting, medications given, and posttreatment care instructions given.

■ In case of other bites, document the patient's reaction to the bite, treatment modalities initiated, and posttreatment care instructions given.

# INTRAUTERINE DEVICE INSERTION AND REMOVAL

### CPT codes
58300  *Insertion of intrauterine device (IUD)*
58301  *Removal of IUD*

## Overview

The intrauterine device (IUD) is a plastic contraceptive device inserted into the uterus through the cervical canal. The IUD is inserted and removed from the uterus most easily during menses, when the cervical canal is slightly dilated. Insertion at menses also reduces the likelihood of inserting an IUD into a pregnant uterus.

Three types of IUDs are available in the United States: the Paragard-T, the Progestasert system, and the Mirena system. The Paragard is a T-shaped, polyethylene device with copper wrapped around the vertical stem. A knotted monofilament retrieval string is attached through a hole in the stem. It's effective for up to 10 years. The Progestasert IUD is a T-shaped device made of an ethylene vinyl acetate copolymer. Progesterone is stored in the hollow vertical stem, suspended in an oil base. A knotted monofilament retrieval string is attached through a hole in the vertical stem. It's effective for up to 1 year. The Mirena is a T-shaped polyethylene device with a cylindrical reservoir containing levonorgestrel. The reservoir is covered by a silicone membrane, and the frame contains barium sulfate, making it radiopaque. A monofilament retrieval thread is attached to a loop in the system. It's effective for up to 5 years.

## Indications

- To be used in women who desire reversible, long-term contraception
- To be used in women who have contraindications to hormonal contraceptives (Paragard-T)
- To be used in women who desire reversible, long-term contraception that offers decreased menstrual flow and relief of dysmenorrhea (Progestasert and Mirena)

## Contraindications

**ABSOLUTE**

- Active, recent, or recurrent pelvic inflammatory disease (PID)
- Infection or inflammation of the genital tract
- Sexually transmitted disease (STD)
- Diseases that suppress immune function, including human immunodeficiency virus
- Unexplained cervical or vaginal bleeding or malignancy
- Previous problems with an IUD
- History of ectopic pregnancy, severe vasovagal reactivity, difficulty obtaining emergency care, valvular heart disease, anatomic uterine deformities, anemia, or nulliparity

**RELATIVE**

- Small uterus

- Wilson's disease

## Preprocedure patient preparation

- Explain the risks, benefits, and effectiveness of this contraceptive method.
- Verify that the patient isn't pregnant and is free from STDs.
- Offer the patient ibuprofen to reduce postinsertion cramping.

## Equipment

### For insertion

Sterile single-toothed tenaculum ◆ sterile uterine sound ◆ sterile scissors ◆ speculum ◆ light source ◆ cotton-tipped applicator ◆ antiseptic cleaning agent, such as povidone-iodine solution or Hibiclens ◆ 4″ × 4″ gauze pads ◆ sterile gloves ◆ drape ◆ gloves ◆ IUD and inserter

### For removal

Sponge forceps ◆ sterile gloves ◆ drape ◆ speculum ◆ tenaculum (optional)

### Equipment preparation

- Review the product documents and instruction for IUD insertion, and ensure that the proper equipment is available before the insertion is scheduled.
- Place the contents of IUD pack on a sterile field close to the lithotomy table.
- Slide the IUD into the insertion tube. Make sure the arms are bent and within the tube just enough to ensure they remain in the tube during insertion. Place the inserter

rod into the barrel of the tube and advance it until it touches the IUD.

➤ **CLINICAL TIP**
*The Mirena system has a different inserter than Paragard-T and Progestasert and doesn't require a sound. Read through the instructions carefully to become comfortable with the process.*

## Procedure

### For insertion of the IUD

■ Explain the procedure to the patient, and address any questions or concerns she may have.

☑ **OBTAIN INFORMED CONSENT**

■ After the patient has removed her clothing from the waist down, voided, and is appropriately draped, assist her to the lithotomy position, with her feet in the stirrups and her buttocks extended slightly beyond the edge of the table. Adjust the light source.

■ Wash your hands, and put on gloves. Tell the patient that you're about to touch her to avoid startling her.

■ Perform a bimanual examination to ascertain uterine position, size, and shape. Evaluate for tenderness suggestive of PID.

■ Insert a warmed, moistened speculum, and visualize the cervix. Put on sterile gloves.

■ Verify the patient isn't allergic to iodine and clean the cervix in concentric circles from the os outward with povidone-iodine or Hibiclens soaked 4″ × 4″gauze. Tell the patient she may notice a cold sensation in the vagina as you complete the preparation. Explain to her

that you'll be applying an instrument to the cervix.

■ Depending on the position of the uterus and cervix, grasp the cervix with the tenaculum at either the anterior or posterior lip and apply traction to align the cervical canal with the uterine cavity. Close the clamp slowly, avoiding jerking motions.

■ Holding the tenaculum in the nondominant hand and the uterine sound in the dominant hand, insert the sound slowly and gently through the cervical canal and into the uterus. Gentle traction on the tenaculum may aid insertion. Tell the patient she may experience cramping during the uterine sounding. When the fundus of the uterus is reached, resistance will be felt.

■ Place a clean, cotton-tipped applicator beside the uterine sound, touching the cervix.

■ Remove the sound and applicator simultaneously. The distance between the tip of the sound and the tip of the swab gives an approximate measure of the depth of the fundus.

■ Note the distance in centimeters. Remove the soiled gloves, and put on sterile gloves.

■ Set the movable flange on the inserter barrel to the depth the uterus sounded. Ensure that the flange and the arms of the T are aligned in the same plane. (See *IUD insertion.*)

■ If needed, use the single-toothed tenaculum to secure the cervix. Introduce the loaded inserter tube through the cervical canal and into the uterus until the flange reaches the cervical opening.

## IUD Insertion

This technique is for the Paragard and Progestasert systems. Set the movable flange on the inserter barrel to the depth the uterus sounded in centimeters. Introduce the loaded inserter tube through the cervical canal and into the uterus while applying gentle, steady traction on the tenaculum. Advance the inserter tube to the flange.

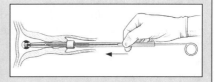

Insert the intrauterine device (IUD) by retracting the inserter slowly about ½″ (1.3 cm) over the plunger, holding the plunger still. This allows the arms to open.

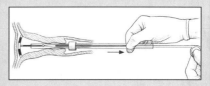

Now gently advance the inserter and plunger until resistance is felt. This action ensures high fundal placement of the IUD and may reduce the potential for expulsion.

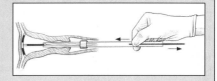

Withdraw the solid rod while holding the insertion barrel stationary. Withdraw the insertion barrel from the cervix. Clip the IUD strings about 1″ to 2″ (3 to 5 cm) from the cervical os. This action leaves sufficient string for the woman to check and for removal of the IUD.

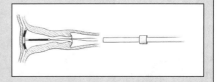

■ Insert the IUD by retracting the inserter as you hold the inserting rod in place.

■ Gently advance the inserter and plunger until resistance is felt.

■ Withdraw the solid rod while holding the insertion barrel stationary and then withdraw the insertion barrel and rod from the cervix.

▶ CLINICAL TIP
*With the Mirena system, the insertion tube is advanced through the cervix until the flange is located ½″ to 1″ (1.5 to 2 cm) from the external os. The arms are released by pulling a slider on the handle back* *until it reaches a specific mark; then the inserter is advanced until the flange touches the cervix. The slider is then pushed down, completely releasing the IUD.*

■ Clip the IUD strings about 1″ to 2″ (3 to 5 cm) from the cervical os with sterile scissors.

■ Remove the speculum, and assist the patient to a seated position. When she feels comfortable, show her how to check for the IUD string.

### For removal of the IUD
■ Explain the procedure for removing the IUD to the patient.

Tell her she'll need another method of birth control after removal of the IUD unless she intends to become pregnant.

■ After the patient undresses from the waist down and drapes herself, assist her to the lithotomy position.

■ Wash your hands, and put on gloves.

■ Insert a speculum for adequate exposure of the cervix.

■ Identify the IUD strings on the surface of the cervix. If the strings are missing, consult a physician.

■ Grasp the IUD strings in the sponge forceps, and apply gentle traction. The IUD should gradually appear at the cervical os. If resistance occurs, a tenaculum may be used to apply gentle traction on the cervix as traction on the string is applied. This action may straighten an anteflexion or retroflexion that's hampering removal.

■ If the IUD can't easily be removed, consult a physician.

■ Remove and discard soiled supplies. Assist the patient to a sitting position.

## Postprocedure patient teaching

■ Tell the patient that she can expect her period to be heavier after an IUD insertion. Cramping may accompany insertion and continue for a time after insertion. Cramping should lessen gradually over the next few days.

■ Instruct the patient to schedule a return visit after the next menses for an IUD check.

■ Tell the patient that if she experiences pain, the best analgesic is a prostaglandin inhibitor such as ibuprofen.

■ Inform the patient that the contraceptive action of the IUD is immediate. Foam and condoms may be used as backup contraception during the first month until retention of the IUD is more certain.

■ Advise the patient that the IUD offers no protection from STDs.

■ Tell the patient to check the strings at least weekly the first month. This action increases confidence in the IUD's presence. Also tell her to check the strings each month after her menses.

■ Instruct the patient to watch for signs of infection, such as fever, pelvic pain, tenderness, severe cramping, and unusual vaginal bleeding or discharge. Tell her to call you or the facility immediately to report infection symptoms. Emphasize to her that untreated infections can progress to PID, which may necessitate a hysterectomy.

■ Emphasize the symptoms of PID:
– Fever of 101° F (38.3° C) or higher
– Purulent vaginal discharge
– Abdominal or pelvic pain
– Dyspareunia

■ Tell the patient to chart her menses. If a period is late, tell her to call you immediately.

■ Tell the patient to report severe cramping or bleeding; if the IUD causes increased menstrual pain and bleeding, it can be removed.

■ Instruct the patient not to attempt to remove the IUD herself or allow her partner to attempt to remove it.

■ Give the patient the mnemonic,

PAINS, to recall the signs of IUD complications:

– **P**: period late, abnormal bleeding, or spotting
– **A**: abdominal pain, pain with intercourse
– **I**: infection, exposure to an STD, abnormal discharge
– **N**: not feeling well, fever, chills
– **S**: string missing, shorter or longer.

## Complications

■ Signs of uterine perforation include pain, loss of strings, or the plastic of the device is felt or visible in the cervix. Ultrasound can help to confirm perforation. If perforation is suspected, refer the patient to a physician or gynecologist.
■ Vasovagal syncopal episodes may accompany IUD insertion. Symptoms are dizziness, flushing, tachycardia, and hypotension. Treatment is immediate removal of the IUD.
■ Anemia secondary to spotting or bleeding requires monitoring. Remove the IUD if the hemoglobin level is less than 9 grams.
■ Pain and cramping may be relieved with nonsteroidal anti-inflammatory drugs after uterine perforation, cervical or pelvic infection, and pregnancy (intrauterine or ectopic) are ruled out.
■ Pregnancy may occur after insertion. There's an increased risk of septic abortion if pregnancy occurs. If menses is delayed, evaluate for pregnancy and infection and remove the IUD if either occurs.
■ Risk for PID increases. Most cases of PID occur during the first 3 months after insertion. After 3 months, the chance of PID is lower unless preinsertion screening failed to identify a person at risk for STDs.

## Special considerations

■ The Paragard IUD can't be used by women with Wilson's disease because of their inability to metabolize copper properly.
■ Remove the IUD during the menstrual period if possible, or during midcycle when the cervix is softer, to minimize trauma to the cervical os.

## Documentation

■ Document the patient's desire for this method of birth control and that a thorough discussion of options, advantages, and disadvantages took place.
■ Record findings of the pelvic examination and that the patient was confirmed not pregnant and free from STDs. Detail the procedure for insertion of the IUD, including the depth of the uterus (sounded) and the depth the IUD was inserted. Include the length of strings protruding from the cervical os after trimming.
■ Note the patient's tolerance of the procedure and any adverse reactions such as a vasovagal reaction and actions taken.
■ Record your instructions related to how to check the strings, symptoms to observe for, and when to return for a follow-up examination.

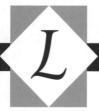

## LASER THERAPY (CO₂ LASER METHOD)

**CPT codes**
17106 *Destruction of cutaneous, vascular, proliferative lesions less than 10 cm² (laser technique)*
17107 *Destruction of cutaneous, vascular, proliferative lesions 10 to 50 cm² (laser technique)*
17108 *Destruction of cutaneous, vascular, proliferative lesions over 50 cm² (laser technique)*
57513 *Laser ablation of the cervix*

## Overview

The use of laser surgery to treat dermatologic and gynecologic lesions is limited now to primarily vascular lesions, as the use of radio frequency surgery has become more widely accepted. The advantages of laser surgery are precision in cutting, vaporizing, or coagulating tissue; better hemostasis; and reduced scarring. Infection is rare and pain may be less as sensory nerve endings are cauterized. Laser surgery has the added advantage of being available on an outpatient basis.

The carbon dioxide ($CO_2$) laser emits an invisible infrared beam of 10,600 nm and can be used in continuous-wave mode, super-pulsed mode, and scanning mode. Water in the tissues nonselectively absorbs laser energy, producing ablative and thermal damage. The results from $CO_2$ laser surgery depend on the laser equipment used and on the skill of the operator. Proper training in the use of $CO_2$ laser equipment and appropriate selection of a patient is essential.

## Indications

- To treat large plantar and peri-ungal warts; cervical dysplasia; ear lobe keloids; actinic cheilitis; rhinophyma; xanthelasma; syringomas; and actinic damage
- To remove extensive lesions in patients with pacemakers
- To remove lesions when a bloodless field is necessary, when electrosurgery is contraindicated, in patients with bleeding disorders, or when other therapies have failed

## Contraindications

**ABSOLUTE**
- Large vascular lesions (other laser modalities preferred in such cases)

**RELATIVE**
- Children and some adolescents and adults may require oral sedation or general anesthesia if they're unable to remain still during the procedure.
- Known HIV-positive status

## Preprocedure patient preparation

- Discuss the results, adverse effects, complications, and cost of therapy. Adverse effects of the test include gross bruising and lid swelling when performed around the eyes.
- Inform the patient that each pulse produces a moderately painful sensation on the skin and immediate bruising. Show him preprocedure photos, immediate postprocedure photos, and photos of results seen at 2- to 4-month intervals.
- Tell the patient that the laser may remove much of a natural tan and freckles in the area treated. This usually isn't permanent.
- Inform the patient that there may be a noxious odor during the procedure.
- Tell the patient that successful therapy may require multiple treatment sessions for each site, depending on the type of lesion being treated.

- Review with the patient that laser treatment may be considered cosmetic treatment and, therefore, not reimbursed by some insurance companies.
- Clarify the method of payment before beginning therapy.

## Equipment

Carbon dioxide laser ◆ face masks ◆ gloves ◆ warm, wet towels ◆ special plume-evacuation devices ◆ protective goggles for the patient, medical assistants, and operator ◆ water or saline solution

## Procedure

- Explain the procedure to the patient, and address any questions or concerns he may have.

☑ **OBTAIN INFORMED CONSENT**

- Wash your hands.
- Assist the patient to a comfortable position.
- Drape normal skin surrounding the surgical field with wet towels.

◀ **CLINICAL TIP**
*Alcohol-containing pads shouldn't be used because residual alcohol on the surface of the skin could ignite when exposed to the CO$_2$ laser beam.*

- Consider using eutectic mixture of local anesthetic. This may reduce skin pain by 25% to 75%.
- As necessary, administer oral sedation and analgesia. In adults, diazepam orally or sublingually can be given. In children less than age 1, chloral hydrate may be administered.

- Put on gloves, a face mask, and protective goggles. Make sure the patient and all assisting personnel put on face masks and protective goggles.
- Perform a patch test on several sites. It's important to select sites that are most sensitive to the laser and least sensitive to the laser.

◥ **CLINICAL TIP**

*Techniques of patch testing vary. Within a single test patch, you may use four separate energy levels. Another technique involves filling an area of approximately 1 cm$^2$ on a specific site with laser pulses at a certain energy level and then increasing or decreasing the energy level on other sites as needed.*

- Pass the laser over the selected site, following the directions and recommendations of the laser equipment manufacturer and taking into account the type of lesion being treated. The slower the laser is passed over the tissue, the deeper and wider the destruction because more energy is delivered to the tissue.
- Schedule the patient to be seen in 7 to 10 days for a wound check and again in 2 to 4 months for additional treatment if necessary. This represents the standard amount of time for complete healing.

## Postprocedure patient teaching

- Tell the patient to avoid sun exposure and local trauma. Emphasize the importance of using sunscreens and wearing protective clothing.

- Inform parents that children must avoid participation in contact sports for the next 5 to 10 days.
- Instruct the patient to keep the treated area lubricated with topical antibiotic ointment. Treated skin is fragile and can easily be peeled off. The patient may apply an ice pack to the site for pain relief as necessary.

## Complications

- The following skin changes may result from the procedure: hypertrophic scarring, hyperpigmentation that usually resolves in 2 to 8 months, cutaneous texture changes, excessive granulation tissue formation, or prolonged erythema and healing times.
- Human papillomavirus (HPV) deoxyribonucleic acid may be present in the smoke plume if the patient is being treated for an HPV infection. Staff should remember to wear face masks during the procedure.
- Unintentional burns to the patient, personnel, and operator may occur.
- Eye injury to personnel may occur to those not wearing protective eyewear.

## Special considerations

- It's better to begin at a lower energy level if you're unsure of the patient's response. Blistering is common, especially around the eyelids, if the energy level is set too high.

- For children and adults with extensively sun-damaged skin, consider starting with energy levels lower than what you think is necessary.
- Continuous-wave mode is an excellent therapeutic choice for very large plantar and periungual warts that have failed to respond to routine facility modalities. Superpulsed mode is useful in the treatment of actinic damage.

## Documentation

- Record the site of treatment, the energy level used, and the number of pulses delivered.
- Take photos before and after the procedure and place in the medical record.
- Document the patient's response to treatment, medications given, and whether analgesia was adequate.
- Document discharge instructions given.

## *LIP LACERATION REPAIR*

### *CPT codes*
40650  *Repair lip, full thickness; vermillion only*
40652  *Up to one-half vertical height*
40654  *Over one-half vertical height, or complex*

## Overview

Lips are vulnerable to injury because of their exposure on the face. Lip injuries commonly result from blows to the face in which the lips are compressed between the object and the teeth, causing bruising and, possibly, laceration. Sports and other contact activities are usually the cause of such blows. The patient's teeth may lacerate or puncture the lips in a fall or blow to the face. Because of their exposure on the face, lip laceration repair must be done cautiously to achieve the best cosmetic results.

## Indications

- To repair a lip laceration

## Contraindications

### ABSOLUTE
- Laceration of the lip extending all the way through, loss of part of the lip, or suspected facial bone fracture (refer the patient to oral, maxillofacial, or plastic surgeon)
- Lacerations that cross the vermillion border — the delineation of the lips from the surrounding skin — need extremely precise repair because the slightest misalignment during repair may be obvious afterward (refer patient to surgeon as above)

## Preprocedure patient preparation

- Ascertain the history of the injury, associated symptoms, and

## Approximating the lip margin

As depicted, be sure to align the margins of the lip before suturing to produce the best cosmetic result.

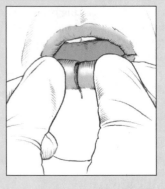

treatments or medications the patient has received.

■ Assess the patient's tetanus immunization status and provide tetanus prophylaxis if necessary.

■ Assess the laceration. A laceration that goes through the lip or crosses the vermillion border, or if a portion of the lip is missing, necessitates referral as above.

## Equipment

Clean and sterile gloves ◆ sterile normal saline solution ◆ 60-ml syringe with a large-bore (18G to 20G) cannula tip ◆ sterile forceps ◆ sterile 4″ × 4″ gauze pads ◆ equipment to administer local anesthesia ◆ equipment to suture, including 6.0 absorbable and 5.0 nonabsorbable suture material ◆ topical antibiotic ointment

## Procedure

■ Explain the procedure to the patient, and address any questions or concerns he may have.

☑ **OBTAIN INFORMED CONSENT**

■ Wash your hands, and put on gloves.

■ Inspect the laceration for foreign material (such as tooth fragments or gravel). Irrigate the laceration using sterile normal saline solution and a 60-ml syringe. A foreign fragment that remains may be removed with sterile forceps. Pat the area with gauze pads to dry.

■ Remove gloves, and put on sterile gloves.

■ Administer local anesthesia. (See "Anesthesia: topical, local, and digital nerve block," page 20.)

■ Suture the laceration using simple interrupted suturing. (See *Suturing of simple lacerations,* page 459.) Suture deeper lacerations in layers from the inside out. Begin by using the 6.0 absorbable material to suture the innermost layers of tissue. Suture the external surface of the lip with the 5.0 nonabsorbable material. Approximate the edges of the laceration as closely as possible to provide the best cosmetic results. (See *Approximating the lip margin.*)

■ Apply a topical antibiotic ointment sparingly to the site.

## Postprocedure patient teaching

■ Tell the patient to return to the facility for suture removal in 3 to 5 days.

■ Instruct the patient to apply ice to the site or take acetaminophen as necessary for pain relief.

■ Teach the patient signs of infection, such as redness, swelling, yellow or green drainage, foul odor, or increase in temperature, and have him notify your facility if any of these occur.

■ Inform the patient that he shouldn't use straws until the sutures are removed.

## Complications

■ Site infection may require topical or systemic antibiotics.

■ Scarring or cosmetically undesirable results may require follow-up care with a plastic surgeon.

## Special considerations

■ For deep lacerations, consider prescribing prophylactic antibiotics to prevent a deeper tissue infection.

■ Dermal adhesives (such as Dermabond) shouldn't be used to close lacerations of the lips.

## Documentation

■ Thoroughly document the location, size, depth, and mechanism of the lip laceration, using illustrations as necessary.

■ Record the type of analgesia and anesthetic used, the type and number of sutures placed, and the patient's toleration of the procedure.

■ Document the patient's scheduled follow-up visit and discharge instructions given.

# LUMBAR PUNCTURE

**CPT code**
62270 *Spinal puncture, lumbar, for diagnostic purposes*

## Overview

Lumbar puncture involves the insertion of a sterile needle into the subarachnoid space of the spinal canal, usually between the third and fourth or fourth and fifth lumbar vertebral spaces. This procedure is used to detect increased intracranial pressure (ICP) or the presence of blood in cerebrospinal fluid (CSF), to obtain CSF specimens for laboratory analysis, and to inject dyes or gases for contrast in radiologic studies. It's also used to administer drugs or anesthetics and to relieve increased ICP by removing CSF.

Before performing a lumbar puncture in a patient with papilledema and focal neurologic deficits, computerized tomography (CT) or magnetic resonance imaging (MRI) must be performed first to help rule out a mass, an abscess, or a lesion. Performing lumbar puncture in the presence of these conditions could worsen the patient's neurologic condition or result in herniation.

## Indications

■ To rule out suspected meningitis or encephalitis (Any patient presenting with fever and altered mental status, severe headache, or nuchal rigidity should have a lumbar puncture to rule out these potentially life-threatening infections.)

■ To investigate the cause of a fever of unknown origin in an immunocompromised patient or neonate younger than age 8 weeks
■ To identify suspected subarachnoid hemorrhage after a negative CT scan
■ To diagnose some neurologic disorders, such as multiple sclerosis, Guillain-Barré syndrome, or tertiary syphilis

## Contraindications

**ABSOLUTE**
■ Cellulitis or evidence of infection over proposed injection site
■ Known supratentorial mass or lesion

**RELATIVE**
■ Coagulopathy or blood dyscrasia

## Preprocedure patient preparation

■ Take a complete history and perform a physical examination.
■ Emphasize to the patient the importance of maintaining a flexed position and remaining still throughout the procedure. The procedure will take approximately 15 minutes.
■ Explain to the patient that there may be discomfort during lidocaine administration as the needle is introduced into the subarachnoid space. Reassure the patient that any additional discomfort

should ease immediately after the procedure ends.

## Equipment

Two pairs of sterile gloves ◆ sterile gown ◆ mask ◆ spinal needles, 20G and 22G ◆ manometer ◆ three-way stopcock ◆ sterile fenestrated drapes ◆ 1% lidocaine without epinephrine in a 5-ml syringe with a 22G ⅝″ needle and a 25G 1½″ needle ◆ Betadine or povidone-iodine ◆ sterile gauze pads (4″ × 4″) ◆ adhesive bandage ◆ sterile collection tubes

Disposable lumbar puncture trays contain most of the sterile equipment needed.

### Equipment preparation

■ Assemble all equipment at the bedside.
■ Wash hands thoroughly.
■ Prepare the equipment or open the disposable lumbar puncture tray, being careful to maintain the sterile field.

## Procedure

■ Explain the procedure to the patient, and address any questions or concerns he may have.

✓ OBTAIN
INFORMED CONSENT
■ Place the patient in either the lateral decubitus or sitting position, as desired.
– For the lateral decubitus position, instruct the patient to lie down on the edge of the bed with his back to you. Place him in the knee-chest position, with the knees and hips flexed maximally.

Flex his head and shoulders downward as much as possible. Rest his head on a pillow to maintain shoulder and pelvis alignment parallel to the bed.

– For the sitting position, instruct the patient to sit down and flex his head and arms over a bedside table.

■ Put on sterile gloves, a gown, and a mask.

■ Prepare the puncture site with sterile gauze pads soaked in Betadine or povidone-iodine, moving in a circular motion outward from the proposed puncture site.

■ Drape the area with the fenestrated drape to provide a sterile field.

■ Remove gloves, and put on another pair of sterile gloves to avoid introducing povidone-iodine into the subarachnoid space with the lumbar puncture needle.

■ Locate the insertion site (L3-L4 or L4-L5 interspace).

■ Palpate the posterior aspect of the iliac crest bilaterally, and palpate the L4 spinous process. The L3-L4 interspace should fall along a line connecting the two iliac crests. Use either this interspace or the one below it. Mark the spot by pressing deeply with your fingernail.

■ Anesthetize the skin and subcutaneous tissue with the 1% lidocaine, using the 25G needle. Change to a 22G needle before anesthetizing between the spinous process.

■ Insert the spinal needle in the midline of the interspace, with the needle parallel to the floor and the point directed toward the patient's umbilicus. Maintain midline alignment. If the patient experiences tingling or an electric shock down one of the extremities, the needle may have migrated from a midline position. If this occurs, withdraw the needle as far as the subcutaneous tissue and redirect it.

■ Advance the needle very slowly about $\frac{3}{4}''$ (2 cm) or until you hear a "pop" (piercing a membrane of the dura). Then withdraw the stylet with every 1- to 2-mm advance of the needle to check for CSF return. If the needle meets the bone or if blood returns, withdraw to the skin and redirect the needle. Bloody return indicates that the needle has entered the venous plexus in the anterior spinal wall. If you can't obtain CSF, don't aspirate. The nerve root may be trapped against the needle and forceful aspiration will cause injury. Instead, try performing the procedure one disk-space below.

■ As CSF begins to flow from the needle, discard the first few drops.

■ Attach the stopcock and manometer to the hub of the needle, and record the CSF pressure (normal pressure: supine, 80 to 150 mm $H_2O$; sitting, 80 to 120 mm $H_2O$). Allow the patient to relax and check for good respiratory variation of the fluid level in the manometer to ensure that the needle is properly positioned.

■ Remove the manometer and allow 2 to 3 ml of CSF to flow into each of the sterile tubes. Collection tubes should be filled as follows:

– 2 to 3 ml for cell count and differential

– 2 to 3 ml for glucose and protein
– 2 to 3 ml for culture and sensitivity and Gram stain
– 2 to 3 ml for viral titer or cultures, india ink preparation, cryptococcus antigen, Venereal Disease Research Laboratory test, or cytology.
■ After the tubes are collected, remove the needle. (See "Special considerations" in this entry for information on the controversy regarding replacing the stylet before removing the needle.)
■ Place an adhesive bandage, and apply slight pressure over the area.

## Postprocedure patient teaching

■ Instruct the patient to lie in a supine position for 2 hours after the procedure.
■ Instruct him to notify you and return to the facility if he experiences severe headache, nausea, vomiting, or signs of infection at the injection site (erythema, increased warmth, fever, swelling, or purulent drainage).
■ Tell him to contact you about additional symptoms that concern him.

## Complications

■ Spinal headache following the procedure is the most common complication. Usually this is a frontal headache that can be quite severe. Using a small-gauge spinal needle and having the patient lie flat for several hours after the procedure can minimize headache incidence. Administration of fluids

and a mild analgesic may also help.
■ Suspect CSF leakage if the patient returns within 36 hours after the procedure with complaints of headache. This can be managed with an epidural blood patch placed by an anesthesiologist.
■ Infection can be minimized by preparing the skin with an antiseptic solution and observing strict sterile technique.
■ Herniation of the spinal cord and brain stem are serious complications that require immediate referral to a neurosurgeon.

## Special considerations

■ Normal CSF is clear and colorless. Any changes in color or consistency must be investigated. Yellow or cloudy fluid indicates an increased concentration of cells in the fluid, signifying infection, jaundice, or increased protein. When bacterial meningitis or encephalitis is suspected, initiate antibiotic therapy as soon as possible. Delaying treatment to wait for the procedure to be performed or results to become available can be more detrimental to the patient.
■ Bloody return on lumbar puncture has several indications. In the event of a traumatic tap, fluid is bloody initially and gradually clears. If a subarachnoid hemorrhage is present, fluid remains uniformly bloody throughout collection. Lumbar puncture can precipitate rebleeding and should be used cautiously with subarachnoid hemorrhage.

- CT scan or MRI should be the first diagnostic tools used to evaluate patients who are potential candidates for lumbar puncture. Lumbar puncture should be performed only if these tests are negative and symptoms persist.

- Controversy exists regarding whether the stylet should be reinserted before the needle is removed to prevent headache after the procedure. According to one theory, a piece of the arachnoid tissue enters the needle during outflow of CSF. If the needle is removed without reinserting the stylet, this strand may thread back into the dura, creating a CSF leak, which is known to cause headache. By reinserting the stylet, this strand is cut off or removed and may reduce incidence of headache. (A study conducted by Strupp and Brandt in 1997 demonstrated that only 5% of 300 patients had a postprocedure headache with stylet reinsertion; 16% experienced a headache when the stylet wasn't reinserted.)

## Documentation

- Review recent or pertinent documentation by other health team members, and then initial their notes to signify you're aware of their findings. This doesn't signify agreement with their comments or reduce your responsibility to conduct your own history and physical examination.

- Before performing this procedure, document abnormal physical findings on the consent form, and have the patient or guardian initial the comments and sign the form,

to signify acknowledgment of preprocedural abnormalities. In the chart, the preprocedural and postprocedural notes should include evaluation of function, range of motion, and neurosensory testing.

- Record all presenting symptoms and indications for lumbar puncture. Be sure to document all allergies to medication or food before administering antibiotics, contrast dye, or lidocaine for local anesthesia.

- Describe the patient's tolerance of the procedure and response to medications, appearance of the injection site, and results of neurovascular checks. Record the CSF pressure, describe the color and characteristics of the CSF, and note which tests were ordered for analysis.

# *Lunelle Injections*

## *CPT code*
90782 *Therapeutic or diagnostic injection (specify material injected); subcutaneous or intramuscular*

## Overview
Lunelle is a monthly injection of medroxyprogesterone acetate (MPA) and estradiol cypionate ($E_2C$) used for contraception. The MPA component suppresses ovulation, while the $E_2C$ promotes a monthly period that simulates normal menses. The hormones in Lunelle are similar to those in a

combined oral contraceptive pill (OCP), but the formulation as an injection provides easier use and higher effectiveness than OCP. It's more than 99% effective when used as directed.

## Indications
- To prevent pregnancy

## Contraindications
### ABSOLUTE
- Carcinoma of the endometrium, breast, or other known or suspected estrogen-dependent neoplasia
- Cerebral vascular disease or coronary artery disease
- Diabetes with vascular involvement
- Headaches with focal neurologic symptoms
- Heavy cigarette smoking (15 or more per day) and age 35 or older
- History of deep-vein thrombophlebitis or thromboembolic disorders
- History of liver dysfunction or disease, such as hepatic adenoma or carcinoma; history of cholestatic jaundice of pregnancy or jaundice with prior hormonal contraceptive use, including severe pruritus of pregnancy
- Known hypersensitivity to ingredients contained in Lunelle Monthly Contraceptive Injection
- Known or suspected pregnancy
- Severe hypertension
- Thrombophlebitis or thromboembolic disorders
- Undiagnosed abnormal genital bleeding

- Valvular heart disease with complications

### RELATIVE
- Breast-feeding (may decrease milk supply)
- Cervical intraepithelial neoplasia
- Gallbladder disease
- Heavy cigarette smoking (15 or more per day)
- History of depression
- Hyperlipidemia
- Use of rifampin, anticonvulsants, antibiotics, St. John's wort, ascorbic acid, or acetaminophen (may reduce effectiveness of Lunelle)

## Preprocedure patient preparation
- Perform a current complete physical examination and cervical cytology before initiating Lunelle. (This is recommended, but not required.)
- Counsel the patient about potential adverse effects, particularly weight gain, menorrhagia, amenorrhea, metrorrhagia, vaginal spotting, emotional lability, acne, breast tenderness or pain, headache, dysmenorrhea, nausea, and depression.

## Equipment
Lunelle 0.5 ml vial or prefilled syringe ♦ 21G to 23G ⅓″ needle ♦ alcohol pad ♦ gloves

### *Equipment preparation*
- Store Lunelle at room temperature.

■ Shake the medication vigorously just before use.

## Procedure

■ Review the patient's history and physical examination findings. Confirm that she's an appropriate candidate for Lunelle.
■ Explain the procedure to the patient, and address any questions or concerns she may have.
■ Wash your hands.
■ Obtain blood pressure measurement.
■ Put on gloves.
■ Prepare the prefilled syringe or draw the medication from the vial into a syringe.
■ Wipe the area to be injected with an alcohol pad.
■ Inject the medication intramuscularly into the deltoid, gluteus maximus, or anterior thigh muscle.
■ Remove the syringe and discard appropriately.

## Postprocedure patient teaching

■ Tell the patient that injections should be repeated monthly (every 28 to 30 days). Receiving injections as scheduled is crucial to the effectiveness of the medication.
■ Inform her that Lunelle doesn't provide protection from sexually transmitted diseases, so condoms should be used in addition to the injection if the patient is at risk for infection.
■ Advise her to contact you if she develops sharp chest pain, coughing up of blood, sudden shortness of breath, pain in the calf, crushing chest pain or heaviness in the chest, sudden severe headache or vomiting, dizziness or fainting, problems with vision or speech, weakness, numbness in an extremity, sudden partial or complete loss of vision, breast lumps, unusually heavy vaginal bleeding, severe pain or tenderness in the abdomen, difficulty sleeping, lack of energy, fatigue, mood changes, jaundice, or persistent pain, pus, or bleeding at the injection site.

## Complications

■ The most common adverse reactions include weight gain, menorrhagia, amenorrhea, metrorrhagia, vaginal spotting, emotional lability, acne, breast tenderness or pain, headache, dysmenorrhea, nausea, and depression.
■ Additional adverse reactions that may occur include abdominal pain, alopecia, asthenia, breast enlargement or secretion, cervical changes, cholestatic jaundice, corneal curvature changes, decreased lactation when given immediately postpartum, decreased libido, dizziness, edema, enlarged abdomen, intolerance to contact lenses, melasma, migraine, nervousness, rash, reduced carbohydrate tolerance, temporary infertility after treatment discontinuation, vaginal moniliasis, vulvovaginal disorder, and weight decrease.
■ Serious complications are rare and include arterial thromboembolism, cerebral hemorrhage, hypertension, myocardial infarction, cerebral thrombosis, gallbladder

disease, hepatic adenomas or benign liver tumors, pulmonary embolism, thrombophlebitis, anaphylaxis, and anaphylactoid reaction.

## Special considerations
■ Follow the recommended schedule for administering doses. (See *Lunelle administration*.)

## Documentation
■ Document the following in the patient's chart, including desire for contraception with Lunelle; counseling about risks and benefits provided; dose, lot number of medication, and site of injection; and date the next injection is due.

---

### Lunelle administration

An initial Lunelle injection should be administered:
■ during the first 5 days of a normal menstrual period.
■ no earlier than 4 weeks postpartum if not breast-feeding.
■ no earlier than 6 weeks postpartum if breast-feeding.
    If more than 33 days have elapsed since a previous injection, determine that the patient isn't pregnant before administering another injection.

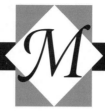

## $\mathcal{M}$AMMAL BITE CARE

***CPT codes***
12001 to 12007   *Simple repair of superficial wounds of scalp, neck, axillae, external genitalia, trunk, and extremities*

## Overview

Although seldom fatal, bites from animals or humans can cause injuries ranging from bruises and superficial scratches to severe crush injuries, deep puncture wounds, tissue loss, and severe damage to blood vessels. In the United States, most mammalian bites involve dogs, with cat bites second and human bites third. Surprisingly, human bites are the most feared because of the great variety of infectious bacteria and viruses normally present in the oral cavity.

A dog bite may cause muscle, tendon, and nerve damage, dislocation of involved joints, and crush injuries, but infection only 2% to 10% of the time. A cat's sharp teeth can cause deep puncture wounds that damage muscles, tendons, and bones; because these tissues have a limited blood supply, the risk of developing infection from a cat bite is 30%.

Infection is more likely to occur if the wound isn't treated promptly, if there is a crush injury, or if the hand is involved. Clenched-fist injuries are the most serious because damaged joint capsules increase the risk of developing osteomyelitis and septic arthritis.

Unfortunately, many animals—usually those in the wild—carry the rabies virus in their saliva and can transmit it by biting or licking an open wound. Rabies is rare in the United States, but it's always fatal unless treated. The risk of getting rabies from a dog is low. Bats cause nearly all cases of rabies in the United States.

Human bites can infect other humans with diseases such as herpes simplex virus, cytomegalovirus, syphilis, tuberculosis and, possibly, human immunodeficiency virus.

Animal bites commonly occur when a sick or injured animal is trying to protect itself or its food, territory, or offspring. Human bites most often result from fights among school-age children and young adults.

## Indications

■ To prevent infection after trauma

## Contraindications

**RELATIVE**

■ Clenched-fist injuries requiring X-rays and often referral to a plastic surgeon or hand surgeon
■ Facial wounds often requiring referral to a plastic surgeon

## Preprocedure patient preparation

■ Obtain a detailed history, and conduct a physical examination.

## Equipment

Sterile basin ◆ antiseptic solution (such as Hibiclens or povidone-iodine) ◆ sterile saline solution ◆ clean gloves ◆ sterile gloves ◆ ice pack ◆ 5- to 10-ml syringe, 60-ml syringe ◆ 27G needle ◆ 18G to 20G needle ◆ 1% or 2% lidocaine ◆ curved hemostat (sterile) ◆ hemostat (sterile) ◆ #3-0 to #5-0 nylon suture material ◆ 4″ × 4″ gauze pads ◆ topical antibiotic (such as bacitracin) ◆ dry, sterile dressing ◆ culture swab with transport medium (optional)

## Procedure

■ Explain the procedure to the patient, and address any questions or concerns he may have.

☑ **OBTAIN INFORMED CONSENT**

■ Wash your hands, and put on gloves.
■ Obtain a wound culture if the bite occurred at least 3 days ago. Insert the culture swab to the wound base and rotate it to collect as much exudate as possible.
■ If the wound is new and isn't bleeding heavily (as with a puncture wound), wash it vigorously with soap and water for 5 to 10 minutes. Let it bleed a bit to help flush out pathogens. You can use a syringe and catheter to create a high-pressure water stream to clean the wound.

➤ **CLINICAL TIP**
*Don't scrub a bite wound; you could bruise the tissue. Also, don't tape the wound or seal it in any way — doing so increases the risk of infection. Apply an ice pack to the wound site for 20 minutes to reduce edema and pain.*

■ Verify that the patient isn't allergic to iodine or local anesthetics.
■ If the wound involves an arm or a leg, place the extremity in an antiseptic bath for 15 to 20 minutes with warm water and antiseptic solution. For other areas, generously irrigate with equal parts of povidone-iodine and sterile saline solution. (The saline solution reduces the harmful effects of the povidone-iodine on healthy tissue.)
■ Draw up lidocaine in the smallest syringe, using a 27G needle.
■ Insert the needle at a 45-degree angle.
■ Ask the patient if he notices any change in sensation. If he reports

pain, indicating direct contact with the nerve, withdraw the needle 1 mm.

- Aspirate to make sure there's no blood return. If there is, the needle is in a blood vessel. Withdraw the needle slightly, and reinsert in another area.
- Inject 1 to 2 ml of lidocaine while partially withdrawing the needle. Then redirect the needle across the surface, advance it, and inject another 0.5 ml while withdrawing the needle. This method distributes the anesthetic uniformly, providing the optimal effect in 5 to 15 minutes.
- Clean the wound using antiseptic solution and 4″ × 4″ gauze pads.
- Irrigate the wound with copious amounts of sterile saline solution, using a 60-ml syringe and a large-gauge (18G or 20G) needle.
- Put on sterile gloves, and have the patient replicate the moment of injury if a joint may be involved, to evaluate internal structures for damage. Then place the affected area in extension. Use the curved hemostat to separate the wound edges and the straight hemostat to thoroughly expose the wound for visualization of potential damage and debris, removing any devitalized tissue and foreign objects.
- Suture the wound as indicated. (Suturing isn't indicated for initial treatment of human bites or if infection is suspected.)
- Apply topical antibiotic ointment and a dry sterile dressing.
- Administer tetanus prophylaxis as indicated.

- Administer rabies prophylaxis, if rabies is possible, without delay after consulting with a physician. (See *Treating rabies,* page 308.)
- Prescribe antibiotics to nullify infection, as indicated.

## Postprocedure patient teaching

- If the bite results in a puncture wound or a tear, advise the patient that bleeding may occur immediately and bruising and swelling may appear later.
- Teach him that signs and symptoms of infection usually appear after 24 hours. Instruct him to call your office for fever higher than 101° F (38.3° C); redness; increased swelling; cloudy, yellow, or green drainage; red streaks in the skin; or a lump in the wound that grows.
- Urge him to schedule and keep a follow-up appointment in 2 days so that you can evaluate his progress and check for infection.
- If he has a hand or foot injury, advise him that the follow-up visit is especially important because you'll need to check his neurovascular status. Tendon injuries aren't always apparent at initial presentation.
- Instruct the patient to urge any witness to the incident to report it to the authorities.

## Complications

- Infection is treated with antiseptic soaks and antibiotics four times per day.

## Treating rabies

When making decisions about how to treat rabies, you'll need to consider several factors, including the details of the exposure, the animal's species and vaccination status, and the prevalence of rabies in your region. The first step is to clean the wound thoroughly with soap and water. The table below provides general guidelines for which actions to take next. Note that the Food and Drug Administration (FDA) considers all three rabies vaccines equally safe and effective.

| SPECIES | ANIMAL'S CONDITION | TREATMENT |
|---|---|---|
| **WILD** | | |
| Skunk<br>Raccoon<br>Bat<br>Other carnivores | Considered rabid unless proven negative (the animal should be euthanized and the head tested immediately; observation isn't recommended) | Rabies immune globulin (RIG), human RIG* and human diploid cell vaccine (HDCV) or rabies vaccine (RVA), absorbed RVA** |
| **DOMESTIC** | | |
| Cat<br>Dog | Healthy and available: 10 days of isolation and observation | None |
| | Unknown (escaped) | Consult public health officials; if treatment is indicated, RIG* and HDCV or RVA** |
| **OTHER** | | |
| Livestock<br>Gnawing animals (such as hamsters, rabbits, and beavers) | Rabies suspected or known | RIG* and HDCV or RVA** (consider individually) |

* RIG should be administered at the beginning of treatment. Administer 20 IU/kg. Infiltrate the wound and then inject the remaining I.M.
** HDCV and RVA are equally effective. Administer 1 ml of vaccine I.M. on days 0, 3, 7, 14, and 28. If using HDCV, divide the dose in half, giving one-half I.M. and one-half infiltrated thoroughly around the wound. HDCV is the only rabies vaccine approved by the FDA for intradermal use.

- Neurovascular compromise may require surgical referral, and repair is possible up to 5 to 7 days after injury.

- Bleeding, pain, tenderness, swelling, and decreased sensation at the injury site are minimized by ice and elevation.

## Special considerations

■ Consult with a physician whenever you suspect that rabies is involved.

■ For temperature elevations, request a complete blood count, erythrocyte sedimentation rate and, possibly, blood cultures.

■ Over-the-counter analgesics (acetaminophen, ibuprofen) are usually adequate for pain relief.

■ If puncture wounds are simple and don't involve the hands, no other treatment is necessary. Debride moderate to severe wounds, and give the patient phenoxymethyl penicillin for 3 to 5 days (or erythromycin if patient is allergic to penicillin). If no signs or symptoms of infection appear after 2 days, close the wound with sutures or tape strips.

■ For all human bites, obtain a wound culture to rule out gram-negative organisms. The patient should receive penicillin and a beta-lactamase-resistant, penicillin-like anti-infective such as amoxicillin (unless allergic to penicillin). Delay wound closure for 2 days; then close the wound if no infection is evident.

■ Splint clenched-fist injuries, elevate them, and order X-rays to rule out fractures. Visualize the wounds fully to detect damage to internal structures and debris such as tooth fragments. Because tendons can retract significantly, the patient must replicate the positioning of the hand when the injury occurred (tight fist). Once damage is ruled out, clean the wound with the hand in extension.

## Documentation

■ Before performing this procedure, document any abnormal physical findings on the consent form. Have the patient initial the comments and sign the form to signify acknowledgment of preprocedural abnormalities.

■ Describe in detail the injury site before and after the procedure, including its location. Record your evaluation of any potentially affected function, range of motion, and sensation. Include the anesthetic type and amount used, any culture taken, the patient's reaction to the procedure, medications ordered, the time frame for follow-up evaluation, and any patient instructions given.

# MECHANICAL DEBRIDEMENT

### CPT codes

11040 *Debridement of the skin, partial thickness*
11041 *Debridement of the skin, full thickness*
11042 *Debridement of skin and subcutaneous tissue*

## Overview

Debridement involves removing dead or devitalized tissue. Wounds can be debrided enzymatically, mechanically, or autolytically to allow underlying healthy tissue to regenerate. Mechanical debridement procedures include irrigation, hydrotherapy, and excision of dead tissue with forceps and scissors. Excision may be done in the office or in a specially prepared room. Depending on the type of wound, a combination of debridement techniques may be used.

Burn wound debridement removes devitalized tissue. This prevents or controls infection, promotes healing, and prepares the wound surface to receive a graft. Frequent, regular debridement guards against possible hemorrhage resulting from more extensive and forceful debridement. It also reduces the need to conduct extensive debridement under anesthesia.

## Indications

■ To remove necrotic or devitalized tissue

## Contraindications

**ABSOLUTE**

■ Closed blisters over partial-thickness burns

## Preprocedure patient preparation

■ Advise the patient that this procedure is painful. Explain that the intensity of pain will depend on the level of injury and the degree of neurologic compromise. Assure him that pain medication will be prescribed. Have him take it 30 to 60 minutes before the procedure.

■ Teach the patient distraction and relaxation techniques to ease pain.

## Equipment

Pain medication (such as morphine) ♦ two pairs of sterile gloves ♦ two gowns or aprons ♦ mask ♦ cap ♦ sterile scissors ♦ sterile forceps ♦ 4″ × 4″ sterile gauze pads ♦ sterile solutions and medications as ordered ♦ hemostatic agent such as silver nitrate sticks ♦ needle holder (optional) ♦ gut suture with needle (optional)

## Procedure

■ Explain the procedure to the patient, and address any questions or concerns he may have.

■ Provide privacy. Administer an analgesic 30 to 60 minutes before debridement begins, or give an I.V. analgesic immediately before the procedure.

■ Keep the patient warm. Expose only the area to be debrided.

■ Put on a gown or apron, gloves, a mask, and a cap. Maintain sterile technique throughout the procedure.

■ Remove the dressings, and clean the wound.

■ Change your gown or apron and dispose of gloves. Put on a fresh set of sterile apparel.

■ Lift loosened edges of eschar with forceps. Use the blunt edge of scissors or forceps to probe the eschar. Cut the dead tissue from the wound with the scissors. Leave a ¼″ (0.6 cm) edge on remaining eschar to avoid cutting into viable tissue.

■ If bleeding occurs, apply gentle pressure on the wound with sterile 4″ × 4″ gauze pads. Then apply the hemostatic agent as needed.

■ Perform additional procedures, such as application of topical medications and dressing replacements, as indicated.

## Postprocedure patient teaching

■ Instruct the patient to schedule a follow-up appointment when you determine, guided by the degree of injury.

## Complications

■ Infection may develop when the protective skin barrier is broken. The use of sterile technique and equipment is mandatory. If infection occurs, obtain a culture and sensitivity specimen of the wound site, and treat the patient with antibiotics.

■ Blood loss may occur if debridement exposes an eroded blood vessel or if a vessel is cut inadvertently. Apply mild to moderate compression until hemostasis is achieved.

■ Fluid and electrolyte imbalances may result from exudate lost during the procedure; order serum electrolyte levels as indicated.

## Special considerations

■ Because debridement removes only dead or devitalized tissue, bleeding should be minimal. Ex-

cessive bleeding or spurting vessels may require ligation using suturing materials (sutures, needle, needle holder).

■ Refer the patient to a specialist if the wound is greater than 4″ (10 cm) and deeper than ⅓″ (1 cm), if infection is present, or if the wound is on the face, hand, or forearm.

■ If possible, work with an assistant and complete the procedure within 20 minutes to limit the patient's pain.

■ Acknowledge the patient's discomfort, and provide emotional support throughout the procedure.

## Documentation

■ Before performing this procedure, document abnormal physical findings on the consent form. Have the patient initial the comments and sign the form to signify acknowledgment of preprocedural abnormalities. In the chart, the preprocedural and postprocedural notes must include an evaluation of potentially affected function, range of motion, and sensation.

■ Record the date, time, and indications for wound debridement, the area debrided, and solutions and medications used. Describe the wound condition, noting signs of infection or skin breakdown. Record the patient's tolerance for the procedure. Note indications for additional therapy.

# METERED DOSE INHALER USE

## CPT code
94640 *Nonpressurized inhalation treatment for acute airway obstruction*

## Overview

A metered dose inhaler (MDI) is a device that consists of a metal canister that is placed in a plastic container with a mouthpiece. It's used to administer medication to the lungs for conditions such as asthma. Children younger than age 9 and some adults may need to use a spacer device with the MDI. The spacer device (which may have a small mask attached to it) attaches to the MDI to increase the amount of medicine that reaches the lungs. The MDI propels the medicine into the spacer; the patient then inhales the medicine into his lungs.

## Indications

■ To improve delivery of asthma, bronchitis, and allergy medication

## Contraindications

### ABSOLUTE
■ Inability to follow directions for MDI use

### RELATIVE
■ Difficulty using proper technique

## Equipment

MDI canister ◆ canister holder ◆ spacer (optional)

## Preprocedure patient preparation

■ Teach the patient about his disorder and how the medication will help him.

## Procedure

■ Explain the procedure to the patient, and address any questions or concerns he may have. If necessary, demonstrate the procedure.
■ Make sure the metal canister is placed securely in the plastic holder.
■ Shake the MDI well.
■ Remove the cap.
■ Have the patient exhale completely.
■ Have the patient hyperextend his head slightly and place the mouthpiece about two fingers' width in front of his mouth.
■ Have the patient start taking long, slow, deep breaths with his mouth open. About one-third of the way into a breath, have him compress the canister and holder to release a puff of medication while he continues to inhale fully. Then have him hold his breath for up to 10 seconds.
■ If the patient needs more than one puff, tell him to wait 30 seconds and repeat the procedure.
■ After the last puff, tell the patient to gargle and rinse his mouth with water. This is especially im-

portant after steroid administration to decrease the risk of thrush.

## Postprocedure patient teaching

▪ Teach the patient how to clean his MDI. Explain that he should remove the canister from the plastic holder every 1 to 2 days and set it aside. He should then rinse the plastic holder and cap with warm water, allow it to dry, and replace the canister. Explain that cleaning the MDI helps prevent clogging.
▪ Teach the patient how to determine the approximate amount of medication remaining in the MDI. He should remove the canister, place a finger on top, and shake it gently to feel the liquid moving inside. If he feels little movement, the MDI is almost empty. Alternatively, he can remove the canister and place it in clean water. The more buoyant it is, the emptier it is; if it floats on its side, it's almost empty.

## Complications

▪ Thrush usually results from steroid inhalation. Prevent this by having the patient gargle and rinse his mouth after using the MDI. If thrush occurs, treat it with an antifungal such as nystatin liquid.

## Special considerations

▪ Each patient's response varies with the medication in the MDI.
▪ A patient who can't master proper MDI technique may benefit from using a spacer device. A spacer may also decrease the risk of thrush for a patient taking steroids with the MDI. Some experts recommend that all patients using an MDI use a spacer device.
▪ If a patient has difficulty taking long, slow, deep breaths and holding his breath, it may help to have him take five breaths before removing the spacer from his mouth.
▪ If mist escapes from the patient's mouth during inhalation, medication is escaping and he isn't receiving the full dose.
▪ The patient must aim the MDI properly or the medication won't reach his lungs. If the patient reports a strong medicinal taste in his mouth after using the MDI, the medicine has only reached his mouth and not his lungs, and he needs to improve his technique.

## Documentation

▪ Document the patient's baseline knowledge, specific instructions he received, his response to the drug, and his ability to use the MDI independently (usually through reverse demonstration).
▪ Note whether the patient needed to use a spacer device.

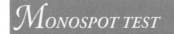

## $\mathcal{M}$ONOSPOT TEST

### CPT code
86308 *Heterophile antibodies; screening*

## Overview

Several screening tests can detect the heterophile infectious mononucleosis (IM) antibody, caused by the Epstein-Barr virus. One of these tests — the Monospot — converts the Paul-Bunnell and the Paul-Bunnell-Davidsohn differential absorption tests into one rapid slide test without titration. Monospot relies on agglutination of horse red blood cells (RBCs) by heterophile antibodies.

Because horse RBCs contain both Forssman and IM antigens, differential absorption of the patient's serum is necessary to distinguish them. This is done by mixing the serum sample with guinea pig kidney antigen (containing only Forssman antigen) on one end of a slide and with beef RBC stroma (containing only IM antigen) on the other end of the slide. Each absorbs only its specific heterophil antibody. After addition of horse RBCs to each spot, agglutination on the beef cell end of the slide indicates the presence of the IM heterophil antibody and confirms IM.

Monospot rivals the classic heterophil agglutination test for sensitivity. False-positives may occur in the presence of lymphoma, hepatitis A and hepatitis B, leukemia, and pancreatic cancer.

## Indications

■ To aid differential diagnosis of viral syndrome, including fever, malaise, pharyngitis, tender lymphadenitis or lymphadenopathy, or splenomegaly

## Contraindications

■ None known

## Preprocedure patient preparation

■ Tell the patient that he may feel a prick as the needle or lancet enters the skin to obtain a blood sample.

## Equipment

Gloves ◆ alcohol pads ◆ lancet or equipment to perform venipuncture ◆ capillary tube or 3-ml syringe ◆ commercially available Monospot test kit ◆ 4″ × 4″ gauze pads

## Procedure

■ Explain the procedure to the patient, and address any questions or concerns he may have.
■ Wash your hands, and put on gloves.
■ Perform a finger stick by cleaning the site with an alcohol pad, wiping away the first drop of blood with a gauze pad, and filling the capillary tube to the appropriate mark. Alternatively, perform a venipuncture (See "Venipuncture," page 525), and collect the sample in a 3-ml syringe. Ask the patient to apply pressure to the puncture site with a gauze pad until bleeding ceases, while you continue with the test.

- Add the blood to the "test" well on the testing device by touching the tip of the capillary tube to the well and using a plunger (provided in the kit) to expel the blood. If venipuncture was performed, expel the blood from the syringe into the test well.
- Add 2 to 3 drops of developer solution to the "sample" well.
- Read test results after the time prescribed in the manufacturer's instructions and according to the reference range provided by the manufacturer. Positive test results may appear sooner than the prescribed time, although negative results can't be confirmed until the prescribed time has expired.

### Postprocedure patient teaching

- Inform the patient that a negative Monospot test doesn't necessarily exclude IM and that further blood testing for antibodies may be necessary.
- Caution the patient on participating in contact sports or doing anything that causes abdominal strain due to the risk of splenic rupture.
- If the test is positive and IM is confirmed, instruct the patient on the treatment plan.
- Teach the patient to inform you of worsening symptoms or if symptoms don't improve over several days to 1 week.

### Complications

- If venipuncture is performed, a hematoma may develop at the venipuncture site. Warm soaks may be applied.

### Special considerations

- Positive test results won't appear until heterophile antibodies are present, which occurs approximately 1 to 2 weeks into the illness.
- Approximately 85% of patients with IM will have a positive Monospot test. Approximately 15% of patients with IM don't produce detectable levels of heterophile antibodies. If the Monospot result is negative but the patient's symptoms correlate with IM, it will be necessary to perform more specific testing.

### Documentation

- Record the indications for the testing, the method of specimen obtainment, the patient's toleration of the procedure, and the result of the testing.
- Document patient instructions given and the patient's understanding of them.

## NASAL PASSAGE EVALUATION

**CPT code**
*No specific code has been assigned.*

### Overview

When a patient presents with nasal symptoms, an evaluation of the nasal passages is necessary. Nasal disorders, such as sinusitis, allergic rhinitis, and deviated septum, can cause changes in facial features and interfere with breathing and taste. Careful assessment is required and, in many cases, recommendations for follow-up treatment may be necessary.

### Indications

■ To examine the interior nares in the presence of nasal stuffiness, suspected perforation or deviation of the nasal septum, or bleeding from the nasal passages

### Contraindications

■ None known

### Preprocedure patient preparation

■ Obtain a complete health history from the patient, including details regarding his present symptoms.

### Equipment

Otoscope with a short, wide-tip attachment or a penlight or small flashlight ◆ nasal speculum ◆ gloves

### Procedure

■ Explain the procedure to the patient, and address any questions or concerns he may have.
■ Wash your hands.
■ Test nasal patency by asking the patient to block one nostril while he inhales through the other. This should cause no respiratory difficulties if the unobstructed nare is patent. Repeat on other nostril. Because most neonates and infants are nose-breathers, obstruct one nostril of these patients with your finger while holding the mouth closed.
■ Inspect the nasal cavity. Ask the patient to tilt his head back slight-

## Inspecting the nostrils

The illustration below shows the proper placement of the nasal speculum during direct inspection as well as the structures that should be visible during this examination.

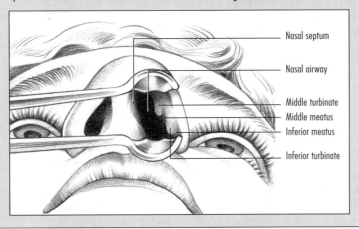

- Nasal septum
- Nasal airway
- Middle turbinate
- Middle meatus
- Inferior meatus
- Inferior turbinate

ly, then push up the tip of his nose. Use the light from the otoscope to illuminate his nasal cavities. Check for severe deviation or perforation of the nasal septum. Examine the vestibule and turbinates for redness, softness, and discharge.

■ Put on gloves. Examine the nostrils by direct inspection, using a nasal speculum, a penlight or small flashlight, or an otoscope with a short, wide-tip attachment. With the patient's head still tilted back, insert the tip of the closed nasal speculum into one nostril to the point where the blade widens. Slowly open the speculum as wide as possible without causing discomfort. Shine the flashlight in the nostril to illuminate the area.

■ Observe the color and patency of the nostril, and check for exudates. The mucosa should be moist, pink to light red, and free from lesions and polyps. After inspecting one nostril, close the speculum, remove it, and inspect the other nostril. (See *Inspecting the nostrils*.)

## Postprocedure patient teaching

■ Explain your examination findings to the patient, and provide follow-up care or teaching as necessary.

## Complications

■ Minimize irritation or bleeding of the nasal lining by inserting the otoscope no farther than necessary to illuminate the nasal cavity and inserting the nasal speculum with gentle technique.

## Special considerations

■ Obstruction of the nasal mucous membranes along with a discharge of thin mucous can signal systemic disorders; such nasal or sinus disorders as a deviated septum; trauma, such as a basilar skull or nasal fracture; excessive use of vasoconstricting nose drops or sprays; or allergies or exposure to irritants, such as dust, tobacco smoke, and fumes.

■ In a neonate or infant, obstruction can signal choanal atresia, a congenital anomaly in which an occlusion blocks the passageway between the nose and pharynx.

## Documentation

■ Record the appearance of the nasal cavity, including color and presence of discharge and nasal patency. Document any abnormal variations.

■ Document follow-up care and teaching that were given as appropriate. Also, record all necessary referrals.

## *N*ASOGASTRIC TUBE *INSERTION AND REMOVAL*

### *CPT codes*
91100 *Intestinal feeding tube, passage, positioning, and monitoring*

91105 *Gastric intubation for aspiration and treatment*

## Overview

Intended for short-term use, a nasogastric (NG) tube has many clinical indications ranging from gastric evacuation to enteral feeding and medication administration. Made of rubber or plastic, NG tubes are passed into the stomach through the nose. Orogastric tubes inserted through the mouth are an option; however, the nose is the preferred route because it minimizes discomfort related to the gag reflex. A patient with a head injury or known septal deviation or who recently had nasal surgery should have the tube inserted orally.

The Levin tube is a single-lumen catheter used for feeding. The Salem sump tube is a double-lumen tube with a separate port for air ventilation. This is commonly used for gastric decompression and lavage. The air vent allows for a constant flow of air to prevent suction of the gastric mucosa. Nasoduodenal tubes (such as the Dobhoff tube) and other soft feeding tubes are available for long-term use. Feeding tubes differ from NG tubes in that the lumens are smaller and more flexible. This helps prevent oropharyngeal and esophageal irritation and pressure necrosis.

## Indications

■ To prevent nausea and vomiting

and to facilitate gastric decompression after surgery
■ To provide a route for feeding and medication administration
■ To remove stomach contents for laboratory analysis
■ To assess GI bleeding
■ To facilitate decompression for paralytic ileus or intestinal obstruction

## Contraindications
**ABSOLUTE**
■ Comatose or obtunded patients with unprotected airway
■ Facial fractures or basilar skull fracture with cribriform plate injury
■ Hypothermic patients (insertion may cause myocardial irritability leading to ventricular fibrillation)

**RELATIVE**
■ History of known caustic ingestions
■ Recent gastrectomy, esophagectomy, or oropharyngeal, gastric, or nasal surgery
■ Known coagulopathies or anticoagulant therapy

## Preprocedure patient preparation

■ Explain possible complications and alternative treatments, if available.
■ Explain that he may feel some discomfort, such as gagging or tearing of the eyes. Request that he cooperate as much as possible with swallowing while the tube is inserted.

■ Place an emesis basin and tissues within his reach.
■ Agree on a signal for the patient to use when he wants to pause before continuing.

## Equipment
Gastric tube (14F to 18F) ◆ lidocaine gel and benzocaine spray (optional) ◆ water-soluble lubricant ◆ phenylephrine spray (optional) ◆ basin filled with warm water or ice (optional) ◆ 20- to 50-ml syringe with adapter ◆ cotton-tipped applicators ◆ emesis basin ◆ 1″ hypoallergenic tape ◆ tincture of benzoin ◆ suction setup ◆ penlight ◆ safety pin and elastic band ◆ linen-saver pad or towel ◆ glass of water and drinking straw ◆ tissues ◆ stethoscope ◆ gloves

### Equipment preparation
■ Inspect the NG tube for defects, such as rough edges or partially closed lumens.
■ Check the tube's patency by flushing it with water.
■ To ease insertion, increase a stiff tube's flexibility by coiling it around your gloved fingers for a few seconds or by dipping it into warm water. Stiffen a limp rubber tube by briefly chilling it in ice.

## Procedure
### Inserting the tube
■ Explain the procedure to the patient, and address any questions or concerns he may have. This will promote his cooperation and reduce his anxiety.

## Determining the length of an NG tube

To determine the length necessary for a nasogastric (NG) tube to reach the stomach, hold the end of it at the tip of the patient's nose. Next, extend the tube to the patient's earlobe, then down to the xiphoid process, as shown here.

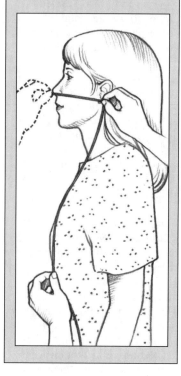

■ Give him a glass of water with a drinking straw to assist with swallowing the tube.

■ Cover his clothing or gown with a towel or linen-saver pad to protect from spillage.

■ Wash your hands, and put on gloves.

■ Provide privacy and maintain clean technique.

■ Assist the patient into a high Fowler's position and support his head with a pillow, if available. This position helps decrease the gag reflex, promotes patient swallowing, and allows gravity to assist with tube insertion.

■ Check for deformity or obstruction of the nostrils. Ask the patient to hyperextend his neck and observe the nares either by using a penlight or by having the patient breathe in while occluding the other nostril. Select the most patent naris for tube insertion.

■ If the patient is unconscious, place him in the left lateral position with his head turned downward and to the side to prevent aspiration.

■ Apply topical lidocaine to the nares with a cotton-tipped applicator and spray benzocaine into the throat as needed.

■ Have the patient blow his nose to clear his nasal passages. If he has a lot of nasal congestion, spray a vasoconstrictor, such as phenylephrine, into each nostril.

■ Determine how far to insert the tube. (See *Determining the length of an NG tube*.) Mark the tube with adhesive tape if the tube doesn't have printed markings on it.

■ Before insertion, curl 4″ to 6″ (10 to 15 cm) of the end of the tube around your finger and then release it. This produces a curve in the tube, which eases insertion around the natural contours in the nose.

■ Generously lubricate the tip of the tube with water-soluble gel or lidocaine gel to decrease mucosal irritation. Unlike a lipid-soluble lubricant, a water-soluble lubricant reduces the risk of aspiration pneumonia if the tube enters the trachea.

■ With the patient's neck hyperextended (if his cervical spine is unaffected), insert the tube with its natural curve toward the patient into the selected nostril and gently advance the tube toward the nasopharynx. (See *Positioning for NG tube placement.*)

■ Direct the tube along the floor of the nostril and toward the ear on the same side. If you meet resistance, withdraw and relubricate the tube and insert it into the other nostril.

■ Once the tube reaches the oropharynx (throat), you'll meet resistance. At this point, have the patient tilt his head forward and continue to pass the tube steadily. (Tilting the head forward helps pass the tube through the esophagus rather than the larynx.) Encourage the patient to swallow water to assist with passing of the tube.

■ If the patient continues to gag, have him rest, take a few deep breaths, and drink water.

■ If the tube doesn't advance with each swallow, withdraw it slightly and inspect the patient's mouth. If the tube is coiled in the back of the mouth or throat, withdraw it until it's straight and then resume insertion.

**CLINICAL TIP**

*If the patient is coughing, choking, or otherwise showing signs of respiratory distress, withdraw the tube until symptoms subside. Once the patient recovers, try again to pass the tube. If you can't pass the tube to*

## Positioning for NG tube placement

Instruct the patient to look straight ahead with her head held upright. Grasp the nasogastric (NG) tube with the end pointing downward, curve it if necessary, and carefully insert it into the nostril. Aim the tube downward and laterally toward the chosen nostril.

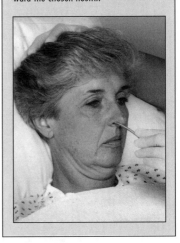

*the measured length, the tube is probably in the trachea. Pull back and try again.*

■ When the tube is inserted to the measured length, verify tube placement by one of these methods, as appropriate:

– Always use radiographic confirmation of tube placement before starting any feedings or medication administration, except in patients undergoing gastric lavage or in an emergency.

– Aspirate contents with a syringe. Gastric contents help determine tube placement.

– Auscultate over the edge of the epigastric area as you inject 10 to 30 cc of air. You'll hear a "whoosh"

## Securing the NG tube

To secure the nasogastric (NG) tube to the patient's nose, you'll need about 4″ (10 cm) of 1″ tape. Split one end of the tape up the center about 1½″ (4 cm). Make tabs on the split ends. Stick the uncut tape end on the patient's nose so that the split in the tape starts about ½″ to 1½″ (1.5 to 4 cm) from the tip of her nose. Crisscross the tabbed ends around the tube. You may apply another piece of tape over the bridge of the nose to secure the tube.

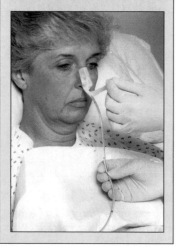

sound if the tube has been placed correctly.
– Ask the patient to talk and hum. If the tube is in his stomach, he'll be able to talk freely.
■ After you've confirmed placement, secure the tube with hypoallergenic tape.
■ Apply benzoin or some type of skin preparation to the patient's face before taping.
■ Use adhesive tape to secure the tube to the bridge of the patient's nose. (See *Securing the NG tube*.)

■ Wrap a rubber band around the tube and pin it to the patient's gown over his shoulder to prevent him from inadvertently moving the tube.

### Inserting the tube via the mouth
■ Place the tube over the patient's tongue instead of through the nasopharynx, if nasal insertion is contraindicated.
■ Remove any dentures before inserting the tube.
■ Ask the patient to lower his chin and open his mouth.
■ Place the tip of the tube on the back of the patient's tongue, give him a cup of water, and tell him to swallow.
■ Advance the tube as he swallows.
■ To advance the tube, follow the same steps for nasal tube insertion.

### Removing the tube
■ Explain the procedure to the patient. Inform him that he may experience discomfort and gagging with tube removal.
■ Assess bowel sounds.
■ Turn off the suction and disconnect the patient from it.
■ Assist him into an upright position and drape a towel over his gown or clothing.
■ Flush the NG tube with air to remove irritating stomach contents before removing the tube.
■ Remove adhesive tape and unpin the tube from the patient's gown.
■ Clamp the tube by folding it in half.
■ Have him take a deep breath and hold it.
■ Gently but quickly remove the

tube to avoid complications (such as aspiration). Tell the patient he can breathe freely. Dispose of the tube appropriately.

■ Provide tissues for the patient to blow his nose.

## Postprocedure patient teaching

■ Caution the patient that he may feel some discomfort from having the NG tube in his nose. Explain that this is common and that the discomfort will be alleviated when the tube is removed.

■ Tell him to avoid food and drink for several hours after the tube is removed to avoid aspiration. (Some health care providers recommend following a soft, bland diet for 12 to 24 hours.)

■ Urge him to report nausea, vomiting, abdominal distention, or increased pain occurring within 48 hours after tube removal.

## Complications

■ Epistaxis can be minimized through gentle handling.

**COLLABORATION**

■ *Pneumothorax requires immediate evaluation and X-ray, possible chest tube placement, and referral to a physician or pulmonologist.*

■ *Perforation of the esophagus and creation of a false passage requires referral to an ear, nose, and throat specialist.*

■ *In rare cases, intracranial tube placement can occur in a head trauma patient, requiring immediate referral to a neurosurgeon.*

■ Aspiration leading to pneumonia requires evaluation, including

X-rays, antibiotics, and supportive therapy.

■ Tube displacement, more common with long-term use, requires reevaluation of the patient's need for the tube. In most cases, another tube is inserted.

■ Necrosis of nasal mucosa or erosion of the esophagus or stomach can occur with long-term placement. Because of this, softer tubes are indicated for long-term therapy.

## Special considerations

■ The nose is the preferred route for temporary gastric tube insertion unless contraindicated by head injury or known nasal deformity.

■ Be aware of respiratory changes during tube insertion. Cyanosis in an unconscious patient and coughing or choking in a conscious patient indicate that the tube may be in the trachea. Withdraw the tube immediately, and try to reinsert it when the patient has recovered.

■ For the unconscious patient, tilt the head forward to close the epiglottis while inserting the tube. Be sure the patient has been evaluated and that he doesn't have a cervical spine injury. Advance the tube gently between respirations to avoid passage of the tube into the airway.

## Documentation

■ Review documentation by other health team members; then initial their notes to signify you're aware of their findings. This doesn't signify agreement with their comments or reduce your responsibility to complete your own history and physical examination. Document abnormal physical findings. (The preprocedural and postprocedural note must include an evaluation of neurologic, respiratory, and GI function.)

■ Record indications for the procedure, the type and size of the NG tube used, and the patient's response to tube insertion.

■ Document any known trauma during tube insertion. If the tube is attached to suction equipment, document the amount of suctioning and whether it's continuous or intermittent. Describe characteristics of aspirated secretions, such as color, amount, consistency, and odor.

■ Record tube removal, the patient's response, and the amount and characteristics of gastric contents.

■ Record the date and time of tube insertion and removal and the patient's tolerance of the procedure.

## *N*EBULIZER THERAPY

### *CPT codes*
94640 *Nonpressurized inhalation treatment for acute airway obstruction*
94664 *Aerosol inhalation, initial*
94665 *Aerosol inhalation, subsequent*

## Overview

An established component of respiratory care, nebulizer therapy aids bronchial hygiene by restoring and maintaining mucous blanket continuity; hydrating dried, retained secretions; promoting expectoration of secretions; humidifying inspired oxygen; and delivering medications. The therapy may be administered through nebulizers that have a large or small volume, are ultrasonic, or are placed inside ventilator tubing.

An ultrasonic nebulizer is electrically driven and uses high-frequency vibrations to break up surface water into particles. The resultant dense mist can penetrate the smaller airways and is useful for hydrating secretions and inducing a cough. A large-volume nebulizer can provide humidity for an artificial airway such as a tracheostomy; a small-volume nebulizer allows delivery of medications such as bronchodilators. (See *Comparing nebulizers.*)

Many questions still exist regarding aerosol therapy, including what type of fluid to use, the type of medications that can be delivered, and the effectiveness of therapy.

## Indications

■ To relieve bronchospasm
■ To provide relief to a symptomatic patient with a hyperresponsive airway
■ Liquefaction and clearance of tenacious secretions

## Comparing nebulizers

Each type of nebulizer has different advantages and disadvantages, as seen in this chart.

| TYPE | DESCRIPTION AND USES | ADVANTAGES AND DISADVANTAGES |
|------|----------------------|------------------------------|
| Ultrasonic 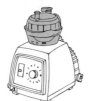 | Uses high-frequency sound waves to create an aerosol mist | *Advantages* <br> ■ Provides 100% humidity <br> ■ About 20% of its particles reach the lower airways <br> ■ Loosens secretions <br> *Disadvantages* <br> ■ May precipitate bronchospasms in the asthmatic patient <br> ■ Increased risk of overhydration in infants |
| Large volume (Venturi jet) 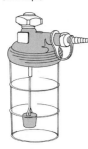 | Supplies cool or heated moisture to a patient whose upper airway has been bypassed by endotracheal intubation or a tracheostomy, or who has recently been extubated | *Advantages* <br> ■ Provides 100% humidity with cool or heated devices <br> ■ Provides oxygen and aerosol therapy <br> ■ Can be used for long-term therapy <br> *Disadvantages* <br> ■ Increased risk of bacterial growth with nondisposable units <br> ■ May collect condensation in its large-bore tubing <br> ■ Requires correct water level in reservoir, or mucosal irritation may result from breathing hot, dry air <br> ■ Increased risk of overhydration from mist in infants |
| Small volume (mini-nebulizer, Maxi-mist) 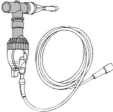 | Delivers aerosolized medication and is handheld | *Advantages* <br> ■ Conforms to patient's physiology, allowing him to inhale and exhale on his own <br> ■ Results in less air trapping than medication administered by intermittent positive-pressure breathing <br> ■ May be used with compressed air, oxygen, or compressor pump <br> ■ Is compact and disposable <br> *Disadvantages* <br> ■ Takes a long time if patient needs assistance <br> ■ Unevenly distributes medication if patient doesn't breathe properly |

# Contraindications

**RELATIVE**
- Tachycardia

# Preprocedure patient preparation

- Explain that slow, deep breaths enhance medication administration and reduce adverse effects.
- Explain that the treatment is complete when the medication and mist disappear.

# Equipment

Air compressor ◆ mask or mouthpiece ◆ medication (typically beta agonists such as albuterol, corticosteroids such as methylprenisolone, or cromoglycates such as cromolyn sodium) ◆ normal saline solution ◆ peak flow meter ◆ pulse oximeter

### For an ultrasonic nebulizer
Ultrasonic gas-delivery device ◆ large-bore oxygen tubing ◆ nebulizer couplet compartment

### For a large-volume nebulizer (such as Venturi jet)
Pressurized gas source ◆ flowmeter ◆ large-bore oxygen tubing ◆ nebulizer bottle ◆ sterile distilled water ◆ heater (if indicated) ◆ in-line thermometer (if using heater)

### For a small-volume nebulizer (such as a mini-nebulizer)
Pressurized gas source ◆ flowmeter ◆ oxygen tubing ◆ nebulizer cup ◆ mouthpiece or mask ◆ normal saline solution or sterile distilled water

# Equipment preparation
### For an ultrasonic nebulizer
- Fill the couplet compartment on the nebulizer to the level indicated.

### For a large-volume nebulizer
- Fill the water chamber to the indicated level with sterile distilled water. Avoid using saline solution to prevent corrosion.
- Add a heating device, if ordered, and place a thermometer in-line between the outlet port and the patient (as close to the patient as possible) to monitor the actual temperature of the inhaled gas and to avoid burning the patient.
- If the unit will supply oxygen, analyze the flow at the patient's end of the tubing to ensure delivery of the prescribed oxygen percentage.

### For a small-volume nebulizer
- Draw up the prescribed medication and inject it into the nebulizer cup.
- Add the prescribed amount of normal saline solution or water.
- Attach the mouthpiece or mask.

# Procedure

- Explain the procedure to the patient, and address any questions or concerns he may have.
- Wash your hands.
- Determine whether to use a mask or mouthpiece. If possible, place the patient in a sitting or high Fowler's position to encourage full lung expansion and promote aerosol dispersion. Obtain baseline data, including vital signs, pulse oximetry, and peak expirato-

ry flow rate (PEFR). Perform screening history and physical, including percussion and auscultation of lung fields.

■ Before beginning, administer an inhaled bronchodilator as indicated, using a metered-dose inhaler or small-volume nebulizer to prevent bronchospasm.

■ Turn on the machine, and check the outflow port to ensure fine misting.

■ Attach the pulse oximeter and monitor throughout treatment.

■ Attach the delivery device to the patient.

■ Encourage the patient to cough and expectorate. Suction as needed.

■ Encourage the patient to take slow, deep breaths.

■ After treatment, auscultate the patient's lungs and repeat the PEFR to evaluate the effectiveness of therapy.

### For an ultrasonic nebulizer

■ Instruct the patient to inhale until the mist disappears and then slowly exhale. Repeat until the medication and the mist disappears.

■ Check the patient frequently during the procedure to observe for adverse reactions. Watch for labored respirations because ultrasonic nebulizer therapy may hydrate retained secretions and obstruct airways.

### For a large-volume nebulizer

■ Attach the delivery device to the patient.

■ Encourage the patient to cough and expectorate. Suction as needed.

■ Check the water level in the nebulizer at frequent intervals and refill or replace as indicated. When refilling a reusable container, discard the old water to prevent infection from bacterial or fungal growth and refill the container to the indicator line with sterile distilled water.

■ Change the nebulizer unit and tubing according to your facility's policy to prevent bacterial contamination.

■ If the nebulizer is heated, tell the patient to report any warmth, discomfort, or hot tubing because these may indicate a heater malfunction. Use the in-line thermometer to monitor the temperature of the gas the patient is inhaling. If you turn off the flow for more than 5 minutes, unplug the heater to avoid overheating the water and burning the patient when the aerosol is resumed.

### For a small-volume nebulizer

■ After attaching the flowmeter to the gas source, attach the nebulizer to the flowmeter and then adjust the flow to at least 10 L/minute to ensure adequate functioning but not more than 14 L/minute to prevent excess venting.

■ Check the outflow port to ensure fine misting.

■ Attach to the delivery device to the patient and remain with him during the treatment, which lasts 15 to 20 minutes. Monitor his vital signs (including pulse and respirations within 5 minutes of treatment initiation) to detect any adverse reaction to the medication.

■ Encourage the patient to cough and expectorate. Suction as necessary. Change the nebulizer cup and tubing according to facility policy to prevent bacterial contamination.

## Postprocedure patient teaching

■ Tell the patient that difficulty breathing, chest tightness, and shortness of breath should ease within 15 minutes of treatment. If he doesn't feel significant relief, the PEFR remains unacceptable, or improvement doesn't last for 4 hours, he may need another treatment or more aggressive action.

■ Tell the patient treated at an emergency department or urgent care center to follow up with his health care provider within 1 to 2 days to evaluate the treatment regimen.

■ Tell the patient to perform nebulizer treatments at home using medications as prescribed. Tell him to notify you of any changes in his condition or if he experiences such adverse effects as nervousness, edginess, rapid heart rate, or palpitations.

■ Tell the patient to seek emergency treatment for nasal flaring, intercostal retractions (the skin between the ribs sinks in during inhalation), or blue nail beds or lips. He should call you for wheezing during inspiration and expiration, breathing out that takes longer than breathing in, and rapid breathing.

■ If the patient is a child who needs to use a compressor-driven nebulizer (a special type of nebu-

lizer), review its use with his parents.

## Complications

■ Airway burns (when heating elements are used) may require further evaluation and treatment depending on the severity of the burn.

■ Adverse reactions from medications require you to stop the medication, decrease the dosage, or wean as soon as possible.

## Special considerations

■ When using a high-output nebulizer (such as an ultrasonic nebulizer) for a child or a patient with a delicate fluid balance, watch for signs of overhydration. These include unexplained weight gain that occurs over several days after the beginning of therapy, pulmonary edema, crackles, and electrolyte imbalance.

■ If the patient is receiving oxygen concomitantly, he may need a higher oxygen flow to maintain his fraction of inspired oxygen ($FIO_2$); increase the oxygen flow if the mist disappears when the patient inhales.

## Documentation

■ Record the time of the treatment, the type and amount of medication given, and the patient's response to treatment.

■ Note the $FIO_2$ or oxygen flow, if administered.

■ Record baseline and posttreatment vital signs, PEFR, pulse oximetry, and breath sounds.

## NORPLANT INSERTION

### CPT codes

11975 *Insertion of implantable contraceptive capsules*
11977 *Removal of implantable contraceptive capsules with reinsertion of implantable contraceptive capsules*

## Overview

The Norplant System (levonorgestrel implants) is the first and only sustained-release subdermal contraceptive delivery system. It provides effective contraception for up to 5 years and consists of six thin, flexible capsules of soft silastic tubing sealed at each end with silicone. Each capsule is 34 mm long and 2.4 mm diameter and contains 36 mg of dry crystalline levonorgestrel. The capsules are very stable; levonorgestrel is released over a period of 5 years. During the first year, approximately 80 mcg/day is released. Gradually, the release of levonorgestrel decreases to 30 to 40 mcg/day.

Norplant is a progestin-only contraceptive and differs from the progestin-only mini-pill by maintaining a constant level of levonorgestrel. It has two possible mechanisms of action: ovulation is suppressed in most of the menstrual cycles because Norplant maintains a consistent low level of progestin; or cervical mucus is thickened, providing a hostile passage for sperm and preventing sperm penetration into the lining of the uterus.

The placement of the Norplant System involves a counseling visit, followed by the office procedure in which the capsules are inserted.

## Indications

- To be used in patients desiring long-term reversible contraception
- To be used in patients who have difficulty remembering to take birth control pills daily
- To be used in patients who can't tolerate other forms of contraception, such as birth control pills and such coitus-dependent techniques as condoms and diaphragms
- To be used in patients who can't tolerate estrogen administration.

## Contraindications

**ABSOLUTE**

- Active thrombophlebitis or thromboembolic disease
- Undiagnosed abnormal genital bleeding
- Possible pregnancy
- Acute liver disease
- Benign or malignant liver tumors
- Known or suspected carcinoma of the breast
- Lack of informed consent
- Unwillingness to accept amenorrhea or metrorrhagia for at least 6 to 9 months
- Excessive concern over the mini-

mal scar that will occur at the site of placement
- Patient who is less than 6 weeks postpartum
- Foreign body carcinogenesis

**RELATIVE**
- Cigarette smokers younger than age 35

## Preprocedure patient preparation

- Emphasize that the Norplant System doesn't provide protection from diseases. As appropriate, review barrier methods, such as a female dam or a male condom.
- Review the history of the Norplant System's effectiveness with the patient. Inform the patient that although this method isn't absolutely foolproof, it has a failure rate of less than 1%.
- Discuss the advantages of the Norplant System, including the absence of estrogen, the long duration of use, its effectiveness combined with its reversibility, and the fact that nothing needs to be remembered and it's independent of coitus. It's effective within 24 hours of insertion if inserted within 7 days of the onset of menses.
- Review the possible adverse effects of the Norplant System, including arm pain, weight gain, headaches, bloating, nausea, depression, dizziness, sore breasts, and acne.
- Tell the patient that irregular bleeding occurs in 60% of women; the patient can expect to experience an alteration of menstrual patterns during the first year. The

menstrual cycle usually becomes more regular within 9 to 12 months.

## Equipment

Norplant System (set of six Norplant System capsules, Norplant System obturator and trocar, #11 scalpel, 5-ml syringe, two 25G needles, package of skin closures, package of three gauze pads, stretch bandage, two sterile drapes, fenestrated surgical drape) ◆ butterfly adhesive strip ◆ 5 ml of 1% or 2% lidocaine without epinephrine ◆ sterile gloves and clean gloves ◆ antiseptic solution such as povidone-iodine solution ◆ normal saline solution ◆ ice pack ◆ Elastoplast (optional) ◆ template to mark the locations for insertion (optional)

## Procedure

- Review the method of insertion with the patient and answer any questions. If there are no contraindications and the patient indicates that she would like to use the Norplant System, obtain an informed consent. (*Note:* The company provides a model arm, so you can show this display, sample capsules, and the site of insertion to the patient.)

☑ **OBTAIN INFORMED CONSENT**
- Verify that the patient isn't pregnant.
- Instruct the patient to lie in a supine position on the examination table with her nondominant arm flexed and the elbow external-

ly rotated so that her hand is lying by her head.

■ Wash your hands, and put on gloves. Verify that the patient isn't allergic to iodine, and clean the patient's upper arm with antiseptic solution. Cover the arm above and below the insertion area with a sterile drape.

■ Open the sterile Norplant System package carefully by pulling apart the sheets of the pouch, allowing the capsules to fall onto a sterile cloth. Count the 6 capsules.

■ Fill a 5-ml syringe with local anesthetic.

■ Anesthetize the insertion area by first inserting the needle under the skin at a 45-degree angle and injecting a small amount of the anesthetic as you withdraw the needle. Then anesthetize 6 areas about $1\frac{1}{2}''$ to $1\frac{3}{4}''$ (4 to 4.5 cm) long, to mimic the fanlike position of the implanted capsules.

▶ CLINICAL TIP
*Because epinephrine can cause cutaneous ulceration, only use lidocaine.*

■ Put on sterile gloves.

■ Use the scalpel to make a small, shallow incision (about 2 mm) through the skin. The optimal insertion area is in the inside of the upper arm about 3″ to 4″ (8 to 10 cm) above the elbow crease.

■ Insert the tip of the trocar subdermally through a small 2-mm incision beneath the skin at a shallow angle. Once the trocar is inserted, it should be oriented with the bevel up toward the skin to keep the capsules in a superficial plane. Correct subdermal place-

ment of the capsules facilitates removal.

■ Advance the trocar gently under the skin to the first mark near the hub of the trocar. The tip of the trocar is now at a distance of about $1\frac{1}{2}''$ to $1\frac{3}{4}''$ (4 to 4.5 cm) from the incision. Don't force the trocar; if resistance is felt, try another direction.

■ The skin should be visibly tented at all times as the trocar is advanced. Keep the trocar superficial even though this typically requires more force than subcutaneous insertion.

■ When the trocar has been inserted the appropriate distance, remove the obturator and load the first capsule into the trocar using the thumb and forefinger.

■ Gently advance the capsule with the obturator toward the tip of the trocar until you feel resistance. Never force the obturator.

■ Hold the obturator steady and retract the trocar until it touches the handle of the obturator.

■ As the trocar is withdrawn, hold the distal tip of the capsule in place through the skin. Proximally, as the trocar is withdrawn to the mark near the tip, you should be able to feel the capsule fall from the tip. Place your index finger over this newly inserted capsule to prevent the trocar from catching on it. If the trocar catches the capsule, it could damage it or force it back under the skin where it will lie in a bent position.

■ Don't remove the trocar from the incision until all capsules have been inserted. The trocar is withdrawn only to the mark close to its

## Checking capsule placement

After insertion, once again identify the six subdermal implants. If the capsules are dropped or if the patient expels a capsule, it can be returned to the company and replaced without cost to the patient or to your facility.

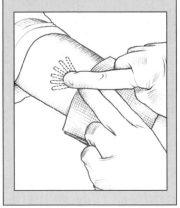

tip. Each succeeding capsule is inserted next to the previous capsule with the forefinger and middle finger of the free hand.

■ Advance the trocar along the tips of the fingers. This action will ensure a suitable distance of about 15 degrees between capsules and keep the trocar from puncturing previously inserted capsules. Leave a distance of about 5 mm between the incision and the tips of the capsules. This action will help to prevent spontaneous expulsions. Ensure the correct position of the capsules by feeling them after the insertion has been completed. (See *Checking capsule placement.*)

■ Press the edges of the incision together, and close the incision with a butterfly adhesive strip.

■ Cover the insertion area with

gauze pads, and wrap the stretch bandage around the arm to ensure hemostasis. Observe the patient for a few minutes for signs of syncope or bleeding from the incision before she's discharged.

■ Apply an ice pack to the site. Instruct the patient to remove the dressing in 1 day and to keep the area clean and dry for 3 days.

## Postprocedure patient teaching

■ Inform the patient that there's a low incidence of thromboembolic phenomena. However, the patient subjected to prolonged immobilization due to surgery or other illness should have the capsules removed before surgery for thrombophlebitis prophylaxis.

■ Tell the patient that she may have arm pain and a large ecchymotic area at the insertion site, which should resolve in approximately 2 weeks.

■ Instruct the patient to ice the area immediately after insertion to decrease bruising.

■ Tell the patient to take acetaminophen (Tylenol) or ibuprofen (Motrin) every 4 to 6 hours as needed for pain.

■ Tell the patient that the gauze may be removed after 1 day. The butterfly bandage may be removed as soon as the incision has healed (normally in 3 days).

■ Advise the patient to keep the insertion area dry for 2 to 3 days.

## Complications

■ Infection near the site of insertion is very uncommon (0.7%);

however, if the site becomes infected, the capsules must be removed and the area must be allowed to heal. The health care provider will decide if all capsules need to be removed.

■ Expulsion of a capsule may occur. This is more common if the placement is too shallow or if infection occurs at the time of insertion. A new, sterile capsule must be placed because fewer than six capsules may provide inadequate contraception.

■ Ulceration over the area is possible and may be more common when the local anesthetic contains epinephrine. Removal of capsules to allow healing is required.

## Special considerations

■ It's important to let women know of the more common adverse effects, such as irregular menses, weight gain, some hair loss, headaches, and hyperpigmentation at the site. Depression and premenstrual symptoms may improve or become worse.

■ Removal of the implants can be difficult because of scar tissue that forms around the implants.

■ Stress the need for annual Pap tests for the patient using long-term contraceptive systems, even though she doesn't need a new prescription.

■ Studies on the Norplant System focused on women ages 18 to 40; however, many health care providers don't impose a lower or upper age limit.

## Documentation

■ Always document that the patient has read the patient education handouts and that you have discussed the risks, benefits, possible complications, and alternatives.

■ Include indications for the procedure, the number of capsules placed, the insertion site, the patient's response to the procedure, site appearance postprocedure, instructions given, and any patient concerns.

# $\mathcal{N}$ORPLANT REMOVAL

## CPT codes
11976  *Removal of implantable contraceptive capsules*
11977  *Removal of implantable contraceptive capsules with reinsertion of implantable contraceptive capsules*

## Overview

Removal of the Norplant System involves incising the area and withdrawing the capsules with forceps, which takes about 20 minutes to perform. It requires more skill and patience than insertion. Removal can be complicated by an initial irregular placement or by a fracture of the silastic capsules.

The modified U technique requires half the time for removal but requires a modified #11 scalpel vasectomy clamp. Local anesthesia is used only at the site of removal.

## Indications

■ To remove capsules due to persistent infection, upon request by the patient, for medical indications, or at the end of 5 years from the time of insertion

## Contraindications

**ABSOLUTE**

■ All 6 capsules aren't palpable. If any of the 6 capsules can't be palpated, they must be located by using ultrasound, X-ray, or compressed mammography before removal can be performed.

## Preprocedure patient preparation

■ Discuss the patient's plan for birth control after the capsules are removed.

## Equipment

Sterile fenestrated drape ◆ sterile gloves ◆ antiseptic solution ◆ local anesthetic with 30G needle ◆ 3-ml syringe ◆ #11 scalpel ◆ forceps (straight and curved mosquito) ◆ butterfly adhesive strips such as Steri-Strips ◆ 4″ × 4″ sterile gauze ◆ Elastoplast or a stretch bandage ◆ sterile skin marker (optional)

## Procedure

■ Explain the procedure to the patient, and address any questions or concerns she may have.
■ Wash your hands, and put on gloves. Draw anesthetic into 3-ml syringe with 30G needle. Clean the area with gauze and antiseptic in a circular motion from the site outward. Apply the fenestrated drape to the insertion area.
■ Locate the implanted capsules by palpation, marking the position with a sterile skin marker if desired. Apply a small amount of local anesthetic under the capsule ends nearest the original incision site by inserting the needle at a 45-degree angle and injecting. This action will serve to raise the ends of the capsules. Anesthetics injected over the capsules will obscure them and make removal more difficult. Additional small amounts of anesthetic can be used for removing each of the capsules, if required.
■ Make a 4-mm incision with the scalpel close to the ends of the capsules — avoid making a large incision.
■ Push each capsule gently toward the incision with the fingers, then grasp it with a mosquito forceps. (See *Removing contraceptive capsules*.)
■ After the procedure is completed, close the incision with a butterfly adhesive strip and bandage as with insertion.

## Postprocedure patient teaching

■ Tell the patient that following removal, a return to the previous level of fertility is usually prompt, and pregnancy may occur at any time.
■ Instruct the patient to keep the upper arm dry for 3 days.

## Complications

- Infection requires evaluation and possible culture and sensitivity study; it's treated with a broad-spectrum antibiotic until laboratory results allow refined treatment. If capsules remain under the skin, refer the patient to a gynecologist.
- Ulceration is avoided by ensuring there is no epinephrine in the anesthetic agent.

## Special considerations

- If the patient wishes to continue using the method, a new set of Norplant System capsules can be inserted through the same incision in the same or opposite direction.
- If the Norplant capsules have been in for a while, there will be a fibrous structure encapsulating them.
- Capsules can sometimes be nicked during removal. However, the incidence of overall difficulties, including damage to capsules, has been 13.2% percent; less than one half of the difficulties occurring during removal cause inconvenience to the patient.
- If the removal of some of the capsules proves difficult, schedule the patient to return for a second visit. The remaining capsules will be easier to remove after the area has healed. If contraception is still desired, a barrier method should be advised until all capsules are removed.

### Removing contraceptive capsules

Push each capsule gently toward the incision with your fingers. When the tip is visible or near the incision, grasp it with a mosquito forceps.

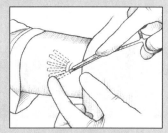

Use the scalpel to gently open the tissue sheath that has formed around the capsule. Remove the capsule from the incision with the straight forceps.

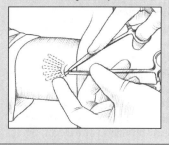

## Documentation

- Record the indications for the procedure, patient education, the patient's response to the procedure, how many capsules were removed, wound appearance, and follow-up plan.

# O

## Obstructed Airway Management

**CPT code**
*No specific code has been assigned.*

## Overview

Sudden airway obstruction may occur when a foreign body lodges in the throat or bronchus; when the patient aspirates blood, mucus, or vomitus; when the tongue blocks the pharynx; or when the patient experiences traumatic injury, bronchoconstriction, or bronchospasm.

An obstructed airway causes anoxia, which in turn leads to brain damage and death in 4 to 6 minutes. Abdominal thrust maneuvers can be performed on a conscious or an unconscious patient. An upper-abdominal thrust maneuver should be used on a conscious adult patient to create diaphragmatic pressure in the static lung below the foreign body sufficient to expel the obstruction. If the patient is unconscious, an abdominal thrust should be used.

However, the abdominal thrust is contraindicated in pregnant women, markedly obese patients, and patients who have recently undergone abdominal surgery. For these patients, a chest thrust to force air out of the lungs, creating an artificial cough, should be used. A finger sweep is then used to manually remove the foreign body from the mouth.

## Indications

- To remove an airway obstruction when the patient is unable to speak, cough, or breathe

## Contraindications

**ABSOLUTE**

- Incomplete or partial airway obstruction, or when the patient can maintain adequate ventilation to dislodge the foreign body by effective coughing
- Don't perform abdominal thrusts on pregnant women, markedly obese patients, and patients who have recently undergone abdominal surgery (use the chest thrust and finger sweep maneuvers)

## Preprocedure patient preparation

- Attempt to relieve the patient's anxiety by speaking calmly while briefly explaining your actions.

## Equipment

- None required

## Procedure

- Determine the patient's level of consciousness by tapping his shoulder and asking, "Are you choking?" If he has a complete airway obstruction, he won't be able to answer due to blocked airflow to his vocal cords. If he makes crowing sounds, his airway is partially obstructed; encourage him to cough. This will either clear the airway or make the obstruction complete. For a complete obstruction, intervene as follows, depending on whether the patient is conscious or unconscious.

### For a conscious adult

- Tell the patient that you'll try to dislodge the foreign body.
- Standing behind the patient, wrap your arms around his waist. Make a fist with one hand, and place the thumb side against his abdomen, slightly above the umbilicus and well below the xiphoid process. Then grasp your fist with the other hand.
- Squeeze the patient's abdomen 6 to 10 times with quick inward and upward thrusts. (See *Performing abdominal thrust maneuvers,* page 338.)

- Make sure you have a firm grasp on the patient because he may lose consciousness and need to be lowered to the floor. Look around the floor for objects that may harm him. If he does lose consciousness, lower him carefully to the floor. Support his head and neck to prevent injury, and continue as described below.

### For an unconscious adult

- If you come upon an unconscious patient, ask any witnesses who are present what happened. Begin cardiopulmonary resuscitation (CPR) and attempt to ventilate the patient. If you're unable to ventilate him, reposition his head and try again.
- If you still can't ventilate the patient, or if a conscious patient loses consciousness during the abdominal thrust maneuver, kneel astride his thighs and give him abdominal thrusts.
- After delivering the abdominal thrusts, open the patient's airway by usint the tongue-jaw lift. Grasp the tongue and lower jaw with your thumb and fingers. Then lift the jaw to draw the tongue away from the back of the throat and away from any foreign body.
- If you can see the object, remove it by inserting your index finger deep into the throat at the base of his tongue. Using a hooking motion, remove the obstruction. Keep in mind that some health care providers object to a blind finger sweep — using your finger when you can't see the obstruction — because your finger acts as a second obstruction. They

## Performing abdominal thrust maneuvers

Abdominal thrust maneuvers may be performed on a patient who is still standing or one who has lost consciousness.

### ON A STANDING PATIENT
The illustration below depicts how to perform the upper-abdominal thrust maneuver on a patient who's standing. Squeeze the patient's abdomen 6 to 10 times with quick inward and upward thrusts. Each thrust should be a separate and distinct movement; each should be forceful enough to create an artificial cough that will dislodge an obstruction.

### ON A SUPINE PATIENT
If you are unable to ventilate the patient or a conscious patient loses consciousness during the abdominal thrust maneuver, position her supine on the floor and perform abdominal thrusts. Place the heel of one hand on top of the other. Then place your hands between the umbilicus and the tip of the xiphoid process at the midline. Push inward and upward with 6 to 10 quick abdominal thrusts.

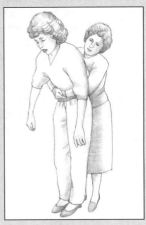

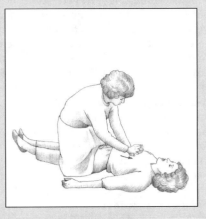

believe that, in most cases, the tongue-jaw lift described above should be enough to dislodge the obstruction.

■ After the object is removed, try to ventilate the patient. Then assess for spontaneous respirations, and check for a pulse. Proceed with CPR if necessary.

■ If the object isn't removed, try to ventilate the patient. If you can't, repeat the abdominal thrust maneuver described above in sequence until you clear the airway.

### For an obese or pregnant adult
■ If the patient is conscious, stand behind her and place your arms under her armpits and around her chest and perform chest thrusts. (See *Performing chest thrusts*.)
■ If the patient loses consciousness, carefully lower her to the floor.
■ Kneel close to the patient's side,

and place the heel of one hand just above the bottom of the patient's sternum. The long axis of the heel of your hand should align with the long axis of the patient's sternum. Place the heel of your other hand on top of that, making sure your fingers don't touch the patient's chest. Deliver each thrust forcefully enough to remove the obstruction.

### For a child

■ If the child is conscious and can stand, perform abdominal thrusts using the same technique as you would with an adult but with less force.

■ If he's unconscious or lying down, kneel at his feet; if he's a large child, kneel astride his thighs. If he's lying on a treatment table, stand by his side. Deliver abdominal thrusts as you would for an adult patient but use less force.

**▶ CLINICAL TIP**
*Never perform a blind finger sweep on a child because you risk pushing the foreign body farther back into the airway.*

### For an infant

■ Regardless of whether the infant is conscious, place him face down so that he's straddling your arm with his head lower than his trunk. Rest your forearm on your thigh and deliver four back blows with the heel of your hand between the infant's shoulder blades.

■ If you haven't removed the obstruction, place your free hand on the infant's back. Supporting his neck, jaw, and chest with your other hand, turn him over onto

## Performing chest thrusts

Provide chest thrusts to a conscious pregnant or obese patient with an obstructed airway. Place the thumb side of your clenched fist against the middle of the sternum, avoiding the margins of the ribs and the xiphoid process. Grasp your fist with your other hand and perform a chest thrust with enough force to expel the foreign body. Continue until the patient expels the obstruction or loses consciousness.

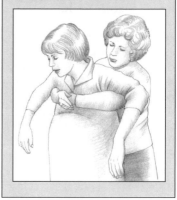

your thigh. Keep his head lower than his trunk.

■ Position your fingers. To do so, imagine a line between the infant's nipples, and place the index finger of your free hand on his sternum, just below this imaginary line. Then place your middle and ring fingers next to your index finger and lift the index finger off his chest. Deliver four chest thrusts as you would for chest compression but at a slower rate. As with a child, never perform a blind finger sweep on an infant.

## Postprocedure patient teaching

■ Once the patient has recovered, determine what caused the airway obstruction and teach the patient how to avoid future episodes.

## Complications

■ Nausea, regurgitation, and achiness may develop after the patient regains consciousness and can breathe independently.
■ Injuries, such as ruptured or lacerated abdominal or thoracic viscera or fractured ribs, may result from incorrect placement of the rescuer's hands or because of osteoporosis or metastatic lesions that increase the risk of fracture. Examine the patient for such injuries, and provide appropriate follow-up care or refer to a health care provider with expertise in these areas as appropriate.

## Special considerations

■ If your patient vomits during abdominal thrusts, quickly wipe out his mouth with your fingers and resume the maneuver as necessary.
■ Even if your efforts to clear the airway don't seem to be effective, keep trying. As oxygen deprivation increases, smooth and skeletal muscles relax, making your maneuvers more likely to succeed.

## Documentation

■ Record the date and time of the procedure, the patient's actions before the obstruction, the approxi-

mate length of time it took to clear the airway, and the type and size of the object removed.
■ Document the patient's vital signs after the procedure, any complications that occurred and follow-up care provided for them, and his tolerance of the procedure.
■ Document postprocedure teaching given and patient's verbalization of understanding.

# *Ophthalmoscopic Examination*

### *CPT codes*
92002  *Ophthalmological services: medical examination and evaluation; intermediate, new patient*
92004  *As above; comprehensive, new patient*
92012  *As above; intermediate, established patient*
92014  *As above; comprehensive, established patient*

## Overview

Disorders that affect the eye generally lead to vision loss or impairment; routine ophthalmic examinations and early treatment can help prevent vision loss through early detection. Ophthalmoscopy allows for magnified examination of the vascular and nerve tissue of the fundus, including the optic disk, retinal vessels, macula, and retina. The ophthalmoscope is a small, handheld instrument consisting of a light source, viewing device, a reflecting device to channel light into the patient's eyes, and spherical lenses to correct refractive error of the patient or the examiner.

Before beginning, practice holding and using the ophthalmoscope until you feel comfortable with it. The "0" lens is glass without any refraction. Set the lens at 0 and then slowly move toward a positive number, such as 6 or 8, or until the patient's optic disk becomes sharply focused. The red, minus numbers may be used to focus on distant structures.

An ophthalmoscopic examination can be used to detect many disorders of the optic disk and retina, but mastering the technique and interpreting abnormalities require skill, experience, and knowledge.

## Indications

■ To examine the internal structures of the eye
■ To detect and evaluate eye disorders as well as ocular manifestations of systemic disease

## Contraindications

**RELATIVE**
■ Insufficient dilation of the pupil, dense cataracts, cloudy media, and gross nystagmus may prohibit a good view of the fundus

## Preprocedure patient preparation

■ Place the patient in a darkened or semidarkened room, with neither the patient nor you wearing glasses (unless you're very myopic

or astigmatic). Contact lenses may be worn.
■ Encourage the patient to remain still throughout the examination and to keep his eye fixated on a point over your shoulder. He shouldn't look directly into the light of the ophthalmoscope.

## Equipment
■ Ophthalmoscope

## Procedure
■ Explain the procedure to the patient, and address any questions or concerns she may have.
■ Wash your hands.
■ Sit or stand in front of the patient with your head about $1\frac{1}{2}'$ (46 cm) in front of and about 15 degrees to the right of the patient's line of vision in the right eye. Hold the ophthalmoscope in your right hand with the viewing aperture as close to your right eye as possible. Place your left thumb on the patient's right eyebrow to prevent hitting the patient with the ophthalmoscope as you move in close. To examine the left eye, perform these steps on the patient's left side. (See *Holding the ophthalmoscope,* page 342.)
■ Instruct the patient to look straight ahead at a fixed point on the wall at eye level. Next, approaching from an oblique angle about 15″ (38 cm) out and with the diopter at 0, focus a small circle of light on the pupil. Look for the orange-red glow of the red reflex, which should be sharp and distinct through the pupil. The red

## Holding the ophthalmoscope

To properly hold the ophthalmoscope, keep your right index finger on the lens selector to adjust the lens as necessary, as shown below.

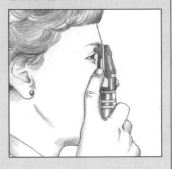

reflex indicates that the lens is free from opacity and clouding.
■ Move closer to the patient, following along the red reflex and changing the lens with your forefinger to keep the retinal structures in focus. (See *Locating the internal structures*.)
■ Change to a positive diopter to view the vitreous humor, observing for any opacity.
■ Next, view the retina, using a strong negative lens. Look for a retinal blood vessel, and follow that vessel toward the patient's nose, rotating the lens selector to keep the vessel in focus. Examine all the retinal structures, including the retinal vessels, the optic disc, the retinal background, the macula, and the fovea.
■ Examine the vessels for their color, the size ratio of arterioles to veins, the arteriole light reflex, and the arteriovenous (AV) crossing.

The crossing points should be smooth, without nicks or narrowing, and the vessels should be free from exudate, bleeding, and narrowing. Retinal vessels normally have an AV ratio of 2:3 or 4:5.
■ Evaluate the color of the retinal structures. The retina should be light yellow to orange and the background free from hemorrhages, aneurysms, and exudates. The optic disc, located on the nasal side of the retina, should be orange-red with distinct margins. The physiologic cup is about one-third the size of the optic disc and is normally yellow-white and readily visible.
■ Examine the macula last and as briefly as possible because it's very light-sensitive. The macula, which is darker than the rest of the retinal background, is free from vessels and located temporally to the optic disc. The fovea centralis is a slight depression in the center of the macula.

### Postprocedure patient teaching

■ Explain your examination findings to the patient and provide follow-up care or teaching as necessary.

### Complications
■ None known

### Special considerations
■ A room that isn't sufficiently dark or an inadequate light source

may interfere with the examination.

- If the patient's pupils aren't sufficiently dilated, mydriatic eyedrops may be used for a clearer examination.

## Documentation

- Document whether the patient was wearing contact lenses during the examination and if he required mydriatic eyedrops, including dosage and patient toleration.
- Record any variations in the retinal appearance or structural abnormalities.
- Document follow-up care and teaching that were given as appropriate. Also, record if any referrals were necessary.

## OROPHARYNGEAL AIRWAY INSERTION AND REMOVAL

***CPT code***
*No specific code has been assigned.*

## Overview

An oropharyngeal airway, a curved rubber or plastic device, is inserted into the mouth to the posterior pharynx to establish or maintain a patent airway. In an unconscious patient, the tongue usually obstructs the posterior pharynx. The oropharyngeal airway conforms to the curvature of the palate, preventing the tongue from becoming an obstruction and allowing air to

### Locating the internal structures

Begin by approaching the patient from a distance of about 15" (38 cm) at an oblique angle, with the diopter of the ophthalmoscope at 0. Focus a small circle of light on the pupil to locate the red reflex, as shown below.

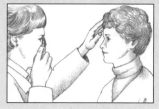

Then, follow the red reflex in toward the patient, moving closer and changing the lens with your forefinger to keep the retinal structures in focus, as shown below.

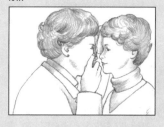

pass around and through the device. It also facilitates oropharyngeal suctioning.

## Indications

- To establish or maintain a patent airway in an unconscious patient, such as after anesthesia, a seizure, or a stroke
- To allow oropharyngeal suctioning
- To help prevent the orally intu-

bated patient from biting the endotracheal tube

## Contraindications

**RELATIVE**
- Loose or avulsed teeth
- Recent oral surgery
- A conscious or semiconscious state

## Preprocedure patient preparation

- Attempt to relieve the patient's anxiety, even though he may not be alert, by speaking calmly as you briefly explain your actions.

## Equipment

Oral airway of appropriate size ♦ regular and padded tongue blades ♦ gloves ♦ suction equipment ♦ handheld resuscitation bag or oxygen-powered breathing device ♦ cotton-tipped applicator

### Equipment preparation

- Select an appropriately sized airway for your patient. Usually, you'll select a small size (size 1 or 2) for an infant or child, a medium size (size 4 or 5) for an average adult, and a large size (size 6) for a large adult.
- Confirm the correct size of the airway by placing the airway flange beside the patient's cheek, parallel to his front teeth. If the airway is the right size, the airway curve should reach to the angle of the jaw.

## Procedure

- Explain the procedure to the patient even though he may not appear to be alert.
- Maintain privacy and standard precautions.
- Put on gloves.
- If the patient is wearing dentures, remove them so they don't cause further airway obstruction.
- Suction the patient if necessary.
- Place the patient in the supine position with his neck hyperextended, if not contraindicated.
- Insert the airway using the cross-finger or tongue blade technique. (See *Inserting an oral airway*.)
- Immediately after inserting the airway, auscultate the lungs to ensure adequate ventilation. If the patient has no respirations or they're inadequate, initiate artificial positive-pressure ventilation using mouth-to-mask technique, a handheld resuscitation bag, or an oxygen-powered breathing device.
- If the patient has adequate ventilation, position him on his side to decrease the risk of aspiration of vomitus.
- Monitor the patient constantly while the airway is in place.
- When the patient regains consciousness and can swallow, remove the airway by pulling it outward and downward, following the mouth's natural curvature.
- After removing the airway, test the patient's cough and gag reflexes to ensure that removal of the airway wasn't premature and that the patient can maintain his own airway. To test the gag reflex, use a

cotton-tipped applicator to touch both sides of the posterior pharynx. To test the cough reflex, gently touch the posterior oropharynx with the cotton-tipped applicator.

## Postprocedure patient teaching

- Patient teaching will have to wait until the patient regains consciousness; specifics will depend on the precipitating event.
- Advise the patient that his throat may be sore for a few days.

## Complications

- Tooth damage or loss, tissue damage, or bleeding may result from insertion of the airway. Remove and save the tooth, suction as needed, and monitor respirations until the patient is stable.
- Complete airway obstruction may result if the airway is too long and presses the epiglottis against the entrance of the larynx. If this happens, remove the airway and insert another airway of the correct size. Improper insertion may block the airway by pushing the tongue posteriorly. Remove and reinsert the airway if this happens.
- To prevent traumatic injury to the lips and tongue, make sure that the patient's lips and tongue aren't between his teeth and the airway. Surgical repair may be needed to repair lacerations.

## Special considerations

- Auscultate for the patient's breath sounds; clear breath sounds

### Inserting an oral airway

Unless this position is contraindicated, hyperextend the patient's head (as shown below) before using either the cross-finger or tongue blade insertion method.

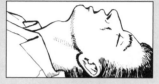

To insert an oral airway using the cross-finger method, place your thumb on the patient's lower teeth and your index finger on his upper teeth. Gently open his mouth by pushing his teeth apart, as shown below.

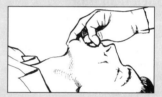

Insert the airway with the end aimed toward the roof of the patient's mouth, to avoid pushing the tongue back toward the pharynx. Rotate the airway as it approaches the back of the pharynx so that it points downward, as shown below.

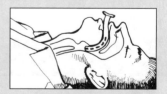

To use the tongue blade technique, open the patient's mouth and depress his tongue with the blade. Guide the airway over the back of the tongue as you did for the cross-finger technique.

indicate that the patient's airway is the proper size and in the correct position.

■ Don't tape the airway in place. The time it takes to remove the tape (as the patient regains consciousness) could delay airway removal, increasing the risk of aspiration.

■ Monitor the patient constantly while the airway is in place, and use the patient's behavior to let you know when to remove the airway. When the patient gags or coughs, he is becoming more alert, indicating that he no longer needs the airway.

## Documentation

■ Record the indications for procedure, the date and time of insertion, and the size of airway used.

■ Document the date and time of airway's removal, the presence of positive gag and cough reflexes, the condition of the patient's mucous membranes, any suctioning performed, any adverse reactions and actions taken, and the patient's tolerance of the procedure. Also document the patient's general condition.

# OTOSCOPY

**CPT code**
*No specific code has been assigned.*

## Overview

Otoscopy is the direct visualization of the external auditory canal and the tympanic membrane through an otoscope. It's a basic part of physical examination of the ear and should be performed before other auditory or vestibular tests. Otoscopy indirectly provides information about the eustachian tube and the middle ear cavity.

## Indications

■ To examine the external auditory canal and the tympanic membrane

■ To detect foreign bodies, cerumen, or stenosis in the external canal

■ To detect external or middle ear pathology, such as infection or tympanic membrane perforation

## Contraindications

**RELATIVE**

■ Painful or tender tragus, which may indicate otitis externa (inserting the speculum could produce severe pain)

## Preprocedure patient preparation

■ Inform the patient that the examination is usually painless and takes less than 5 minutes to perform.

■ Tell him that his ear will be pulled upward and backward to straighten the canal in facilitating insertion of the otoscope.

## Equipment

Otoscope ◆ ear speculums of various sizes (use largest speculum possible for a comfortable examination) ◆ curette, ear syringe, or forceps

## Procedure

■ Explain the procedure to the patient, and address any questions or concerns he may have.

■ Wash your hands.

■ Have the patient sit in a comfortable position or lie down on the side opposite the ear you wish to examine.

■ Hold the otoscope's handle in the space between your thumb and index finger.

■ Assist the patient in tilting his head toward the shoulder opposite the ear you're examining. While envisioning how the ear canal curves in an adult, gently grasp the auricle and pull it up and back to straighten the ear canal before inserting the speculum. (See *Inserting the speculum.*)

> **CLINICAL TIP**
> *Keep in mind the sensitivity of the skin in the ear canal. Using an improper technique at this time can cause the patient considerable discomfort or even pain.*

■ If you're examining a child's ear, utilize a child restraint technique, if necessary. (See "Child restraint techniques," page 95.) Then pull the auricle gently downward to straighten the ear canal before inserting the speculum.

■ Grasp the otoscope in your dominant hand with the handle parallel to the patient's head and the speculum at the patient's ear. Holding the otoscope with the handle facing up allows you to

---

### Inserting the speculum

Before inserting the speculum into the patient's ear, straighten the ear canal by grasping the auricle and pulling it up and back, as shown below.

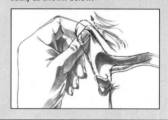

---

brace your hand against the patient's head to stabilize the instrument. This helps to prevent injury if the patient moves his head quickly. (See *Positioning the otoscope,* page 348.)

■ Inspect the auditory canal for cerumen, redness, or swelling. You'll see hairs and cerumen in the distal two-thirds of the ear canal. Note if excessive cerumen obstructs your view; you may need to remove it using a curette, ear syringe, or forceps to complete your inspection.

■ Inspect the tympanic membrane. Typically, middle ear problems are evident from the appearance of the tympanic membrane. Focus on the membrane's color and contour; it should be pearly gray and appear concave at the umbo. Then move the otoscope to identify landmarks on the tympanic membrane, including the umbo, handle of malleus, and cone of light. Be alert for perforations,

## Positioning the otoscope

To examine the auditory canal and tympanic membrane, hold the otoscope with the handle parallel to the patient's head, as shown below. Bracing your hand firmly against his head keeps you from hitting the canal with the speculum.

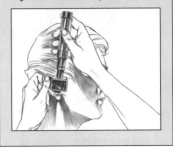

bulging, missing landmarks, or a distorted cone of light.

## Postprocedure patient teaching

■ Explain your examination findings to the patient and provide follow-up care or teaching as necessary.

## Complications

■ The otoscope should be advanced slowly and gently through the medial portion of the ear to avoid irritation of the canal lining, especially if an infection is suspected.
■ Bleeding may occur while cleaning the fragile ear canal. This may be minimized by gently removing the obstructing material and using care to avoid irritating the ear canal.

■ Continuing to insert an otoscope against resistance may cause perforation of the tympanic membrane.

## Special considerations

■ Scarring, discoloration, or retraction or bulging of the tympanic membrane indicates a pathologic condition.
■ Use a speculum that fits comfortably in the patient's external ear canal. Speculums range in diameter from 2 to 9 mm. Use the largest speculum possible for a comfortable examination.
■ Perform the otoscopic examination before testing the patient's hearing. Ear canals that are impacted with cerumen may cause hearing loss.

## Documentation

■ Record the appearance of or any structural variations in the external auditory canal or the tympanic membrane, including color, landmarks, and presence of fluid.
■ Document follow-up care and teaching that were given as appropriate. Also, record if any referrals were necessary.

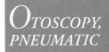

*O*TOSCOPY,
*P*NEUMATIC

***CPT code***
*No specific code has been assigned.*

## Overview

Pneumatic otoscopy is highly effective for diagnosing disorders of the middle ear, particularly those involving infants and children. It's an assessment of the movement of the tympanic membrane while increasing or decreasing the pressure in the external auditory canal. All health care providers who treat children should be skilled in performing and interpreting the results of pneumatic otoscopy.

## Indications

■ To evaluate the mobility of the tympanic membrane when an abnormality of the membrane is observed upon routine inspection or when the patient presents with signs or symptoms of a disorder of the middle ear

## Contraindications

### ABSOLUTE

■ Inability to see the tympanic membrane (obscured by blood, pus, cerumen, or a foreign body)
■ Immediately following a tympanoplasty

### RELATIVE

■ Presence of an obviously tense, bulging tympanic membrane
■ Presence of an obviously perforated tympanic membrane

### Preprocedure patient preparation

■ It's imperative that the head remains still during the procedure. If necessary, instruct the parent on assisting in a child restraint technique or have an assistant available. (See "Child restraint techniques," page 95.)
■ In the older child or adult, explain that they will feel an odd sensation and perhaps even a little pain in the ear during insufflation but they should remain still.

## Equipment

Otoscope ◆ insufflator ◆ ear speculums of various sizes (use largest speculum to comfortably create a seal between the speculum and the canal) ◆ curette, ear syringe, or forceps

## Procedure

■ Explain the procedure to the patient, and parents if necessary, and address any questions or concerns they may have.
■ Wash your hands.
■ With the patient's head secured, introduce the speculum into the canal to form a snug seal. (See "Otoscopy" for procedure recommendations, page 346.) Hold the otoscope and insufflator in one hand to allow you to position the ear properly with your free hand. (See *Holding the otoscope and insufflator,* page 350.)
■ If necessary, remove any obstructing material, such as cerumen, with the curette, ear syringe, or forceps. While visualizing the tympanic membrane, gently and slowly squeeze the insufflator and then release it. Squeezing the insufflator will produce positive pressure in the external auditory

## Holding the otoscope and insufflator

Position your hands as shown below to hold the otoscope and insufflator in one hand. Use your thumb and forefinger to squeeze and release the bulb. Your other hand should be used to position the auricle and further secure the patient's head.

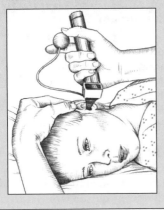

canal; releasing the insufflator will produce negative pressure in the canal.

■ Observe the mobility of the tympanic membrane.

■ Repeat on the opposite side.

▶ **CLINICAL TIP**
*The two most difficult portions of the procedure are creating a proper seal and properly interpreting the movement of the drum. Health care providers who are new to pneumatic otoscopy should perform the procedure on every patient's ear they examine. This will help to hone the skill and help with the subtleties of interpretation.*

### Postprocedure teaching

■ Explain your findings from the examination to the patient and provide follow-up care or teaching as necessary.

### Complications

■ Perforation of the tympanic membrane is the most serious complication.

■ Bleeding may occur while cleaning the fragile ear canal. This may be minimized by gently removing the obstructing material and using care to avoid irritating the ear canal.

### Special considerations

■ Diminished or absent movement of the tympanic membrane with pneumatic otoscopy may occur with acute or chronic otitis media.

■ In young, crying children the results may be very difficult to interpret. A tympanogram may serve as a useful adjunct in these patients.

■ Many people have sensitive ears, and all ears are sensitive if the speculum is introduced too deeply into the canal. Choose a speculum that will form a seal in the outer third of the canal.

### Documentation

■ Document your observations of the tympanic membrane prior to insufflation (color, presence of fluid, and landmarks).

■ Record the movement of the

drum with both positive and negative pressure.

# Oxygen Administration, Neonatal

***CPT code***
99440 *Newborn resuscitation*

## Overview

The neonate with signs and symptoms of respiratory distress will probably need oxygen. Because of his small size and respiratory requirements, he'll need special equipment and administration techniques.

In an emergency, a handheld resuscitation bag and a small oxygen mask may be sufficient until more permanent measures can be initiated, such as using an oxygen hood, nasal prongs, or a ventilator.

Oxygen administration is potentially hazardous to the neonate no matter which system delivers the oxygen. The gas must be warmed and humidified to prevent hypothermia and dehydration. Oxygen can cause retinopathy of prematurity (which may result in blindness) in high concentrations over prolonged periods. With insufficient oxygen concentrations, hypoxia and central nervous system damage may occur. Additionally, oxygen can contribute to bronchopulmonary dysplasia, depending on how it's delivered.

## Indications

■ To treat signs and symptoms of respiratory distress, such as cyanosis, pallor, tachypnea, nasal flaring, bradycardia, hypothermia, retractions, hypotonia, hyporeflexia, and expiratory grunting

## Contraindications

■ No contraindications exist when indications are present

## Preprocedure patient preparation

■ Speak calmly to the parents to decrease their anxiety and provide explanations as appropriate.

## Equipment

Oxygen source (wall, cylinder, or liquid unit) ◆ compressed air source ◆ flowmeters ◆ blender or Y-connector ◆ large- and small-bore oxygen tubing (sterile) ◆ warming-humidifying device ◆ sterile water ◆ thermometer ◆ stethoscope ◆ nasogastric (NG) tube ◆ specially sized mask with manual resuscitation bag ◆ manometer with connectors (the resuscitation bag must have a pressure-release valve)

### Equipment preparation

■ Wash your hands. Gather the necessary equipment and assemble it conveniently, to allow a quick setup.
■ Place the resuscitation bag and mask in the crib. Connect the large-bore oxygen tubing to the

mask outlet. Then use connectors and small-bore tubing to connect a manometer to the bag.

■ Next, connect the free end of the oxygen tubing to the warming-humidifying device, and fill the device with sterile water.

■ Turn on the device when ready to use it, or prepare the device according to the manufacturer's instructions.

■ Connect another piece of small-bore tubing to the inlet of the warming-humidifying device.

■ Attach a Y-connector to the opposite end of the small-bore tubing.

■ Place a piece of small-bore tubing on each end of the Y-connector, and connect the pieces of tubing to the flowmeters. Place an in-line thermometer as close as possible to the delivery end of the apparatus.

## Procedure

■ Explain the procedure to the parents or caregivers to reduce their anxiety and to ensure cooperation.

■ Turn on the oxygen and compressed air flowmeters to the prescribed flow rates.

■ Place the mask on the neonate's face. Don't cover the neonate's eyes. Check pressure settings and mask size to ensure that air doesn't leak from the mask's edges.

■ Provide 40 to 60 breaths/minute. Use enough pressure to cause a visible rise and fall of the infant's chest. Provide enough oxygen to maintain pink nail beds and mucous membranes. Deliver the oxy-

gen percentage defined by your facility's protocol.

■ Continuously watch the neonate's chest movements, and listen to breath sounds. Avoid overventilation, which will blow off too much carbon dioxide and cause apnea. If the neonate's heart rate falls below 100 beats/minute and doesn't rise, continue to use the handheld resuscitation bag until the heart rate rises to 100 beats/minute or higher.

■ Insert an NG tube to vent air from the infant's stomach.

## Postprocedure patient teaching

■ As soon as possible, explain the situation and the procedures to the parents or caregivers. Explain measures to keep the infant warm because hypothermia impedes respiration.

## Complications

■ Hypothermia and increased oxygen consumption can result from administering cool oxygen.

■ Metabolic and respiratory acidosis may follow inadequate ventilation.

■ A pulmonary air leak (pneumothorax, pneumomediastinum, pneumopericardium, interstitial emphysema) may develop spontaneously with respiratory distress or result from forced ventilation.

## Special considerations

■ Perform neonatal chest auscultation carefully to hear subtle respiratory changes. Also, be alert for respiratory distress signs, and be prepared to perform emergency procedures. If required, perform chest physiotherapy and percussion. Follow with suctioning to remove secretions. You'll generally discontinue oxygen when the infant's fraction of inspired oxygen reaches room air level and his arterial oxygen stabilizes between 60 and 90 mm Hg.

## Documentation

■ Note any respiratory distress that requires oxygen administration, the oxygen concentration given, and the delivery method.

■ Record each change in oxygen concentration. Note all checks of oxygen concentration.

■ Document all arterial blood gas values, the times that samples were obtained, the infant's condition during therapy, times suctioned, the amount and consistency of mucus, the type of continuous oxygen monitoring (if any), and any complications.

■ Note respiratory rate, and describe breath sounds and any signs of additional respiratory distress.

■ List any patient instructions given to the parents or caregivers and their understanding.

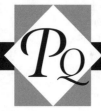

## $\mathcal{P}$APANICOLAOU TEST

### CPT codes
88142 *Cytopathology, cervical or vaginal, collected in preservative fluid, automated thin layer preparation; manual screening under physician supervision*
88144 *Cytopathology, cervical or vaginal, collected in preservative fluid, automated thin layer preparation; with manual screening and computer assisted rescreening under physician supervision*
88147 *Cytopathology, cervical or vaginal; screening by automated system under physician supervision*
88150 *Cytopathology, cervical or vaginal; manual screening under physician supervision*

### Overview

The Papanicolaou test, also known as the Pap test or Pap smear, was developed in the 1920s by George N. Papanicolaou and allows early detection of cervical cancer. This cytologic test involves scraping secretions from the cervix. The cells are then spread on a slide and im-

mediately coated with fixative spray or solution to preserve specimen cells for nuclear staining. Alternatively, the ThinPrep system may be used, in which the collection device is rinsed in a vial of preservative solution and sent to the laboratory. Cytologic evaluation outlines cell maturity, morphology, and metabolic activity. Although cervical scrapings are the most common test specimen, the Pap test also permits cytologic evaluation of the vaginal pool, prostatic secretions, urine, gastric secretions, cavity fluids, bronchial aspirations, and sputum.

### Indications

- To perform annual screening
- To rule out cervical dysplasia or malignancy noted on previous Pap test
- To evaluate history of sexually transmitted diseases or multiple sexual partners

### Contraindications
**RELATIVE**
- Current menses, acute infection, or inflammation

■ Douching or intercourse within previous 72 hours

## Preprocedure patient preparation

■ Advise the patient to abstain from intercourse, douching, or using any vaginal medications, spermicidal foams, creams, or gels for 2 days prior to the appointment. These activities may wash away cells or alter test results.

## Equipment

Bivalve vaginal speculum of appropriate size ◆ gloves ◆ cervical sampling device (wooden or plastic spatula and endocervical brush such as Cytobrush, or ThinPrep broom device) ◆ glass microscope slides or ThinPrep vial ◆ fixative for slide (a commercial spray or 95% ethyl alcohol solution) ◆ adjustable lamp ◆ drape ◆ laboratory request forms

### *Equipment preparation*

■ If preparing smear specimens, label the frosted end of the glass slides with the patient's name and "E" or "C" to indicate endocervical or cervical. If the patient has had a hysterectomy, label one slide "V" to differentiate a vaginal specimen.

## Procedure

■ Explain the procedure to the patient, and address any questions or concerns she may have.
■ Instruct the patient to void. This will relax the perineal muscles

and facilitate bimanual examination of the uterus, which will be performed after the Pap test.
■ Provide privacy, and instruct the patient to undress below the waist. Then instruct her to sit on the examining table and drape her genital region.
■ Wash your hands.
■ Assist the patient to the lithotomy position, with her feet in the stirrups and her buttocks extended slightly beyond the edge of the table. Adjust the drape.
■ Adjust the lamp so that it fully illuminates the genital area. Then fold back the corner of the drape to expose the perineum.
■ Put on gloves. Examine the vulva, including Bartholin's and Skene's glands, and assess for inflammation or lesions. Note the pattern of hair growth for Tanner scale evaluation, any discharge, and any abnormal anatomy.
■ Take the speculum in your dominant hand and moisten it with warm water to ease insertion. Avoid using water-soluble lubricants, which can interfere with accurate laboratory testing.
■ Warn the patient that you're about to touch her to avoid startling her. Then gently separate the labia with the thumb and forefinger of your nondominant hand.
■ Instruct the patient to take several deep breaths, and insert the speculum into the vagina, applying gentle pressure posteriorly as you advance it. Make sure you can see the entire cervix as you open the speculum. If you can't, remove the speculum, insert your index finger into the vagina, and locate

the cervix; then reinsert the speculum. Once it's in place, slowly open the blades to expose the cervix; lock the blades in place.

➤ **CLINICAL TIP**
*If the cervix is difficult to visualize, ask the patient to place her fists under her sacrum, causing a pelvic tilt. This works best with females who have a very posterior cervix.*

■ Note any signs of inflammation, infection, dysplasia, or structural abnormalities. Identify the transformation zone. Note the appearance of any cervical mucus and gently blot mucus or discharge to permit a full view.

■ Being careful not to traumatize the cervix, insert the endocervical brush through the speculum no farther than three-quarters of the length of the brush into the cervical os. Rotate the applicator 360 degrees to obtain an endocervical specimen. Then remove the endocervical brush and, if using slides, gently roll it in a circle across the slide marked "E." Refrain from rubbing the applicator on the slide to prevent cell destruction. Immediately place the slide in a fixative solution or spray it with a fixative to prevent drying of the cells.

■ Insert the small curved end of the wooden or plastic spatula through the speculum and place it directly over the cervical os. Rotate the spatula gently but firmly to scrape cells loose from the ectocervix. Remove the spatula, spread the specimen across the slide marked "C," and fix it immediately, as before. It's important to obtain cells from both the endocervix

and the transformation zone. (See *Obtaining an adequate Pap test specimen.*)

■ If using the ThinPrep system, rotate the broom device 360 degrees on the cervix five times to obtain specimens from the endocervix and ectocervix at the same time. Then insert the brush into the vial and rinse the broom in the liquid medium for the recommended amount of time, discard the brush, and close the lid of the vial.

■ If the patient has had a hysterectomy and there is no cervix, insert the wooden or plastic spatula through the speculum, and scrape the posterior fornix or vaginal pool, an area that collects cells from the endometrium, vagina, and cervix. Remove the spatula, spread the specimen across the slide marked "V," and fix it immediately, as before. If any abnormalities are seen in this area, another specimen should be obtained and sent as a separate specimen.

■ Unlock the speculum to ease removal and avoid accidentally pinching the vaginal wall. Then examine the vaginal walls as you slowly withdraw the speculum.

■ Remove the glove from your nondominant hand and lubricate the glove on your dominant hand. Perform the bimanual examination, which usually follows the Pap test. Note the mobility of the cervix as well as the size, position, and mobility of the uterus, and any tenderness or abnormalities of these areas.

■ Instruct the patient to bear down and then cough as you assess for urinary leakage and prolapse of the uterus or cervix. Insert a lubricated gloved finger rectally to check for masses and, if the woman is over age 40, to obtain a specimen for fecal occult blood testing if any stool is obtained from the rectal vault.

■ Remove your other glove and discard both gloves. Gently remove the patient's feet from the stirrups and assist her to a sitting position. Provide privacy for her to dress. Fill out the appropriate laboratory request forms, including the date of the patient's last menses, any clinical findings, and risk factors.

### Postprocedure patient teaching

■ Tell the patient that minor bleeding after the procedure is common.

■ Advise the patient that a Pap smear is a screening test and that further testing may be necessary for diagnosis.

■ Inform the patient that results should be available within 10 days of the procedure. If she isn't contacted within that time, she should call the facility.

### Complications

■ Discomfort, bleeding, and flashbacks of trauma or abuse require supportive care and cessation of the procedure if the adverse reaction is severe.

## Obtaining an adequate Pap test specimen

It's important to obtain cells from the endocervix and the transformation zone in order to have an adequate Papanicolaou (Pap) test specimen. First, insert the endocervical brush into the endocervix, turning it 360 degrees, as shown below. If you obtain a great deal of mucus, wipe it away without swabbing the endocervix.

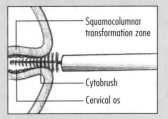

Squamocolumnar transformation zone

Cytobrush

Cervical os

Then take the wooden or plastic spatula and lightly scrape around the ectocervix.

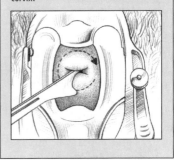

### Special considerations

■ In addition to the Pap test and bimanual examination, a breast examination should be performed. While doing so, self-breast examination should be reviewed with the patient.

■ False negative results and incomplete results are minimized by ensuring an adequate specimen and routine follow-up testing.

■ Look for lesions on the cervix and in the vaginal area and include cells from this area on the Pap smear, making a note of it on the Pap slip that's sent to the laboratory. Also note on the slip if any bleeding occurred and note "contact bleeding" in the patient's chart.

■ Any lesions that are seen or palpated may require colposcopy, which may be performed at the time of the Pap smear. If an infection is suspected, a wet mount may also be performed at the time of the Pap smear.

■ If the patient appears anxious or upset during the pelvic examination, stop at once, make eye contact, and ask if she wants you to stop. If she does, stop the examination, but discuss the importance of having a pelvic examination and Pap test at the next visit or with another provider. When the patient has dressed, discuss your observations (for example, hands balled into fists, pallor, tears, and changes in breathing pattern) and ask if she wants to discuss anything. Think about your response in advance; you don't want to respond with hesitancy or silence if the patient discloses trauma or abuse.

## Documentation

■ Document indications for and details of the procedure, including a detailed description of any abnormalities noted.

■ Note specimens sent, the patient's reaction to the procedure, medications ordered, time frame for follow-up evaluation, and instructions given to the patient.

# PARACENTESIS, ABDOMINAL

### CPT codes
49080  *Abdominal paracentesis, initial*
49081  *Abdominal paracentesis, subsequent*

## Overview

Abdominal paracentesis is one of the quickest and most cost-effective methods for diagnosing the cause of ascites. It involves inserting a needle into the peritoneal space of a patient with ascites and withdrawing a fluid sample. Samples of the fluid can be sent to the laboratory for diagnosis. In the patient with large-volume ascites, therapeutic paracentesis helps relieve the pressure in the abdominal wall, makes him feel more comfortable, and avoids the complications of respiratory compromise, abdominal pain, and abdominal hernias.

## Indications

■ To relieve intra-abdominal pressure causing respiratory distress
■ To evaluate ascites fluid for signs of infection

# Contraindications

**ABSOLUTE**

- Acute abdomen requiring immediate surgery
- Disseminated intravascular coagulation
- Inability of health care provider to demonstrate presence of ascites on physical examination

**RELATIVE**

- Coagulopathy that can't be corrected with fresh-frozen plasma or vitamin K
- Bowel distention or intestinal obstruction
- Infection or surgical scar at the needle entry site
- History of multiple abdominal surgeries
- Poor patient cooperation (patient movement could lead to serious injury)

# Preprocedure patient preparation

- Assure the patient that he'll probably feel little if any pain after the procedure. Explain that breathing will be easier if a significant amount of fluid is withdrawn, because it will relieve pressure on the diaphragm.
- Obtain a recent prothrombin time/partial thromboplastin time to assess for coagulopathy.

# Equipment

Commercially prepared paracentesis kit or the following supplies: Skin cleansing solution (povidone-iodine) and alcohol ◆ gown ◆ mask ◆ eyeshield ◆ sterile gloves ◆ sterile marking pen ◆ sterile drapes ◆ 1% or 2% lidocaine with or without epinephrine (epinephrine helps decrease unwanted abdominal wall bleeding) ◆ 10-ml syringe ◆ 50-ml sterile syringe ◆ 18G 1½″ needle ◆ 1 L vacuum bottles ◆ sterile specimen tubes (optional if infection is suspected) ◆ two blood culture bottles ◆ I.V. tubing and additional 22G needle ◆ adhesive bandage

# Procedure

- Explain the procedure to the patient, including its risks, benefits, and alternatives.

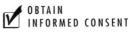 **OBTAIN INFORMED CONSENT**

**CLINICAL TIP**
*When obtaining informed consent, assess whether the patient has hepatic encephalopathy; in this case, the patient's designated power of attorney will probably need to sign for consent.*

- Ask the patient to empty his bladder immediately before the procedure.
- Wash your hands.
- Obtain baseline vital signs.
- Place the patient in the supine position, with the head of the bed slightly elevated. (Patients with less ascites can be placed in the lateral decubitus position.)
- Identify the site of paracentesis and mark it with a sterile pen. You may use the lower left or right quadrant, about ¾″ to 1¼″ (2 to 3 cm) lateral to the rectus muscle border for large-volume paracentesis. This site offers a thin abdomi-

nal wall. The linea alba, 1¼″ to 1½″ (3 to 4 cm) below the umbilicus, is an alternative site. The midline site is avascular and has less risk of bleeding. Place midline needles caudal to the umbilicus.

■ Avoid the following areas:
– rectus muscle, which has an increased risk of hemorrhage from epigastric vessels.
– surgical scars because of the increased risk of perforation caused by adhesion of the bowel wall to the wall of the peritoneum.
– areas of skin infection because of the increased risk of intraperitoneal infection.
– areas cephalic to the umbilicus in a patient with portal hypertension because a large venous collateral is usually located midline.

■ Put on gloves, a gown, a mask, and an eyeshield.

■ Clean the area with povidone-iodine followed by alcohol; then drape the abdomen.

■ Using 1% to 2% lidocaine, anesthetize the puncture site by infiltrating the skin and deeper tissues down to and including the peritoneum.

■ Attach an 18G needle to a 10-ml syringe. In patients with a large adipose panniculus, spinal needles (3½″) may be necessary.

■ Retract the skin at the site caudally (Z-track technique). Insert the needle, attached to a sterile syringe, initially at a 45-degree angle, then perpendicular to the skin; advance the needle slowly in 5-mm increments. You'll feel a "pop" as the needle advances through the anterior and posterior muscular fasciae and a "give" when the needle enters the peritoneal cavity. (See *Tapping the peritoneal cavity*.)

◢ **CLINICAL TIP**
*A slow, incremental insertion allows you to observe for a flash of blood if entering a blood vessel and to withdraw the needle to avoid further damage.*

■ When ascites fluid returns freely, hold the needle in place. Don't advance the needle further to avoid bowel perforation.

■ Gently aspirate 10 ml of fluid; then attach the 50-ml syringe. Aspirate further quantities of fluid as needed for analysis (usually 100 to 200 ml).

■ Obtain fluid for diagnostic purposes. Common tests include lactate dehydrogenase, glucose, albumin, protein, specific gravity, complete blood cell count and differential, Gram stain, cytology (requires 50 ml), amylase, lipase, pH, cholesterol, triglycerides, carcinoembryonic antigen, and special cultures for tuberculosis by acid-fast bacillus (AFB), bacteria, viruses, or fungi.

■ After removing the fluid needed for pathology, remove additional fluid as needed to alleviate symptoms. To do this, attach the I.V. tubing to the needle and place a second needle on the opposite end. Insert the free needle end into the vacuum bottle, and fluid will collect spontaneously.

■ If no fluid returns after several attempts, use ultrasound-directed aspiration.

◢ **CLINICAL TIP**
*When performing therapeutic paracentesis in a patient with signif-*

*icant peripheral edema, remove no more than 6 L of fluid. In a patient without peripheral edema, remove no more than 1,500 ml. If paracentesis is strictly for diagnostic purposes, 100 ml of fluid should be adequate.*

■ When the desired amount of fluid has been collected, withdraw the needle in a quick motion and release the skin retraction. This technique forms a Z-track and helps minimize leakage.

■ Apply pressure to the site for several minutes and apply an adhesive bandage. If fluid leaks from the site, keep the patient supine with the site upward until leakage stops.

■ If a large-volume paracentesis was performed (4 to 6 L), monitor the patient's vital signs according to your facility's protocol (usually, every hour for 2 to 4 hours).

■ Label all samples for analysis according to your facility's policy. Send to the laboratory for analysis.

■ Review results. (See *Interpreting peritoneal drainage results,* page 362.)

## Postprocedure patient teaching

■ Tell the patient to remain on his back with the site facing upward until fluid stops leaking and you tell him he can stand.

■ Teach him to monitor for and immediately report signs of infection, such as elevated temperature, increased or prolonged abdominal pain, and bleeding.

## Tapping the peritoneal cavity

After administering a local anesthetic to numb the area near the patient's navel, insert the needle (about ¾" [2 cm]) through the skin and subcutaneous tissues of the abdominal wall. Then advance the needle slowly into the pelvic midline until it enters the peritoneum (feeling for a little pop as it enters the peritoneum and carefully watching for a flash of blood, which would indicate inadvertent entry into a blood vessel).

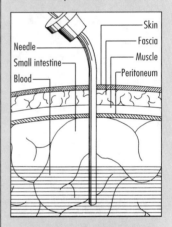

Using a syringe attached to the catheter, aspirate fluid from the peritoneal cavity and look for blood or other abnormal findings.

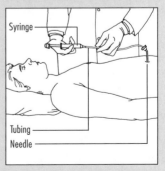

## Interpreting peritoneal drainage results

The most common abnormal findings associated with peritoneal drainage include:
- unclotted blood, bile, or intestinal contents in aspirated peritoneal fluid (20 ml in an adult or 10 ml in a child)
- bloody or pinkish-red fluid, dark enough to prevent the reading of newsprint through it (If you can read newsprint through the fluid, test results are considered negative, although more testing may be indicated.)
- green, cloudy, turbid, or milky peritoneal fluid return (Normal peritoneal fluid appears clear to pale yellow.)
- red blood cell count over 100,000/µl
- white blood cell count exceeding 500/µl
- bacteria in fluid (identified by culture and sensitivity testing or Gram stain)

If the patient's condition is stable, borderline positive results may suggest the need for additional tests, such as ultrasonography and arteriography. If the test results are questionable or inconclusive, consider leaving the catheter in place to repeat the procedure.

- Have him schedule a follow-up appointment within 48 hours for review of fluid analysis results.

## Complications

- Persistent leakage of ascitic fluid can be treated by having the patient lie flat while you apply pressure to the site. Place a suture if leakage persists.
- Hypotension and shock require monitoring and fluid management. Transport to an acute care center may be required if the condition doesn't stabilize.
- Perforated bowel requires urgent surgical referral. This occurs rarely; the risk is 0.8%.

✿ **COLLABORATION**
*Abscess formation at the puncture site may require antibiotic therapy and collaboration with a specialist in infectious diseases. Peritonitis may require collaboration with a specialist in infectious diseases and a surgical consult.*

- Abdominal wall hematoma must be monitored. Risk of hematoma requiring transfusion is 0.2% to 1.6% despite coagulopathy.

## Special considerations

- If you performed large-volume paracentesis (4 to 6 L), monitor the patient's vital signs frequently to detect possible hypotension. If vital signs remain stable, have the patient ambulate as tolerated.
- Colloid replacement with albumin is recommended after large-volume paracentesis (4 to 6 L), at a rate of 6 to 8 grams of albumin per liter of ascitic fluid removed.
- Bare steel needles are preferable to plastic sheathed cannulas because plastic sheaths tend to kink or collapse after the metal trocar is removed.

## Documentation

- Review documentation by other health team members; then initial their notes to signify you're aware of their findings. This doesn't signify agreement with their comments or reduce your responsibility to complete your own history and physical examination. Document abnormal physical findings. (The preprocedural and postprocedural note must include an evaluation of respiratory and GI function.)

- Note indications for the procedure and the amount and appearance of fluid removed.
- Record laboratory requests regarding specimens sent for diagnostic paracentesis.
- Note the patient's vital signs and tolerance of the procedure.
- Record any complications, actions taken, and final outcome.
- Record albumin replacement per facility guidelines.

## 𝒫EAK FLOW METER USE

### CPT code
94150 *Vital capacity, total*

### Overview

Peak expiratory flow rate (PEFR) is the maximum force and speed that a patient can exhale air from his lungs. It's a valuable measurement because it can demonstrate a decrease in lung function 1 to 3 days before other respiratory signs become apparent. It's measured with a spirometer or a peak flow meter (PFM). Although not as accurate as a spirometer, a PFM is a simple, portable, and inexpensive device. (See *Peak flow meter*.)

### Peak flow meter

Once your patient uses a particular brand of flow meter, make sure she sticks with that brand. If she must switch to a new brand, she'll need to establish a new "personal best" because different brands assign different values to the results. This illustration shows a typical peak flow meter, with a bar graph on the top where the sliding indicator stops after the patient reaches her peak expiratory flow rate.

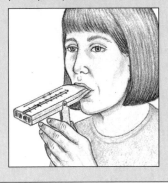

The health care provider can use a PFM to determine the patient's individual range of PEFR values and customize it to define a patient's "personal best." Individualized guidelines can be developed in conjunction with his health care provider to allow the patient to adjust the dose according to his PEFR. Using a system that divides the patient's PEFRs into three ranges (green, yellow, and red zones), the health care provider defines the treatment according to the patient's current PEFR. Using a PFM can reduce the frequency, duration, and severity of asthma attacks as well as the number of visits to the emergency department.

## Indications
- To determine the severity of asthma
- To check response to treatment during an acute episode
- To detect unrecognized decrease in lung function
- To diagnose asthma triggers such as exercise

## Contraindications
**ABSOLUTE**
- Respiratory distress
- Asthma attack

## Preprocedure patient preparation

- Make sure the patient remains inactive for 5 minutes before testing, to obtain a baseline, resting measurement. Activity of the patient can affect PEFR readings, especially if he gets exercise-induced asthma.

## Equipment
- PFM

## Procedure
- Explain the procedure to the patient, and address any questions or concerns he may have.
- Wash your hands.
- Check that the PFM indicator is set to the zero mark.
- Have the patient stand up, if possible. If he can't, have him as-

sume a position that allows maximal chest expansion. Keep him in that position for all maneuvers.
- Tell the patient to inhale as deeply as possible.
- Have the patient bring the PFM to his mouth, hold it in the proper direction (according to the manufacturer's instructions), and form a tight seal around the mouthpiece with his lips. Remind the patient not to cough or let his tongue block the mouthpiece.
- Tell the patient to exhale as hard and fast as possible for 1 to 2 seconds.
- Note the PEFR.
- Have the patient repeat the procedure twice more.
- Record the highest of the three values obtained, and note it in the patient's medical records. If the patient keeps his own diary to chart progress, record results there as well.
- Determine the zone of lung function, and instruct the patient on which medications to take based on PEFR values obtained. (See *Lung function zones,* pages 366 and 367.)
- Clean the PFM according to the manufacturer's instructions to prevent bacterial and fungal growth and to ensure accuracy.

## Postprocedure patient teaching

- Teach the patient proper technique for obtaining his PEFR, and have him demonstrate his ability to use the PFM.
- If the patient is a child, tell his parents or caregivers to obtain

three roughly similar readings to ensure that the child made a good effort each time.

■ Tell the patient he'll need to determine his PEFR twice daily for 2 to 3 weeks to perfect his technique and develop guidelines with his health care provider based on those values.

■ Explain what individualized treatment steps the patient should follow for each of the three ranges of PEFR.

■ Explain to the patient that he can expect a significant decline in acute exacerbations within 1 month of using PEFR-guided treatment. He'll know his asthma is controlled when he has no more asthma symptoms (including nocturnal symptoms) and can maintain a normal activity level.

■ Tell the patient to follow up with you within 2 days of an emergency department visit for a physical examination and to assess his technique, diary, and treatment protocol.

■ Tell the patient to call you for persistent, changing, worsening, or anxiety-producing signs and symptoms. Explain the guidelines he should follow if his PEFRs are in the yellow and red zones. (See *Lung function zones,* pages 366 and 367.)

■ Tell the patient to measure his PEFR twice daily (upon awakening and between noon and 2 p.m.) after exposure to asthma triggers, when he has a respiratory infection, and when his asthma management plan changes.

■ To identify asthma triggers, tell the patient to write down his PEFR before and after exposure to allergens, irritants, exercise, and other suspected triggers. Once identified, triggers should be avoided at all times.

■ Tell the patient to wash the PFM in soapy water every 2 weeks or according to the manufacturer's instructions.

## Complications

■ If left untreated, acute respiratory distress can cause hypoxia, brain damage, or death. If signs of respiratory distress occur, stop the procedure and institute emergency medical procedures as needed. This procedure can exacerbate respiratory distress in a patient already short of breath.

## Special considerations

■ The patient doesn't need to wear nose-clips during the procedure.

■ If the patient can't achieve 80% of PEFR during the initial 2 to 3 weeks, he'll need a course of oral corticosteroids to help determine his personal best measurement.

■ The patient doesn't have to wake up at night to determine if nocturnal asthma occurred. If the morning reading is 15% or more below the reading from the night before, he experienced nocturnal asthma.

■ Evaluating the PEFR during different seasons can help identify such seasonal triggers as pollen, cold, and dry air.

■ A child's PEFR shouldn't decrease; he should undergo reevaluation every 6 months to assess changes that occur with growth.

## Lung function zones

The following three charts can help you to determine appropriate lung function zones for your patient. The first two charts list expected normal peak expiratory flow rates (PEFRs) that you can use to evaluate your patient's PEFR. The first chart includes values for both sexes under age 20 based on height.

### NORMAL PEFR FOR THOSE UNDER AGE 20

| HEIGHT (IN.) | PEFR (L/MINUTE) | HEIGHT (IN.) | PEFR (L/MINUTE) | HEIGHT (IN.) | PEFR (L/MINUTE) |
|---|---|---|---|---|---|
| 43 | 147 | 51 | 254 | 59 | 360 |
| 44 | 160 | 52 | 267 | 60 | 373 |
| 45 | 173 | 53 | 280 | 61 | 387 |
| 46 | 187 | 54 | 293 | 62 | 400 |
| 47 | 200 | 55 | 307 | 63 | 413 |
| 48 | 214 | 56 | 320 | 64 | 427 |
| 49 | 227 | 57 | 334 | 65 | 440 |
| 50 | 240 | 58 | 347 | 66 | 454 |

The second chart lists the different values for men and women at age 20. After age 20, the normal predicted PEFR decreases from 5 to 15 L/minute every 5 years. Keep in mind that a "normal" PEFR can vary widely among individuals.

### NORMAL PEFR AT AGE 20

| HEIGHT (IN.) | | PEFR (L/MINUTE) | HEIGHT (IN.) | | PEFR (L/MINUTE) |
|---|---|---|---|---|---|
| *Males* | 60 | 554 | *Females* | 55 | 390 |
| | 65 | 602 | | 60 | 423 |
| | 70 | 649 | | 65 | 460 |
| | 75 | 693 | | 70 | 496 |
| | 80 | 740 | | 75 | 529 |

■ To simplify reading the PFM for a child or visually impaired patient, colored tape or lines can indicate the green, yellow, and red zones on the PFM.

## Documentation

■ Record the patient's current PEFR.

■ Record whether the patient demonstrated proper technique and described appropriate actions for each range of PEFR.
■ Document the management plan for each zone of lung function.

This last chart uses the patient's personal best to determine his lung function zones. A patient's personal best is the highest value he can reach in the middle of a good day after inhaling a bronchodilator (if prescribed). Once you and your patient have established his personal best, this chart can help him maintain 80% or more of that value or intervene as needed if he falls below that. The chart uses a familiar color-coded system — green for go, yellow for caution, and red for danger — to help keep the patient on track, even when he's under stress.

| ZONE | RANGE OF PEFR VALUES | TREATMENT GUIDELINES |
| --- | --- | --- |
| Green: All systems GO | 80% to 100% of personal best | ■ Continue current management plan.<br>■ If on chronic medications and constantly in the green zone with minimal variation, consider gradually decreasing daily medication. |
| Yellow: Lung function decreasing, CAUTION | 50% to 80% of personal best | ■ Temporarily increase asthma medication; refer to individualized guidelines for the patient (for instance, use bronchodilator, inhaled steroid, or oral steroid burst).<br>■ Have the patient notify the health care provider.<br>■ If PEFR is constantly in the yellow zone using chronic medications, increase maintenance therapy. |
| Red: Asthma control is failing, DANGER | Below 50% of personal best | ■ Instruct the patient to use an inhaled bronchodilator. If PEFR doesn't return to yellow or green zone, the patient requires medically supervised aggressive therapy. If the patient is unable to contact the health care provider, he should go to an urgent care center or walk-in clinic.<br>■ Adjust maintenance therapy. |

# PESSARY INSERTION

### CPT code
57160 *Fitting and insertion of pessary or other intravaginal support device*

## Overview

A pessary is a device that's worn internally, such as a diaphragm, and supports the uterus, bladder, or rectum. Vaginal supportive pessaries are helpful in managing uterine prolapse, uterine retrodisplacement, and stress urinary incontinence as well as pathology associated with these conditions.

## Indications

■ To alleviate uterine prolapse, cystocele, genital hernias, dysmenorrhea, dyspareunia, retroverted incompetent cervix (the pessary tilts the cervix, promoting fertility)
■ To treat bladder incontinence
■ To be used when surgery is contraindicated for the patient
■ To be used as an intermediate measure while awaiting surgery

## Contraindications

**ABSOLUTE**
■ Genital infection
■ Atrophic vaginitis
■ Adherent uterus

## Preprocedure patient preparation

■ Teach the patient about the specific type of pessary to be inserted, including its purpose (for instance, to maintain the position of the uterus or bladder). Show her the device.

## Equipment

Sterile pessary (Gehrung for cystocele; ring, ball, inflatable, or other option for cystocele or rectocele; and Gelhorn, Hodge, Cube, or Napier for uterine prolapse) ◆ drape ◆ sterile gloves ◆ antiseptic such as povidone-iodine ◆ sterile basin ◆ sterile ring forceps or claw forceps ◆ water-soluble lubricant such as K-Y gel ◆ mirror

## Procedure

■ Explain the procedure to the patient, and address any questions or concerns she may have.
■ Have the patient void, then undress from the waist down. Assist the patient into the lithotomy position.
■ Drape the patient, wash your hands, and put on gloves.
■ Measure the internal dimensions to determine the size of the pessary. For length, measure from the introitus to the top of the posterior vaginal vault and then subtract ⅓″ (1 cm) from this measurement. For the width, insert the ring forceps into the vagina to the level of the cervix, open them until they touch the walls, and note the distance between the handles of the forceps. Remove the forceps, open them to the same distance between the handles, and measure the distance between the tips. Average these two measurements to determine the pessary diameter.
■ Soak the pessary in a basin of povidone-iodine.
■ Lubricate the pessary with water-soluble gel.
■ Apply gentle pressure to the pelvic opening with your nondominant hand to enlarge the introitus. (See *Pessary insertion*.)
■ After insertion, instruct the patient to urinate, walk, and squat to evaluate placement. Adjust the pessary if the patient reports discomfort or if the pessary becomes displaced.
■ Teach the patient how to insert and remove the pessary herself. Then leave her with the pessary in

place so that she can practice removing and inserting the pessary in private. Instruct her to leave it in place when finished. Then examine her to check for proper placement.

## Postprocedure patient teaching

- Instruct the patient to schedule a follow-up appointment in 2 weeks to evaluate for proper fit, infection, irritation, and technique for its insertion and removal.
- Explain that she should remove the pessary daily or monthly as appropriate for that type of pessary, and clean it with soap and water. If any vaginal infection is detected, the patient should soak the pessary in alcohol for 20 minutes, then dry and insert.
- Instruct her to never use powder or perfume on the pessary.
- Tell the patient she can douche using a 1:1 solution of vinegar and water to lower the risk of infection and decrease odor. Tell her to follow up as appropriate but not to wait more than 3 months. She should bring the pessary to her routine gynecologic exams so fit can be reevaluated and it can be replaced annually.
- Tell the patient to call you if she experiences urinary retention, frequency, and urgency; dysuria; foul odor; and unusual vaginal discharge.

## Complications

- Vaginal and urinary tract infections are treated with cessation of

### Pessary insertion

To insert a pessary, apply gentle pressure to the patient's pelvic opening with your nondominant hand to enlarge the introitus. Grasp the pessary with the forceps and squeeze them to minimize the pessary. Insert the pessary toward the back of the vagina behind the suprapubic bone, stopping when you feel resistance. Release the pessary and close and remove the forceps.

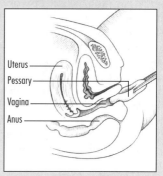

Assess fit — there should be a finger's width on all sides and the pessary shouldn't be visible at the introitus. To maintain the position of the uterus or bladder, the pessary should support the posterior vaginal fornix and push the cervix slightly backward and upward into the pelvis, as shown below.

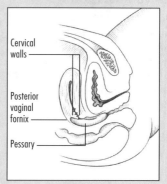

pessary use, which may be reinstituted after completion of antimicrobial treatment.

■ Vaginal burning and itching, dysuria, and urinary retention, frequency, and urgency are indications for cessation of pessary use and may be indications for referral.

## Special considerations

■ The patient may find a pessary that doesn't exert pressure on the bowel or bladder (such as the Cube) more comfortable, but because suction holds such a pessary in place, the patient needs to remove it daily to prevent erosion of vaginal mucosa. The Gelhorn and ring-type pessaries exert pressure on the bowel or bladder, but they may be left in for up to 3 months at a time.

■ Strongly consider using estrogen vaginal cream with the pessary.

■ Provide routine follow-up, focusing on inspecting for lacerations and ulcerations.

## Documentation

■ Document indications for and details of the procedure, including the patient's reaction to the procedure and ability to demonstrate proper technique, time frame for follow-up evaluation, and patient instructions given.

# PHOTOTHERAPY, BILIBLANKET

**CPT code**
96900  *Actinotherapy (ultraviolet light)*

## Overview

Phototherapy is an effective, easy-to-use treatment for physiologic hyperbilirubinemia (jaundice). It reduces bilirubin levels and the risk of bilirubin toxicity without any major short- or long-term adverse effects. Most healthy infants over 24 hours of age with non-pathologic jaundice may be safely managed as outpatients, using a biliblanket, which is a fiber-optic blanket that can be used at home for phototherapy.

## Indications

■ To treat hyperbilirubinemia for the infant 25 to 48 hours old with a total serum bilirubin (TSB) greater than 15 mg/dl (consider treatment if the TSB is greater than 12 mg/dl)

■ To treat hyperbilirubinemia for the infant 49 to 72 hours old with a TSB greater than 18 mg/dl (consider treatment if the TSB is greater than 15 mg/dl)

■ To treat hyperbilirubinemia for the infant greater than 72 hours old with a TSB greater than 20 mg/dl (consider treatment if the TSB is greater than 17 mg/dl)

## Contraindications

**ABSOLUTE**

- The presence of a direct (or conjugated) hyperbilirubinemia
- A rapidly rising bilirubin in which an exchange transfusion may be necessary for the removal of antibodies

## Preprocedure patient preparation

- Teach parents about jaundice, what causes it, and how to evaluate the baby for it.

◥ **CLINICAL TIP**
*In neonates, jaundice can be detected by blanching the skin with digital pressure, which reveals the underlying color of the skin and subcutaneous tissue. The clinical assessment of jaundice must be done in a well-lighted room. Jaundice (dermal icterus) always proceeds in a cephalocaudal manner. Once phototherapy has begun, however, the skin color no longer is a reliable indicator of serum bilirubin levels.*

- Explain the need for phototherapy and how the equipment is used.
- Educate the mother on the need for frequent breast feedings (8 to 10 times every 24 hours) to decrease the likelihood of problems with jaundice due to dehydration.

◥ **CLINICAL TIP**
*The interruption of breastfeeding hasn't been shown to significantly reduce bilirubin and isn't recommended. Supplementing nursing with water or dextrose water also doesn't lower the bilirubin in jaundiced, healthy breast-feeding infants.*

- Emphasize normal care and development of the infant.

## Equipment

Fiberoptic phototherapy blanket with disposable covers ◆ eyepatches

## Procedure

- Explain the procedure to the parents, and address any questions or concerns they may have.
- Evaluate the infant's need for phototherapy using the indications listed above as criteria.
- Demonstrate how to use the biliblanket to the parents so they'll be able to use it independently at home.
- Cover the blanket panel with a disposable covering.
- Place the illuminator unit on a secure surface less than 4 feet from the infant.
- Place the covered blanket panel around the infant's back or chest and secure it into position. Be careful not to wrap the blanket too tightly.
- Allow as much skin to be exposed to the panel as possible.
- Swaddle the infant in the receiving blanket, covering both the infant and the fiberoptic panel. The infant may also be dressed in a sleeper.
- Use eye patches only if the infant has direct exposure to the lights in the blanket panel.

■ Attach the blanket panel to the illuminator. Turn on the illuminator to the highest possible irradiance level.

> **CLINICAL TIP**
> *By using a fiberoptic blanket, the baby can be cuddled and held, and the blanket can remain on during feedings.*

■ Tell the parents that the biliblanket needs to be on the infant to be effective — encourage them to keep it on as much as possible to reduce the infant's bilirubin level. Allow the parents to practice applying and removing the biliblanket, and be available for questions and assistance.

■ Discontinue phototherapy when the TSB falls below 14 to 15 mg/dl. A rebound increase in the serum bilirubin level of 1 mg/dl is normal following the discontinuation of phototherapy.

■ If the TSB level doesn't decline with the use of conventional phototherapy or with a TSB above 20 mg/dl, intensive phototherapy should be instituted, requiring the infant's admission to the hospital. Further investigation and treatment is warranted.

## Postprocedure patient teaching

■ Have the parents return with the infant daily for examination and bilirubin level assessments.

■ Reassure the parents that the bilirubin isn't likely to rebound to a significant level that would require further therapy, and that the infant won't suffer adverse effects from the phototherapy.

## Complications

■ Dehydration secondary to insensible water loss can be avoided by ensuring adequate fluid intake.

■ Hyperthermia is possible from having the infant wrapped in the biliblanket, clothing, and a blanket. Have the parents monitor the infant's temperature every 4 hours initially. Blankets or clothing may need to be loosened or removed.

■ Skin changes, such as increased pigmentation, erythema, rash, or burns, can be avoided by not using topical ointments during phototherapy or allowing plastic to come into contact with the baby's skin.

## Special considerations

■ There are several instruments on the market to measure transcutaneous bilirubin levels. No system has proved to be useful as of yet because they must be calibrated to a given laboratory as well as calibrated for different skin types and color.

■ A direct Coombs' test, a blood type, and Rh(D) type on the infant's blood is recommended when the mother hasn't had prenatal blood grouping or is Rh negative.

■ A fractionated bilirubin, measuring both direct and indirect bilirubin, should be obtained to rule out pathologic causes of hyperbilirubinemia.

## Documentation

- Document the indications for initiating home phototherapy, including all serum bilirubin levels.
- Document the infant's weight to monitor for fluid losses and to assess intake (time spent nursing, frequency of feedings, or amount of formula consumed) and output (number of wet diapers and stools daily).
- Document parental coping.

# POSTCOITAL TEST

**CPT code**
89300 *Semen analysis; presence and motility of sperm including Huhner test (postcoital)*

## Overview

The postcoital test (PCT) involves obtaining a specimen that's used to evaluate the cervical mucus following intercourse. Often used early in the infertility workup, the PCT determines:

- if the ejaculate is delivered appropriately during intercourse
- the quantity and quality of preovulatory cervical mucus
- the character of the cervical os
- the sperms' ability to survive in the cervical mucus
- the adequacy of the number of the sperm
- the presence of an immunologic incompatibility.

A PCT is performed during the late follicular phase—before ovulation, which occurs in the prolif-erative phase of the menstrual cycle—when cervical mucus is most receptive to sperm. It's performed a minimum of 3 hours but no more than 12 hours following intercourse.

## Indications

- To evaluate the interaction between sperm and cervical mucus

## Contraindications

**RELATIVE**
- Any condition that would preclude unprotected sexual intercourse
- Bacterial cervicitis or vaginitis

## Preprocedure patient preparation

- Before the PCT is scheduled, explain the purpose, procedure, and timing of the test:
  – Carefully review the ovulation determination technique she'll use, and instruct her to schedule the postcoital test 1 to 2 days before the expected ovulation.
  – Advise her to have intercourse 4 to 12 hours before the appointment and not to use lubricants, douche, or take a tub bath after intercourse.
  – She may shower before the appointment.
- The postcoital test involves the insertion of a speculum and the removal of cervical mucus and takes approximately 15 minutes.
- Tell the patient that no complications are commonly associated

with this procedure and it shouldn't be painful.

## Equipment

Glass slides and coverslips (two) ◆ tuberculin syringe without needle or endometrial biopsy device such as a Pipelle ◆ speculum ◆ gloves ◆ drape ◆ 4″ × 4″ gauze ◆ microscope

## Procedure

■ Explain the procedure to the patient, and address any questions or concerns she may have.

■ Have the patient undress from the waist down, and apply drape.

■ Assist the patient into a dorsal lithotomy position.

■ Wash your hands and put on gloves.

■ Insert a vaginal speculum lubricated with warm water.

■ Gently swab the vagina with 4″ × 4″ gauze.

■ Assess the cervical os (it should be open and hyperemic) along with the quality and quantity of cervical mucus (it should be watery, clear, abundant and stretchy; also known as spinnbarkeit).

■ Insert a tuberculin syringe without a needle or a Pipelle 2 to 3 mm into the cervix.

■ Pull back on the suction applicator and withdraw about 2 ml of cervical mucus, then cap the syringe or Pipelle.

■ On the first slide, place a drop of cervical mucus; immediately cover with a coverslip to view under a microscope.

■ Evaluate the mucus for clarity and volume. Perform the spinnbarkeit test to determine how far the mucus will stretch without breaking. This may be done with forceps as they're withdrawn from the vaginal opening or by placing mucus between the gloved index finger and thumb.

■ Spinnbarkeit greater than 10 cm indicates a high level of estrogen and mucus conducive to ovulation. Spinnbarkeit less than 3 cm isn't conducive to ovulation as sperm are unlikely to be capable of penetrating the mucus.

■ On the second slide, spread remaining mucus on the pipette tip uniformly across the slide and allow to air-dry to evaluate the ferning pattern (present with high estrogen levels).

■ View the first slide and evaluate sperm, cell characteristics, and pH:
– 20 or more sperm is generally associated with a sperm count above 20 million/ml.
– A finding of 5 to 15 motile sperm with good linear progression is interpreted as a good PCT.
– The presence of white blood cells, clue cells, or trichonomads may indicate an infection.

■ View the second slide for a ferning pattern; if present, it indicates adequate estrogen production.

## Postprocedure patient teaching

■ Inform the patient that test results are known immediately and can be used to guide the next step in the infertility evaluation.

## Complications

■ None known

## Special considerations

- A pH below 7 may be treated with a precoital baking soda douche.
- Some couples may find the PCT to be intrusive and interfering with the privacy of their sexual relationship. Also, some women may feel self-conscious and uncomfortable seeing a health care provider so soon after intercourse.

## Documentation

- Before scheduling the PCT, document that patient education and counseling have taken place, and that the patient verbalizes an understanding of ovulation determination technique and importance of proper timing for the postcoital test.
- On the day of the PCT, document the cycle day and when intercourse occurred. Document the appearance of the cervical os, the quality and quantity of cervical mucus, and the presence and quality of spinnbarkeit and ferning. Document the number and motility of the sperm. Document the patient counseling that was provided after the procedure and the plan for further evaluation.

# *P*OSTPARTUM *FUNDAL ASSESSMENT*

**CPT code**
59430 *Postpartum care only*

## Hand placement for fundal palpation and massage

A full-term pregnancy stretches the ligaments supporting the uterus, placing the uterus at risk for inversion during palpation and massage. To guard against this, use your hands to support and fix the uterus in a safe position.

Place one hand against the patient's abdomen at the symphysis pubis level. This steadies the fundus and prevents downward displacement. Place the other hand at the top of the fundus, cupping it, as shown below.

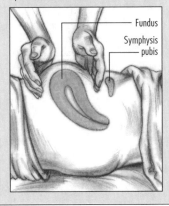

Fundus

Symphysis pubis

## Overview

After delivery, the uterus gradually shrinks and descends into its prepregnancy position in the pelvis — a process known as involution. You'll evaluate normal involutional progress by palpating and massaging the uterus to identify uterine size, firmness, and descent. (See *Hand placement for fundal palpation and massage.*)

Involution normally begins immediately after delivery, when the firmly contracted uterus lies midway between the umbilicus and

## Fundal height measurement

Involution normally begins immediately after delivery, when the firmly contracted uterus lies midway between the umbilicus and the symphysis pubis. Soon, the uterus rises to the umbilicus; after the first postpartum day, it begins returning to the pelvis.

The average descent rate is 1 cm or fingerbreadth daily — slightly slower if the patient had a cesarean section. By the 10th postpartum day the now unpalpable uterus lies deep in the pelvis, at or below the symphysis pubis.

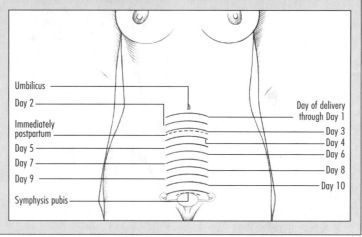

Umbilicus
Day 2
Immediately postpartum
Day 5
Day 7
Day 9
Symphysis pubis

Day of delivery through Day 1
Day 3
Day 4
Day 6
Day 8
Day 10

the symphysis pubis. (See *Fundal height measurement*.)

When the uterus fails to contract or remain firm during involution, uterine bleeding or hemorrhage can result because placental separation after delivery exposes large uterine blood vessels, which uterine contractions close off (like a tourniquet). Fundal massage, synthetic oxytocic delivery, or natural oxytocic substances released during breast-feeding help to maintain or stimulate contractions.

Typically, fundal palpation and massage are performed while you're caring for the perineum and evaluating healing. (See *Postpartum perineal care*.)

### Indications

■ To evaluate the position of the uterus in the postpartal period

### Contraindications

■ None known

### Preprocedure patient preparation

■ Tell the patient that you're measuring the height of the fundus to make sure it's dropping toward a

## Postpartum perineal care

Vaginal birth (which stretches and sometimes tears the perineal tissues) and episiotomy (which may minimize tissue injury) usually leave the patient with perineal edema and tenderness. Postpartum perineal care aims to relieve this discomfort, promote healing, and prevent infection.

Performed after the patient eliminates, perineal hygiene involves cleaning and drying the perineum and assessing the wound area and the lochia (blood and debris sloughed from the placental site and the decidua). Red immediately after delivery, the lochia turns pinkish brown in 4 to 7 days and appears white during the second and third weeks after delivery. This discharge decreases gradually but may continue for up to 6 weeks.

### CLEANING THE PERINEUM

Teach the patient to use a water-jet irrigation system or a peri-bottle to clean the perineum. Here are the basic steps:

■ If using a water-jet irrigation system, insert the prefilled cartridge containing antiseptic or medicated solution into the handle, and push the disposable nozzle into the handle until it audibly clicks into place. While sitting on the commode, place the nozzle parallel to the perineum and turn on the unit. Rinse the perineum for at least 2 minutes from front to back. Then turn off the unit, remove the nozzle, and discard the cartridge. Dry the nozzle, and store it appropriately for later use.

■ If using a peri-bottle, fill it with cleaning solution, and pour it over the perineal area.

■ Stand up before you flush the commode to avoid spraying the perineum with contaminated water.

■ Apply a new perineal pad before returning to bed. Apply the pad front to back to avoid infection.

■ Be alert for such signs of infection as unusual swelling, pain, and foul-smelling drainage.

prepregnancy level. Fundal massage will help the uterus contract and decrease bleeding and is done if the fundus is above the umbilicus in the first hour after delivery or feels soft and boggy.

■ Teach the patient relaxation techniques (such as deep breathing) to help her cope with the discomfort associated with fundal palpation and massage. Advise the patient who has had a cesarean section there will be some discomfort because you're touching near the incision, but it will resolve quickly.

## Equipment

Gloves ◆ analgesics ◆ perineal pad ◆ urinary catheter (optional)

## Procedure

■ Explain the procedure to the patient, and address any questions or concerns she may have. Provide privacy. Wash your hands and put on gloves.

■ Generally, schedule fundal assessments every 15 minutes for the first hour after delivery, every 30 minutes for the next 2 to 3 hours, every hour for the next 4 hours, every 4 hours for the rest of the first postpartum day, and every 8 hours until the patient's discharge. Offer analgesics before fundal checks if indicated.

■ Encourage the patient's efforts to urinate because bladder distention impairs uterine contraction by pushing the uterus up and aside. You may need to catheterize the patient if she can't urinate or if the uterus becomes displaced with increased bleeding.

■ Lower the head of the bed until the patient lies supine. If this position causes discomfort — especially if she has had cesarean surgery — keep the head of the bed slightly elevated.

■ Expose the abdomen for palpation and the perineum for observation. Watch for bleeding, clots, and tissue expulsion while massaging the fundus.

■ Gently compress the uterus between both hands to evaluate uterine firmness. Note the level of the fundus above or below the umbilicus in fingerbreadths or centimeters.

■ If the uterus seems soft and boggy, gently massage the fundus with a circular motion until it becomes firm. Simply cupping the uterus between your hands may also stimulate contraction. Alternatively, massage the fundus with the side of the hand above the fundus. Without digging into the abdomen, gently compress and release, always supporting the lower uterine segment with the other hand. Observe for lochia flow during massage.

■ Massage long enough to produce firmness. The sensitive fundus needs only gentle pressure.

This should produce the desired results without causing excessive discomfort.

### ✦ COLLABORATION

*Notify the collaborating physician immediately if the uterus fails to contract and if heavy bleeding occurs. If the fundus becomes firm after massage, keep one hand on the lower uterus, and press gently toward the pubis to expel clots.*

■ Clean the perineum, and apply a clean perineal pad. Help the patient into a comfortable position.

## Postprocedure patient teaching

■ Demonstrate fundal massage so the patient can perform it herself. She supports the lower aspect of the uterus with one hand while gently massaging the top, sides, and front of the fundus by moving the loose abdominal tissues over the fundus.

■ Teach the patient about the amount, color, and consistency of lochial flow she can expect during the postpartal period.

■ Advise the patient of the importance of emptying her bladder at regular intervals to prevent urinary retention and promote uterus contraction.

## Complications

■ Pain is the most common complication of fundal palpation and massage because the uterus and its supporting ligaments are usually tender after delivery. Avoid excessive massage, which can stimulate premature uterine contractions, causing undue muscle fatigue and leading to uterine atony or inversion.

## Special considerations

■ Because incisional pain makes fundal palpation uncomfortable for the patient who has had a cesarean section, provide pain medication beforehand as ordered. If the lochia flow diminishes after 4 hours, consider performing fewer fundal checks than usual, especially if the patient is receiving oxytocin.
■ If the patient has had a vertical abdominal incision for a cesarean section, palpate the uterus from the sides to determine tone.
■ Beware if no lochia appears. This may signal a clot blocking the cervical os. Subsequent heavy bleeding may result if a position change dislodges the clot. Take vital signs to assess for hypovolemic shock. If vital signs are stable, massage with slightly increased pressure to help expel any clots and to help the uterus contract further.

## Documentation

■ Record vital signs, fundal height in centimeters or fingerbreadths, and position (midline or off-center) and tone (firm or soft and boggy) of the uterus.
■ Document massage and note the passage of any clots.
■ Note how the patient tolerated the procedure.
■ Record excessive bleeding or other complications, your actions, and the outcome.

# *PROSTATE MASSAGE*

## CPT code
*No specific code has been assigned.*

## Overview

Prostate massage is performed as part of supportive therapy for treatment of symptomatic chronic prostatitis, the most common cause of recurrent urinary tract infections in men that typically result from bacterial invasion from the urethra. This procedure may promote drainage of prostatic secretions and lead to relief of symptoms.

It's also used to collect part of the samples required for the Meares and Stamey technique, a test that can provide a firm diagnosis of prostatitis. This test requires four specimens: one collected when the patient starts voiding (voided bladder one [VB1]); another midstream (VB2); another after the patient stops voiding and the health care provider massages the prostate to produce secretions (expressed prostate secretions); and a final voided specimen (VB3). A significant increase in colony count in the prostatic specimens confirms prostatitis.

## Indications

■ To promote drainage of prostate secretions for symptomatic relief or to collect prostate secretion specimens

## Palpating the prostate gland

To palpate the prostate gland, insert your gloved, lubricated index finger into the rectum. Palpate the prostate on the anterior rectal wall, just past the anorectal ring, as shown below.

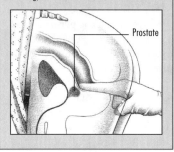

Prostate

## Contraindications

**ABSOLUTE**
- Acute bacterial prostatitis
- Prostate gland abscess
- Significant urinary symptoms, such as dysuria, urinary frequency, or urinary urgency.

## Preprocedure patient preparation

- Warn the patient that he'll feel some pressure or urgency during this procedure as well as for a short time afterward (approximately 30 minutes to 1 hour).

## Equipment

Gloves ◆ water-soluble lubricant ◆ microscope slide or sterile container for specimen collection

## Procedure

- Explain the procedure to the patient, and address any questions or concerns he may have.
- Wash your hands and put on gloves.
- Position the patient comfortably for access to the prostate gland. He may stand and lean over the examination table or lie on his left side, with his right knee and hip flexed or with both knees drawn toward his chest.
- Generously lubricate the gloved index finger of your dominant hand and the anus with water-soluble lubricant.
- Place the finger on the anal orifice and gently press until the anal sphincter relaxes. Gently advance the finger, keeping the finger pad facing the anterior rectal wall.
- To ease the passage of the finger through the anal sphincter, tell the patient to relax or have him perform Valsalva's maneuver during finger insertion.
- With your finger pad, palpate the prostate gland on the anterior rectal wall just past the anorectal ring. (See *Palpating the prostate gland*.)
- Begin to massage the gland. Start on one side of the prostate and apply gentle pressure with your finger from the lateral aspect of the gland medially, promoting drainage of secretions to the urethra. Massage several times on this side, covering the entire side of the prostate. Then repeat on the other side of the prostate, applying pressure laterally to medially.

■ Once both sides of the prostate are massaged, gently massage the medial aspect of the gland up and down to promote drainage of secretions through the urethra. (See *Massaging the prostate gland.*)

■ Collect any secretions in the sterile specimen container (quantity may vary from scant drops to 2 ml), and apply to slide for microscopic examination; send remainder to laboratory for culture if necessary.

## Postprocedure patient teaching

■ Tell the patient to notify you of fever, chills, rash, nausea, vomiting, or gastrointestinal irritation, or if symptoms worsen.

■ Teach patient other supportive therapies that may be utilized, such as sitz baths, adequate hydration, and stool softeners.

## Complications

■ Sepsis can be avoided by not massaging the prostate in a patient with suspected acute bacterial prostatitis or an abscess on the prostate gland.

## Special considerations

■ The prostate should be palpated gently because excessive manipulation can cause bacteremia.

■ In addition to prostate massage, regular ejaculation may also help promote drainage of prostatic secretions. Frequent participation in sexual activity may be helpful.

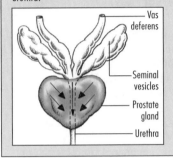

### Massaging the prostate gland

Massage the prostate by applying gentle pressure with your finger from the lateral aspect of the gland medially; repeat on other side. Then massage the medial aspect of the gland up and down to promote drainage of secretions through the urethra.

— Vas deferens
— Seminal vesicles
— Prostate gland
— Urethra

## Documentation

■ Document the indications and purpose for the procedure and the patient's toleration of it.

■ Record the amount of secretions collected and tests performed on the secretions.

■ Chart follow-up care and patient teaching as well as his understanding.

# $\mathcal{P}$ULMONARY FUNCTION TESTING

## *CPT code*
94010 *Spirometry (includes graphic record, total and timed vital capacity, expiratory flow rate measurements [including calculation of*

*forced vital capacity and forced expiratory volume] and interpretation)*

94060 *Spirometry before and after bronchodilator (or before and after exercise)*

94150 *Vital capacity screening test*

94375 *Respiratory flow volume loop*

## Overview

Pulmonary function testing (PFT) uses standardized measures to evaluate lung function. Complete PFT includes static and dynamic lung volumes, diffusing capacity, flow volume loop, maximal voluntary ventilation, and maximal inspiratory and expiratory pressures.

PFT uses spirometry to obtain measurements. Spirometry can classify processes as normal, restricted, or obstructive, but it can't yield specific diagnoses. Airflow measurements reflect airway patency, elasticity of the respiratory muscles, and the conscious muscular effort exerted by the patient. However, these measurements don't indicate the adequacy of gas exchange — diffusing capacity and arterial blood gas measurements indicate gas exchange. Electronic spirometers produce flow volume loops by generating continuous recordings of flow and volume during forced inspiration and expiration. (See *Understanding pulmonary function test results,* pages 384 and 385.)

To obtain accurate, reproducible results (based on the standards set by the American Thoracic Society [ATS]), the patient must exert his maximal inspiratory effort. Because the results depend on the patient's effort, active coaching increases the likelihood of obtaining valid results.

## Indications

- To evaluate lung function
- To detect obstructive or restrictive lung disease
- To assess the presence and extent of reversibility of airway obstruction
- To evaluate and monitor therapeutic interventions (for instance, to evaluate the success of bronchodilators)
- To determine the presence and extent of drug-induced toxicity (for instance, from chemotherapy)
- To assess patients at risk for respiratory complications before surgery
- To screen for occupational lung disease
- To motivate a patient to stop smoking
- To screen for disability

## Contraindications

**RELATIVE**

- Severe shortness of breath or bronchoconstriction related to effort
- Severe fatigue
- Recent myocardial infarction and acute illness, including viral infection in the past 2 to 3 weeks
- Large pulmonary blebs or bullae
- History of marked vasovagal responsiveness
- History of spontaneous pneumothorax
- Uncontrolled hypertension

## Preprocedure patient preparation

■ At least 6 hours before the test, withhold bronchodilators (if possible), unless the purpose of the test is to evaluate the bronchodilator's effectiveness.

■ Make sure the patient understands that he shouldn't smoke, drink beverages, or eat a heavy meal for at least 1 hour before the test or he won't be able to produce his maximal breathing effort.

## Equipment

Volume-based spirometer (spirometer meets ATS accuracy standards and fulfills National Institute of Occupational Safety and Health requirements; it must have at least a 7-L and 15-second strip capacity and be regularly checked for leaks) or flow-based pneumotachygraph ◆ nose clip

## Procedure

■ Explain the purpose of the specific test to the patient and what he'll need to do, and address any questions or concerns he may have.

■ Make sure the patient is alert enough to follow directions.

■ Record the patient's age, gender, height, and race. If the patient can't stand or has a spinal deformity, you can approximate his height from his arm span.

■ Have the patient sit or stand. If he sits, make sure that his legs aren't crossed and that he has both feet solidly on the floor.

■ Have the patient remove poorly fitting dentures and loosen or remove any constricting clothing, such as a belt or necktie.

■ Tell the patient to slightly elevate his chin, with his neck slightly extended; he shouldn't have his chin down toward the chest.

■ Calibrate the machine based on instructions from the manufacturer.

■ Put the nose clips on the patient and have him make sure that he can't pass any air through his nose.

■ Tell the patient to seal his lips tightly around the mouthpiece with his teeth around the outside. For a cardboard mouthpiece, tell the patient not to bite down so that he doesn't obstruct the hole in the tubing. Tell him not to protrude his tongue into the mouthpiece.

■ Tell the patient to exhale forcibly into the tube. If necessary, demonstrate how to do this.

■ Actively coach the patient to blow out all his air as hard and as fast as possible.

■ Make sure the patient exhales for at least 6 seconds, up to 20 seconds.

■ Repeat the procedure until you achieve three acceptable trials, but don't do more than eight trials or the patient may become fatigued.

■ Record the measurements on the spirometer. Note the measurement on the spirometer recording at 1 second as forced expiratory volume in 1 second ($FEV_1$).

■ Evaluate the strips. The tracing needs to last at least 6 seconds with at least 2 seconds of plateau.

*(Text continues on page 386.)*

## Understanding pulmonary function test results

These graphs show the results of pulmonary function testing (PFT). However, to understand the results, you first need to understand the terminology.

■ Total lung capacity (TLC): The total volume of air remaining in the lungs after maximum inspiration.

■ Vital capacity (VC): The maximum volume of air an individual can completely (and slowly) exhale after a maximum inspiration; normal is 3.88 to 5 L.

■ Forced vital capacity (FVC): The same as VC but using maximum forceful expiration. The FVC may be less than the VC because of premature closure of the terminal airways, reflecting obstructive disease. A reduced FVC may also indicate the presence of restrictive disease.

■ Tidal volume (TV): Airflow in a resting individual; normal is 500 ml.

■ Forced expiratory volume in 1 second ($FEV_1$): The FVC volume exhaled in 1 second; normal is 3.12 to 3.96 L; it primarily reflects the condition of the large airways.

■ Percentage of $FEV_1$ ($FEV_1$/FVC): $FEV_1$ compared to FVC; normal is at least 75%; less than 75% suggests obstruction.

FIGURE 1: NORMAL SPIROMETRY
(VOLUME-BASED)

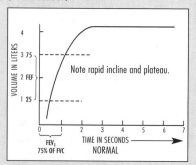

FIGURE 2: NORMAL SPIROMETRY
(FLOW-BASED)

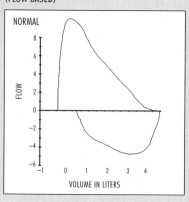

FIGURE 3: SPIROMETRY REFLECTING
OBSTRUCTIVE DISEASE

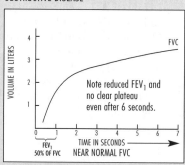

FIGURE 4: SPIROMETRY REFLECTING
RESTRICTIVE DISEASE

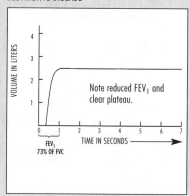

■ Mean forced expiratory flow (FEF$_{25\%-75\%}$): Formally called midexpiratory flow; a sensitive indicator of the condition of the small airways. Decreased values are an indication of obstruction disease, especially in asthma and bronchitis.

When interpreting PFT results, keep in mind the criteria for acceptable results and reproducibility.

### ACCEPTABLE RESULTS
■ The tracing doesn't reflect coughing, early glottic closure (see figure 7), a hesitant start, or problems with equipment.
■ Forceful expiration occurs with 6 seconds of smooth, continuous exhalation or a plateau of at least 2 seconds or both.

### REPRODUCIBILITY
■ The largest FVC is within 0.2 L of the next largest FVC.
■ The largest FEV$_1$ is within 0.2 L of the next largest FEV$_1$.

FIGURE 5: ABRUPT DECREASES IN TRACING BECAUSE OF COUGHING

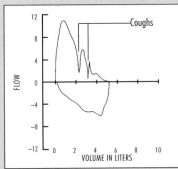

FIGURE 6: HESITANT START

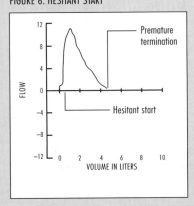

FIGURE 7: EARLY GLOTTIC CLOSURE

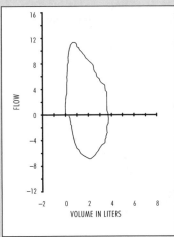

■ Make sure the two best tracings don't vary by more than 100 ml, or 5%; this suggests consistent best effort. Note whether the patient coughed, which could interfere with some tests.

■ If you didn't obtain any acceptable tracings after eight trials, select the best one, noting its limitations.

■ Compare the patient's results (and previous test results if available) with standardized norms. Norms vary according to race, height, age, and gender.

***Bronchodilator evaluation***

■ If you're evaluating the patient's response to bronchodilators, administer the medication after selecting the initial two tracings.

■ Wait 15 minutes and then repeat the procedure until you've obtained three acceptable trials.

■ Interpret the two best tracings. A positive response to bronchodilators is generally considered to be an increase in forced vital capacity (FVC) of at least 15% and an increase in $FEV_1$ of at least 12%.

> ◥ **CLINICAL TIP**
> *Keep in mind that exceptionally fit lungs might have to deteriorate by as much as 40% of their capacity to fall out of normal range.*

## Postprocedure patient teaching

■ Tell the patient he may experience some fatigue but no other adverse effects.

■ Demonstrate how to blow out hard right at the start of the test and repeat the trial, coaching the patient. (See Figure 6 in *Understanding pulmonary function test results,* page 385.)

■ Tell the patient he should try to keep the flow as fast and as consistent as possible and repeat trials as necessary.

■ Tell the patient to follow up based on his indication for PFT.

■ Make sure the patient contacts you if he experiences persistent fatigue or any breathing difficulties. Explain that this may stem from the pulmonary disorder rather than the testing.

## Complications

■ Prevent fainting by allowing the patient to decrease expiration after the initial 3 seconds and continue exhaling without forcing it. If the patient faints, ease him to the floor and elevate his legs until consciousness returns. Defer testing, if possible, for another day.

■ Test-induced bronchospasm (each subsequent effort demonstrates declining airflow) may occur. Select the best effort, and note the problem. The patient is usually scheduled for further testing after administration of a bronchodilator.

■ If the machine malfunctions, check for air leaks and recalibrate.

## Special considerations

■ Children younger than age 5 typically can't cooperate well enough to ensure valid results.

- Blacks and Asians have spirometry and lung volumes 15% lower than Whites.
- A cough peak expiratory flow rate (PEFR) approximates the peak flow you should observe during testing. For this measurement, the patient should take a deep breath and then cough into the mouthpiece. If the observed PEFR isn't more than 1 L/second more than cough PEFR, the patient may not be exerting his best effort.
- Normal $FEV_1$ values peak for women at age 20 and for men at age 22. Such values then decrease approximately 20 to 30 ml per year and shouldn't demonstrate more than a 15% change per year.
- FVC and $FEV_1$ values greater than 80% of the predicted values are considered normal. The highest FVC and $FEV_1$ should be reported, even if they're from two separate trials. Forced expiratory flow$_{25\%-75\%}$, however, must be reported from the most acceptable test curve with the largest sum of FVC and $FEV_1$.
- If the patient coughs during testing, repeat the trial if possible, especially if the coughing occurs during the first second of testing. If the patient can't control coughing, note that in the comments. (See Figure 5 in *Understanding pulmonary function test results,* page 385.)
- If the patient puts forth a poor effort, explain once again the importance and purpose of the test, and repeat the trial as necessary.
- If the patient stops exhaling too early, explain the problem and its significance and increase your coaching as you repeat the trial.
- If the results show variable peak flow rates, repeat the trial as necessary and increase your coaching during each trial (for example, say, "Keep blowing; don't stop!").

## Documentation

- Document the patient's age, gender, height, and race.
- Note the patient's position during trials and the number of trials.
- Record the patient's effort.
- Note whether you administered any bronchodilator, including the dose and timing.
- Record the spirometry results.
- Note the patient's appearance after testing.

## RAPID ANTIGEN DETECTION TEST (RADT)

### CPT code
87430 *Infectious agent antigen detection by enzyme immunoassay technique, qualitative or semiquantitative, multiple step method—Streptococcus, Group A*

### Overview
The rapid antigen detection test (RADT) for group A streptococcus, also known as the rapid strep test, can be done quickly in an office setting with a simple throat swab stick. The test has a sensitivity of 80% to 95% and a specificity of 95%. Because of the lower sensitivity, a negative test should be confirmed with throat cultures of specimens taken from the posterior pharynx or tonsillar fossae. In the face of a negative test, current recommendations suggest that antibiotic therapy be withheld unless the subsequent culture is positive. However, in actual practice, many patients are treated with antibi-

otics based on the clinical presentation despite a negative RADT.

### Indications
- To identify group A beta-hemolytic streptococci in a patient presenting with pain on swallowing, myalgia, fever, rhinorrhea, lymphadenopathy, and pharyngeal edema (with or without exudative pharyngitis)

### Contraindications
- None known

### Preprocedure patient preparation
- Check the patient's history for recent antimicrobial therapy.
- Tell the patient that a specimen will be collected from his throat. Warn him that he may gag during the swabbing.

### Equipment
Commercially available RADT test kit ◆ gloves

## Procedure

- Explain the procedure to the patient, and address any questions or concerns he may have.
- Wash your hands and put on gloves.

➤ **CLINICAL TIP**
*There are several commercially available RADT test kits. The following procedure is representative, but care should be taken to follow the manufacturer's directions carefully.*

- Position the patient comfortably.
- Using the sterile swab provided in the kit, swab the posterior pharynx and tonsils. Avoid touching the teeth, gums, and buccal mucosa with the swab.
- Add sufficient extraction reagent to the test tube.
- Place the swab in the test tube.
- Vigorously mix the solution by rotating the swab against the side of the test tube at least 10 times.
- Let the specimen stand for 2 minutes.
- Express liquid from the swab by squeezing the tube as the swab is removed.
- Discard the swab according to your facility's protocol.
- Remove a test stick from the kit and place the absorbent end in the test tube.
- Let the test stick stand for 5 minutes.
- Read the results from the test stick. A positive result may appear prior to 5 minutes; however, negative results can't be confirmed before 5 minutes.

## Postprocedure patient teaching

- Inform the patient of the results. For positive results, antibiotic and supportive therapy is indicated. Emphasize the importance of completing the full course of antibiotics.
- Tell the patient that if results are negative, a throat culture will need to be obtained and that this result will be available in 2 to 3 days.
- Instruct the patient to follow up with you if symptoms worsen or don't improve over several days to a week.

## Complications

- Laryngospasm may occur after the swab specimen is obtained if the patient has epiglottitis or diphtheria. Keep resuscitation equipment nearby.

## Special considerations

- Store the test kits according to the manufacturer's instructions. Check the expiration date on individual test packages before using.
- The patient with throat pain can minimize sources of throat irritation in the environment by using a bedside humidifier.

## Documentation

- Document the indications for the test, the time and date of specimen collection, and any recent or current antibiotic therapy.
- Record the results of the test along with follow-up care as pro-

vided (throat culture or initiation of antibiotics). Document patient teaching and the patient's understanding of instructions.

# RECTAL PROLAPSE REDUCTION

*CPT code*
*No specific code has been assigned.*

## Overview

Rectal prolapse is the circumferential protrusion of one or more layers of the mucous membrane through the anus. Prolapse may be complete (with displacement of the anal sphincter or bowel herniation) or partial (involving only the mucosal layer). (See *Types of rectal prolapse.*)

Rectal prolapse usually occurs in men under age 40, in women around age 45 (three times more often than in men), and in children ages 1 to 3 (especially those with cystic fibrosis). Rectal prolapse reduction can help to alleviate symptoms until the prolapse spontaneously resolves or until treatment interventions (such as injection of a sclerosing agent or surgical repair) take place.

## Indications

■ To replace prolapsed rectal tissue back into the rectum

## Contraindications

**ABSOLUTE**
■ Strangulation, which requires surgical intervention
■ Gangrene or rupture of the anterior rectal wall with extrusion of the small bowel
■ Signs of uncontrolled bleeding
■ Signs of infection
■ Rectal mass or tumor

## Preprocedure patient preparation

■ Educate the patient about underlying causes of rectal prolapse, such as straining during defecation and weak sphincter muscles.
■ Inform the patient that you'll need him to produce the rectal prolapse so that you can examine it and rule out hemorrhoids, rectal polyps, or other conditions that produce similar symptoms.

## Equipment

Gloves ◆ water-soluble lubricant

## Procedure

■ Explain the procedure to the patient, and address any questions or concerns he may have.
■ Position the patient in the left lateral decubitus position with knees bent up toward the chest.
■ Wash your hands and put on gloves.
■ Drape the patient so that only the perianal area is exposed to promote privacy.
■ Inform the patient that you're going to touch his rectal area.

- Spread the gluteal fold and examine the external anal structure.
- Instruct the patient to bear down as if having a bowel movement; observe for prolapse of rectal tissue. If the prolapse isn't obvious, have the patient strain while standing or squatting to produce the prolapse, then assist him back to the left lateral decubitus position.
- Visually differentiate rectal prolapse from hemorrhoids, rectal polyps, or other conditions that produce similar symptoms.
- Apply lubricant to your fingers and gently push the prolapsed rectal tissue back through the anal sphincter.
- Perform anoscopy if indicated. (See "Anoscopy," page 25.)
- Instruct the patient to remain reclined for a short time following the procedure.

## Postprocedure patient teaching

- Teach the patient to perform prolapse reduction at home, using gauze pads or toilet tissue to gently push the rectal tissue back into the rectum.
- Help the patient to prevent constipation by teaching him the correct diet and stool-softening regimen. Advise the patient with severe prolapse and incontinence to wear a perineal pad.
- Teach perineal strengthening exercises. Instruct the patient to lie supine on a mattress, pull in his abdomen, and squeeze while taking a deep breath. Alternatively, instruct the patient to repeatedly

### Types of rectal prolapse

Partial rectal prolapse involves only the rectal mucosa and a small mass of radial mucosal folds. In complete rectal prolapse (also known as procidentia), the full rectal wall, sphincter muscle, and a large mass of concentric mucosal folds protrude. Ulceration is possible after complete prolapse.

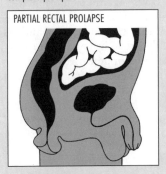

PARTIAL RECTAL PROLAPSE

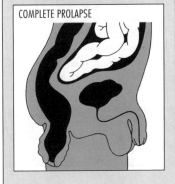

COMPLETE PROLAPSE

squeeze and relax his buttocks while sitting on a chair.
- Inform the patient to notify you of any rectal bleeding, pain, or bloody diarrhea.

## Complications

■ Irritation of rectal tissue from manipulation during reduction may be decreased by using a gauze pad soaked in normal saline solution.

## Special considerations

■ Severe or chronic prolapse requires surgical repair by strengthening or tightening the sphincters with wire or by anterior or rectal resection of prolapsed tissue. The patient needs referral to a surgeon.
■ The patient should be seen monthly unless surgery has been done or the prolapse is resolved.

## Documentation

■ Document the patient's history of symptoms, the appearance and type of prolapse, and the patient's toleration of the procedure.
■ Record patient teaching and his understanding of instructions.

# $R$HOGAM ADMINISTRATION

### CPT codes

90384 *Rh$_o$(D) immune globulin (RhIG), human (with principal code 90782)*
90782 *Therapeutic injection, intramuscular (specify medication injected)*

## Overview

Rh$_o$(D) human immune globulin (RhoGAM) is a concentrated solution of immune globulin containing Rh$_o$(D) antibodies. Intramuscular injection of RhoGAM keeps the Rh-negative mother from producing active antibody responses and forming anti-Rh$_o$(D) to Rh-positive fetal blood cells and endangering future Rh-positive infants. It should be given within 72 hours of precipitating event to prevent future maternal sensitization. Maternal immunization to the Rh antigen commonly results from transplacental hemorrhage during gestation or delivery. If unchecked during gestation, incompatible fetal and maternal blood can lead to hemolytic disease in the neonate. RhoGAM is indicated for the Rh-negative mother with a neonate having Rh$_o$(D)-positive or D$^u$-positive blood and Coombs'-negative cord blood.

## Indications

■ To treat an Rh-negative patient with low Rh-positive antibody titers
■ To protect the fetus of an Rh-negative mother
■ To treat Rh-positive exposure resulting from full-term pregnancy, termination of pregnancy, amniocentesis, threatened abortion (uterine bleeding with a closed cervix), abruptio placentae, or abdominal trauma during pregnancy
■ To treat blood transfusion exposure

## Contraindications

**ABSOLUTE**
- $Rh_o(D)$-positive
- Previously immunized to $Rh_o(D)$ blood factor
- History of hypersensitive response to human globulin

**RELATIVE**
- Immunoglobulin A deficiency
- More than 72 hours has passed since indication for RhoGAM occurred

## Preprocedure patient preparation

- Discuss with the patient the Rh factor, antibodies, and how Rh can affect pregnancy.
- Advise the patient on the importance of RhoGAM administration.
- Explain to her the adverse effects of RhoGAM, such as some discomfort at the injection site and a slight chance of mildly elevated temperature.

## Equipment

3-ml syringe ◆ 22G 1½″ needle ◆ RhoGAM vial ◆ alcohol pads ◆ triplicate form and patient identification (from the blood bank or laboratory)

## Procedure

- Identify the patient. Explain RhoGAM administration to the patient, and address any questions or concerns she may have.

- Obtain a history of allergies and reaction to immunizations.
- Two health care providers must check the vial's identification numbers and sign the triplicate form that comes with the RhoGAM. Complete the form as indicated. Attach the top copy to the patient's chart. Send the remaining two copies, along with the empty RhoGAM vial, to the laboratory or blood bank.
- Wash your hands and put on gloves.
- Withdraw the appropriate dose of RhoGAM from the vial with the needle and syringe. Clean the gluteal injection site with an alcohol pad, and administer the RhoGAM I.M.

## Postprocedure patient teaching

- Give the patient a card that identifies her Rh-negative status, and instruct her to carry it with her or keep it in a convenient location.

## Complications

- Fever, myalgia, lethargy, discomfort, splenomegaly, or hyperbilirubinemia may occur after multiple injections (for example, those given after Rh mismatch). Complications rarely occur after a single RhoGAM injection; when they do, they're mild and confined to the injection site.

## Special considerations

■ After the procedure, watch for redness and soreness at the injection site.

■ Provide an opportunity for the patient to voice any guilt or anxiety she may feel if she perceives her body is acting against the fetus.

■ Administration of RhoGAM at approximately week 28 of gestation can also protect the fetus of the Rh-negative mother. The dose is determined according to the fetal packed red blood cell (RBC) volume that enters the mother's blood. A volume under 15 ml usually calls for one vial of RhoGAM; a significant fetal-maternal hemorrhage calls for more than one vial if the fetal packed RBC volume is greater than 15 ml.

## Documentation

■ Record the date, the time, and the site of the RhoGAM injection.
■ If applicable, note the patient's refusal to accept a RhoGAM injection and a summary of the risks that were explained to the patient inherent in that refusal. Follow the policy of your facility for documenting this refusal (the patient and witnesses may need to sign a waiver form).
■ Document patient teaching about RhoGAM.
■ Note that the patient received a card identifying her Rh-negative status.

# RING REMOVAL

### CPT code
26989 *Unlisted procedure, hands or fingers*

## Overview

Many patients come to the office, clinic, or emergency department for removal of a ring or other constricting band from an edematous finger or toe when they can't remove the object at home. Trauma, weight gain, fluid retention, arthritic changes, I.V. infusion infiltration, general soft-tissue swelling from sunburn, dependent edema, or allergic reaction may cause a ring to constrict the digit, resulting in pain, hypoxia, and neurovascular compromise. Children may also cause neurovascular compromise by placing circular or oval objects, such as pull tabs or toys, on a finger or toe.

The least invasive means of ring removal remains lubrication and circular traction. If this method fails, the string wrap method may be attempted; although this procedure can be painful and is time-consuming, it does retain the integrity of the ring. If all other attempts fail, the ring should be removed by cutting the band with a ring cutter, orthopedic pin cutter, or hand-operated circular saw. All cutting methods pose an additional risk to the patient, involving potential cuts or abrasions from the equipment and the possibility of metal shavings, which may lead to foreign-body granuloma if left undetected.

## Indications

■ To relieve chronic or acute edema and prevent vascular compromise in a finger or toe from constriction by a ring or other metal band

## Contraindications

**RELATIVE**

■ Open wound or finger fracture
■ Deeply embedded ring erosion
■ Lack of appropriate cutting tools

## Preprocedure patient preparation

■ Warn the patient that either method will cause some pain due to the edema in the digit and the nature of the removal technique.

## Equipment

2% lidocaine without epinephrine (optional) ◆ water-soluble lubricant (optional) ◆ 3-ml syringe and 27G needle (optional) ◆ 3′ (0.9 m) of string (polyester fiber strip, such as No. 1 Mersilene, umbilical tape or 1-0 silk suture) ◆ small hemostat ◆ manual or electric ring cutter with new blade ◆ two large hemostats ◆ 20-ml syringe filled with water

## Procedure

◢➔ CLINICAL TIP
*Even if the patient tells you he has tried to remove the object from the finger at home, it's generally worthwhile to attempt removal with a water-soluble lubricant before trying other techniques. The pain from constriction often prevents the patient from applying adequate circular traction to remove the ring. Placing the patient's finger or toe in a cup of icy water for 10 minutes may reduce the edema enough to effect removal with lubrication and circular traction.*

■ Explain the procedure to the patient. If the ring is to be cut off, obtain written consent for cutting and removing the ring. Lubrication and string removal don't require written consent.
■ Wash your hands.

◢➔ CLINICAL TIP
*Some health care providers advocate using a digital block before these procedures to reduce pain and make the patient more comfortable and cooperative. However, remember that lidocaine will cause additional edema. If it's necessary to use a digital block, use the least amount of lidocaine necessary to obtain anesthesia. Never use any product containing epinephrine in a finger or toe because epinephrine exerts a vasoconstrictive effect.*

### String wrap method

■ Lubricate the ring finger lightly with water-soluble lubricant.
■ Use the string wrap method to remove the ring. (See *Using the string method,* page 396.)

## Using the string method

If lubrication and circular traction are ineffective in removing a patient's ring, your next option is to use the string method. Advise the patient that this procedure will be uncomfortable and that injecting an anesthetic can cause additional problems due to vasoconstriction.

Lubricate the ring finger lightly with water-soluble lubricant. Grasp one end of the string in the jaws of the hemostat. Slide the tip of the hemostat under the ring on the palmar surface with the jaws pointing proximally. Pull enough string through so that you'll be able to grasp it firmly later. Tape the string in place.

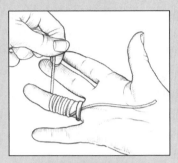

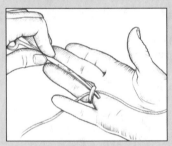

Wrap the string firmly around the finger, beginning adjacent to the ring margin. Wrap the string in a smooth, single layer, progressing from proximal to distal until it covers the area of greatest swelling, compressing the edematous tissue as you progress.

Place a small amount of lubricant over the string to facilitate sliding the ring. Remove the tape from the proximal end and pull the string distally, sliding the ring over the wrapped string and off the finger. If the ring hasn't traversed the entire area of edema, repeat the string wrapping process until the ring is removed.

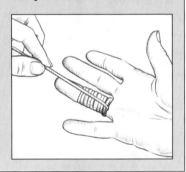

■ Reassess neurosensory and neurovascular function.

### Ring cutter removal

■ Place the small hook of the ring cutter (called the ring cutter guard) under the ring on the palmar surface. (See *Using a ring cutter.*)

■ Hold the ring cutter firmly in your nondominant hand and apply steady, firm downward pressure on the handle while turning the cutter blade with your dominant hand.

▶ **CLINICAL TIP**
*Inexpensive rings are generally the most difficult to cut because they are composed of a number of alloys with traces of silver or gold. They usually require extensive cutting and*

*may require more than one blade to complete the procedure.*

▶ **CLINICAL TIP**
*Some hard rings require extensive cutting. The friction caused by the cutting may produce an uncomfortable amount of heat in the ring and the patient's hand. Ask the patient if he's comfortable, and regularly check the temperature of the ring and cutter blade with your own fingers. Stop briefly to allow the ring and cutter to cool down if necessary.*

■ When cutting is complete, grasp each of the cut ends with a large hemostat and spread the ring edges with a steady opposing force.

■ Irrigate the skin with high-pressure water to remove any metal particles.

■ Reassess neurovascular and neurosensory function.

## Postprocedure patient teaching

■ Tell the patient that pain should resolve within 1 to 2 hours and edema should resolve within 24 hours or as indicated by initial trauma to the digit. All symptoms should resolve within 48 hours.

■ Tell the patient that no follow-up is needed unless complications arise.

■ Instruct the patient to apply an ice pack to the digit for 20 minutes four times daily for 36 to 48 hours to relieve edema and pain.

■ Advise the patient to take ibuprofen or acetaminophen for pain relief every 4 to 6 hours as needed.

### Using a ring cutter

Whether you use a manual, a battery-operated, or an electric ring cutter, you'll follow the same procedure. Place the ring cutter guard under the ring on the palmar surface of the patient's hand to protect the tissue from the cutting blade. Then turn the "key" that causes the blade to cut through the ring, as shown below.

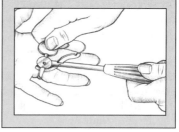

■ Caution the patient to avoid constricting objects on fingers and toes and to remove rings when edema is possible.

■ Instruct the patient to contact you promptly if he experiences signs and symptoms of infection, such as warmth, increased edema, and pain.

## Complications

■ Infection may be treated with an appropriate topical antibiotic. Soak the area in warm salt water 4 or 5 times daily. Oral antibiotics may be needed for extensive infection.

■ Skin abrasion or a cut from a cutting tool may be treated by washing with an antimicrobial and then applying an antibiotic ointment.

## Special considerations

■ Inability to remove a ring requires immediate referral to emergency care. Have the patient hold an ice pack over the digit and elevate it as much as possible while in transit.

■ Explain to the patient that the cut is a straight line that a jeweler can usually repair. Carefully clean the ring, store it safely in a container, and return it to the patient or significant other as soon as possible. Most rings, such as wedding bands, family heirlooms, or gifts from loved ones, typically hold great sentimental value to patients. Treat the ring with respect while cutting and removing it.

■ When removing rings or other objects from children, use age-appropriate language. Allow the parent to stay with and hold the child during the procedure. Allow the child to examine the equipment if appropriate.

■ When you suspect a fracture, order X-ray studies to be performed before or after the ring removal.

■ The patient may request that the ring not be removed. If edema is expected to be transient and vascular compromise isn't expected, conservative management may be tried. Instruct the patient to elevate the affected area and intermittently apply ice or cold compresses to the site until he is able to slide the ring off. Review with the patient signs and symptoms that indicate vascular compromise and the risk for losing his finger.

## Documentation

■ Before performing this procedure, document any abnormal physical findings on the consent form. Have the patient initial the comments and sign the form to signify acknowledgment of preprocedural abnormalities. In the chart, the preprocedural and postprocedural notes must include an evaluation of potentially affected function, range of motion, and sensation. Be certain to document evidence of skin breakdown or concomitant injury.

■ Note that you obtained written consent for removal with a cutter and that you discussed options and risks at length.

■ Indicate the disposition of the ring.

■ If the patient declines ring removal, document that you informed him of the risks of losing his finger, the warning signs and symptoms indicating he should seek emergency ring removal, and care measures for his finger.

# SELF-INJECTION THERAPY FOR ERECTILE DISORDER

## CPT code

54235 *Injection of the corpora cavernosum with medication*

## Overview

Erectile disorder, or impotence, refers to a male's inability to attain or maintain penile erection sufficient to complete intercourse. The patient with primary impotence has never achieved a sufficient erection; secondary impotence, which is more common and less serious than the primary form, implies that, despite present inability, the patient has succeeded in completing intercourse in the past.

Transient periods of impotence aren't considered dysfunction and probably occur in half of adult males. Erectile disorder affects all age groups but increases in frequency with age. The prognosis depends on the severity and duration of impotence and the underlying cause.

Treatment options are usually presented in a stepwise approach, according to preferences of the individual patient. Attempts should be made to include the patient's sexual partner in the decision-making process, as appropriate. Simple, safe, and noninvasive options include oral medications, such as sildenafil citrate (Viagra) and vacuum constriction device therapy. Intracavernosal injections (given by the patient as a self-injection) are considered a second-line option. The most invasive treatment options include penile prostheses and penile revascularization therapy. Intracavernosal injection therapy is the most effective of the nonsurgical treatment options currently available.

Alprostadil, a prostaglandin derivative, is the medication commonly used for intracavernosal injections. It induces erection by relaxing trabecular smooth muscle and dilating cavernosal arteries. This leads to expansion of lacunar spacers and entrapment of blood by compressing venules against the tunica albuginea, a process referred to as the corporal veno-occlusive mechanism. Because injection of alprostadil will produce erection 5

## Location for injections

Self-injections for the treatment of erectile disorder are to be administered into the corpus cavernosum, indicated by the arrows in the illustration below. The patient should place the needle on either side of the lateral shaft of the penis to inject medication into the space.

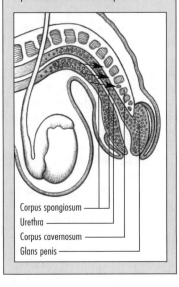

Corpus spongiosum —
Urethra —
Corpus cavernosum —
Glans penis —

to 20 minutes after administration, the patient must be taught how to do self-injections.

### Indications

■ To treat erectile dysfunction due to vasculogenic, psychogenic, neurogenic, or mixed etiology

### Contraindications

■ Hypersensitivity to alprostadil
■ History of priapism
■ Conditions associated with pre-disposition to priapism (sickle cell anemia or trait, multiple myeloma or leukemia) or penile deformation (angulation, cavernosal fibrosis, Peyronie's disease)
■ Penile implants
■ Patient's for whom sexual activity is inadvisable or contraindicated

### Preprocedure patient preparation

■ Obtain a complete history and perform a physical examination.
■ Provide the patient with his treatment options, including rates of effectiveness and risks and benefits for each option.
■ Tell the patient that you'll need to teach him how to administer the self-injections in your facility and that he'll need to stay for evaluation after the injection to determine proper dosage.

### Equipment

Gloves ♦ alcohol pads ♦ 30G ½″ needle with 1 to 3 cc syringe

### Procedure

■ Explain the procedure to the patient, and address any questions or concerns he may have. Show him a picture of penile anatomy and the area to be utilized for self-injections. (See *Locations for injections.*)
■ Teach the patient how to prepare and administer the drug before he begins treatment at home. Stress the importance of reading and following the patient instructions in each package insert.

- Determine the appropriate dose, and have the patient draw up the medication into a syringe.
- Wash your hands and put on gloves.
- Examine the penis, checking the penile shaft and glans for lesions, nodules, inflammations, and swelling.
- Show the patient appropriate injection sites along the penis. Then clean the site with an alcohol pad. The patient should inject into the corpora cavernosum by directing the 30G ½″ needle perpendicular to the penile shaft. The needle should be advanced ¼″ to ½″ before the medication is injected. If resistance is felt during injection, the medication can be administered while slowly withdrawing the needle. He should then massage the injection site for 2 to 3 minutes.
- If there is no erectile response after the initial injection, additional dosages may be given in increments until the patient achieves a suitable erection.
- Monitor the patient every 15 minutes in your facility to evaluate erectile response. The patient may be discharged once the erection subsides.

## Postprocedure patient teaching

- Inform the patient that he can expect an erection 5 to 20 minutes after administration, with a preferable duration of no more than 1 hour. If his erection lasts more than 6 hours, tell him to notify you immediately.

- Tell the patient to discard vials with precipitates or discoloration. Reconstituted vials are designed for single use only and should be discarded after withdrawal of proper volume of the solution.
- Remind the patient to take the drug as instructed — generally, no more than three times weekly, with at least 24 hours between each use. Warn him not to change dosage without consulting you.
- Review possible adverse reactions. Tell the patient to inspect his penis daily and to report redness, swelling, tenderness, curvature, priapism, unusual pain, nodules, or hard tissue.
- Remind the patient to keep regular follow-up appointments so you can evaluate drug safety and effectiveness.

## Complications

- Fibrosis of penile tissue can occur over injection sites. Tell the patient to massage the site after every injection and to use a different site along the penile shaft for each injection.
- Penile pain is a common adverse reaction of alprostadil. It may be relieved by using a lower dose.
- Priapism, or prolonged erection, occurs if the erection doesn't subside within 1 hour. Interventions to relieve the erection may be considered, such as aspirating blood from the penis or administering an antidote.
- Discontinuation of the drug is warranted if the patient develops penile angulation, cavernosal fibrosis, or Peyronie's disease.

## Special considerations

- The patient must have any underlying treatable medical causes of erectile dysfunction diagnosed and treated before initiation of therapy.
- Regular follow-up care with thorough examination of the penis is strongly recommended to detect signs of penile fibrosis.
- Alprostadil may also be administered as a urogenital suppository. Dosage may still be adjusted to achieve desired response.

## Documentation

- Record the indications for the procedure and patient counseling before the initiation of therapy.
- Document the dosage, site, and patient response to the injection.
- Record the patient's understanding of proper dosage, storage, handling, and administration of the medication. Document return demonstrations given by the patient.
- Document patient instructions given and provide the patient with a written copy of the instructions.

## SIGMOIDOSCOPY, FLEXIBLE

### CPT codes

45330  *Sigmoidoscopy, flexible; diagnostic, with or without collection of specimens by brushing or washing (separate procedure)*

45331  *Sigmoidoscopy, flexible; with biopsy, single or multiple*
45332  *Sigmoidoscopy, flexible; with removal of foreign body*

## Overview

Flexible sigmoidoscopy is the direct visualization of the distal colon using a fiberoptic or video endoscope. As a colorectal cancer screening technique, it detects from 50% to 60% of colon cancers. With flexible sigmoidoscopy, the inner lining of the rectum and the last 2′ (61 cm) of the distal colon can be visualized.

## Indications

- To evaluate rectal bleeding, new onset or persistent diarrhea or constipation, mass on digital examination, lower left quadrant abdominal pain and cramping, anal or perianal itching or pain, suspected colitis or proctitis, or radiographic lesions identified in the sigmoid region
- To screen for colon cancer
- To remove a foreign body in the rectum

## Contraindications

**ABSOLUTE**
- Acute abdomen
- Diverticulitis
- Cardiovascular or pulmonary disease (acute)
- Ileus
- Suspected perforation
- Megacolon
- Pregnancy
- Fulminant colitis

■ Uncooperative patient

**RELATIVE**
■ Recent pelvic or abdominal surgery
■ Coagulation disorders
■ Severe inflammatory bowel disease
■ Change in bowel habits (usually requires colonoscopy)

## Preprocedure patient preparation

■ Ensure that the patient performed proper bowel preparation before the procedure: clear liquid diet the night before and the morning of the procedure, one bottle of citrate of magnesia the evening before the procedure, and two small-volume hypertonic phosphate enemas (such as Fleet) 60 minutes before the procedure. If the patient can't complete the enemas at home, two Fleet enemas may be given in the office before the procedure.

■ To allay apprehension and anxiety, explain why and how the procedure will be performed. Review the equipment used, the anatomy of the colon to be examined, associated discomforts (cramping and distention), potential complications (perforation, bleeding, and infection), possible findings (polyps, colitis, diverticulosis, or hemorrhoids), and the potential for tissue sampling, biopsy, or photography.

## Equipment

Flexible sigmoidoscope, 60 cm

◆ light source ◆ three gloves ◆ water-resistant gown ◆ face shield ◆ suction ◆ suction tubing ◆ water-soluble lubricant (K-Y jelly or 2% lidocaine jelly) ◆ drape ◆ prepared 10% formalin or saline specimen collection jars obtained from pathology laboratory ◆ biopsy forceps

## Procedure

■ Explain the procedure to the patient, and address any questions or concerns he may have.

☑ **OBTAIN INFORMED CONSENT**

■ Wash your hands and obtain baseline vital signs.
■ Complete the patient history and physical examination. Confirm that the patient meets the indications specified for flexible sigmoidoscopy.
■ Administer an enema if the patient didn't do this at home.
■ Test the sigmoidoscope for light, water, air, and suction.
■ Drape the rectal area and place the patient in the left lateral decubitus position with the knees bent up toward the chest. (Some health care providers prefer to have the patient's right leg flexed at the hip and knee to facilitate ease of entry.)
■ Put on a faceshield, a gown, and gloves (wear two on your dominant hand).
■ Using a gloved, lubricated finger, perform a digital examination to dilate the anal sphincter. If stool is present, administer another enema.
■ Lubricate the anus and the tip

of the sigmoidoscope. Be sure not to get gel on the lens because this will distort the view.

■ Separate the gluteal folds and observe the rectal area for hemorrhoids, fissures, or inflammation.

■ Insert the scope obliquely 3″ to 4″ (8 to 10 cm) by pressing the curved surface of the tip against the sphincter rather than straight in.

■ Remove the contaminated top glove from the dominant hand.

■ With the dominant hand, advance the scope. With the nondominant hand, work the controls on the scope.

■ Open the colon by instilling a small amount of air, angulate the tip to locate the lumen, and advance the instrument gently. Note that the tip must be constantly maneuvered to keep the lumen in view as the instrument is passed.

■ When the lumen isn't seen, pull the scope back. Don't advance blindly. If the colon is in spasm, apply gentle bursts of air to open puckered folds. Then continue advancing the instrument toward the dark center of the lumen.

▶ **CLINICAL TIP**
*Don't use too much air; this causes discomfort and can increase the risk of perforation.*

■ Advance the scope using one of the following techniques:

– The hook and pullout method straightens the colon. Hook the mucosal fold with the tip of the scope and pull it back gently to straighten the colon.

– The dither and torque method shortens the colon. Alternate insertion with slow, partial withdrawal to pleat the colon. Then twist the instrument shaft clockwise or counterclockwise with a forward or backward motion to straighten it before advancing the scope again.

▶ **CLINICAL TIP**
*The goal is to provide a safe, thorough, comfortable examination, not to insert the instrument to its full length.*

■ If the instrument won't advance beyond the rectosigmoid junction (around 6″ [15 cm]), gentle pressure may permit the instrument to pass. This is safe even if the lumen isn't clearly seen, as long as the mucosa slides by. If the patient is uncomfortable or the instrument doesn't advance, withdraw the scope, torque it, and try again.

■ Also be careful when advancing in a patient with diverticulosis. The mouth of a diverticulum may appear to be the lumen. Inserting the scope into a diverticulum can result in perforation.

■ Observe for natural landmarks and abnormalities.

■ Take a biopsy of all abnormal-appearing areas or polyps. The biopsy forceps can be passed through the biopsy channel of the scope. When the forceps are visible and in the area of interest or pathology, open the forceps and grasp a small sample of tissue with the prongs. Close the forceps and, with a tugging motion, retrieve the tissue sample. Remove the forceps through the channel. Place the tissue sample in a specimen jar for pathology and label it according to your laboratory's guidelines, particularly noting location from the anal verge, either anatomically or numerically (in centimeters).

▲ **CLINICAL TIP**
*Polypectomy or removal of colon lesions should be performed during a colonoscopy to minimize complications from the procedure. For example, the combination of electrocautery and incomplete bowel preparation has caused explosions of bowel gases in the colon.*

■ On reaching 60 cm (or the greatest distance tolerated by the patient), withdraw the sigmoidoscope slowly, reinspecting the mucosa. This provides the best view of the mucosa. Be sure to examine behind each mucosal fold.

■ When in the rectal vault, retroflex the tip of the scope to visualize the distal rectum (twisting the knob until the tip of the scope flexes 180 degrees). Retroflection is used to diagnose and stage internal hemorrhoids or other pathology in the distal rectum.

■ Straighten the tip and gently withdraw the scope.

■ Clean, sterilize, and store the sigmoidoscope according to the manufacturer's instructions.

## Postprocedure patient teaching

■ Review the findings with the patient.

■ Tell him that he can resume normal activity shortly after the procedure (in 5 to 15 minutes) and that no special diet is needed.

■ Review common complications, such as abdominal cramping with air insufflation (relieved with passage of flatus or suction from

scope); feeling of fullness, distention, or flatus; lack of bowel movement for several days; and minor bleeding (if a biopsy is taken in the low rectum). For a vasovagal reaction, such as vertigo, diaphoresis, hypotension, and mild malaise, tell the patient to remain supine and monitor his vital signs until the feeling passes.

■ Urge the patient to promptly report signs of infection (elevated temperature, diarrhea, or increased or prolonged abdominal pain), bloody diarrhea, or bleeding that persists for more than 2 days.

## Complications

■ Complications are rare. Their incidence is higher in the patient with previous abdominal surgery or irradiation, which can cause adhesions. Bowel adhesions can fixate the bowel and cause tethering, which predisposes the colon to perforation.

❋ **COLLABORATION**
*Bowel perforation requires emergency surgical referral. Bleeding may require referral or collaboration with a gastroenterologist.*

■ Abnormal distention and pain require evaluation and treatment, depending on findings.

■ Infection may require antibiotics and referral, depending on whether the infection is local or systemic.

■ Vasovagal symptoms are treated with rest, with the patient in a supine position until symptoms resolve.

■ Undetected disease is minimized with periodic screening.

# Sample documentation form for flexible sigmoidoscopy

## OFFICE FLEXIBLE SIGMOIDOSCOPY

Date: _6/28/02_      Chart #/ID #: _82995150_

Patient name: _Ian Mansfield_

DOB: _08/14/49_      Age: _53_

### Signs and symptoms

FOBT results: _Positive_      Date: _6/10/02_

Previous sigmoidoscopy: _None_      Date:

### PMH

Allergies: _PCN_

Medications: _Denies_

Bacterial endocarditis prophylaxis: _No_

Blood pressure: _136/88_

### Bowel preparation used

- ☑ Clear liquids / Citrate of magnesia
- ☑ 2 Fleet enemas at home
- ☐ 2 Fleet enemas in office

**Adequacy of preparation:** _Optimal cleansing_

**Type of scope:** _Flexible 35-cm scope with video pathway system_

**Depth of visualization:** _35 cm_

**Preoperative diagnosis:** _N/A_

**Postoperative diagnosis:** _Internal hemorrhoids_

**Findings:** _Lining of sigmoid colon, rectal mucosa, rectum, and anus appear normal in color, texture, and size except for painless bluish, engorged veins near anus seen on retroversion._

**Location of biopsies:** _N/A_

**Plan:** _Advised patient to engage in physical activity for 30 minutes daily. Recommended increasing intake of low-fat and high-fiber foods (at least five servings of fruits and vegetables daily plus six servings of other high-fiber foods, such as whole-grain breads, rice, and pasta). Discussed smoking cessation._

SIGNATURE: _Megan Frenz, PA-C_    CC: _Rick Gill, MD_

## Special considerations

■ GI discomfort usually resolves in 24 to 48 hours. A feeling of pressure is generally greatest immediately after the procedure. The patient may feel a need to evacuate stool with no results or may experience increased flatulence for a few days after the procedure.

■ Provide the patient with written instructions to reinforce your teaching.

■ The American Cancer Society recommends the use of flexible sigmoidoscopy to screen the patient at average risk for colon cancer. The current recommendation is that males and females age 50 and over should have a flexible sigmoidoscopy every 3 to 5 years and participate in yearly fecal occult blood testing. Average-risk individuals are those without a family history of colon cancer, personal history of adenoma polypectomy, personal history of pancolitis within the previous 8 years, and currently without anemia, heme-positive stools, or change in bowel habits. Because only 60% of colon cancer can be detected with a sigmoidoscopy, the patient with a family history of colon cancer or colon polyps, symptoms of blood mixed in his stool, or a change in the pattern or characteristic of his stools should undergo a complete colonoscopy rather than a sigmoidoscopy.

## Documentation

■ Document findings in the patient's chart. (See *Sample documen-tation form for flexible sigmoi-doscopy.*)

■ Be sure to document the type and adequacy of bowel preparation, type of scope used, depth of visualization, appearance of mucosa, biopsy locations (if taken), complications, the patient's tolerance of the procedure, and instructions given to the patient for follow-up and treatment (if required).

# *Skin Scraping, KOH Preparation*

### *CPT code*
87220 *Tissue examination by KOH slide of specimens from skin, hair, or nails for fungi or ectoparasites*

## Overview

A skin scrape involves the gentle removal of a skin specimen that's then placed on a microscope slide for evaluation. This procedure is commonly performed using potassium hydroxide (KOH) on the slide to reveal a superficial fungal infection or arthropod infestation.

## Indications

■ To verify the presence of a superficial fungal infection or arthropod infestation

## Contraindications

■ None known

## Preprocedure patient preparation

■ Before beginning, tell the patient that you're about to scrape the skin but that it shouldn't cause pain.
■ Explain that the scraping will help ensure proper diagnosis and treatment.

## Equipment

Surgical blade such as #15 Bard-Parker blade (if unavailable, use the edge of a glass microscope slide) ◆ gloves ◆ alcohol pad ◆ microscope slide and coverglass ◆ 5% to 20% KOH solution ◆ match ◆ lens paper

## Procedure

■ Explain the procedure to the patient, and address any questions or concerns he may have.
■ Position the patient comfortably, leaving the area to be scraped easily accessible.
■ Wash your hands and put on gloves.
■ If necessary, clean the area with an alcohol pad.
■ Lightly run the surgical blade perpendicular to the skin. When the blade has collected enough of the superficial skin layer, wipe it across the microscope slide. Make sure you use a gentle technique; the patient shouldn't bleed or experience pain.
■ Place the coverglass on the slide.
■ If you suspect a dermatophyte infection, apply KOH to the edge of the coverglass, allowing capillary action to draw the solution under it.
■ Gently heat the slide with a match until bubbles begin to expand.
■ Blot excess KOH solution with lens paper.
■ Look for hyphae (septated, tubelike structures), dermatophytes, pseudohyphae (tubelike structures without septa), and budding yeast forms to identify candidiasis.

## Postprocedure patient teaching

■ Tell the patient when to schedule a follow-up appointment based on the diagnostic findings.

## Complications

■ None known

## Special considerations

■ If KOH results are negative, collect a culture specimen and send it to the microbiology laboratory for growth and species identification.

## Documentation

■ Record indications for testing, the location and appearance of the specimen site, results of testing, and the patient's tolerance for the procedure.
■ Note the prognosis, patient instructions given, and follow-up appointment information.

# SKIN SCRAPING, SCABIES

## CPT code

87220 *Tissue examination of the skin, hair, and nails for ectoparasites (scabies)*

## Overview

Scabies — an age-old, highly transmissible skin infestation — is characterized by burrows, pruritus, and excoriations with secondary infections. It occurs worldwide, typically associated with overcrowding and poor hygiene, and can be endemic. The mites that cause this disorder, *Sarcoptes scabiei* var. *hominis* (itch mite), can live their entire life cycles in human skin, causing chronic infection. The female mite burrows into the skin to lay eggs, from which larvae emerge to copulate and then reburrow under the skin.

Rapid diagnosis and treatment of this condition is essential to prevent spreading. A skin scraping of the burrows can reveal adults, mite feces (called scybala), and eggs.

## Indications

■ To determine the cause of any rash that's suspicious for scabies (itchy, threadlike lesions that are approximately ⅜″ [1 cm] long that generally occur between fingers, on flexor surfaces of the wrists, on elbows, in axillary folds, at the waistline, on nipples and buttocks in females, and on genitalia in males)
■ To detect a scabies infection in the patient who has been exposed to scabies or who has already begun treatment for an itchy rash that hasn't improved

## Contraindications

■ None known

## Preprocedure patient preparation

■ Obtain a medical history from the patient, including any known exposure to or history of scabies, the length of time his symptoms have been present, and any treatments or medications he has tried.

## Equipment

Gloves ♦ #15 scalpel ♦ microscope slide ♦ cover slip ♦ mineral oil ♦ microscope

### Equipment preparation

■ Ensure that the microscope slide is clean and free of debris.

## Procedure

■ Explain the procedure to the patient, and address any questions or concerns he may have.
■ Wash your hands and put on gloves.
■ Identify a burrow in the skin. If a burrow isn't obvious, select a papule or the roof of a vesicle to use as a scraping site. Place a small amount of mineral oil over the burrow, papule, or vesicle.

## Identifying the scabies mite

Infestation with *Sarcoptes scabiei* — the itch mite — causes scabies. This mite (shown enlarged below) has a hard shell and measures a microscopic 0.1 mm.

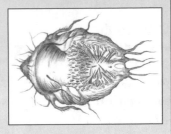

■ Using the scalpel, vigorously scrape the area to remove the top of the burrow, papule, or vesicle. Don't scrape so vigorously that you cause bleeding to occur. Scraping may cause the tissue to "roll up" or crumble, which can make interpretation difficult. Alternately, shave a very thin layer (3 to 5 mm) off the top of the papule or burrow. Tissue can be gathered from several sites, increasing the chance to identify the organisms.

■ Transfer the scraping to a clean microscope slide and apply a cover slip.

■ View the slide with a microscope looking for mites. (See *Identifying the scabies mite*.) Also look for eggs, oval structures that are one-third to one-half the size of the mite, and feces, numerous, tiny dark flecks that are one-tenth the size of the egg. Mites, eggs, and feces are sometimes seen with a potassium hydroxide prep or saline mount.

## Postprocedure patient teaching

■ Inform the patient of his test results.

■ If the diagnosis of scabies is confirmed and treatment is initiated, teach the patient to apply the pediculicide cream or lotion from the neck down, covering his entire body. (He may need assistance to reach all body areas.) Tell him to wait about 15 minutes after application before dressing and to avoid bathing for 8 to 12 hours. Stress the importance of meticulous handwashing to prevent the infection's spread and recurrence.

## Complications

■ None known

## Special considerations

■ If the patient has scabies, his family members and other close personal contacts should be checked for possible symptoms.

■ If the skin scraping yields no positive identification of the mite and if scabies is still suspected (for example, if family members and close contacts also report itching), skin clearing that occurs after a therapeutic trial of a pediculocide will confirm the diagnosis.

## Documentation

■ Document the indications for performing the procedure, the findings of your microscopic analysis, and any treatments prescribed in the patient's chart.

■ Record all patient education given.

---

## SKIN SCRAPING, TZANCK SMEAR

### CPT code
87207 *Smear, primary source with interpretation, special stain for inclusion bodies (herpes viruses)*

### Overview

Herpes simplex I and II and herpes zoster (shingles) can be painful diseases that significantly alter the life of a patient. Because there is no cure for herpes simplex, lifelong control of herpes simplex is a long-term goal that requires correct identification of the initial infection. Only then can a patient be offered medical modalities that alleviate symptoms, decrease disease duration, and hopefully prevent transmission to others. Herpes zoster, a reactivation of the varicella-zoster virus, can have long-lasting painful consequences (such as postherpetic neuralgia), especially in the elderly or debilitated patient. Although most patients may recover completely, early treatment with proper antiviral medications may help decrease the extent of the initial infection as well as the incidence of this complication.

A Tzanck smear can provide useful information for early diagnosis of a herpes or varicella infection, but it should be followed by a culture of the lesion for confirmation.

### Indications
■ To evaluate the cause of vesicular skin lesions suspicious for herpes

### Contraindications
■ None known

### Preprocedure patient preparation

■ Obtain a medical history from the patient, including when the symptoms started, if there are any associated symptoms, if he had known contact with a person with herpes simplex virus, if he had chicken pox (when suspecting herpes zoster), and what medications or treatments the patient has tried.
■ Examine the skin lesions and their distribution.

### Equipment
Alcohol pads ◆ #15 scalpel blade ◆ microscope slide ◆ Bunsen burner or other flame source (optional) ◆ Wright's stain or Giemsa stain ◆ methyl alcohol fixing (if using Giemsa stain) ◆ microscope (optional)

#### Equipment preparation
■ Make sure the microscope slide is clean and free from debris.

### Procedure
■ Explain the procedure to the pa-

tient, and address any questions or concerns he may have.

- Wash your hands and put on gloves.

- Determine the skin lesion for scraping

◢◣ **CLINICAL TIP**
*Choose a vesicle that appears fresh, slightly dimpled, and unmanipulated.*

- Gently wipe the site with an alcohol pad.

- Using the scalpel, unroof the vesicle being careful not to disturb its base.

- Then gently scrape the base of the vesicle with the scalpel and smear the scrapings onto the microscope slide.

- Air dry the slide or gently heat to fix the smear on the slide using a Bunsen burner or other flame source. If Giemsa stain is to be used, the slide must be fixed with methyl alcohol for 10 to 15 minutes initially.

- Submit the specimen to the laboratory in a cardboard container that protects the specimen and order a Tzanck smear. The laboratory will stain the slide and send test results.

- If your office is certified and OSHA compliant to perform this test using Wright's stain: Add a drop or two of fresh Wright's stain and allow to sit for 1 minute. Add an equal amount of water and gently blow on the slide to mix the stain and water. Look for formation of a scum on the surface that appears shiny. Once this occurs, allow the stain to set for 4 minutes. Rinse gently with tap water. Dry off the back of the slide. Ex-

amine the smear under a microscope using low power to choose a good area to study. Use the high-power oil-immersion lens to look for multinucleated giant cells (containing 10 to 12 nuclei) or giant epithelial cells.

- If your facility is certified and OSHA compliant to perform this test using Giemsa stain: Add a drop or two of fresh Giemsa stain and allow to dry. Rinse the slide gently with water and dry off the back of the slide. Continue with microscopic examination as above.

## Postprocedure patient teaching

- If the specimen was sent to the laboratory, inform the patient of when the results will be available.
- If you're able to perform the smear, discuss the results with the patient, and explain any treatment or further testing that's necessary.

## Complications

- None known

## Special considerations

- Patients diagnosed with genital herpes will need emotional support and counseling. Elderly patients with herpes zoster may need home assistance with dressing changes.

## Documentation

- Document the indications for performing the procedure. Note whether you sent the specimen to a laboratory for analysis or if you did the microscopic analysis yourself, including the method of staining, your findings, further testing done, and treatments prescribed.

■ Record all patient education given.

## $S$OFT-TISSUE ASPIRATION

### CPT codes

20600 *Arthrocentesis, aspiration, or injection: small joint, bursa, or ganglionic cyst (for example, fingers or toes)*

20605 *Arthrocentesis, aspiration, or injection: intermediate joint or bursa (for example, wrist, elbow, ankle, olecranon bursa)*

20610 *Arthrocentesis, aspiration, or injection: major joint or bursa (for example, shoulder, hip, knee joint, subacromial bursa)*

### Overview

Soft-tissue aspiration involves removing fluid or exudate from an area of soft tissue for evaluation and palliative care.

### Indications

■ To relieve pain or swelling in soft tissue
■ To evacuate a hematoma resulting from trauma

### Contraindications

**ABSOLUTE**
■ Broken skin at the site

**RELATIVE**
■ Coagulopathies
■ Swelling of the face
■ Cellulitis
■ Prosthetic joint

### Preprocedure patient preparation

■ Advise the patient that discomfort is minimal after the procedure (except in patients with fibromyalgia).

### Equipment

Povidone-iodine solution or alcohol swabs ◆ sterile gloves ◆ drape (optional) ◆ hemostat (optional) ◆ 10-ml syringe with 18G to 20G 1″ needle ◆ red-topped collection tube (optional) ◆ elastic bandage ◆ sterile 3″ × 3″ or 4″ × 4″ gauze pads ◆ tape

### Procedure

■ Explain the procedure to the patient, and address any questions or concerns that he may have.

**☑ OBTAIN INFORMED CONSENT**
■ Assemble the equipment before beginning.
■ Wash your hands.
■ Place the patient in as comfortable a position as possible to allow performance of the procedure. Drape as appropriate for the site to be aspirated.

- Verify that the patient isn't allergic to iodine.
- Clean the area with povidone-iodine solution or with an alcohol swab.
- Put on sterile gloves and maintain aseptic technique throughout the procedure.
- Attach an 18G or a 20G 1″ needle to a 10-ml syringe.
- Insert the needle with the bevel (the sloped edge) down, into the leading edge of the swelling. Aspirate as you advance the needle.
- If the syringe becomes full and needs to be changed, attach the hemostat to the needle hub to avoid needle rotation, remove the first syringe, replace it with an empty syringe, and continue aspirating.
- Place the aspirated fluid into a red-topped collection tube, and send it to the laboratory for analysis, if indicated.
- Apply a pressure dressing and compression device such as an elastic bandage.

## Postprocedure patient teaching

- Urge the patient to keep the pressure dressing intact for 24 hours before removing it.
- Suggest applying ice or heat for the first 24 hours to relieve discomfort.
- Emphasize the need to rest the affected area to ensure proper healing, even after pain is relieved.
- Instruct the patient to notify you promptly if he experiences signs and symptoms of infection, such as red streaking; increased

pain, redness, or warmth at the site; purulent drainage; fever; and chills.

## Complications

- Infection may be treated with local or systemic antibiotics and antiseptic soaks. It may also require consultation with a physician, a surgeon, or an infectious disease specialist.

## Special considerations

- Aspiration of cloudy fluid doesn't necessarily indicate infection; sebaceous fluid will also appear cloudy. As long as no other signs of infection are evident, treatment with antibiotics isn't indicated.

## Documentation

- Before performing this procedure, document abnormal physical findings on the consent form. Have the patient initial the comments and sign the form to signify acknowledgment of preprocedural abnormalities. In the chart, the preprocedural and postprocedural notes must include an evaluation of potentially affected function, range of motion, and sensation.
- Note whether a culture was sent to the laboratory.
- Describe the site before and after the procedure, the characteristics of the aspirated fluid, the patient's reaction to the procedure, medications ordered, the time frame for follow-up evaluation, and any instructions given to the patient.

# SPLINTING/ FRACTURE IMMOBILIZATION

### CPT codes
29105  *Application of long arm splint*
29125  *Application of short arm splint, static*
29130  *Application of finger splint, static*
29505  *Application of long leg splint*
29515  *Application of short leg splint*
29550  *Strapping: toes*
99070  *Splinting: supplies and material beyond those usually included for the office visit or service rendered*

## Overview

Splinting can temporarily stabilize and immobilize acute injuries and provide symptomatic relief of chronic conditions, increasing patient comfort and preventing further injury. Acute injuries — such as sprains, strains, and fractures — typically require immediate joint stabilization; at the scene of the trauma, any rigid object can function as a splint. A temporary measure, splinting is initially preferred over circumferential casting for acute injuries because increased swelling within a circumferential cast can lead to vascular compromise, compartment syndrome, and distal swelling.

Inversion injuries with plantar flexion, the most common cause of acute ankle injuries, typically occur in young adults who take part in recreational activities and sports. Fractures are more common in older adults. Sprains vary based on the level of injury, disability, pain, and swelling.

Chronic conditions typically occur in the upper extremities and can usually be managed in a primary care setting or by an orthopedic specialist. Chronic injuries typically affect the wrists and hands and usually result from tenosynovitis and can occur with repetitive-motion injuries, such as carpal tunnel syndrome and tennis elbow. Splints increase the patient's comfort by keeping the joint immobilized and in proper alignment.

Consider referrals for an unstable joint, a fracture, potential limb loss, suspected internal derangement (indicated by clicking, popping, or locking of the joint), persistent pain, or unresolved injury.

## Indications

■ To stabilize an acute strain, sprain, or fracture
■ To relieve repetitive-motion disorders and overuse disorders
■ To immobilize a joint after dislocation reduction

## Contraindications
**ABSOLUTE**
■ Neurovascular compromise
■ Soft-tissue compression
■ Open injury

## Ottawa ankle rules

Use the following Ottawa ankle rules to determine if X-rays are needed:
- If the patient is between ages 18 and 55 and can walk four steps immediately after the injury or when being evaluated, X-rays aren't required.
- If the patient feels pain on ambulation immediately after the injury and on evaluation, plus tenderness within 2½″ (6 cm) of the posterior edge of the malleoli, order ankle X-rays.
- If the patient feels pain on ambulation immediately after the injury and on evaluation, plus tenderness of the fifth metatarsal or navicular, order foot X-rays.

## Preprocedure patient preparation

■ Take a complete history and perform a physical examination. Obtain a description of the injury and the joint involved, how and when it occurred, the patient's level of activity right after the injury and at the time of evaluation, and previous history of injury to the joint. Physical assessment should focus on the joint involved and its physical appearance, including swelling, obvious deformity, bleeding, and ecchymosis as well as a comparison with the other uninjured extremity, if possible. Also assess the patient's neurovascular status and ability to the move the extremity.

## Equipment

Tube stockinette in various diameters ◆ casting material in various widths ◆ 4″ or 6″ elastic wraps ◆ bucket of water ◆ soft padding ◆ scissors (optional) ◆ 1″ to 2″ adhesive tape (optional) ◆ sling (optional) ◆ aluminum splints (optional) ◆ wrist and finger splints (optional) ◆ knee immobilizer (optional)

## Procedure

■ Explain the procedure to the patient, and address any questions or concerns he may have.

### Ankle splinting

■ Perform X-rays as appropriate to rule out fracture. (See *Ottawa ankle rules*.)
■ After the X-ray has been read and fracture has been ruled out, prepare the patient for immobilization. Place him in a comfortable position that permits splinting or taping. The joint must be in a neutral position while ensuring adequate stretching of the tendons.
■ Measure the casting material against the patient and then add about 1½″ (3.8 cm) to the length of the splint to ensure a proper fit. After measuring out 10 to 15 lengths of material and cutting it, fold the material into overlapping layers to form the desired length.
■ Put on the stockinette; it should be approximately 2″ to 3″ (5 to 7.5 cm) above and below the area to be splinted.
■ Alternatively, apply a soft cotton padding, such as Webril, to the extremity to protect the skin (with extra layers over bony promi-

nences as needed) before applying the splint. Make sure the material doesn't bunch up and cause a pressure area.

■ Holding the ends of the overlapping layers of material, submerge the material for 5 to 10 seconds in cool water. Shear off excess water before applying to the patient and molding to the limb.

■ Allow the casting material to harden for 10 minutes; then wrap an elastic bandage around the extremity and splint while maintaining the extremity in the proper position.

■ Secure the elastic bandage with tape or clips.

### Finger splinting

■ Although several types of finger splints exist, the aluminum finger splint is most commonly used for isolated proximal and distal interphalangeal joint injuries. Place it on both sides of the injured finger and secure it with tape.

■ If this isn't the first injury to the finger, incorporate the finger splint into a volar arm splint for added support.

### Arm splinting

■ Obtain a volar arm splint for grades 2 and 3 wrist sprains.

■ Have the patient extend his wrist slightly, with the metacarpophalangeal joint flexed 60 to 70 degrees and the fingers flexed 10 to 20 degrees.

■ Put on the stockinette; it should be at least 3″ longer than the intended casting area. Cut a hole for the thumb.

■ Cut the casting material to the

length needed; then submerge the material for 5 to 10 seconds in cool water.

■ Maintain this position as you mold the casting material and as it hardens. Fold the excess stockinette over the casting material. Secure it with an elastic bandage. The splint should extend from the tip of the fingers to about 1¼″ to 1½″ (3 to 4 cm) distal to the elbow joint.

### Thumb splinting

■ Obtain an aluminum thumb splint.

■ Flex the thumb slightly at the distal interphalangeal joint.

■ Measure the aluminum splint to fit 1″ to 2″ (2.5 to 5 cm) beyond the wrist.

■ Bend the splint to the position of the thumb, and apply it to the dorsal side of the thumb.

■ Wrap the splint with an elastic wrap; include the thumb in the wrap.

### Below-the-knee splinting

■ Obtain an ankle fracture brace for injury to the tibiofibular, lateral collateral, or deltoid ligament to limit inversion and eversion.

■ Place the patient in a prone position (if possible), making sure the knee and ankle are flexed 90 degrees. Help him maintain this position as you apply the splint, which should extend from the metatarsal joint to about 1½″ below the popliteal fossae. Secure the splint with an elastic bandage (usually 4″ to 6″ [10 to 15 cm] wide).

■ Alternatively, you can use a stirrup ankle splint for such injuries. Place a 5″ (12.7 cm) plaster splint over the plantar aspect of the foot and up both the medial and the lateral sides of the foreleg to the level of the fibula head.

### Toe splinting

■ To "buddy tape" the injured toe, use 1″ (2.5 cm) of silk tape to tape the toe to the neighboring toe; this stabilizes and immobilizes the fracture or sprain.

■ Help the patient put on his shoe and lace it securely to provide support and immobilization. Recommend that the patient wear hard-sole shoes that lace to ease putting on the shoe and to provide extra support.

## Postprocedure patient teaching

■ Teach the patient the RICE regimen — rest, ice, compression, and elevation.

■ Tell him to apply ice every 2 to 3 hours for 20 to 30 minutes for the first 24 hours. Then he can switch to moist heat (without wetting the dressing) for the next 24 to 48 hours.

■ Tell him to wear the splint except when sleeping or showering until he's reevaluated and to avoid activities that cause pain.

■ Instruct him to watch for signs of neurovascular compromise, such as coolness, swelling, pain, darkness, or pallor in the area around the splint or tape. If he notes any, he should rest at once with the extremity elevated above his heart. Emphasize that swelling

can occur swiftly with activity, but it will take much longer to subside. Urge him to contact you if swelling doesn't improve within 30 minutes.

■ Tell him to take acetaminophen, a nonsteroidal anti-inflammatory drug, or both to relieve pain as directed.

■ Instruct the patient to follow up with you 48 hours after the initial taping or splinting and then as indicated.

■ Tell him to remove the splint or tape and immediately call you if he experiences signs of neurovascular compromise, such as peripheral pallor or blue-purple color, pain, coldness, swelling, or numbness and tingling, that don't resolve.

## Complications

■ Vascular compromise, ischemia, and compartment syndrome of the affected extremity can result from a splint that's wrapped too tightly. To prevent this, make sure the elastic bandage is snug but not tight, and use a linear splint rather than a circular splint.

■ Pressure ulcers can result from the splint rubbing against bony prominences. Soft cotton padding applied directly to the skin beneath the splint can help minimize this complication.

## Special considerations

■ For chronic injuries, consider taping to stabilize and support the joint, particularly for an athlete. Taping immobilizes the area and provides support, allowing the athlete to continue activities with minimal interference. Make sure the tape isn't too tight, and keep in mind that most taping loosens after activity, placing the joint at risk for further injury. Several methods of taping exist; a skilled professional, such as a trainer or sports medicine health care provider, should perform such taping.

✦ **COLLABORATION**
*As appropriate, refer the patient to an orthopedic specialist for a custom-made splint, which may be more comfortable than standard-sized splints.*

## Documentation

■ Review recent or pertinent documentation by other health team members; then initial their notes to signify you're aware of their findings. This doesn't signify agreement with their comments or reduce your responsibility to conduct your own history and physical examination.

■ Before performing this procedure, document any abnormal physical findings on the consent form and have the patient initial the comments as well as sign the form to signify acknowledgment of preprocedural abnormalities. In the chart, the preprocedural and postprocedural note must include an evaluation of function, range of motion, and such neurosensory testing as 2-point discrimination.

■ Record indications for and details of the procedure, including a detailed description of the site, the type of splint used, the patient's re-action to the procedure, medications ordered, the time frame for follow-up evaluation, and any instructions given to the patient.

## SPUTUM CULTURE

**CPT codes**
87070 *Bacterial culture, any source except urine, blood, or stool, with isolation and presumptive identification of isolates*
87205 *Gram stain*

## Overview

Sputum is a viscid secretion raised from the trachea, bronchi, bronchioles, and lungs. It may consist of a variety of substances, including mucus, epithelial cells, cellular debris, white blood cells, red blood cells, normal respiratory bacteria, and pathogenic organisms.

Bacteriologic examination of sputum is an important aid to the management of lung disease. The usual method of specimen collection is deep coughing and expectoration, but it may occasionally require assistance by induction.

## Indications

■ To identify the cause of pulmonary infection, thus aiding diagnosis of respiratory diseases (most frequently bronchitis, tuberculosis, lung abscess, and pneumonia)

## Contraindications

■ None known

## Preprocedure patient preparation

■ Explain to the patient that this test is used to identify the organism causing respiratory tract infection.

■ Teach the patient how to expectorate by taking three deep breaths and forcing a deep cough; emphasize that sputum isn't the same as saliva, which is unacceptable for culturing. Advise the patient that if necessary, a steam-like mist may be provided to assist in raising sputum.

■ Encourage fluid intake the night before collection to help sputum production, unless contraindicated by a fluid restriction. A first-morning specimen is optimal, before eating or drinking, as sputum will have accumulated overnight.

■ Tell the patient to remove his dentures, as necessary.

■ Have the patient rinse his mouth well with plain water prior to specimen collection to decrease the potential for specimen contamination by food particles or oropharyngeal flora. Toothpaste and mouthwash shouldn't be used, as these may alter the flora.

## Equipment

Sterile, disposable, impermeable container with a tight-fitting cap ♦ specimen label, including patient name and other information as required by individual facility or policy ♦ gloves ♦ facial tissues

### For induction
Nebulizer and tubing ♦ 20 to 25 ml of sterile normal saline solution for aerosol inhalation

## Procedure

■ Explain the procedure to the patient, and address any questions or concerns he may have.

■ The patient should be in a sitting or high Fowler position.

■ Wash your hands and put on gloves. Uncap the sterile specimen container.

■ Instruct the patient to take three deep breaths and force a deep cough, raising sputum; he should then expectorate into the specimen container.

■ Avoid touching the inside of the container to decrease risk of contamination.

■ A minimum sample of 1 ml of sputum is necessary. The patient should continue coughing and expectorating until an adequate amount is collected.

■ If the patient has difficulty raising sputum, induction of sputum may be indicated. Instruct the patient to breathe a sample of sterile normal saline solution via nebulizer, then cough and expectorate. (Note that this may produce a thinner sample of sputum.)

■ Replace the cover on specimen container and clean exterior if necessary.

■ Attach or inspect for appropriate label, including whether the specimen was expectorated or induced. Send immediately to laboratory. Don't refrigerate the specimen.

■ Offer the patient facial tissue and water to rinse his mouth.

## Postprocedure patient teaching

■ Advise the patient that the sputum will be cultured to identify pathogenic organisms, with preliminary results on this available in 24 hours; final results in 48 to 72 hours; and up to 6 weeks if fungal organisms are suspected.

■ If a gram stain will be performed, explain that additional preliminary information regarding the potential presence of pathogens in the sputum will be available within about 1 hour.

■ Instruct the patient to take antibiotics or other medications as prescribed following the procedure.

## Complications

■ Complications are rare during or following this procedure.

■ Observe for respiratory difficulty precipitated by coughing, especially in patients with asthma or chronic obstructive pulmonary disease.

■ Patients with cardiac disease may be at increased risk of arrhythmia during coughing.

## Special considerations

■ Saliva or spit is unsatisfactory and won't yield adequate results. This should be suspected if the

sample (non-induced) appears thin like saliva and the patient's cough effort was weak.

■ Immediate Gram stain testing in the laboratory will also yield information regarding the adequacy of the sample: sputum contains a maximum of 25 epithelial cells per low power field on microscopy; a greater number suggests saliva, a suboptimal sample, and the need to consider repeating the collection procedure.

■ If the suspected organism is *Mycobacterium tuberculosis,* the patient may need to provide as many as 3 morning sputum specimens.

■ Respiratory viruses usually require serologic or histologic diagnosis rather than diagnosis by sputum culture.

## Documentation

■ Record collection technique (expectorated or induced), how the patient tolerated the procedure, color and consistency of the specimen, and note antibiotics the patient is currently receiving or will be prescribed (if necessary).

## *S*TAPLE REMOVAL

***CPT code***
*No specific code has been assigned. (Removal is included as part of the staple insertion procedure.)*

## Overview
Skin staples or clips may be used in place of standard sutures to

close lacerations and surgical wounds. They can secure a wound more quickly than sutures, making them useful in areas such as the abdomen where cosmetic results are less important. When properly placed, staples and clips distribute tension evenly along the suture line with minimal tissue trauma and compression, promoting healing and minimizing scarring. Because staples and clips are made from surgical stainless steel, tissue reaction to them is minimal.

## Indications

■ To remove staples once a wound is fully healed

## Contraindications

■ None known

## Preprocedure patient preparation

■ Obtain a detailed history, and conduct a physical examination.
■ Assess the wound and confirm the appropriateness of staple removal.
■ Inform the patient that he may feel a slight pulling or tickling sensation but little discomfort during staple removal.
■ Reassure him that because his incision is healing properly, removing the supporting staples or clips won't weaken the incision line.

## Equipment

Waterproof trash bag ◆ adjustable light ◆ gloves if wound is dressed; otherwise, sterile gloves ◆ sterile gauze pads ◆ sterile staple or clip extractor (prepackaged, sterile disposable staple or clip extractors are available) ◆ povidone-iodine solution or other antiseptic cleaning agent ◆ sterile cotton-tipped applicators ◆ adhesive butterfly strips or Steri-Strips (optional) ◆ compound benzoin tincture or other skin protectant (optional)

### Equipment preparation
■ Assemble all equipment.
■ Check the expiration date on each sterile package and inspect for tears.
■ Open the waterproof trash bag and place it near the patient, forming a cuff by turning down the top of the bag.

## Procedure

■ Explain the procedure to the patient, and address any questions or concerns he may have.
■ Verify that the patient isn't allergic to latex and iodine.
■ Position the patient so that he's comfortable without placing undue tension on the incision line. Because some patients experience nausea or dizziness during the procedure, have the patient recline if possible.
■ Adjust the light so that it shines directly on the suture line.
■ Wash your hands thoroughly.
■ If the patient's wound has a dressing, put on gloves to remove and discard the dressing and gloves.
■ Observe the wound for gaping,

drainage, inflammation, signs of infection, and embedded staples. Absence of a healing ridge under the suture line 5 to 7 days after insertion indicates that the line needs continued support and protection during healing. Either postpone suture removal for up to 3 days or consider the use of adhesive butterfly strips.

■ Establish a sterile work area with all the equipment and supplies you'll need for staple removal and wound care. Open the supplies and put on sterile gloves.

■ Wipe the incision gently with sterile gauze pads soaked in an antiseptic cleaning agent or with sterile cotton-tipped applicators to remove surface encrustations.

■ Pick up the sterile staple or clip extractor. Then, starting at one end of the incision, remove the first staple or clip. Dislodge an embedded staple by gently rocking it from side to side.

■ Hold the extractor over the trash bag and release it to discard the staple or clip.

■ Repeat the procedure for each staple or clip until all are removed. (See *Removing staples*.)

■ Apply a sterile gauze dressing, if applicable, to prevent infection or provide comfort and protection from rubbing. Discard gloves.

■ Make sure that the patient is comfortable.

## Postprocedure patient teaching

■ Inform the patient that he may shower in 1 to 2 days if the incision is dry and healing well.

### Removing staples

Removing a staple from a wound involves changing the shape of the staple before pulling it out of the skin. These illustrations show how to properly remove a staple using a staple extractor.

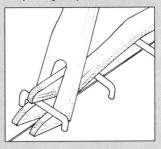

Position the extractor's lower jaws beneath the span of the first staple, as shown above. Squeeze the handles until they're completely closed.

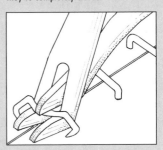

Then lift the staple away from the skin, as shown above. The extractor changes the shape of the staple and pulls the prongs out of the intradermal tissue.

■ Teach him how to remove the dressing, if applicable, and care for the wound.

■ Advise him that the redness surrounding the incision should gradually disappear and that after a few

## Using Steri-Strips or butterfly strips

Steri-Strips, shown below, are used as a primary means of keeping a wound closed after suture removal. They're made of thin strips of sterile, nonwoven, porous fabric tape.

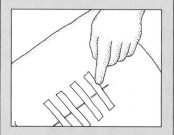

Butterfly closures, shown below, consist of sterile, waterproof adhesive strips. A narrow, nonadhesive "bridge" connects the two expanded adhesive portions. These strips are used to close small wounds and to assist healing after suture or staple removal.

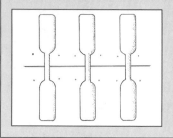

ness, swelling, pain, and warmth; cloudy yellow, green, or brown drainage; opening of wound; foul odor; a red streak from the site; or fever.

## Complications

■ Infection may be treated with local or systemic antibiotics and antiseptic soaks. It may also require consultation with a physician, a dermatologist, or an infectious disease specialist.

■ Dehiscence requires additional wound support and may require referral. If the wound dehisces during staple removal, apply butterfly adhesive strips or Steri-Strips to support and approximate the edges until the wound can be repaired. Repair depends on the extent of the dehiscence. Consult your collaborating physician as indicated. Options include using Steri-Strips alone or with an elastic bandage to relieve tension on the wound edges or monitoring the wound as it heals by secondary intention.

■ Scarring and keloids are minimized with gentle handling and the use of such techniques as undermining and layered suturing.

## Special considerations

■ If the incision appears to need additional support, consider removing only alternate staples or clips initially and leaving the others in place for 1 or 2 more days. When removing a staple or clip, place the extractor's jaws carefully

weeks only a thin line should show.

■ Inform him that Steri-Strips or butterfly strips will fall off in 3 to 5 days, frequently in the shower. Instruct him not to pull them off.

■ Urge the patient to notify you promptly if he experiences signs of infection, such as increasing red-

between the patient's skin and the staple or clip to avoid pinching the patient. Staples or clips that have been placed too deeply within the skin or left in place too long may resist removal.

■ If the wound dehisces after staples or clips are removed, apply butterfly adhesive strips or Steri-Strips to approximate and support the edges and repair the wound. (See *Using Steri-Strips or butterfly strips*.)

■ You may also apply butterfly adhesive strips if the wound is healing normally to give added support to the incision and prevent lateral tension from forming a wide scar. Use a small amount of compound benzoin tincture or other skin protectant to ensure adherence. Leave the strips in place for 3 to 5 days.

## Documentation

■ Record the date and time of staple or clip removal, the number of staples or clips removed, dressings or butterfly strips applied, signs of wound complications, and the patient's tolerance for the procedure.

■ Include a detailed description of the site before and after the procedure; any abnormalities in potentially affected function, range of motion, or sensation before the procedure; medications ordered; the time frame for follow-up evaluation; and any instructions given to the patient.

# STRAIGHT CATHETERIZATION

**CPT codes**
53670 *Simple urethra catheterization*
53675 *Complicated urethra catheterization*

## Overview

Straight urinary catheterization is used most often to obtain sterile urine specimens for laboratory testing or to aid in the diagnosis of urologic dysfunction.

Catheter insertion should be performed using sterile technique, and should be performed with extreme care to prevent injury and infection.

## Indications

■ To obtain sterile urine specimens

■ To relieve bladder distension caused by urine retention

■ To measure the volume of residual urine

■ To allow for urine drainage when the urinary meatus is swollen from child-birth, surgery, or local trauma

## Contraindications

■ Recent urologic surgery
■ Infection of the prostate gland or urethra

## Preprocedure patient preparation

■ Explain the purpose of the procedure to the patient.

■ Ask the patient when he voided last. Percuss and palpate the bladder to establish baseline data. Ask if he feels the urge to void.

■ Advise the patient that he may experience some discomfort while the catheter is inserted (pressure).

## Equipment

Sterile catheter (latex or silicone #10 to #22 French [average adult sizes are #16 to #18 French]) ◆ washcloth ◆ towel ◆ soap and water ◆ two linen-saver pads ◆ gloves ◆ sterile gloves ◆ sterile drape ◆ sterile fenestrated drape ◆ sterile cotton-tipped applicators (or cotton balls and plastic forceps) ◆ povidone-iodine or other antiseptic cleaning agent ◆ sterile urine receptacle or sterile urine-specimen collection container ◆ sterile water-soluble lubricant (Prepackaged sterile disposable kits that contain all the necessary equipment are available.)

## Procedure

■ Explain the procedure to the patient, and address any questions or concerns he may have.

■ Have a coworker hold a flashlight or place a gooseneck lamp next to the patient's bed so that you can see the urinary meatus clearly in poor lighting.

■ Wash your hands.

■ Place the female patient in the supine position, with her knees flexed and separated and her feet flat on the bed, about 2′ (61 cm) apart. If she finds this position uncomfortable, have her flex one knee and keep the other leg flat on the bed.

■ You may need an assistant to help the patient stay in position or to direct the light. Place the male patient in the supine position with his legs extended and flat on the bed. Ask the patient to hold the position to give you a clear view of the urinary meatus and to prevent contamination of the sterile field.

■ Put on gloves and use the washcloth to clean the patient's genital area and perineum thoroughly with soap and water. Dry the area with the towel. Then discard the gloves and wash your hands.

■ Place the linen-saver pads on the bed between the patient's legs and under the hips. To create the sterile field, open the prepackaged kit or equipment tray and place it between the female patient's legs or next to the male patient's hip. If the sterile gloves are the first item on the top of the tray, put them on. Place the sterile drape under the patient's hips. Then drape the patient's lower abdomen with the sterile fenestrated drape so only the genital area remains exposed. Take care not to contaminate your gloves.

■ Open the rest of the kit or tray. Put on the sterile gloves if you haven't already done so.

■ Make sure the patient isn't allergic to iodine solution; if he is allergic, another antiseptic cleaning agent must be used.

■ Open the packet of povidone-iodine or other antiseptic cleaning agent, and use it to saturate the sterile cotton balls or applicators. Be careful not to spill the solution on the equipment.

■ Open the packet of water-soluble lubricant and apply it to the catheter tip; place the other end of the catheter into the sterile urine receptacle or sterile urine-specimen container. Make sure all tubing ends remain sterile.

◆ **CLINICAL TIP**

*Some health care providers use a syringe prefilled with water-soluble lubricant and instill the lubricant directly into the male urethra, instead of on the catheter tip. This method helps prevent trauma to the urethral lining as well as possible urinary tract infection. Check your facility's policy.*

■ Before inserting the catheter, inspect it for resiliency. Rough, cracked catheters can injure the urethral mucosa during insertion, which can predispose the patient to infection.

■ For the female patient, separate the labia majora and labia minora as widely as possible with the thumb, middle, and index fingers of your nondominant hand so you have a full view of the urinary meatus. Keep the labia well separated throughout the procedure.

■ With your dominant hand, use a sterile, cotton-tipped applicator (or pick up a sterile cotton ball with the plastic forceps) and wipe one side of the urinary meatus with a single downward motion.

■ Wipe the other side with another sterile applicator or cotton ball

## Female catheter insertion

For the female patient, keep the labia well separated throughout the procedure, as shown below, to avoid obscuring the urinary meatus or contaminating the area when it's cleaned. After properly cleaning, advance the catheter 2" to 3" (5 to 7.6 cm), while continuing to hold the labia apart, until urine begins to flow.

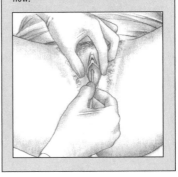

in the same way. Then wipe directly over the meatus with still another sterile applicator or cotton ball. Take care not to contaminate your sterile glove.

■ For the male patient, hold the penis with your nondominant hand. If he's uncircumcised, retract the foreskin. Then gently lift and stretch the penis to a 60- to 90-degree angle. Hold the penis this way throughout the procedure.

■ Use your dominant hand to clean the glans with a sterile cotton-tipped applicator or a sterile cotton ball held in the forceps. Clean in a circular motion, starting at the urinary meatus and working outward.

■ Repeat the procedure, using an-

## Male catheter insertion

For the male patient, hold the penis with your nondominant hand. Then gently lift and stretch the penis to a 60- to 90-degree angle. Hold the penis this way throughout the procedure to straighten the urethra and maintain a sterile field, as shown below. After properly cleaning, insert the catheter 5" to 7½" (13 to 19 cm) and check for urine flow.

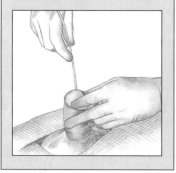

other sterile applicator or cotton ball and taking care not to contaminate your sterile glove.

■ Pick up the catheter with your dominant hand and prepare to insert the lubricated tip into the urinary meatus. To facilitate insertion by relaxing the sphincter, ask the patient to cough as you insert the catheter. Tell him to breathe deeply and slowly to further relax the sphincter and spasms. Hold the catheter close to its tip to ease insertion and control its direction.

➤ **CLINICAL TIP**
*Never force a catheter during insertion. Maneuver the catheter gently, angling it slightly toward the symphysis pubis as the patient bears down or coughs. If you still meet re-*sistance, stop the procedure. Sphincter spasms, strictures, misplacement in the vagina (in females), or an enlarged prostate (in males) may cause resistance.*

■ For the female patient, advance the catheter 2" to 3" (5 to 7.6 cm) — while continuing to hold the labia apart — until urine begins to flow. (See *Female catheter insertion,* page 427.) If the catheter is inadvertently inserted into the vagina, leave it there as a landmark. Then begin the procedure over again using new supplies.

■ For the male patient, advance the catheter 5" to 7½" (13 to 19 cm) and check for urine flow. (See *Male catheter insertion.*) If the foreskin was retracted, replace it to prevent compromised circulation and painful swelling.

■ Hold the catheter in place until urine stops flowing, then gently withdraw it from the urethra. Carefully handle the urine specimen to avoid spillage or contamination. Measure the volume of urine obtained and place the lid on securely.

■ Clean off any remaining povidone-iodine solution from the patient and pat dry with the towel. Dispose of all used supplies properly.

### Postprocedure patient teaching

■ Inform the patient of when test results (diagnostic or laboratory) will be available, and provide follow-up care, teaching, and support as necessary.

■ Instruct the patient to notify

you if he experiences any signs or symptoms of a urinary tract infection.

## Complications

- Urinary tract infection, resulting from the introduction of bacteria into the bladder, can be avoided by adhering to strict aseptic technique.
- Improper insertion can cause traumatic injury to the urethral and bladder mucosa. Insert gently with adequate lubricant, and don't force the catheter if resistance is met.
- Bladder atony or spasms can result from rapid decompression of a severely distended bladder. Observe the patient carefully for reactions caused by removing excessive volumes of residual urine.

## Special considerations

- If necessary, ask the female patient to lie on her side with her knees drawn up to her chest during the catheterization procedure. This position may be especially helpful for elderly or disabled patients such as those with severe contractures.

## Documentation

- Record the date, time, and size of catheter used. Also, describe the amount, color, and other characteristics of urine emptied from the bladder.
- If large volumes of urine have been emptied, describe the patient's tolerance for the procedure.

Note whether a urine specimen was sent for laboratory analysis.

# STRESS ECHOCARDIOGRAPHY WITH DOBUTAMINE

### CPT code
93350    *Echocardiography, transthoracic, real-time with image documentation, pharmacologically induced stress test with interpretation and report*

## Overview

Stress echocardiography with dobutamine is an imaging technique used for patients who can't exercise and for whom adenosine or dipyridamole procedures aren't appropriate. Dobutamine produces hemodynamic changes similar to those produced by exercise. This imaging technique allows assessment of myocardial wall motion abnormalities, ejection fraction, and valvular disease at rest and during exercise.

## Indications

- To assess cardiac function in patients taking drugs, such as beta-adrenergic blockers or calcium channel blockers, that would interfere with adenosine or dipyridamole testing but can't be stopped prior to testing
- To assess cardiac function in patients who can't ambulate easily (due to prosthetic limbs, obstruc-

tive lung disease, severe peripheral vascular disease, or severe peripheral neuropathy)
■ To assess the progression of coronary artery disease (CAD)
■ To assess the significance of known CAD
■ To evaluate the results of revascularization
■ To evaluate high-risk patients before surgery

## Contraindications

**ABSOLUTE**
■ Hypersensitivity to dobutamine
■ Hypertrophic cardiomyopathy
■ Uncontrolled hypertension
■ Uncontrolled atrial fibrillation
■ Malignant ventricular arrhythmia

**RELATIVE**
■ Hypovolemia (correct with volume expanders before initiating infusion)
■ Poor echogenic window because of funnel chest from emphysema or other conditions (poor visualization of the endocardium prevents accurate identification of myocardial wall motion abnormalities)
■ Recent myocardial infarction
■ Hemodynamically significant left ventricle outflow tract obstruction
■ Large aneurysm

## Preprocedure patient preparation

■ Instruct the patient not to eat for 4 hours before the procedure.
■ Tell the patient that he'll have

an I.V. line inserted into an arm vein and that he may feel his heart racing after the dobutamine infusion starts. Explain that these feelings will resolve shortly after the procedure ends (dobutamine has a half-life in plasma of about 2 minutes).

## Equipment

Echocardiography machine ◆ cardiac stress monitor (such as the Quinton 4000) ◆ electrodes ◆ cable ◆ alcohol pads ◆ clippers ◆ sphygmomanometer and blood pressure cuff ◆ emergency crash cart ◆ emergency medications ◆ infusion pump and tubing ◆ dobutamine ◆ normal saline solution ◆ 20-ml syringe ◆ peripheral I.V. access devices, tape, and gauze

### *Equipment preparation*

■ Enter complete patient information on the protocol stress-test sheet, including history, medications, current signs and symptoms, age, predicted stress time to achieve target heart rate, cardiac risk factors, and weight in kilograms.
■ Enter demographic data into the echocardiography machine and cardiac stress monitor.

## Procedure

■ Explain the procedure to the patient, and address any questions or concerns he may have.

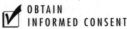 **OBTAIN INFORMED CONSENT**
■ Wash your hands.
■ Wipe the area for electrode

placement with alcohol, allow it to dry, and lightly abrade the skin with the electrode pad. If necessary, clip excess hair.

- Obtain a baseline electrocardiogram (ECG).
- Obtain resting vital signs.
- Initiate continuous monitoring with the cardiac stress monitor.
- Obtain a resting two-dimensional echocardiograph.
- Insert an I.V. catheter or heparin lock.
- Prepare the dobutamine solution with normal saline solution in a 20-ml syringe to the appropriate concentration.
- Enter the patient's weight in kilograms on the volumetric pump.
- Enter the starting dobutamine rate.
- Using the volumetric pump, begin the dobutamine infusion and increase every 3 minutes to a maximum of 40 mcg/kg/minute if the patient doesn't meet the target heart rate. (A high dose of dobutamine helps to achieve a maximal heart rate.)
- Monitor vital signs every 3 minutes.
- Assess for adverse effects, such as angina and arrhythmias.
- Obtain and record a two-dimensional echocardiogram every 3 minutes.
- If the patient doesn't reach the target heart rate, inject atropine every minute up to a maximum of 1 mg over 4 minutes. Ultrasound is performed after 1 mg of atropine is given or when the maximal heart rate is achieved.

## Postprocedure patient teaching

- Tell the patient that he should resume normal activities after the procedure.
- Advise the patient to schedule an appointment with you a couple of days after the procedure to discuss the results.

## Complications

- Reduce the rate of administration or discontinue the drug if any of the following occur: a decrease in systolic blood pressure of more than 20 mm Hg, angina, development of or increase in ventricular arrhythmia, excessive tachycardia, or ST-segment depression of 2 mm or more. If necessary, administer esmolol, an antagonist to dobutamine, to reverse symptoms.

## Special considerations

- Coronary steal — uncommon with adenosine or dipyridamole — can occur with dobutamine administration.
- Emergency equipment, such as a crash cart and emergency medications, should be readily available.
- Depending on results, referral to a cardiologist may be necessary.

## Documentation

- Before the procedure, document underlying comorbidities, medications, allergies, previous history of and risk factors for CAD, baseline ECG, presenting symptoms, physical examination results, and differential diagnoses.

■ During the procedure, document the amount of dobutamine infused, the heart rate achieved and blood pressure response, manifestation of symptoms, and any use of atropine or antagonistic medication.

■ After the procedure, document complications, ECG evaluation, diagnosis, results of the echocardiogram, and the amount of dobutamine and atropine administered, if necessary.

# STRESS TEST

### CPT codes
93015 *Cardiovascular stress test using maximal or submaximal treadmill or bicycle exercise, continuous electrocardiograph monitoring and/or pharmacological stress; with physician supervision, with interpretation and report*
93017 *Cardiovascular stress testing with continuous electrocardiograph monitoring, tracing only, without interpretation and report*
93350 *Stress echocardiography, real time with image documentation, interpretation, and report*

## Overview

Stress testing, also known as exercise electrocardiography (ECG), evaluates the heart's action during physical stress, when the demand for oxygen increases. It provides important diagnostic and prognostic information about patients with ischemic heart disease. It's also performed immediately before a stress echocardiogram.

During testing, ECG and blood pressure measurements are recorded while the patient walks on a treadmill or pedals a stationary bicycle. Each type of device has its advantages and disadvantages. (See *Comparing exercise testing devices.*)

The patient's response to a constant or increasing workload is monitored; the test continues until the patient reaches a target heart rate, as determined by an established protocol such as Borg's rate of perceived exertion, or until he experiences chest pain or fatigue. (See *Borg's rate of perceived exertion,* page 434.)

Exercise stress testing allows indirect determination of maximum oxygen uptake ($VO_2$), the greatest amount of oxygen that a person can extract from inspired air. Maximum $VO_2$ is described in terms of metabolic equivalents (METS), with 1 MET equaling 3.5 ml/kg/minute. A moderately active young man walking 2 miles per hour on level ground uses about 2 METS. The patient's maximum $VO_2$ is determined by comparing the number of METS used during exercise stress testing to normal values. Maximum $VO_2$ varies with age, body weight, heredity, gender, and conditioning.

During testing, the patient should have a gradual increase in heart rate to a maximum target rate, an increase in systolic pressure, and minimal change in diastolic pressure. After exercise stops, the patient's systolic blood pressure

# Comparing exercise testing devices

When the patient uses a treadmill or stationary bicycle, information can be gathered about the heart's action during physical stress. Each device has advantages and disadvantages, listed below.

## TREADMILL

### Advantages
■ Is standardized and provides the most reproducible results
■ Requires the patient to walk, a familiar activity
■ Maintains a constant pace of activity
■ Attains the highest maximum oxygen uptake
■ Involves commonly used muscles, decreasing the chance of fatigue

### Disadvantages
■ May result in the patient losing balance and falling off
■ Results in increased workload with increased weight
■ Makes obtaining blood pressure readings and electrocardiogram (ECG) readings more difficult because the upper body is in motion
■ Is more expensive
■ Is noisy, making communication with the patient more difficult

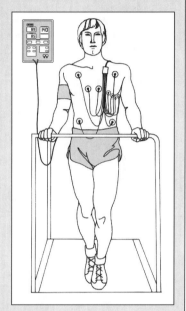

## STATIONARY BICYCLE

### Advantages
■ Doesn't result in increased workload with increased weight
■ Makes obtaining blood pressure and ECG readings easy because the upper body remains relatively still
■ Is less expensive

### Disadvantages
■ Requires a constant rate of pedaling to maintain power
■ Requires frequent calibration
■ Induces more stress
■ Attains a lower maximum oxygen uptake
■ Involves less commonly used muscles, increasing the chance of fatigue

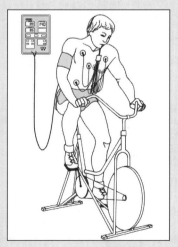

## Borg's rate of perceived exertion

Borg's rate of perceived exertion (RPE), developed by Dr. Gunnar Borg, is a scale that assigns a numeric value (ranging from 6 to 20) to subjective feelings of exercise exertion, as shown in the table below. The scale allows the patient to express his perception of fatigue based on all the factors — psychological, musculoskeletal, and environmental — that affect his sense of exertion.

For example, an RPE of 12 to 13 corresponds to about 60% to 80% of maximal

heart rate; an RPE of 16, about 90% of maximal heart rate. A patient typically meets his maximal, or target, heart rate at a level of 12 to 16.

The revised 10-grade scale rates exercise intensity on a scale of 0 to 10. It was developed to simplify terms and make the scale easier to understand.

| ORIGINAL 15-GRADE SCALE | REVISED 10-GRADE SCALE |
|---|---|
| 6 No exertion at all | 0 Nothing at all |
| 7 Extremely light | 0.5 Very, very light (just noticeable) |
| 8 | 1 Very weak |
| 9 Very light | 2 Weak (light) |
| 10 | 3 Moderate |
| 11 Light | 4 Somewhat strong |
| 12 | 5 Strong (heavy) |
| 13 Somewhat hard | 6 |
| 14 | 7 Very strong |
| 15 Hard (heavy) | 8 |
| 16 | 9 |
| 17 Very hard | 10 Extremely strong (maximal) |
| 18 | |
| 19 Extremely hard | |
| 20 Maximal exertion | |

should return to its resting value within about 6 minutes.

To administer such testing, a health care provider should be familiar with exercise protocols and have advanced cardiac life support (ACLS) certification. The test carries a mortality of approximately 1 in 10,000, and complications from the test — including prolonged chest pain, arrhythmias, and myocardial infarction (MI) — result in about 4 in 10,000 patients requiring hospital admission.

## Indications

- To aid in the diagnosis of coronary artery disease (CAD)
- To determine functional capacity in a patient with known CAD or in a patient who has had an MI, cardiac surgery, or coronary angioplasty
- To screen for asymptomatic CAD in a patient who requires a physical examination for his occupation (pilots, air traffic controllers, police officers, and fire

fighters) or who is at high risk for developing CAD

- To determine a patient's exercise tolerance before he begins an exercise regimen
- To evaluate the functional capacity of a patient with congenital or valvular heart disease
- To evaluate the functioning of a patient's rate-responsive pacemaker
- To determine the presence of exercise-induced arrhythmias in a symptomatic patient
- To evaluate the response to medical therapy of a patient with CAD or heart failure
- To evaluate blood pressure response in a patient undergoing treatment for hypertension who wishes to begin an exercise program

## Contraindications

### ABSOLUTE
- Unstable angina
- Recent acute MI (generally within previous 6 days)
- Recent significant change in resting ECG suggesting infarction or other acute cardiac event
- Third-degree atrioventricular block
- Intracardiac thrombi
- Symptomatic severe left ventricular dysfunction
- Potentially life-threatening cardiac arrhythmias
- Acute pericarditis, myocarditis, or endocarditis
- Severe aortic stenosis or suspected dissecting aortic aneurysm
- Uncontrolled hypertension
- Acute pulmonary edema or heart failure

- Pulmonary embolism
- Acute deep vein thrombosis or thrombophlebitis
- Orthopedic, musculoskeletal, neuromuscular, or arthritic conditions that interfere with or impede exercise
- Acute systemic illness
- Severe hypertrophic obstructive cardiomyopathy
- Unavailability of ACLS equipment or an individual certified to perform ACLS

## Preprocedure patient preparation

- Describe the procedure and the reason for it to the patient. Explain that he'll have ECG and blood pressure monitoring during and for a short time after the test. Tell him the entire test usually takes about 30 minutes to complete.
- Tell the patient not to eat, drink, smoke, or take any caffeine products for 3 to 12 hours (depending on your preference) before the test. Clarify which medications the patient may take before the test. Patients with diabetes should be instructed regarding food intake and medications that may be taken before the test.
- Instruct the patient to wear comfortable clothes and shoes suitable for walking and jogging.
- As appropriate, teach the patient how to use the treadmill. To obtain more accurate results, show him how to stay erect and close to the front of the treadmill with his hands resting lightly on the handrail.

- Tell the patient to report symptoms — such as chest, arm, or jaw pain; leg cramping; shortness of breath; dizziness; light-headedness; or fatigue — that he may experience during the test.

## Equipment

Treadmill with adjustable speed and grade or bicycle ergometer with adjustable resistance and pedal frequency ◆ cardiac stress monitor with 12-lead ECG recorder and continuous tracing capability (such as the Quinton 4000) ◆ electrodes and cables ◆ sphygmomanometer and stethoscope ◆ emergency equipment (including a defibrillator, oxygen, handheld oxygen resuscitation bag, intubation equipment, suction equipment and catheters, and emergency drug kit with those drugs recommended by ACLS protocols)

### Equipment preparation

- Enter complete information on the protocol stress-test sheet, including history, medications, current signs and symptoms, age, predicted time exercising to achieve target heart rate, and cardiac risk factors.
- Enter demographic data into the machine.

## Procedure

- Explain the procedure to the patient, including using the treadmill (if applicable) and Borg's rate of perceived exertion.

### ✔ OBTAIN INFORMED CONSENT

- Assess the patient for the appropriate testing protocol (treadmill, bicycle, or arm ergometry). If you use the treadmill protocol, make sure it's consistent with the patient's physical capacity and the purpose of the test. Treadmill testing typically uses the Bruce protocol. (See *The Bruce protocol.*) If the patient would better tolerate it, you can use a modified Bruce protocol with a more gradual workload progression.
- Have the assistant prepare the patient, and connect the exercise 12-lead ECG cables.
- If the patient is also having a stress echocardiogram, obtain a resting two-dimensional echocardiogram. (See *Stress echocardiography,* page 438.)
- Obtain a baseline blood pressure, heart rate, and 12-lead ECG tracing with the patient in supine and standing positions.
- Begin the exercise testing.
- Encourage the patient to continue with the testing as long as possible.
- Record a 12-lead ECG and blood pressure at the end of each stage of the testing (every 3 minutes), at any indication of a complication, whenever the ECG monitor shows an abnormality, immediately upon ending the testing, and every minute for the first 4 to 10 minutes after exercise stops.
- Continuously monitor the patient's ECG, vital signs, signs and symptoms, and heart rate. Tell the

patient to report any symptoms and to let you know when he feels he needs to stop the test. If indicated, stop the test early. (See *Indications for stopping stress testing,* page 439.) Otherwise, end the test when the patient reaches the target heart rate or completes the protocol. Rather than abruptly stopping the exercise, allow the patient to walk for approximately 1 minute to allow his heart rate to decrease gradually.

■ If the patient is also undergoing echocardiography, ask him to return immediately to the imaging table for a two-dimensional echocardiogram. These images must be obtained within seconds of stopping the treadmill, so the patient can have no cooling-off period.

■ Monitor the patient's blood pressure and heart rate, and note any symptoms he may experience during recovery. Continue monitoring until all symptoms disappear, the ECG returns to baseline, or for 4 minutes after ending the testing phase.

## Postprocedure patient teaching

■ Tell the patient he can resume normal activities after the resolution of any unusual feelings, which should occur within a few minutes after the test ends.

■ Clarify for the patient medication instructions as appropriate

■ Advise the patient to schedule an appointment with you a couple of days after the procedure to discuss the results.

## The Bruce protocol

The Bruce protocol is the most commonly used treadmill protocol for adults. The patient progresses in 3-minute stages from a slow walk at a 10% grade to a slow run at a 16% to 20% grade. The health care provider administering the test takes the patient's heart rate, blood pressure, and electrocardiogram (ECG) readings at the end of each stage and throughout the 4- to 10-minute recovery period.

Before the procedure begins but after monitoring starts, the patient hyperventilates to allow the health care provider to assess the effect of body movement on ECG readings.

| STAGE | SPEED (KM/HOUR) | GRADE (%) |
|-------|-----------------|-----------|
| 1 | 2.7 | 10 |
| 2 | 4 | 12 |
| 3 | 5.4 | 14 |
| 4 | 6.7 | 16 |
| 5 | 8 | 18 |
| 6 | 8.8 | 20 |
| 7 | 9.6 | 22 |

## Complications

■ Chest pain or signs of distress, such as dizziness, headache, nausea, and dyspnea, require monitoring and possible admission for inpatient monitoring and treatment.

# Stress echocardiography

Stress echocardiography is an imaging technique that allows detection of resting and ischemia-induced wall motion abnormalities, ejection fraction, and valvular disease. It's comparable in sensitivity to stress thallium and sestambi nuclear studies. The patient either exercises or receives a pharmacologic agent to reach the target heart rate and then undergoes imaging. If the patient has severe coronary artery disease, pharmacologic stress echocardiography may be safer because it allows careful titration of the amount of stress.

Stress echocardiography is especially useful in patients with an intermediate or high likelihood of cardiovascular disease; resting ECG abnormalities, such as digitalis effect, severe left ventricular hypertrophy with strain, left bundle-branch block, or Wolff-Parkinson-White syndrome; cardiomyopathy; previous coronary artery bypass surgery or myocardial infarction; or electrolyte abnormalities.

In women, stress echocardiography is preferred because it offers much higher specificity than graded exercise stress testing. It's believed that the similar chemical structures of digoxin and estrogen result in the high false-positive rate in graded stress testing.

## INDICATIONS
- To determine exercise-induced abnormalities in left ventricular wall motion
- To differentiate viable from nonviable myocardial tissue

## CONTRAINDICATIONS
### Absolute
- Acute MI
- Unstable angina pectoris
- Uncontrolled ventricular arrhythmias
- Symptomatic severe aortic stenosis
- Known or suspected dissecting aneurysm

- Active or suspected myocarditis
- Thrombophlebitis
- Acute systemic or pulmonary embolism
- Active infection
- Acute pericarditis
- Decompensated heart failure
- Resting diastolic blood pressure over 120 mm Hg
- Severe arthritis or other orthopedic condition that prevents the patient from positioning his arms above his head

### Relative
- Aortic stenosis
- Suspected left main coronary artery narrowing
- Idiopathic hypertrophic subaortic stenosis
- Compensated heart failure
- Severe ST-segment depression at rest
- Hypertension (systolic blood pressure greater than 200 mm Hg or diastolic blood pressure over 110 mm Hg or both)
- Poor echogenic window because of funnel chest from emphysema or other condition (poor visualization of the endocardium prevents accurate identification of myocardial wall motion abnormalities)
- Diffuse cardiomyopathy associated with left bundle-branch block

## PROCEDURE
- Have the patient follow the same steps as he would for stress testing, but tell him not to eat for 4 hours before the procedure, and tell him not to take any beta-adrenergic blockers unless otherwise directed by the cardiologist.
- Before beginning the procedure, show the patient the ECG machine and demonstrate how to dismount from the treadmill and get on the table for the echocardiogram. Emphasize that the patient should move to the table as quickly as possible.

■ Arrhythmias require monitoring. For lethal arrhythmias, initiate ACLS protocols.

## Special considerations

■ Current guidelines for periodic screening (per the U.S. Preventive Services Task Force) don't recommend routine stress testing as a screening tool for the general public.

■ Performing stress testing on patients with known cardiac disease or cardiac risk factors increases the sensitivity of the test as well as the likelihood of complications during testing.

■ A patient who feels anxious about the test may have an initial overreaction of heart rate and systolic blood pressure, but this should stabilize after 1 to 2 minutes.

■ Patients taking digoxin and those with certain conditions, such as left ventricular hypertrophy or left bundle-branch block, are also required to undergo nuclear imaging.

■ Patients being evaluated for effort–chest pain syndromes may not need to stop their cardiac medications (including drugs such as beta blockers) because the cardiac symptoms (such as breathlessness and epigastric or chest discomfort) are predictably occurring during effort while they're taking their medications. As long as the angina presents, the test can determine if it has ischemic or flow-related etiology.

■ Stress testing shows changes that occur with increased myocardial

---

## Indications for stopping stress testing

You would normally end exercise stress testing when the patient reaches the target heart rate or completes the protocol. However, consider ending the test early if the patient develops:
■ increasing chest pain
■ fatigue, shortness of breath, wheezing, leg cramps, or worsening intermittent claudication
■ a hypertensive response with systolic blood pressure greater than 240 mm Hg or diastolic blood pressure greater than 120 mm Hg
■ problematic ST-segment changes or increasing QRS changes, QT prolongation, or abnormal beats
■ bundle-branch block that isn't distinguishable from ventricular tachycardia.

You must end the test early for:
■ systolic blood pressure that drops below resting values during the exercise portion of the test
■ appearance of or worsening chest pain
■ light-headedness, dizziness, presyncope, or syncope
■ signs of poor perfusion, such as pallor and cyanosis
■ signs of severe intolerance to the workload, such as dyspnea and hyperventilation
■ serious arrhythmias
■ electrocardiogram (ECG) readings that show ST-segment depression of more than 3 mm or ST-segment elevation of more than 2 mm
■ patient's request to stop
■ technical difficulties in monitoring ECG activity or blood pressure
■ progressive, reproducible increase in systolic blood pressure.

---

vasospasm, ST changes, pulsus alternans, T-wave inversion, early onset of myocardial ischemia (onset in under 3 minutes), prolonged duration of ischemic changes during the recovery phase, and hypotension associated with the ischemic changes.

■ Imaging tests, such as echocardiography and nuclear imaging, depict ischemia and cardiac defects (such as which vessels are involved). Angiography detects coronary artery changes but doesn't detect ischemia.

■ A patient with an effort–chest pain syndrome may have a negative angiogram but a positive stress test. This combination of results reveals ischemic effects without large vessel disease and is frequently associated with Syndrome X. Though unresponsive to nitrates, this type of angina may respond favorably to angiotensin-converting enzyme inhibitors as well as aggressive reduction of coronary risk factors.

■ Emergency equipment and medications should be readily available.

■ Depending on results, referral to a cardiologist may be necessary.

## Documentation

■ Document the indications for exercise stress testing, what medications the patient is presently taking, and medications the patient was told to avoid or take before the test.

■ Before the test, record baseline vital signs (including blood pressure and heart and respiratory rates), cardiac and pulmonary assessment, and a baseline 12-lead ECG.

■ Describe the protocol and exercise mode used for testing.

■ Maintain a log of blood pressures, heart rates, ECG tracings, and symptoms that the patient experienced during the different phases of the exercise stress test.

■ Note the length of time the patient tolerated the test, stage of the stress test the patient achieved, peak heart rate, and reason for stopping the test.

■ Document the occurrence of any absolute or relative symptoms or conditions that require the test to be aborted, the time they occurred, the treatment or management of these symptoms, and the patient's response.

■ List any medications administered during and after the test.

■ Note the patient's condition at the end of the test.

■ Record the patient's vital signs and 12-lead ECG tracing at the end of the stress test, results of testing, and recommendations made to the patient.

## *S*TRESS TEST WITH ADENOSINE

### CPT codes

78460  *Myocardial perfusion imaging; (planar) single study, at rest or stress (exercise or pharmacologic), with or without quantification*

78461  *Myocardial perfusion imaging; multiple studies, at rest or stress (exercise or pharmacologic) and redistribution or rest injection, with or without quantification*

## Overview

A two-part imaging procedure, adenosine stress testing uses adenosine, radioactive tracers, and a camera connected to a computer to produce pictures of heart muscle perfusion. The adenosine infusion causes vasodilation, decreasing coronary vascular resistance and increasing blood flow to three to four times the normal rate (compared with exercise, which increases blood flow to twice the normal rate). The nuclear imaging reveals areas of hypoperfusion distal to the lesion in stenosed arteries. These regional disparities in blood flow that result from coronary stenosis are called perfusion defects.

## Indications

■ To evaluate patients who have a limited (if any) ability to exercise (qualifying conditions include disabling arthritis, severe peripheral vascular disease, severe peripheral neuropathy, a prosthetic limb, systemic muscular disease, aortic aneurysm, aortic stenosis, severe hypertension, or left bundle-branch block) for the following:
– atypical cardiac symptoms
– the significance of known coronary artery disease (CAD)
– the progression of CAD
– the likely outcome (if the patient is symptomatic)
– the results of surgical revascularization

– before major surgery (if the patient is at a high risk for impaired cardiac perfusion).

## Contraindications

### ABSOLUTE

■ Second-degree or third-degree heart block, except in patients with a functioning atrial pacemaker (adenosine can induce first-degree and second-degree atrioventricular block)
■ Sinus node disease, except in patients with a functioning atrioventricular pacemaker
■ Known or suspected bronchoconstrictive or bronchospastic lung disease (adenosine may induce bronchospasm)
■ Hypersensitivity to adenosine
■ Systolic blood pressure lower than 90 mm Hg

### RELATIVE

■ Recent myocardial infarction (caution required)
■ Unstable angina (caution required)
■ Resting hypotension
■ History of asthma

## Preprocedure patient preparation

■ Before the day of testing, tell the patient to take nothing by mouth for 4 hours before testing, to discontinue nitrates 12 hours before testing, to avoid caffeine for at least 48 hours before testing (caffeine has properties similar to aminophylline), and to discontinue dipyridamole 48 hours before testing.

■ Before the procedure, inform the patient that he'll have an I.V. line inserted in his arm and undergo continuous cardiac monitoring during the infusion of adenosine. Tell him the effects of the medication will last only a few seconds. After the adenosine has been infusing for 3 minutes, the radioisotope will be injected. After the infusion, he'll need to wait for 35 to 40 minutes and then undergo the first scan. For the second part of the procedure (which may take place on the following day, depending on the facility), the patient will have a radioisotope injected and wait about 45 minutes for the tracer to circulate. Then he'll undergo a scan of the tracer.

■ Inform the patient that the radioactive exposure received from the procedure is about the same as the average background radiation exposure received in 8 years, or less than half the annual radiation exposure allowed for X-ray and nuclear medicine technologists.

# Equipment

Cardiac stress monitor (such as the Quinton 4000) ◆ gamma camera ◆ sphygmomanometer and blood pressure cuff ◆ cable and electrodes ◆ alcohol pads ◆ clippers (if needed) ◆ emergency crash cart with defibrillator, emergency medications, airway, handheld resuscitation bag, oxygen, and suction equipment ◆ aminophylline (direct antagonist to adenosine) ◆ peripheral I.V. access supplies ◆ volumetric infusion pump and tubing ◆ adenosine and dose calibrator ◆ radioisotope

### Equipment preparation

■ Enter complete information on the stress-test sheet, including history, medications, current signs and symptoms, age, predicted test time to achieve target heart rate, stress time, and cardiac risk factors.

■ Enter demographic data into the machine.

# Procedure

■ Explain the procedure to the patient, and address any questions or concerns he may have.

### ✓ OBTAIN INFORMED CONSENT

■ Before the procedure, verify that the patient has had nothing by mouth for the past 4 hours and has refrained from medications as directed.

■ Wipe the skin with alcohol, abrade it lightly by scraping skin with the electrode, and apply the electrodes. If necessary, clip excess hair.

■ Obtain a baseline electrocardiogram (ECG) and resting vital signs.

■ Initiate continuous cardiac monitoring.

■ Insert an I.V. line into the patient's arm.

■ Instruct the nuclear technologist to start the infusion. (The nuclear technologist calculates the dose of adenosine per kilogram of body weight and prepares the volumetric pump for infusion.)

- Once the infusion has started, record vital signs every minute.
- Monitor the patient's ECG rhythm, blood pressure, heart rate, and symptoms. If necessary, stop the test early. (See *Indications for decreasing or stopping adenosine infusion*.)
- After waiting 3 minutes to ensure the patient doesn't receive a bolus dose, the nuclear technologist slowly injects the radioisotope (such as thallium) without stopping the adenosine infusion.
- The patient undergoes nuclear imaging 30 to 45 minutes after injection of the radioisotope.
- The next day, the patient undergoes the second part of the procedure. The nuclear technologist injects the radioisotope into a peripheral vein, and the patient undergoes nuclear imaging about 45 minutes later.

## Postprocedure patient teaching

- Clarify for the patient medication instructions as appropriate
- Advise the patient to schedule an appointment with you a couple of days after the procedure to discuss the results.

## Complications

- Chest pain, ST-segment depression, atrioventricular heart block, dizziness, headache, nausea, flushing, dyspnea, and hypotension are adverse effects of medication and require monitoring.
- Arrhythmias require monitoring

---

### Indications for decreasing or stopping adenosine infusion

Certain signs and symptoms call for you to decrease or stop the adenosine infusion.
- Chest pain: Decrease the infusion rate.
- ST-segment depression of 2 mm or more with angina: Stop the infusion and administer sublingual nitroglycerin.
- Atrioventricular heart block, dizziness, or headache accompanied by hypotension or worsening nausea or dyspnea: Decrease the infusion rate. If the adverse effect worsens, stop the infusion but complete the imaging.

---

and treatment as indicated by the rhythm.

## Special considerations

- Preliminary results may be available within 2 hours after completion of the test.
- Severe ischemia may cause a persistent defect up to 4 hours after the test is completed.
- Delayed images at 6 to 24 hours may reveal the reversible pattern of ischemia.
- Thallium imaging can't differentiate scarring from acute infarction, therefore it can't reveal the age of a persistent defect. For further information regarding a defect, a technetium scan or cardiac catheterization should be considered.
- Emergency equipment and medications should be readily available.
- Referral to a cardiologist may be necessary if the test is abnormal.

## Documentation

■ Before the procedure, document underlying comorbidities, medications, allergies, risk factors for CAD, baseline ECG, presenting symptoms, physical examination results, and differential diagnoses.

■ During the procedure, document the amount of adenosine infused, heart rate achieved and blood pressure response, manifestation of symptoms, any use of antagonistic medication, and ECG changes.

■ After the procedure, document blood pressure and heart rate response, ECG interpretation, arrhythmias, heart block, tolerance to the procedure, complications, dissipation of symptoms, diagnosis, and results of the nuclear scan. Normal findings are homogenous distribution of isotope throughout all segments of the left ventricle, with no transient or fixed regional perfusion defects.

# STRESS TEST WITH THALLIUM

### CPT codes

78464   *Myocardial perfusion imaging tomographic (SPECT), single study*
78465   *Myocardial perfusion imaging tomographic (SPECT), multiple studies*

## Overview

This procedure uses nuclear scanning to assess ischemic heart disease and myocardial perfusion. It differentiates areas of infarction from areas of ischemia in the ventricle and is useful in evaluating the health and function of the myocardium. The procedure works by distributing the nuclear agent thallium or radioactive technetium 99m to the myocardial cells in proportion to the blood supply they receive. Nuclear scanning then reveals myocardial perfusion by displaying the radioisotopes attached to cell proteins.

## Indications

■ To help diagnose ischemic heart disease in asymptomatic or symptomatic patients

■ To assess the efficacy of various medical and surgical procedures and therapies

■ To further evaluate cardiac perfusion in a patient whose resting electrocardiogram (ECG) exhibits paced rhythm or who has left bundle-branch block, digoxin effect, severe left hypertrophy with strain, or baseline ST-T wave abnormalities

■ To determine risk in a patient with known coronary artery disease

## Contraindications

**ABSOLUTE**

■ Pregnancy
■ Acute myocardial infarction (MI)

- Unstable angina pectoris
- Uncontrolled ventricular arrhythmia
- Symptomatic severe aortic stenosis
- Suspected or known dissecting aneurysm
- Active or suspected myocarditis
- Thrombophlebitis
- Active infection
- Acute pericarditis
- Decompensated heart failure
- Resting diastolic blood pressure higher than 120 mm Hg
- Weight of more than 325 lb (147.4 kg) (weight limit depends on the camera or table being used and should be checked before scheduling the procedure)
- Severe arthritis or other orthopedic condition that prevents the patient from positioning his arms above his head
- Extreme claustrophobia
- Hypersensitivity to thallium

**RELATIVE**
- Left main coronary stenosis (caution required)
- Moderate to severe stenotic valvular heart disease (caution required)
- Electrolyte abnormalities
- Severe arterial hypertension (systolic blood pressure above 200 mm Hg or diastolic blood pressure above 110 mm Hg or both)
- Tachyarrhythmias or bradyarrhythmias
- Hypertrophic cardiomyopathy and other forms of outflow obstruction
- Mental or physical impairment

that leads to inability to exercise adequately
- High-degree atrioventricular block

## Preprocedure patient preparation

- Tell the patient that the whole procedure takes 2 days. On the first day, he'll undergo the stress portion of the procedure, in which he'll ambulate on the treadmill before injection of the radioisotope. After the injection, he'll wait 20 minutes and undergo nuclear imaging. On the second day, he'll receive the injection while resting, wait 45 minutes for the isotope to circulate, and then undergo imaging.
- Instruct the patient to discontinue beta-adrenergic blocking and calcium channel blocking agents 48 hours before the procedure so that they don't interfere with reaching the target heart rate. Tell him to take nothing by mouth after midnight the night before the test (with the exception of patients with diabetes, who may need to fast for only 4 hours before the test and may have juice if needed).
- Tell the patient to wear comfortable, loose-fitting clothing, along with sneakers or rubber-soled walking shoes.
- Tell the patient you'll need to weigh him before scheduling the procedure.
- Explain to the patient that he'll have to ambulate for at least 1 minute after injection of the radioisotope; this means that 1 minute before he reaches peak ex-

ercise or fatigue, he'll need to inform the test supervisor or nuclear technologist so that he can receive the injection. Indications include angina; feeling dizzy, fatigued, or short of breath; or leg cramps.

## Equipment

Cardiac stress monitor (such as the Quinton 4000) ◆ treadmill ◆ sphygmomanometer and blood pressure cuff ◆ electrodes ◆ alcohol pads ◆ clippers (optional) ◆ peripheral I.V. supplies ◆ thallium supplies ◆ emergency cart

### Equipment preparation

■ Enter complete information on the stress-test sheet, including history, medications, current signs and symptoms, age, predicted time to achieve the target heart rate, and cardiac risk factors.

■ Enter demographic data into the machine.

## Procedure

■ Explain the procedure to the patient, including Borg's rate of perceived exertion. (See *Borg's rate of perceived exertion,* page 434.)

☑ OBTAIN
INFORMED CONSENT

■ If the patient is a woman under age 50, also have her sign the pregnancy release form.

■ Wipe the chest area with alcohol and abrade the skin lightly with the electrode. Clip excess hair if necessary.

■ Apply the electrodes, and obtain a baseline ECG and blood pressure.

■ With the patient lying down, ask him to hyperventilate for 30 seconds and record a second ECG.

■ Set the cardiac monitor to leads II, $V_1$, and $V_5$.

■ Program the standard Bruce protocol (you can use an accelerated or modified protocol, depending on the patient's needs).

■ Demonstrate how to use the treadmill.

■ The nuclear technologist will insert an I.V. line into a peripheral vein.

■ Instruct the patient to tell you about dizziness, leg cramping, chest pain, dyspnea, or other symptoms that occur during the test, and instruct the patient to begin walking on the treadmill.

■ Record the patient's blood pressure every 2 minutes or if symptoms occur.

■ Instruct the nuclear technologist to inject the isotope when the patient reaches the target heart rate.

■ Instruct the patient to ambulate for 1 minute after the injection.

■ After the procedure, monitor the patient's blood pressure, rhythm, and heart rate for 4 minutes or until the ECG readings return to baseline.

■ Have the patient wait 20 minutes and then lie under the nuclear camera so that the technologist can take the perfusion images.

■ The following day, the patient will receive an injection of the radioisotope while he is at rest, wait about 45 minutes, and then undergo nuclear imaging again.

## Postprocedure patient teaching

■ Instruct the patient to resume normal activities after the procedure.

■ Advise the patient to schedule a follow-up appointment with you to discuss results.

## Complications

■ Mild headache and chest discomfort may be experienced but can be relieved with aminophylline.

■ MI or signs of cardiac distress may require inpatient evaluation and treatment.

■ Arrhythmias are treated as indicated by the rhythm.

## Special considerations

■ If necessary, modify the stress portion of the test by adjusting the Bruce protocol to meet the patient's needs.

■ Keep in mind that, if necessary, the injection of the radioisotope can be made within 10% of the target heart rate.

■ Absolute indications for terminating the exercise portion of the test include:
– patient request to stop
– failure of monitoring system
– moderate to severe angina
– increasing nervous symptoms (ataxia, dizziness, or near syncope)
– drop in systolic blood pressure of more than 10 mm Hg from baseline despite an increase in workload, when accompanied by other evidence of ischemia
– sustained ventricular tachycardia
– indications of poor perfusion, including pallor, dyspnea, and dizziness
– ST elevation (greater than 1 mm) in leads without diagnostic Q waves (other than $aV_R$ or $V_1$).

■ Relative indications for terminating the exercise portion of the test include:
– ST or QRS changes, such as excessive ST depression (greater than 2 mm of horizontal or downsloping ST-segment depression) or marked axis shift
– fatigue, shortness of breath, wheezing, or leg cramps
– development of bundle-branch block that can't be distinguished from ventricular tachycardia
– arrhythmias other than sustained ventricular tachycardia, including multifocal premature ventricular contractions (PVCs), triplets of PVCs, supraventricular tachycardia, and onset of second-degree or third-degree heart block
– drop in systolic blood pressure of more than 10 mm Hg from baseline in the absence of ischemia
– hypertensive response (systolic blood pressure greater than 250 mm Hg or diastolic blood pressure greater than 115 mm Hg or both).

■ Emergency equipment and medications should be readily available.

■ Referral to a cardiologist may be necessary depending on results.

## Documentation

■ Before the procedure, document underlying comorbidities, medications, risk factors, previous history of coronary artery disease, baseline ECG and blood pressure, presenting symptoms, physical examination results, differential diagnoses, predicted heart rate, stage, and average time to achieve target heart rate correlated with gender and age.

■ During the procedure, document Borg's rate of perceived exertion, test duration, heart rate achieved at completion of the procedure, blood pressure response (blunted, paradoxical, or hypertensive), indications for terminating the procedure, and arrhythmias.

■ After the procedure, document any arrhythmias or symptoms that occurred and the length of time for symptoms to resolve, referral to a cardiologist for an equivocal or positive test, results of the nuclear scan, and diagnosis.

# *S*UBUNGUAL HEMATOMA EVACUATION

### *CPT code*
11740   *Evacuation of subungual hematoma*

## Overview

A subungual hematoma is the accumulation of blood between the nail and the nail bed, generally secondary to trauma. The expanding collection of blood causes pain and pressure and, if not relieved, future nail deformity by compress-

ing the underlying nail matrix. The primary indication for release of a subungual hematoma is pain management.

Hematoma release may be affected either by handheld cautery or by a heated paper clip. Although both are equally effective, use of a handheld cautery is preferred when the equipment is available.

## Indications

■ To evacuate a visible, painful hematoma involving less than 50% of the nail bed

## Contraindications

**RELATIVE**

■ Crushed or fractured nail
■ Fracture of the distal phalanx without laceration of the nail bed
■ Already split nail (allows blood to evacuate)
■ Presence of tumor under the nail
■ Hematoma involving more than 50% of the nail

## Preprocedure patient preparation

■ Instruct the patient that the nail has no nerve endings and the procedure should be painless. No anesthesia is required.
■ Alert the patient to the fact that the burning nail may have an irritating or unpleasant smell.

## Equipment

Handheld battery or electric

## Subungual hematoma release

Although a cautery needle looks more professional, a heated paper clip is just as effective in subungual hematoma release. The important point is to apply just enough pressure to penetrate the nail, then immediately release and encourage drainage by lowering the extremity and wicking away blood as it appears.

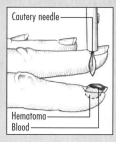
Cautery needle
Hematoma
Blood

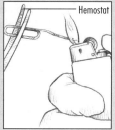
Hemostat

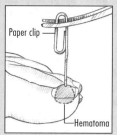
Paper clip
Hematoma

cautery unit or large needle or paper clip ◆ heat source, such as matches or a lighter ◆ hemostat to hold the hot paper clip ◆ antiseptic solution such as povidone-iodine ◆ finger splint (optional) ◆ hydrogen peroxide ◆ gloves ◆ alcohol wipes ◆ adhesive bandage ◆ eye protection (optional)

## Procedure

■ Explain the procedure and rationale to the patient, and address any questions or concerns that he has.

☑ **OBTAIN INFORMED CONSENT**

■ Wash your hands and put on gloves. Then examine the digit and assess neurovascular and neurosensory function.

■ Consider X-ray of the digit to rule out distal phalanx fracture.

■ Assess the patient's level of pain, using a pain scale.

■ Verify that the patient isn't allergic to iodine.

■ Soak the digit in antiseptic solution for 5 minutes.

■ Clean the nail with an alcohol wipe and allow to dry.

■ Heat the handheld cautery or the tip of the paper clip until it's red hot.

■ Apply firm, gentle pressure over the nail, holding the cautery or paper clip at a 90-degree angle to the nail. A hole should develop in the nail almost instantly. (See *Subungual hematoma release*.)

▸ **CLINICAL TIP**
*A glowing red tip is necessary for rapid, effective evacuation. If a hole doesn't appear in the nail plate within 2 seconds of heat application, the cautery or paper clip isn't hot enough. Reheat the tool and reapply to the nail.*

■ As soon as a hole appears in the nail, quickly withdraw the heat source and observe for fluid drainage. Sometimes a second heat application is necessary to enlarge the hole to a size sufficient for the hematoma to evacuate (1 to 2 mm).

■ Soak the digit in an antiseptic solution (approximately 50 ml povidone-iodine with 20 ml of hydrogen peroxide) for 5 to 10 minutes to complete evacuation.

■ Reassess neurovascular and neurosensory function.

■ Clean the nail with an alcohol wipe, and apply a loose dressing or adhesive bandage.

■ The digit may be splinted for 24 hours for comfort, as necessary.

## Postprocedure patient teaching

■ Tell the patient to expect almost immediate improvement in his level of pain, with continued resolution over the next 24 hours. Pain and throbbing can be relieved by acetaminophen or ibuprofen (assuming no fracture). The digit will feel normal in 2 to 3 days.

■ Tell the patient that complete healing of the nail and resolution of the remaining ecchymosis will take 5 to 7 months (the length of time for the new nail to grow out).

■ Inform him that no follow-up is necessary unless complications develop.

■ Explain that there is a possibility of nail deformity, even with new nail growth, if the nail matrix was damaged at the time of trauma.

■ Tell the patient to keep the digit elevated above the level of the heart for 24 hours after the procedure, if possible.

■ Remind the patient to soak the finger in warm salt water three times a day for the next 3 days.

■ Advise him to keep the open nail area loosely covered with an adhesive bandage.

■ Explain that small amounts of serosanguineous drainage are likely for the next 24 to 48 hours.

■ If a splint was applied, tell the patient to remove it for soaks and then to reapply it; he can use the splint for 24 to 48 hours to promote comfort.

■ Tell the patient that he may return to normal activity as tolerated.

■ Urge the patient to notify you promptly if he experiences signs and symptoms of infection, such as chills, temperature higher than 101° F (38.3° C), redness, purulent drainage, increased pain, and red streaking of the digit.

## Complications

■ Infection needs to be assessed; the patient may be placed on antibiotic therapy and soaks continued four times a day.

✤ **COLLABORATION**
*Edema resulting in vascular compromise (usually as a result of the trauma, not the subungual hematoma evacuation) requires assessment of neurosensory and neurovascular function and referral to the emergency department immediately for a surgical consultation.*

## Special considerations

■ Assess for indications of domestic, elder, or child abuse during the history and physical examination. Remember that striking the hands and nails with a blunt object or compressing the fingers or toes can cause subungual hematoma.

■ Subungual hematoma evacuation should be a painless procedure that results in immediate pain improvement for the patient. It's important that you make sure you have a very hot cautery or paper clip tip and apply enough pressure for the tip to "pop" through the nail. The release feels very similar to the "pop" of going through a vein wall for venipuncture or I.V. insertion. Beware of a fountain of blood when the nail is penetrated and the hematoma is large. If this is a possibility, wear eye protection.

■ A subungual hematoma involving more than 50% of the nail may indicate a laceration of the underlying nail bed. Some experts recommend leaving the nail in place to act as a splint; others recommend total nail removal to effect laceration repair. In either case, the patient should be informed that without nail bed examination and possible laceration repair, there may be future nail deformity.

## Documentation

■ Before performing this procedure, document any abnormal physical findings on the consent form. Have the patient initial the comments and sign the form to signify acknowledgment of preprocedural abnormalities. In the chart, the preprocedural and postprocedural notes must include an evaluation of potentially affected function, range of motion, sensation, and evaluation for further injury.

■ This patient must be assessed for domestic, elder, or child abuse, and you must document notification of appropriate authorities for any suspicion of child or elder abuse. This notification is mandatory. However, you can't report domestic violence without the patient's consent.

■ Include in your notes that options and risks associated with the procedure were discussed at length and that the patient agreed that the procedure should be done.

■ Relate the cause of injury, the type of X-rays and results as indicated, the type of heat source used, the size and resultant release of the hematoma, the quantity of blood evacuated, and improvement in the patient's level of pain (using a pain scale).

■ Record the patient's understanding of all patient teaching.

## SUPRAPUBIC BLADDER ASPIRATION

### CPT code
51000  *Aspiration of bladder by needle*

### Overview
The objective of this procedure is to obtain a sterile urine specimen

from an infant (neonate) or young child (up to age 2). Until age 2, the bladder is located in the abdomen, and as the child reaches age 2, the bladder is much lower in the pelvis and thus more difficult to penetrate with this approach.

This procedure is indicated in neonates and young children who present with vague yet worrisome symptomatology where there is concern of urinary tract infection or to rule out sepsis. Infants and young children don't tend to localize infection well and their ability to verbally tell the health care provider how they feel is limited. In addition, individuals in this age group don't tend to have well-developed immune systems and thus are at increased risk for urinary tract infections and subsequent bacteremias.

## Indications

- To obtain urine from infants who can't void on command
- To collect urine from infants who are severely ill and need definitive diagnosis immediately
- To obtain urine from children who have had several urine specimens that equivocally show bacturia

## Contraindications

### ABSOLUTE

- Infants with skin infections, especially located at or near the site of the needle insertion point

### RELATIVE

- Infants and young children with a history of a bleeding abnormality, an abnormal coagulopathy, or leukopenia.
- Infants or young children with known genitourinary or abdominal tract abnormalities, such as ileus, peritonitis, necrotizing enterocolitis, or obstruction

## Preprocedure patient preparation

- Explain to the parents or caregivers the steps in the procedure for obtaining a sterile urine specimen. Discuss the need to make a definitive diagnosis so that the child can be treated appropriately and quickly.
- Be sure to check the child's record for any history of allergy to iodine products prior to using these products.

## Equipment

EMLA cream anesthetic (eutectic mixture of lidocaine 2.5% and prilocaine 2.5% in an emulsion) ◆ 4″ × 4″ transparent dressing (such as Tegaderm) ◆ povidone-iodine solution ◆ 70% rubbing alcohol ◆ 4 sterile 4″ × 4″ gauze pads ◆ 2 pairs of sterile gloves ◆ 3-ml sterile syringe ◆ 22G 1″ needle ◆ sterile urine container ◆ restraining board with arm and leg restraints ◆ radiant warmer, if the infant is very young ◆ 1 or 2 small sterile towels ◆ sharps container

### Equipment preparation

- Assemble all of the equipment

in the room. Place the infant under a radiant warmer to decrease loss of heat during the procedure.

## Procedure

■ Answer any questions the parents or caregivers may have.

☑ **OBTAIN INFORMED CONSENT**

■ If desired apply a liberal amount of EMLA cream just above where the needle is to be inserted. Apply the sterile transparent dressing over the creamed area. Allow area to remain untouched for at least 30 minutes. Tell the parents or caregivers that you'll perform the procedure when the area is numb in 30 minutes.

■ Place infant on the restraining board, and restrain his arms and legs, making sure that the straps are secure but not overly tight. The infant should be in the supine, frog-legged position. Make sure that the board is padded to decrease the chance of burns from the heating of the restraining board.

■ Wash and dry hands thoroughly, and put on two pairs of gloves. The first pair will be used during the percussion and prepping phase of the procedure. Inspect the skin for any irritations or sores. Place the small sterile towel across the legs and perineum of the infant or child to ensure maintenance of the sterile field during the procedure. If the umbilical cord is oozing or moist, another sterile towel should be placed over the abdomen, exposing only the lower abdomen.

■ Determine that the child hasn't voided in the last hour. The typical infant's kidneys produce 1 to 2 ml/kg/hr of urine.

■ To ensure that the infant doesn't void during the procedure, an assistant can gently apply pressure to the urethra (female) through the rectum or by gentle pressure directly to the male penis.

■ Locate the symphysis pubis. Then move your gloved hand approximately 1 to 2 cm in midline. You should feel a full bladder.

■ Moisten one 4″ × 4″ gauze pad with povidone-iodine solution and another one with the 70% alcohol solution. Using a circular motion, wipe with the povidone-iodine solution, from the most medial to approximately 2″ to 4″ on all sides from the site, cleaning the area with a gentle touch. Remember infant skin is often thin and friable. Allow the area to air dry.

■ Next take the 4″ × 4″ gauze pad that's moistened with alcohol and repeat the procedure. Allow the skin surface to dry. Remove the first pair of gloves.

■ Take the 1″ needle and attach it to the 3-ml syringe, and pull back slightly on the plunger. Using your sterile gloved hand, relocate the bladder. (See *Performing suprapubic bladder aspiration*, page 454.)

■ Hold the syringe with the needle perpendicular or slightly caudally to the bladder. Penetrate the skin at the selected site of the bladder, and begin to draw back on the plunger, using gentle, slow pressure.

■ Stop advancing the needle once the urine has begun to flow. This will decrease the possibility of

## Performing suprapubic bladder aspiration

To locate the bladder, first find the symphysis pubis. Palpate 1 to 2 cm above the symphysis pubis in midline to detect the bladder. Often there is a transverse crease at the exact location where you'll be penetrating the skin, as shown below. Take the 1″ needle and attach it to the 3-ml syringe and pull back slightly on the plunger. Using your sterile gloved hand, relocate the bladder by palpating 1 to 2 cm above the symphysis pubis in midline.

Hold the syringe with the needle perpendicular or slightly caudally to the bladder. Penetrate the skin and begin to draw back on the plunger, using gentle, slow pressure. Stop advancing the needle when the urine begins to flow.

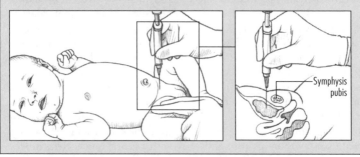

Symphysis pubis

puncturing the posterior bladder wall. In a small infant you may get only 1 to 2 ml of urine as your sample. Insert the urine in the sterile urine container.

◆ CLINICAL TIP

*If no urine appears on aspiration, withdraw the needle slightly while steadily pulling back on the plunger. If urine still doesn't appear, change the angle of the needle in the bladder by 10- to 20-degrees caudally and aspirate again.*

■ If no urine is obtained, remove the needle and wait 30 minutes or longer before repeating the procedure.

■ After removing the needle, remove the transparent dressing (if used) and cover the entry site with a sterile 4″ × 4″ gauze, and apply gentle pressure for 1 to 2 minutes.

Discard the syringe and needle in the sharps container.

■ Remove gloves and wash and dry your hands. Then remove the bindings from the restraining board, diaper the infant, and gently swaddle him in a receiving-type or small blanket.

## Postprocedure patient teaching

■ Reassure the parents or caregivers that the infant should have little pain and no limitation in activity after the procedure. They may hold the infant immediately afterwards.

■ After the procedure is completed, explain what will be done to care for the infant and treat him until the results of the culture are obtained (in 24 to 48 hours).

■ Show the parents or caregivers how to change the diaper and check the bladder area after the procedure. Tell them that they can remove the dressing with the next diaper change.

■ Instruct parents or caregivers to contact you for any signs of infection, such as fever greater than 100° F (37.8° C) or low temperature less than 96° F (35.6° C), extreme irritability, somnolence or lethargy, lack of desire to eat as usual, or bleeding at the site of the puncture.

■ Tell the parents or caregivers that they may see a slight darkening of the urine (microscopic hematuria), but this should clear within 12 to 24 hours after the procedure.

## Complications

■ Transient microscopic hematuria (resolves without treatment) can develop from the procedure.

■ Infection secondary to needle puncture may be caused by this procedure; this is minimized with good sterile technique.

■ Rare perforation of the bowel may require antibiotics or rare hematoma or damage to retroperitoneal structures may develop. Both require consultation with a specialist.

## Special considerations

■ Infants and young children do experience some pain from any needle puncture. The infant may receive liquid acetaminophen or liquid ibuprofen if able to take oral medication.

■ Infants and young children at an age indicated for this procedure are in the formative stages of developing trust. Be sure to talk to them and handle them in a kind and loving manner.

## Documentation

■ Document the indication for the procedure as well as the date and time the procedure started.

■ Record the vital signs of the infant; the preprocedure activities, such as placing on the restraining board under an infant warmer; and the actual draping, skin cleaning, and chemicals used to clean the area.

■ Record the actual procedure by noting where and how deep the needle was inserted into the abdomen. Be sure to chart how deep the needle was (approximately) when urine was obtained and any signs of bleeding that occurred at the time of the procedure.

■ Chart the appearance and quantity of urine obtained from the bladder.

■ Document the appearance of the site and the dressing application when procedure was completed. Note in charting that the infant was covered or dressed and returned to his parents or caregivers.

■ List any complications such as bleeding at the site or swelling over the area.

■ Note the time the procedure was terminated.

■ Document any patient instructions given to the parents or care-givers if child is being seen in the office and sent home afterward.

## SUTURE REMOVAL

### CPT code
*No specific code has been assigned. (Removal is included as part of suture insertion.)*

## Overview

The goal of suture removal is to remove skin sutures from a healed wound without damaging newly formed tissue. More can be learned about suture technique and final results at the time of suture removal than at the end of the original suture placement. If sutures are placed too tightly, resulting in ischemic skin margins, the detrimental results of ischemia are readily apparent at the time of suture removal. Only by seeing the wound after suture removal can a health care provider modify techniques that will influence the final result.

## Indications

■ To promote complete wound healing and minimize the occurrence of inflammation and scarring

## Contraindications

**RELATIVE**

■ Skin edges that require support

## Preprocedure patient preparation

■ Inform the patient that discomfort should be minimal unless granulation has occurred over the sutures. Assure him that redness surrounding the incision should gradually disappear, leaving only a thin line.

## Equipment

Waterproof trash bag ◆ adjustable light ◆ gloves ◆ sterile forceps or hemostat ◆ normal saline solution ◆ sterile gauze pads ◆ antiseptic cleaning agent ◆ sterile curve-tipped suture scissors ◆ povidone-iodine pads ◆ adhesive butterfly strips or Steri-Strips (optional) ◆ compound benzoin tincture or other skin protectant (optional) ◆ prepackaged, sterile suture-removal trays (optional) ◆ hydrogen peroxide or sterile water (optional) ◆ cotton-tipped applicators

### Equipment preparation

■ Assemble all the equipment.
■ Check the expiration date on each sterile package and inspect for tears.
■ Open the waterproof trash bag, and place it near the patient. Form a cuff by turning down the top of the trash bag.

## Procedure

■ Obtain a detailed history, and conduct a physical examination as indicated.
■ Verify that the patient isn't allergic to adhesive tape and povidone-

iodine or other topical solutions and medications.

■ Explain the procedure to the patient, and answer any questions he has. Remind him that this procedure is typically painless but that he may feel a tickling sensation as the sutures are removed.

■ Place the patient in a comfortable position that doesn't put undue tension on the suture line. Because some patients experience nausea or dizziness during the procedure, have the patient recline, if possible.

■ Adjust the light so that it shines directly on the suture line.

■ Wash your hands thoroughly. If the patient's wound has a dressing, put on gloves and carefully remove the dressing. Discard the dressing and gloves in the waterproof trash bag.

■ Observe the wound for gaping, drainage, inflammation, signs of infection, and embedded sutures. Absence of a healing ridge under the suture line 5 to 7 days after insertion indicates that the line needs continued support and protection during healing. Either postpone suture removal for up to 3 days or consider the use of adhesive butterfly strips.

■ Establish a clean work area with all the equipment and supplies you'll need for suture removal and wound care.

■ Put on gloves.

■ Remove crusts from the wound with cotton-tipped applicators and hydrogen peroxide or sterile water. Then gently lift the suture with the forceps, cut at the edge close to the skin surface, and pull the suture across the wound to remove it. Use gentle traction to avoid breaking the suture material.

■ Remove the sutures according to the suture type. (See *Removing sutures,* page 458.)

■ After removing the sutures, wipe the incision gently with gauze pads soaked in an antiseptic cleaning agent. Rinse clean with gauze pads and normal saline solution.

■ Apply a light, sterile gauze dressing or adhesive butterfly strips, if needed (optional).

## Postprocedure patient teaching

■ Teach him how to remove the dressing (if applicable) and care for the wound.

■ Tell him that he may shower in 1 to 2 days if the incision is dry and heals well.

■ Instruct him to notify you promptly if he experiences signs and symptoms of infection, such as increasing redness, swelling, pain, and warmth; cloudy yellow, green, or brown drainage; opening of wound; foul odor; a red streak from the site; or fever.

## Complications

■ Infection may be treated with local or systemic antibiotics and antiseptic soaks. It may also require consultation with a physician, a dermatologist, or an infectious disease specialist.

■ Scarring and keloids are minimized with gentle handling and the use of such techniques as undermining and layered suturing.

# Removing sutures

For all suture types, you should grasp and cut sutures in the correct place to avoid pulling the exposed — and thus contaminated — suture material through subcutaneous tissue. The illustrations and text below demonstrate the individual techniques involved in removing four common suture types.

## SIMPLE INTERRUPTED SUTURES

Using sterile forceps, grasp the knot of the first suture and raise it off the skin. This will expose a small portion of the suture that was below skin level. Place the rounded tip of sterile curved-tip suture scissors against the skin and cut through the exposed portion of the suture. Then, still holding the knot with the forceps, pull the cut suture up and out of the skin in a smooth continuous motion to avoid causing the patient pain. Discard the suture. Repeat the process for every other suture. If the wound doesn't gape, remove the remaining sutures.

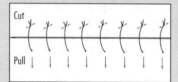

## MATTRESS INTERRUPTED SUTURES

If possible, remove the small visible portion of the suture opposite the knot by cutting it at each end and lifting the small piece away from the skin to prevent pulling it through and contaminating subcutaneous tissue. Then remove the rest of the suture by pulling it out in the direction of the knot, as shown top right. If the visible portion is too

small to cut twice, cut it once and pull the entire suture out in the opposite direction. Repeat for the remaining sutures. Monitor the incision carefully for signs of infection.

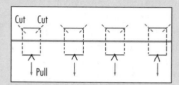

## SIMPLE CONTINUOUS SUTURES

Cut the first suture on the side opposite the knot. Next, cut the same side of the next suture in line. Lift the first suture out in the direction of the knot. Proceed along the suture line, grasping each suture where you grasped the knot on the first one.

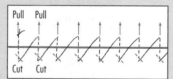

## MATTRESS CONTINUOUS SUTURES

Follow the procedure for removing mattress interrupted sutures. First remove the small visible portion of the suture, if possible, to prevent pulling it through and contaminating subcutaneous tissue. Then extract the rest of the suture in the direction of the knot.

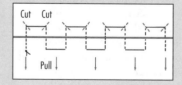

✦ COLLABORATION

*Dehiscence requires additional wound support and may require a referral. If the wound dehisces during suture removal, apply butterfly adhesive strips or Steri-Strips to support and approximate the edges until the wound can be repaired. Repair depends on the extent of the dehiscence. Consult with the collaborating physician as indicated. Options include using Steri-Strips alone or with an elastic bandage to relieve tension on the wound edges or monitoring the wound as it heals by secondary intention.*

## Special considerations

■ The blood supply and healing times vary with location, requiring that sutures be removed at different times in different locations. In general, remove face, neck, and scalp sutures in 3 to 5 days and trunk and extremity sutures in 7 to 14 days.

## Documentation

■ Document indications for and details of the procedure, including a detailed description of the site before and after the procedure, any abnormalities in function before the procedure, the patient's reaction to the procedure, medications ordered, the time frame for follow-up evaluation, and any instructions given to the patient.

# SUTURING OF SIMPLE LACERATIONS

## CPT codes

Note: *Precise code depends on wound size.*
12001 to 12007   *Simple repair of superficial wounds on the scalp, neck, axillae, external genitalia, trunk, and extremities*

12011 to 12018   *Simple repair of superficial wounds on the face, ears, eyelids, nose, lips, and mucous membranes*
12020   *Treatment of superficial wound dehiscence and simple closure*
12031 to 12037   *Intermediate repair with layered closure of wounds of the scalp, axillae, trunk, and extremities (excluding hands and feet)*
12041 to 12047   *Intermediate layered closure of wounds of the neck, hands, feet, and external genitalia*
12051 to 12057   *Intermediate repair with layered closure of wounds of face, ears, eyelids, nose, lips, and mucous membranes*

## Overview

Wounds may require the use of absorbable and nonabsorbable sutures, such as polypropylene (for example, Prolene) and nylon (for example, Monosof). Usually placed deep within a wound, absorbable sutures are absorbed into the body over time; nonabsorbable sutures are used at the wound surface and require removal. Some wounds may be closed with a skin adhesive (for example, Dermabond), which can reduce pain, shorten the time spent on wound closure, and provide a more aesthetically pleasing outcome. (See *Using a skin adhesive,* page 460.)

Suturing typically starts with a dermal layer of interrupted absorbable sutures. Such sutures are especially important in high-tension areas, where the risk of pulling apart is greatest.

## Using a skin adhesive

Many lacerations can be treated without sutures, using a skin adhesive such as Dermabond. It's quicker and less painful than suturing and may achieve better cosmetic results.

To use a skin adhesive, you must approximate the wound edges. While maintaining well-approximated closure, apply thin layers (usually three) of adhesive, with light brushstrokes of the applicator. Moisture on the skin's surface activates the adhesive. Full strength is achieved in about 2½ minutes.

Be sure to review appropriate wound care with the patient. Instruct him not to rub or scrub the wound area. Tell him to wet the site only briefly during showering and to pat it dry. If you applied a protective dressing, remind the patient not to let the tape touch the site or adhesive. Advise him to avoid prolonged sunlight and tanning lamps, particularly while the wound is fresh and the

adhesive is in place. Similarly, advise him to avoid activities or environments likely to cause heavy perspiration and to refrain from applying other medications, lotions, or creams to the site; these actions can cause premature separation of the adhesive.

Follow up with the patient to check for infection and neurovascular compromise. Urge him to contact you if the wound edges separate. Advise him that the adhesive will wear off by itself in 5 to 10 days.

Don't apply a skin adhesive if the wound involves subcutaneous approximation or if the patient has an infection, pressure sores, or hypersensitivity to cyanoacrylate or formaldehyde. Also, consider a different method if the patient has deep wounds (the adhesive can penetrate below the dermal layer), wounds involving tension areas (knuckles, elbows, and knees), or wounds of the scalp, mucosa, or periorbital area.

Nonabsorbable sutures are used on the epidermal layer; these sutures allow for improved approximation and eversion of the wound edges, producing optimal cosmetic results.

A simple interrupted suture for the epidermal layer completely closes the wound. This type of suture offers the advantages of properly everting skin edges so that the wound lies flat when it spreads, lining up unequal wound edges, and allowing for regional variations of tension. It takes longer to close a wound, however, with this suture than with a running suture.

Wounds closed by approximation of the skin edges heal by primary intention. Wounds heal

faster under an occlusive or semi-occlusive dressing, which prevents crust formation.

## Indications

■ To repair surgical and traumatic disruptions of skin or tissue that won't heal naturally

## Contraindications

**RELATIVE**
■ Clinical risk factors for poor healing
■ Dirty and infected wounds
■ Contaminated wounds
■ Malnutrition
■ Diabetes
■ Sepsis

- Chemotherapy
- Immunosuppression
- Peripheral vascular disease
- Obesity
- Radiation therapy
- Edema
- Foreign bodies
- Tension on wound edge
- Pressure over a bony prominence
- Dog and cat bites
- Human bites

## Preprocedure patient preparation

- Inform the patient that he'll feel a "pinch" as the local anesthesia is injected, but afterward pain should be minimal.

## Equipment

20- to 60-ml syringe with a 20G plastic I.V. cannula ◆ sterile saline solution ◆ antiseptic solution (such as povidone-iodine) ◆ smooth or multitooth forceps ◆ needle holder ◆ scissors ◆ scalpel, if needed ◆ sterile gloves ◆ sutures ◆ needles (round and tapered for mucosa, fascia, and muscle) ◆ injectable anesthetic (such as lidocaine) ◆ 4″ × 4″ gauze dressings ◆ nonadherent dressing ◆ antibiotic ointment ◆ tape

## Procedure

- Explain the procedure to the patient, and address his questions or concerns.

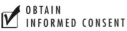
**OBTAIN INFORMED CONSENT**

- Place the patient in a comfort-able position that allows full wound visualization.

- Wash your hands and put on gloves.

- Verify that the patient isn't allergic to iodine or local anesthetics.

- Clean the wound with povidone-iodine solution in a circular pattern from the wound edges outward.

- Anesthetize the skin along each side of the wound. First on one side, and then the other, insert the needle containing the anesthetic at a 45-degree angle. Ask the patient if he notices any change in sensation. If he reports pain, indicating direct contact with the nerve, withdraw the needle 1 mm. Aspirate to make sure there is no blood return. If there is, the needle is in a blood vessel. Withdraw the needle slightly and redirect it to another area. Inject lidocaine slowly along the length of the wound as you partially withdraw the needle. Then redirect the needle across the surface, advance it, and inject while withdrawing the needle. This method distributes the anesthetic uniformly, providing the optimal effect in 5 to 15 minutes.

- Examine the wound to its base for foreign bodies or injury to underlying structures, such as a tendon or joint capsule.

- Use the syringe and I.V. cannula to irrigate the wound with antiseptic or sterile saline solution. Some health care providers recommend equal parts antiseptic and sterile saline solution to decrease tissue toxicity except for very dirty wounds.

- Trim and undermine wound

edges as needed to provide effective approximation.

■ Using your dominant hand, grasp the suture needle securely with the needle holder. Use a toothed forceps in your other hand to stabilize the wound edge in a slightly everted position.

■ Insert the needle at a right angle through the skin about ¼″ to ¾″ (0.5 to 2 cm) from the wound edge. Grasp the needle from the exterior with the needle holder. Before inserting the needle again, be sure the tissue layers are well approximated with minimal tension.

■ Repeat the process and then tie the suture, being careful not to pull the suture edges too taut.

■ Use scissors to trim jagged edges from the wound.

■ As appropriate, place a vertical mattress suture in the middle of the wound and bisect each half sequentially with vertical mattress sutures. (See *Choosing a suture technique*.)

■ After approximating skin edges, fill in the remaining gaps with simple interrupted stitches.

■ Remove redundant cones of skin (called "dog ears") to optimize the cosmetic result. Excise the residual skin by making a small ellipse that extends the defect or by making an incision that lifts the dog ear with the skin hook and drapes excess tissue over the side of the wound.

■ To help equalize tension on wound edges, make a "hockey stick" incision, an angled incision that extends one end of the wound in the shape of a hockey stick.

This incision creates a curvilinear line that allows for approximation of skin edges without placing undue tension on any specific point along the line.

■ After suturing the wound, compress the wound gently and look for residual bleeding. Use direct pressure for 5 minutes to minimize swelling and bleeding from the wound edge.

■ Cover the site with a three-layer pressure dressing by applying a thin layer of antibiotic ointment, a nonadherent dressing, and 4″ × 4″ gauze pads with tape to secure it. Apply pressure to the site. Leave this in place for 24 hours.

■ Splint if necessary.

■ Prescribe an antibiotic (such as cephalexin) if the area is infected.

■ Administer tetanus prophylaxis if the patient hasn't been immunized within the past 5 years.

## Postprocedure patient teaching

■ Instruct the patient to keep the sutures dry.

■ Tell him to remove the initial dressing in 24 hours.

■ Teach him to clean the wound site twice daily with soap and water (no rubbing or scrubbing of the wound) and to cover it with antibiotic ointment.

■ Teach him how to apply the nonadherent dressing, the 4″ × 4″ gauze pads, and the tape to form a pressure dressing.

■ Tell him to switch to a thin layer of antibiotic ointment and a smaller gauze bandage when drainage no longer appears on the

## Choosing a suture technique

The most commonly used suture techniques include the simple continuous, simple interrupted, and horizontal and vertical mattress sutures. The type of suture technique used depends on the site, shape, size, and depth of the wound.

The space left between sutures also varies, according to the wound's location or the amount of tension applied to the wound. For instance, the space between sutures in most wounds is about 0.25 cm, but you should place sutures even closer for facial wounds or those associated with high tension — for example, those on the elbow or knee.

### SIMPLE CONTINUOUS
Simple continuous sutures provide even tension across the incision and are used for quick repair.

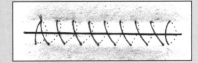

### SIMPLE INTERRUPTED
Simple interrupted sutures allow precise approximation of wound edges.

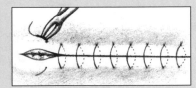

### HORIZONTAL MATTRESS
Horizontal mattress sutures reduce dead space within the wound and reinforce subcutaneous tissue.

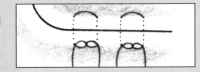

### VERTICAL MATTRESS
Vertical mattress sutures also reduce dead space within the wound and reinforce subcutaneous tissue. They're used in thick skin, such as in the palms or the soles, and in lax skin. These sutures are difficult to approximate and take more time to place.

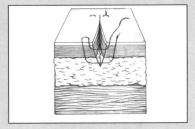

large dressing. Caution him not to place the gauze itself directly over the wound. (Fibers in the gauze can get trapped in the wound edge, become matted, and delay healing.)

■ Advise him to use over-the-counter analgesics, such as acetaminophen or ibuprofen, to manage pain.

■ Instruct him to notify you promptly if he experiences signs and symptoms of infection, such as increasing redness, swelling,

## Selecting nonabsorbable suture materials

Nonabsorbable suture materials are commonly chosen based on the type of tissue surrounding the wound site. The following chart shows which type of suture works best in each type of tissue.

| TISSUE TYPE | SUTURE MATERIAL |
|---|---|
| Skin | Nylon (Ethilon), polypropylene (Prolene), silk, or polyester fiber (Mersilene) |
| Subcutaneous tissue | Chromic gut or polyglycolic, polylactic acid (such as Dexon or Vicryl) |
| Subcuticular tissue | Nylon (Ethilon) |
| Fascia | Polyglactin 910 (coated Vicryl) or silk |
| Mucosa | Plain gut |

pain, and warmth; cloudy yellow, green, or brown drainage; opening of wound; foul odor; a red streak from wound area; or fever.

■ Have him schedule a follow-up appointment to remove the sutures and check for signs of infection or nerve damage.

## Complications

■ Infection may be treated with local or systemic antibiotics and antiseptic soaks. It may also require consultation with a physi-

cian, a dermatologist, or an infectious disease specialist.

■ Scarring and keloids are minimized with gentle handling and the use of such techniques as undermining and layered suturing.

## Special considerations

✴ COLLABORATION
*Refer the patient to a plastic surgeon for debridement or if the wound has a large amount of dead space, which may require drain placement.*

■ Lidocaine with epinephrine at a concentration of 1:100,000 may be used, except in wounds involving an appendage (such as the nose, the penis, or a digit).

■ Scalp sutures should be removed in 6 to 8 days; face sutures, in 3 to 5 days; abdomen and chest sutures, in 7 to 10 days; upper-extremity sutures, in 7 to 8 days; lower-extremity sutures, in 7 to 14 days; and back sutures, in 10 to 14 days.

■ To avoid infection, the wound should be closed within 6 hours of injury.

■ For embedded sutures, absorbable material is required because it dissolves over time. Absorption rate varies according to the material selected, based on the patient's needs: plain gut, 7 to 14 days; chromic gut, 20 to 40 days; and polyglycolic acid synthetic and polyglactin 910, 60 to 90 days.

■ For nonabsorbable sutures, selection is usually based on the suture site. (See *Selecting nonabsorbable suture materials*.)

## Documentation

- Before performing this procedure, document any abnormal physical findings on the consent form. Have the patient initial the comments and sign the form to signify acknowledgment of preprocedural abnormalities. In the chart, the preprocedural and postprocedural notes must include an evaluation of potentially affected function, range of motion, and sensation.

- Record indications for and details of the procedure. Describe the wound site before and after the procedure, any preprocedural abnormalities in function, the type and amount of anesthetic used, the patient's reaction to the procedure, medications ordered, the time frame for follow-up evaluation, and any patient instructions given.

## *SWAB SPECIMEN COLLECTION*

### *CPT code*
87070   *Culture, bacterial; any other source except urine, blood, or stool*

## Overview

Correct collection and handling of swab specimens helps the laboratory staff identify pathogens accurately with a minimum of contamination from normal bacterial flora. Collection normally involves sampling inflamed tissues and exudates from the nasopharynx, wounds, eye, ear, or rectum with sterile swabs of cotton or other absorbent material.

After the specimen has been collected, the swab is immediately placed in a sterile tube containing a transport medium and, in the case of sampling for anaerobes, an inert gas.

## Indications
- To identify pathogens
- To identify asymptomatic carriers of certain easily transmitted disease organisms

## Contraindications
**RELATIVE**
- Must be performed before initiating antibiotic therapy

## Preprocedure patient preparation

- Explain to the patient the purpose of obtaining the specimen. Emphasize the importance of obtaining a sterile specimen to encourage patient cooperation.

## Equipment
### *For a nasopharyngeal specimen*
Gloves ◆ penlight ◆ sterile, flexible cotton-tipped swab ◆ tongue blade ◆ sterile culture tube with transport medium ◆ label ◆ laboratory request form ◆ nasal speculum (optional)

### For a wound specimen

Sterile gloves ♦ sterile forceps ♦ alcohol or povidone-iodine pads ♦ sterile cotton-tipped swabs ♦ sterile 10-ml syringe ♦ sterile 21G needle ♦ sterile culture tube with transport medium (or commercial collection kit for aerobic culture) ♦ labels ♦ special anaerobic culture tube containing carbon dioxide or nitrogen ♦ fresh dressings for the wound ♦ laboratory request form ♦ rubber stopper for needle (optional)

### For an ear specimen

Gloves ♦ normal saline solution ♦ two 2″ × 2″ gauze pads ♦ sterile swabs ♦ sterile culture tube with transport medium ♦ label ♦ laboratory request form

### For an eye specimen

Sterile gloves ♦ sterile normal saline solution ♦ two 2″ × 2″ gauze pads ♦ sterile swabs ♦ sterile wire culture loop (for corneal scraping) ♦ sterile culture tube with transport medium ♦ label ♦ laboratory request form

### For a rectal specimen

Gloves ♦ soap and water ♦ washcloth ♦ sterile swab ♦ normal saline solution or sterile broth medium ♦ sterile culture tube with transport medium ♦ label ♦ laboratory request form

## Procedure

■ Explain the procedure to the patient, and address any questions or concerns he may have.

### Collecting a nasopharyngeal specimen

■ Tell the patient that he may gag or feel the urge to sneeze during the swabbing but that the procedure takes less than 1 minute.

■ Have the patient sit erect at the edge of the bed or in a chair, facing you. Then wash your hands and put on gloves.

■ Ask the patient to blow his nose to clear his nasal passages. Then check his nostrils for patency with a penlight.

■ If the nostril appears narrow, use a nasal speculum to have better access to the specimen.

■ Tell the patient to occlude one nostril first and then the other as he exhales. Listen for the more patent nostril because you'll insert the swab through it.

■ Ask the patient to cough to bring organisms to the nasopharynx for a better specimen.

■ While it's still in the package, bend the sterile cotton-tipped swab in a curve and then open the package without contaminating the swab.

■ Ask the patient to tilt his head back and gently pass the swab through the more patent nostril about 3″ to 4″ (7.5 to 10 cm) into the nasopharynx, keeping the swab near the septum and floor of the nose. Rotate the swab quickly and remove it. (See *Obtaining a nasopharyngeal specimen*.)

■ Alternatively, depress the patient's tongue with a tongue blade and pass the bent swab up behind the uvula. Rotate the swab and withdraw it.

- Remove the cap from the sterile culture tube, insert the swab, and break off the contaminated end. Then close the tube tightly.
- Remove and discard your gloves and wash your hands.
- Label the specimen for culture, complete a laboratory request form, and send the specimen to the laboratory immediately. If you're collecting a specimen to isolate a possible virus, check with the laboratory for the recommended collection technique.

### Collecting a wound specimen

- Wash your hands, prepare a sterile field, and put on sterile gloves. With sterile forceps, remove the dressing to expose the wound. Dispose of the soiled dressings properly.
- Clean the area around the wound with an alcohol or a povidone-iodine pad to reduce the risk of contaminating the specimen with skin bacteria. Then allow the area to dry.
- For an aerobic culture, use a sterile cotton-tipped swab to collect as much exudate as possible, or insert the swab deeply into the wound and gently rotate it. Remove the swab from the wound and immediately place it in the aerobic culture tube. Label the tube and send it to the laboratory immediately with a completed laboratory request form. Never collect exudate from the skin and then insert the same swab into the wound; this could contaminate the wound with skin bacteria.
- For an anaerobic culture, insert

---

### Obtaining a nasopharyngeal specimen

After you've passed the swab into the nasopharynx, quickly but gently rotate the swab to collect the specimen. Then remove the swab, taking care not to injure the nasal mucous membrane.

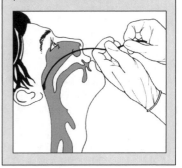

---

the sterile cotton-tipped swab deeply into the wound, rotate it gently, remove it, and immediately place it in the anaerobic culture tube. (See *Anaerobic specimen collection,* page 468.) Or insert a sterile 10-ml syringe, without a needle, into the wound, and aspirate 1 to 5 ml of exudate into the syringe. Then attach the 21G needle to the syringe, and immediately inject the aspirate into the anaerobic culture tube. If an anaerobic culture tube is unavailable, obtain a rubber stopper, attach the needle to the syringe, and gently push all the air out of the syringe by pressing on the plunger. Stick the needle tip into the rubber stopper, remove and discard your gloves, and send the syringe of aspirate to the laboratory immediately with a

## Anaerobic specimen collection

Because most anaerobes die when exposed to oxygen, they must be transported in tubes filled with carbon dioxide or nitrogen. The anaerobic specimen collector shown here includes a rubber-stoppered tube filled with carbon dioxide, a small inner tube, and a swab attached to a plastic plunger.

Before specimen collection, the small inner tube containing the swab is held in place with the rubber stopper (as shown on the left). After collecting the specimen, quickly replace the swab in the inner tube and depress the plunger to separate the inner tube from the stopper (as shown on the right), forcing it into the larger tube and exposing the specimen to a carbon dioxide–rich environment.

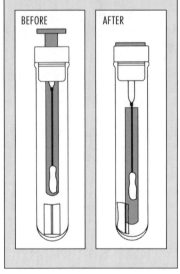

BEFORE    AFTER

completed laboratory request form.

Put on sterile gloves.

■ Apply a new dressing to the wound.

### Collecting an ear specimen

■ Wash your hands and put on gloves.
■ Gently clean excess debris from the patient's ear with normal saline solution and gauze pads.
■ Insert the sterile swab into the ear canal and rotate it gently along the walls of the canal to avoid damaging the eardrum.
■ Withdraw the swab, being careful not to touch other surfaces to avoid contaminating the specimen.
■ Place the swab in the sterile culture tube with transport medium.
■ Remove and discard your gloves and wash your hands.
■ Label the specimen for culture, complete a laboratory request form, and send the specimen to the laboratory immediately.

### Collecting an eye specimen

■ Wash your hands and put on sterile gloves.
■ Gently clean excess debris from the outside of the eye with sterile normal saline solution and gauze pads, wiping from the inner to the outer canthus.
■ Retract the lower eyelid to expose the conjunctival sac. Gently rub the sterile swab over the conjunctiva, being careful not to touch other surfaces. Hold the swab parallel to the eye, rather than pointed directly at it, to prevent corneal irritation or trauma due to sudden movement. (If a corneal scraping is required, this procedure is performed using a wire culture loop.)
■ Immediately place the swab or

wire loop in the culture tube with transport medium.
- Remove and discard your gloves and wash your hands.
- Label the specimen for culture, complete a laboratory request form, and send the specimen to the laboratory immediately.

### Collecting a rectal specimen
- Wash your hands and put on gloves.
- Clean the area around the patient's anus using a washcloth and soap and water.
- Insert the sterile swab, moistened with normal saline solution or sterile broth medium, through the anus and advance it about ⅜″ (1 cm) for infants or 1½″ (3.8 cm) for adults. While withdrawing the swab, gently rotate it against the walls of the lower rectum to sample a large area of the rectal mucosa.
- Place the swab in a culture tube with transport medium.
- Remove and discard your gloves and wash your hands.
- Label the specimen for culture, complete a laboratory request form, and send the specimen to the laboratory immediately.

## Postprocedure patient teaching

- Inform the patient of when laboratory results will be available, and provide follow-up care, teaching, and support as necessary.

## Complications
- None known

## Special considerations
- Note recent antibiotic therapy on the laboratory request form

### For a wound specimen
- Although you would normally clean the area around a wound to prevent contamination by normal skin flora, don't clean a perineal wound with alcohol because this could irritate sensitive tissues. Also, make sure that antiseptic doesn't enter the wound.

### For an eye specimen
- Don't use an antiseptic before culturing to avoid irritating the eye and inhibiting growth of organisms in the culture. If the patient is a child or an uncooperative adult, ask an assistant to restrain the patient's head to prevent eye trauma resulting from sudden movement.

## Documentation
- Record the time, date, and site of specimen collection and any recent or current antibiotic therapy. Also, note whether the specimen has an unusual appearance or odor.

## THORACENTESIS

***CPT codes***
32000  *Thoracentesis, puncture of pleural cavity for aspiration, initial or subsequent*
32002  *Thoracentesis with insertion of tube*

### Overview

In thoracentesis, a needle is inserted into the pleural space to remove abnormal fluid or air. It's done therapeutically to relieve pulmonary restriction and respiratory distress and diagnostically to help determine the etiology of pleural effusion.

### Indications

■ To assess a pleural fluid of unknown etiology
■ To provide relief from and assess a large symptomatic effusion
■ To treat a stable spontaneous pneumothorax

### Contraindications

**ABSOLUTE**
■ Bleeding dyscrasias
■ Lack of patient cooperation

**RELATIVE**
■ Anticoagulant use

### Preprocedure patient preparation

■ Explain to the patient that analgesics and sedatives provide comfort that encourages fuller chest expansion during the procedure.
■ Instruct the patient on the importance of not moving during the procedure.
■ Tell the patient to expect feelings of pressure that may elicit the need to cough. Tell him to let you know when he feels the need to cough or experiences shortness of breath so that you can momentarily stop the procedure to avoid puncturing lung tissue.
■ Tell him he should feel relief from respiratory distress after the procedure. Explain that he may cough briefly during and after the procedure but should recover shortly after the procedure. Tell

him that chest X-rays after the procedure should demonstrate less effusion or pneumothorax.

# Equipment

Prepackaged thoracentesis tray, which typically includes: povidone-iodine and isopropyl alcohol solution ♦ 1% or 2% lidocaine ♦ 5-ml syringe with 21G and 25G needles for anesthetic injection ♦ 15G (for fluid) or 18G (for air) thoracentesis needles for aspiration ♦ 50-ml syringe ♦ 3-way stopcock ♦ tubing ♦ sterile specimen containers ♦ sterile hemostat ♦ 4″ × 4″ pads

*Additional supplies*

Adhesive tape ♦ shaving supplies ♦ fenestrated drape or sterile towels ♦ sphygmomanometer ♦ stethoscope ♦ sterile gloves, gown, and mask ♦ 500- to 1,000-ml vacuum collection bottles ♦ Teflon catheter (18G for air, 15G for fluid) if not included in the kit ♦ specimen tubes, including one red-top tube, one lavender-top tube, culture tubes (aerobic and anaerobic), one green-top tube, and a 10-ml tube ♦ povidone-iodine ointment ♦ 4″ × 4″ sterile gauze pads ♦ analgesia such as fentanyl and sedative such as lorazepam (optional)

### *Equipment preparation*

■ Assemble all equipment at the patient's bedside or in the treatment area.

■ Check the expiration date on each sterile package, and inspect for tears.

■ Prepare the necessary laboratory request forms. Be sure to list current antibiotic therapy on the forms because this will be considered in analyzing the specimens.

■ Have the patient's chest X-rays available.

# Procedure

■ Explain the procedure to the patient, and address any questions or concerns he may have. Verify allergies, such as latex, iodine, and lidocaine.

☑ **OBTAIN INFORMED CONSENT**

■ Inform the patient that he'll feel some pressure and discomfort during needle insertion.

■ Assess the patient's vital signs and respiratory status before the procedure. If appropriate, administer analgesia and a sedative.

■ Confirm the location and extent of effusion or air by percussion, auscultation, and assessment of chest X-rays (posterior-anterior and lateral films). Use a lateral decubitus film to differentiate fluid effusion from consolidation. Review the film with a collaborating physician or radiologist if needed and document clinical findings.

■ Position the patient upright if possible. Typically, the patient sits leaning forward on the bed, with his feet down and his head and folded arms supported on a pillow on the overbed table. (See *Positioning the patient for thoracentesis,* page 472.)

■ If the patient can't sit, turn him onto his unaffected side, with the arm of the affected side raised over his head and his palm against the

## Positioning the patient for thoracentesis

Before you can perform thoracentesis, you need to help the patient find a position he can maintain in reasonable comfort. Typically, he'll sit on the bed and lean forward on the overbed table, as shown below.

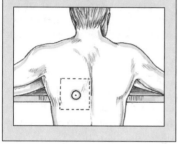

back of his head. Then elevate the head of the bed to at least 30 degrees but as close as possible to 90 degrees. (Proper positioning stretches the chest or back, allowing easier access to the intercostal spaces.) For air removal, position the patient supine at a 30- to 45-degree angle.

■ Apply oxygen for supplemental support because it's common for arterial saturation to drop transiently during and after the procedure.

■ Wash your hands, and maintain aseptic technique.

■ Select the insertion site. To remove air, choose a site at the second or third intercostal space at the midclavicular line or more laterally. To remove fluid, choose a site one to two intercostal spaces below the level of the fluid (but not below the eighth intercostal space) and 5 to 10 cm lateral to the spine.

■ Clip hair close to the site if necessary.

■ Put on sterile gloves, gown, and mask; open the thoracentesis tray; and set up the equipment. Keep the specimen containers nearby. Set up the three-way stopcock with the 50-ml syringe on one end and tubing for vacuum collection bottles on the other end. Turn the stopcock off to the vacuum collection bottle tubing.

■ Clean the skin with povidone-iodine solution, working outward in concentric circles. Allow the area to dry.

■ Drape the area with the fenestrated drape or sterile towels.

■ Draw up the 1% to 2% lidocaine into a 5-ml syringe with a large-gauge needle. Switch to the 1½" 23G or 25G skin needle, and inject a wheal of solution under the skin and deeper into the tissue on the superior edge of the rib.

**▲ CLINICAL TIP**
*Never insert a needle under the rib because the intercostal nerve bundles and blood vessels that run on the inferior rib borders could be damaged.*

■ Infiltrate the area through the wheal with a downward angle. The needle should rub against the superior edge of the rib. Alternate aspiration and injection to prevent inadvertently administering lidocaine into the circulation. Continue infiltrating the anesthetic into the intercostal space and intercostal muscle. When you enter the parietal pleura, you may feel a pop, and air or fluid may rush into the syringe. The patient may feel an uncomfortable sensation at this point; encourage him to remain still. (See *Injecting local anesthesia*.)

■ Place a clamp on the needle at the level of the skin to mark the depth of needle penetration. Withdraw the needle and observe the depth of penetration necessary to enter the pleural space.

■ There are several methods to drain the thoracic cavity: needle, catheter-within-a-needle, and needle-within-a-catheter.

■ No matter which method you use, support the patient verbally through the procedure.

■ Watch for signs of distress during the procedure, including pallor, vertigo, weak or rapid pulse, hypotension, dyspnea, tachypnea, diaphoresis, chest pain, blood-tinged mucus, and excessive coughing. If any of these signs or symptoms occur and are sustained, suspend the procedure and provide symptomatic treatment.

■ After the procedure, dress the site with povidone-iodine ointment, 4″ × 4″ sterile gauze pads, and adhesive tape. Order a chest X-ray to assess the degree of removal and to check for complications, such as pneumothorax or hemothorax.

■ Place the patient into a comfortable position. Order vital signs and respiratory assessment every 15 minutes for 1 hour after the procedure, with instructions to call you immediately if there is any change in condition.

■ Send sterile fluid specimens for analysis. Diagnostic studies include cell count, Gram stain, tuberculin and fungal smears, aerobic and anaerobic cultures, cytology, cell block for immunochemi-

---

## Injecting local anesthesia

When you're injecting anesthesia for thoracentesis, alternate injecting and aspirating anesthetic as you advance the needle. This allows the anesthetic to infiltrate the area, prevents injecting anesthesia into a vessel, and confirms correct placement when you observe fluid during aspiration. At this point, you should mark the proper depth for thoracentesis needle insertion by clamping the needle with hemostats, as depicted below.

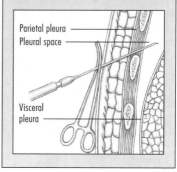

---

cal staining, and protein, glucose, pH, lactate dehydrogenase, and amylase levels.

### Needle method

■ Attach the clamp to the 15G or 18G needle and mark it at the depth of the first needle. This prevents you from penetrating too deeply into the thoracic cavity, which can lead to pneumothorax. (See *The needle method,* page 474.)

■ Attach the three-way stopcock to the needle, a 50-ml syringe, and tubing for connection to vacuum collection bottles.

■ With the stopcock off to the tubing, insert the procedure needle through the anesthetized zone, ad-

## The needle method

As you advance the needle, it slides over the superior end of the rib and then into the pleural space, as shown, while the patient exhales.

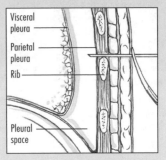

Visceral pleura
Parietal pleura
Rib
Pleural space

Fluid can then travel from the pleural space and through the needle to the three-way stopcock. From there, you can draw it into a syringe or allow it to drain into the collection bottle, as shown.

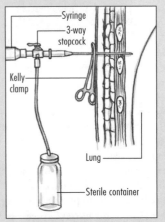

Syringe
3-way stopcock
Kelly clamp
Lung
Sterile container

You can also draw fluid up into a syringe, reposition the stopcock, and then inject the fluid into the collection bottle.

vancing the needle over the rib to the level of the clamp.
■ Withdraw fluid with the sy-

ringe, and then turn the stopcock off to the patient. Push fluid into the specimen tubes and vacuum collection bottles from the syringe. Set aside the first specimen to send to the laboratory, if appropriate. Continue the process until you can't remove much more fluid or until you've withdrawn 1,000 to 1,500 ml (the amount depends on the patient's size). Alternatively, allow fluid to drain from the needle directly into the vacuum collection bottles, and use the syringe once to withdraw a fluid sample for specimens. With the stopcock turned off to the patient, withdraw the needle.

### Catheter-within-a-needle method
■ Place a 10-ml syringe onto an introducer needle. Mark the depth of insertion with a clamp, and insert the needle to the level of the clamp, bevel down, over the anesthetized site. Use the syringe to withdraw fluid and confirm proper placement of the needle.
■ Remove the syringe. Use your gloved finger to cover the needle hub when changing equipment to prevent air from entering the pleural space.
■ While the patient exhales, insert the catheter through the needle; then remove the needle.
■ Attach the end of the catheter to a three-way stopcock turned off to the patient, and attach a syringe and collection bottle tubing to the other end.
■ Drain fluid from that half of the thorax.

### Needle-within-a-catheter method
■ Attach the 10-ml syringe to the

needle and insert it throughout the anesthetized zone, (as previously described), until you withdraw fluid.

■ Advance the catheter into the pleural space and remove the needle during exhalation. Place a gloved finger over the catheter hub until you can attach the three-way stopcock, 50-ml syringe, and vacuum collection bottle tubing.

■ Drain fluid into the vacuum collection bottles.

## Postprocedure patient teaching

■ Have the patient report shortness of breath or chest discomfort after the procedure; this requires reassessment and another chest X-ray.

■ Continue to provide supplemental oxygen, if needed, after the procedure.

## Complications

■ Pleuritic or shoulder pain indicates that the needle's point is causing pleural irritation. The pain isn't clinically significant and resolves spontaneously.

■ Pneumothorax occurs in 5% to 20% of patients undergoing thoracentesis and can result from the needle puncturing the lung. About 20% of patients with this complication will need a chest tube inserted. Observe for tachypnea, shortness of breath, decreased arterial saturation, tracheal shift from the midline, or clinical deterioration. Order a portable chest X-ray and evaluate it.

■ Hemothorax can result from

laceration of thoracic vasculature and requires that a chest tube be inserted. Evaluate and provide the same treatment that you would for a pneumothorax.

■ Faulty low-needle entry into the thorax can result in laceration of the liver, spleen, or diaphragm, which requires immediate surgical consultation. Prevent this complication by inserting needles only above the level of the eighth rib.

■ Reexpansion pulmonary edema and hypotension result from excessive fluid removal. Prevent this by removing no more than 1,000 to 1,500 ml of fluid depending on the size of the patient. Provide supportive therapy, including oxygen therapy, I.V. fluid replacement, pressors if needed, and diuretics if persistent.

■ Avoid infection by using aseptic technique during the procedure.

■ Hypoxia results from a ventilation-perfusion mismatch in the reexpanded lung. Administer oxygen temporarily during and after the procedure until pulse oximetry levels stabilize.

## Special considerations

■ If the patient coughs, briefly halt the procedure and withdraw the needle slightly to prevent puncture.

■ The diagnostic pleural fluid tests needed for each patient vary with the clinical situation. Some health care providers recommend sending fluid for basic testing (such as cell counts) and storing remaining fluid for further testing as indicated by those results.

■ To minimize the risk of hypoxia,

the patient should have his oxygenation monitored after the procedure with pulse oximetry and arterial blood gas levels. He may benefit from prophylactic oxygen administration for several hours after the procedure.

## Documentation

- Document informed consent.
- Note the date, time, and location of the insertion site.
- Document the indication for the procedure, describe the fluid withdrawn, indicate the amount withdrawn, and note specimens you sent to the laboratory.
- Record the patient's vital signs and respiratory status before and after the procedure, chest X-ray results, the patient's reaction to the procedure, and any complications, including actions taken to remedy the situation.

# THROAT CULTURE

### CPT code
87070 *Culture, bacterial; any source except urine, blood, or stool, with isolation and presumptive identification of isolates*

## Overview

A throat culture is used primarily to isolate and identify group A beta-hemolytic streptococci (*Streptococcus pyogenes*), allowing early treatment of pharyngitis and prevention of sequelae, such as rheumatic heart disease and glomerulonephritis. It's also used to screen for asymptomatic carriers of pathogens, especially *Neisseria meningitides*. In rare instances, a throat culture may be used to identify *Corynebacterium diphtheriae, Bordetella pertussis, Staphylococcus aureus, Streptococcus pneumoniae,* or *Haemophilus influenzae.* Although a throat culture may be used to identify *Candida albicans,* direct potassium hydroxide preparation usually provides the same information faster.

A throat culture requires swabbing the throat, streaking a culture plate, and allowing the organisms to grow for isolation and identification of pathogens. A Gram-stained smear may provide preliminary identification, which may guide clinical management and determine the need for further tests.

## Indications

- To isolate and identify group A beta-hemolytic streptococci
- To screen asymptomatic carriers of pathogens, especially *Neisseria meningitides*

## Contraindications
**RELATIVE**
- Antibiotic therapy already initiated

## Preprocedure patient preparation

- Explain to the patient the reason for this test.
- Inform him that he need not restrict food or fluids before the test.
- Tell the patient that he may gag during the swabbing but that the

procedure typically takes less than one minute.

■ Check the patient's history for recent antimicrobial therapy.

## Equipment

Gloves ◆ tongue blade ◆ penlight ◆ sterile cotton-tipped swab ◆ sterile culture tube with transport medium (or commercial collection kit) ◆ label ◆ nasal speculum (optional)

## Procedure

■ Explain the procedure to the patient, and address any questions or concerns he may have.

■ Instruct the patient to sit erect at the edge of the bed or in a chair, facing you. Then wash your hands and put on gloves.

■ Ask the patient to tilt his head back. Depress his tongue with the tongue blade and illuminate his throat with the penlight to check for inflamed areas.

■ If the patient starts to gag, withdraw the tongue blade and tell him to breathe deeply. When he's relaxed, reinsert the tongue blade but not as deeply as before.

■ Using the sterile cotton-tipped swab, wipe the tonsillar areas from side to side, including any inflamed or purulent sites. Make sure you don't touch the tongue, cheeks, or teeth with the swab to avoid contaminating it with oral bacteria.

■ Withdraw the swab and immediately place it in the sterile culture tube. If you're using a commercial kit, crush the ampule of culture medium at the bottom of the tube and then push the swab into the medium to keep the swab moist.

■ Remove and discard your gloves and wash your hands.

■ Label the specimen. On the laboratory request form, indicate which organism is strongly suspected, especially *Corynebacterium diphtheriae, Bordetella pertussis,* and *Neisseria meningitides* because they require specific preparations.

## Postprocedure patient teaching

■ Inform the patient of when laboratory results will be available, and provide follow-up care, teaching, and support as necessary.

## Complications

■ Laryngospasm may occur after the culture is obtained if the patient has epiglottiditis or diphtheria. Keep resuscitation equipment nearby.

## Special considerations

■ Culture results must be interpreted in light of clinical status, recent antimicrobial therapy, and amount of normal flora.

■ Normal throat flora include nonhemolytic and alpha-hemolytic streptococci, *Neisseria* species, staphylococci, diphtheroids, some *Haemophilus* species, pneumococci, yeasts, and enteric gram-negative rods.

■ Pathogens that may be cultured include group A beta-hemolytic streptococci (*S. pyogenes*), which can cause scarlet fever and pharyngitis; *C. albicans,* which can cause thrush; *C. diphtheriae,* which can cause diphtheria; and *B. pertussis,* which can cause whooping cough. The laboratory report should indicate the prevalent organisms and the quantity of pathogens cultured.

■ Failure to use the proper transport medium can interfere with the results of the test.

## Documentation

■ Record the time, date, and site of specimen collection and any recent or current antibiotic therapy. Also, note whether the specimen has an unusual appearance or odor.

## *TICK REMOVAL*

### CPT codes
10120  *Removal of superficial foreign body, skin*
10121  *Incisional removal of foreign body, complex*

## Overview

Ticks are arachnids common in woods and fields throughout the United States. A tick can attach to its host in any of its life stages (larva, nymph, or adult) by fastening to the host with its mouthparts, then secreting a cementlike material to reinforce the attachment. A bite from a tick may cause nothing more than a local reaction; however, significant disease can occur from infectious agents transmitted by ticks. All ticks should be re-

moved from the body as soon as possible. The longer a tick is attached and feeding, the higher the chance to pass infectious organisms on to the patient. There are several acceptable methods to remove ticks.

## Indications

■ To remove a tick attached to the skin
■ To remove a tick unable to be removed by nonsurgical methods or if the mouth parts separate from the body

## Contraindications

■ None known

## Preprocedure patient preparation

■ Obtain a medical history from the patient. Determine how long the tick has been attached to the patient, the location where the patient may have acquired the tick, and any removal attempts the patient has already made.
■ Inform the patient of the removal options available, and discuss which one is appropriate for his circumstances.

## Equipment

Gloves ◆ antiseptic solution such as povidone-iodine ◆ sterile water or normal saline solution

### Option 1
Petrolatum jelly or 70% isopropyl alcohol ◆ small specimen cup (optional)

### Option 2
Blunt tip forceps or tweezers

### Option 3
Tick remover tool

### Option 4
Lidocaine 1% or 2% ◆ 1-ml syringe ◆ 28G or 30G needle ◆ scalpel larger than size of tick ◆ sterile 4″ × 4″ gauze pads ◆ tape ◆ suture equipment (optional)

### Option 5
Lidocaine 1% or 2% ◆ 1-ml syringe ◆ 28G or 30G needle ◆ punch biopsy tool ◆ sterile 4″ × 4″ gauze pads ◆ tape ◆ suture equipment (optional)

### Equipment preparation
■ If surgical removal or punch biopsy is necessary, the instruments should be properly sterilized before use.

## Procedure

■ Explain the procedure to the patient, and address any questions or concerns he may have.
■ Wash your hands and put on gloves.

### Option 1
■ Although unreliable (because ticks have a very low respiratory rate), these suffocation methods are occasionally used.
■ Cover the entire tick with a large amount of petrolatum jelly. The goal is to completely seal the tick in the jelly and cause suffocation. This alone may make the tick back itself out of the skin.
■ Alternatively, cover the tick with

gauze and soak with 70% isopropyl alcohol. Or, if it is possible to form a tight seal with a small specimen cup, put alcohol in the cup and place over the tick, covering all body parts. Invert while maintaining a seal so that tick is completely encased in the alcohol. This is noxious to the tick and also causes suffocation; the tick may back itself out of the skin.
■ Inspect the site to be sure all parts, including the mouth, have been removed. Clean the site with an antiseptic solution such as povidone-iodine, rinse with water or normal saline solution, and allow to dry.

### Option 2
■ Clean the area around tick gently with povidone-iodine solution.
■ Gently grasp the tick as close to the skin surface as possible with forceps, tweezers, or your fingers; be sure to wear gloves.
■ Apply gentle continuous traction to the mouth parts. Take care not to use a jerking or twisting motion, which may separate the mouth parts from the body. Don't squeeze or crush the tick because infectious agents may be present in its body fluids.
■ Inspect the site to be sure all parts, including the mouth, have been removed. Clean the site with antiseptic solution such as povidone-iodine, rinse with water or normal saline solution, and allow to dry.

### Option 3
■ Use the tick remover tool, a small plastic bowl with a notch cut in it, to gently, slowly scrape along

the skin where the mouth is attached. As the tool progresses, the angle of the plastic causes the tick to release its grasp on the skin.

■ Inspect the site to be sure all parts, including the mouth, have been removed. Clean the site with topical antiseptic solution such as povidone-iodine, rinse with water or normal saline solution, and allow to dry.

### Option 4
■ Clean the area with povidone-iodine solution.
■ Infiltrate around the mouth parts with 1% or 2% lidocaine solution in a 1 ml syringe with a 28G or 30G needle. Lidocaine with epinephrine may be used if the tick isn't on the fingers, toes, penis, or ears.
■ Using a scalpel larger than the size of the tick, cut at a 30- to 45-degree angle toward the lesion to facilitate undermining the mouth parts, and make an elliptical incision, completely encasing the mouth parts.
■ Remove and submit the specimen including the body for analysis. Apply pressure with sterile gauze to control bleeding.

◢➤ CLINICAL TIP
*If bleeding can't be controlled, close the wound with one or two interrupted sutures.*
■ Inspect the site to be sure all parts, including the mouth, have been removed. Clean the site with topical antiseptic solution such as povidone-iodine, rinse with water or normal saline solution, and allow to dry.

■ Cover with a loose dressing of gauze and tape.

### Option 5
■ Clean the area with povidone-iodine solution.
■ Infiltrate around the mouth parts with 1% or 2% lidocaine solution in a 1 ml syringe with a 28G or 30G needle. Epinephrine may be used if tick isn't on the fingers, toes, penis, or ears.
■ Apply the punch biopsy tool to cover the tick, perpendicular to the skin.
■ With your fingers, tighten the skin on opposite sides of the tool.
■ With continuous downward pressure, rotate the tool from right to left until you have penetrated through the dermis. You'll note a decrease in resistance at this point.
■ Remove the punch and lift the specimen with forceps.
■ Snip the base of the tissue.
■ Remove and submit the specimen, including the body, for analysis. Apply pressure with sterile gauze to control bleeding.

◢➤ CLINICAL TIP
*If bleeding can't be controlled, close the wound with one or two interrupted sutures.*
■ Inspect the site to be sure all parts, including the mouth, have been removed. Clean the site with topical antiseptic solution such as povidone-iodine, rinse with water or normal saline solution, and allow to dry.
■ Cover with a loose dressing of gauze and tape.

## Postprocedure patient teaching

■ Educate the patient about the possibility of a local infection. Tell him to watch for signs of infection, such as warmth, redness, or drainage, and to notify you if these symptoms arise.

■ Inform the patient that systemic infection (such as Lyme disease) may be caused by organisms transmitted by the tick. Tell him to watch for rash, fever, myalgia, or arthralgias and to return for evaluation should any of these occur.

■ If necessary, the patient should return for suture removal in approximately 7 days, depending on location.

■ Teach the patient how to avoid getting ticks; for example, by wearing long sleeves and pants, tucking pants into socks, and applying an insect repellent such as diethyltoluamide in high-risk locations.

## Complications

■ Complications are rare from the removal procedure. Local or systemic infection can be avoided by making sure all parts of the tick are removed and by cleaning with povidone-iodine solution.

■ Systemic infection can be transmitted from the tick bite itself or by body parts left in the skin after removal. The pathogens that cause several diseases in the United States are transmitted by ticks of the Ixodes species. These ticks have become the most common carriers of vector-transmitted diseases. Deer ticks carry the organisms that cause Lyme disease, babesiosis, and ehrlichiosis. Other ticks are vectors for Rocky Mountain spotted fever, tularemia, and Colorado tick fever.

## Special considerations

■ To preserve the tick for analysis, place it in a labeled bottle with alcohol or follow your laboratory's instructions. In most cases, keep any ticks for future identification and possible analysis for infectious disease.

## Documentation

■ Record the local reaction seen at the time of visit.

■ Document in the record the date and site of removal as well as the method or methods used and medications needed.

■ Chart patient education along with postprocedure instructions given.

# *TONGUE LACERATION REPAIR*

### *CPT codes*

41250 *Repair of laceration 2.5 cm or less; floor of mouth and/or anterior two-thirds of tongue*

41251 *Repair of laceration 2.5 cm or less; posterior one-third of tongue*

41252 *Repair of laceration of the tongue; floor of mouth, over 2.6 cm or complex*

## Overview

Tongue lacerations can occur from a variety of mechanisms, such as penetrating injuries or falls, where the teeth perforate the tongue on impact. Small lacerations of the tongue are typically considered minor as long as the wound edges remain in approximation. Large or extensive lacerations require repair in order to ensure appropriate wound edge approximation. If this isn't accomplished, epithelialization will occur downward, producing a "cleft" that can be a problem functionally and cosmetically.

## Indications

■ To repair any laceration of the tongue, regardless of size, in which the wound edges aren't in good approximation

## Contraindications

**ABSOLUTE**

■ Partial or complete traumatic amputation of a portion of the tongue

■ Lesions to the posterior one-third of the tongue in which local regional anesthesia won't be effective

■ Large lacerations of the tongue in which patient cooperation or aspiration may be an issue

■ Lacerations that will necessitate general anesthesia

## Preprocedure patient preparation

■ Explain the injury in detail, using anatomic illustrations (if possi-ble), and discuss treatment options.

■ Assess the patient's tetanus immunization status. Appropriate immunization should be administered, if warranted.

## Equipment

Clean and sterile gloves ◆ linen-saver pad ◆ oral suction equipment ◆ sterile 4″ × 4″ gauze pads ◆ normal saline solution ◆ 20- or 60-ml syringe (without needle) ◆ equipment to administer regional nerve block ◆ equipment for suturing

## Procedure

■ Explain the procedure to the patient, and address any questions or concerns he may have.

☑ **OBTAIN INFORMED CONSENT**

■ Wash your hands and put on gloves.

■ Cover the patient with a linen-saver pad to protect his clothes.

■ Have the patient tell you if he needs to use the oral suction equipment at any time during the procedure to avoid aspiration. You may need to suction if the field becomes obscured with saliva or blood.

■ Insert rolled gauze into both sides of the patient's mouth to prevent him from biting down.

■ Remove gloves and put on sterile gloves.

■ Administer a regional block to the lingual nerve, which will anesthetize the anterior two-thirds of the tongue, and assure that proper anesthesia has occurred before proceeding. (See "Anesthesia: Topical, local, and digital nerve block," page 20.)

◢◣ CLINICAL TIP
*Don't attempt to infiltrate local anesthesia directly into a sensate, moving tongue; it's very painful and ineffective.*

■ Stabilize the tongue by having the patient or an assistant hold it with gauze. Alternatively, two suture loops may be placed and left untied for the patient or assistant to hold.

■ Gently irrigate the laceration with normal saline solution in a 20- or 60-ml syringe.

■ Approximate the wound edges using the simple interrupted suturing technique with absorbable suture material. (See "Suturing simple lacerations," page 459.)

■ Once completed, make sure there's no leftover suture material in the oral cavity.

## Postprocedure patient teaching

■ Inform the patient to return if he has swelling of the tongue, increasing pain, fever and chills, or difficulty swallowing.

■ Instruct the patient to have nothing by mouth until the anesthesia has worn off. For local pain relief, he may apply ice to the site and take acetaminophen or ibuprofen.

■ Tell the patient that the sutures will dissolve in approximately 5 to 10 days (depending on the suture material used — chromic gut takes longer to dissolve than plain gut) and won't need to be removed. Also, inform the patient that he'll

feel the sutures in place, and instruct him to try not to pick at them or rub them against his teeth.

■ Have the patient return in approximately 1 week for follow-up evaluation.

## Complications

■ Inappropriate approximation of the wound edges may require revision for functional and cosmetic reasons.

■ Infection may require treatment with systemic antibiotics.

## Special considerations

■ Treatment with antibiotics typically isn't indicated unless the wound is very extensive (large tongue laceration or lacerations of the tongue and adjacent mucosal surfaces) or penetration has occurred with a "dirty" object. If penetration has occurred, the patient's tetanus immunization status must be assessed.

## Documentation

■ Thoroughly document the location, size, depth, and mechanism of the tongue laceration; an illustration is best.

■ Record the type of analgesia and anesthetic used, the type and number of sutures placed, and the patient's toleration of the procedure.

■ Document the patient's scheduled follow-up visit and discharge instructions given.

# TONOMETRY

## CPT codes
92100 *Serial tonometry with multiple measurements of intraocular pressure over an extended time period with interpretation and report*
92120 *Tonography with interpretation and report, recording indentation tonometer*

## Overview
Tonometry allows indirect measurement of intraocular pressure and serves as an effective screen for early detection of glaucoma, a common cause of blindness. Intraocular pressure rises when the production of aqueous humor — the clear fluid secreted continuously by the ciliary process in the eye's posterior chamber — exceeds the rate of drainage. This rise in pressure causes the eyeball to harden and become more resistant to extraocular pressure.

Indentation tonometry tests this resistance by measuring how deeply a known weight depresses the cornea; applanation tonometry provides the same information by measuring the amount of force required to flatten a known area of the cornea. (See *Applanation tonometry*, and *Schiøtz tonometer,* page 486.) Both procedures necessitate corneal anesthetization and careful examination technique.

The diagnostic significance of tonometry is readily apparent because glaucoma — which can be treated if detected early enough — is the second leading cause of permanent blindness in the United States and the leading cause of blindness in blacks. This test should be performed routinely on people over age 40 because glaucoma strikes 2% of people past this critical age.

## Indications
- To measure intraocular pressure
- To aid diagnosis and follow-up evaluation of glaucoma

## Contraindications
ABSOLUTE
- Trauma or suspected anatomical abnormalities

## Preprocedure patient preparation
- Explain to the patient that this test measures the pressure within his eyes. Tell him the test takes only a few minutes and requires that his eyes be anesthetized. Reassure him that the test is painless.
- If the patient wears contact lenses, instruct him to remove them before the procedure and leave them out for 2 hours after the test or until the anesthetic wears off completely.
- Explain that his cooperation during the test will ensure accurate test results.

## Equipment
Indentation tonometer (the Schiøtz tonometer is the most popular), sterilized or used with disposable sterile tonofilms ◆ topi-

cal ophthalmic anesthetic such as 0.5% proparacaine hydrochloride

## Procedure

### Indentation tonometry

■ Explain the procedure to the patient, and address any questions or concerns he may have.

■ Ask the patient to assume a supine position. Avoid any elevation in his intraocular pressure by ensuring he's relaxed and having him loosen or remove restrictive clothing around his neck.

■ Instruct him not to cough or squeeze his eyelids together.

■ Ask the patient to look down. Raise his superior eyelid with your thumb, and place one drop of the topical ophthalmic anesthetic at the top of the sclera. The solution spreads over the entire sclera when the patient blinks.

■ Check the tonometer for a zero reading on the steel test block that comes with the instrument. Make sure the plunger moves freely. The first measurement on each eye is obtained with the 5.5-g weight.

■ Have the patient look up and stare at a spot on the ceiling. Then ask him to open his mouth, take a deep breath, and exhale slowly. This distracts him, preventing forceful closure of the lids. After this initial breath, tell the patient to breathe normally during the test.

■ With the thumb and forefinger of one hand, hold the lids of his right eye open against the orbital rim. Hold the tonometer vertically with the thumb and forefinger of the other hand, and rest the footplate on the apex of the cornea. Be

---

## Applanation tonometry

Applanation tonometry, the most precise test of intraocular pressure, measures the force required to flatten a certain area of the cornea. The applanation tonometer (usually the Goldmann tonometer) is mounted on a slit-lamp biomicroscope.

This test is performed with minimal corneal trauma and may be done after a routine slit-lamp examination. However, because the slit-lamp biomicroscope is used only by an ophthalmologist, applanation tonometry is less available than indentation tonometry for large-scale screening of the general population.

To perform this test, instill a topical anesthetic and stain the tear film with fluorescein drops or insert a moistened fluorescein paper strip into the lower conjunctival sac. Seat the patient as for a slit-lamp examination and instruct him to look straight ahead. Move the slit-lamp forward until the tonometer comes in contact with the cornea. Through the eyepiece of the slit lamp, you should see two fluorescein semicircles. Adjust the tension dial on the tonometer until the inner, straight-edged margins of the semicircles touch.

The reading on the tension dial provides a direct indication of the patient's intraocular pressure.

---

especially careful to avoid resting your fingers on the cornea or pressing on the cornea, because this increases intraocular pressure. With the footplate in place, check the indicator needle for a rhythmic transmission caused by the ocular pulse. Then record the calibrated scale reading that converts to a measurement of intraocular pressure. If the reading doesn't exceed 4, add an additional weight (7.5,

## Schiøtz tonometer

The Schiøtz tonometer, depicted below, is the most popular type of indentation tonometer. It consists of a concave footplate that rests on the cornea, a plunger to apply pressure to the cornea, and a calibrated scale to measure the amount of pressure applied by the plunger.

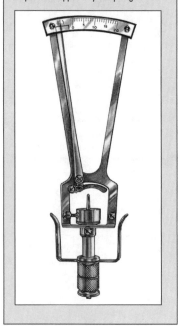

10, or 15 g) to obtain a reliable result.

■ Repeat the procedure on the left eye, and record the time when the test was performed.

### Postprocedure patient teaching

■ Because an anesthetic was instilled, tell the patient not to rub his eyes for at least 20 minutes after the test to prevent corneal abrasion. If the patient wears contact lenses, tell him not to reinsert them for at least 2 hours.

■ If the tonometer moved across the cornea during the test, tell the patient he may feel a slight scratching sensation in the eye when the anesthetic wears off. This sensation should disappear within 24 hours because most corneal abrasions resulting from tonometry affect only the corneal epithelium, which regenerates within 24 hours without scarring.

### Complications

■ To avoid corneal abrasion, hold the tonometer still. Don't touch the lashes because this could trigger a blink response or Bell's phenomenon (upward movement of the eyes with forced closure of the lids), which can cause the footplate to move and scratch the cornea.

### Special considerations

■ Intraocular pressure normally ranges from 12 to 20 mm Hg, with diurnal variations. The highest point is reached at the time of waking; the lowest point, in the evening.

■ Elevated intraocular pressure requires further testing for glaucoma. Because intraocular pressure varies diurnally, findings must be supplemented with serial measurements obtained at different times on different days.

■ Findings must be confirmed by visual field testing and opthalmoscopy.

## Documentation

- Record the indications for the test, the time the procedure was performed, and the measurement of intraocular pressure. Document the ophthalmic anesthetic used, number of drops instilled, and how the patient tolerated it.
- Document follow-up care and instructions given, and any referrals made, if necessary.

## Tooth, Avulsion and Fracture Management

### CPT code
*No specific code has been assigned.*

## Overview

Dental trauma involving an avulsed or fractured tooth is a common facial injury. Traumatic injuries to a tooth may be successfully repaired, but they require timely and appropriate management and healthy pretrauma dentition. Therefore, knowledge of basic dental anatomy and management of basic dental trauma is crucial for primary care providers.

A tooth consists of three layers: enamel (outer), dentin (middle), and pulp (inner). Dentin, the major portion of the tooth, appears slightly yellowish compared to the white enamel, and is harder than bone. It surrounds and protects the dental pulp, which consists of connective tissue, nerve endings, capillaries, and lymph vessels. Ver-

tically, only one-third of the tooth is visible above the gingiva; this portion is called the crown. Beneath this, the root is embedded in the alveolus, or socket, of the jaw bone. Between these two levels is a thin neck, or cervix, at the level of the gingiva. Below the crown, a periodontal membrane surrounds the root and holds the tooth in its alveolus.

## Indications

- To replace an avulsed permanent tooth without significant damage to pulp, root, or periodontal tissue
- To replace an avulsed tooth resulting from recent trauma (less than 1 hour) with proper tooth storage
- To determine management for a fractured permanent tooth that isn't avulsed (may require professional dental evaluation to assess potential viability for repair or salvage)

## Contraindications

### ABSOLUTE

- Deciduous (milk) tooth involved (this will eventually be replaced by a permanent tooth)
- Preexisting tooth decay or caries in the affected tooth
- Concurrent fracture of an avulsed tooth
- Preexisting periodontal disease in the area of the affected tooth, indicating loss of periodontal support
- Prolonged duration (more than 1 hour) of tooth avulsion out of its socket without proper tooth stor-

age — root dries and is rendered nonviable beyond this time frame

## Preprocedure patient preparation

■ Discuss the intent of tooth salvage for reimplantation or repair. Explain that an avulsed tooth has a greater likelihood of successful reattachment if it's reimplanted within an hour.

■ Explain proper tooth storage medium. Saliva is an excellent temporary storage medium. Advise the patient, if off-site, to rinse the mouth with warm water, and to clean the tooth in water and store it in the mouth under the tongue or within the cheek pouch until he gets to your facility or to a dentist. If the patient is unconscious, has an altered level of consciousness, has impaired swallowing or gag reflex, or has significant oral trauma, the tooth may be stored in the mouth of another person. Other acceptable tooth storage mediums include milk, blood, or normal saline. Universal precautions should always be taken into consideration. If no other medium is available, advise storage in water, however this is the least optimal medium. Emphasize the importance of not allowing the tooth to dry out.

■ Explain that initial treatment isn't definitive and will require dental follow-up.

■ Explain potential complications and the potential for nonsuccessful tooth salvage despite treatment.

■ Review the history of the traumatic event: How, where, and when did the trauma occur? Was there a loss of consciousness? Are there any other presenting complaints suggesting additional facial, neck, or neurological injury?

■ Advise the patient that a fractured tooth doesn't typically require emergency treatment.

## Equipment

Sterile normal saline solution ◆ large syringe (60-ml) without a needle for irrigation ◆ sterile 4″ × 4″ gauze pads ◆ tissue or tooth forceps ◆ for a fractured tooth, dental or orthodontic wax ◆ radiographic equipment for X-rays, if available ◆ equipment to administer local anesthesia (optional)

## Procedure

■ Explain the procedure to the patient, and address any questions or concerns he may have.

■ Wash your hands and put on gloves.

### For management of avulsed tooth

■ Clean the avulsed tooth in water or normal saline solution, and place in normal saline solution as quickly as possible. Avoid handling the root surface.

■ Inspect the oral cavity and dentition, assessing for concurrent lacerations, foreign bodies, or other dental trauma. Observe dental alignment for bite disturbances caused by the avulsed tooth or additional trauma. Assess for periodontitis of the affected area.

■ If available, obtain dental and mandibular radiographs; obtain additional facial films, if indicated, based upon evidence of facial trauma.

■ Inspect the avulsed tooth socket for debris and tissue; irrigate with sterile normal saline. Remove any clotted blood collected within the socket.

■ Holding the tooth with cotton gauze or tooth forceps, re-implant it into the socket, approximating its original position as closely as possible. Use only finger pressure in insertion. Avoid contact with the root surface.

■ Prescribe antibiotic prophylaxis with penicillin.

■ Administer tetanus toxoid if not updated within previous 5 years.

### *For management of fractured tooth*

■ Inspect the involved tooth for degree of fracture. This may range from minor (chipping of enamel only) to severe or comminuted (may require dental radiographs and professional dental evaluation for determination). If comminuted, save the pieces in an appropriate storage medium because the dentist may be able to temporarily cement them together.

■ Clean the affected tooth or fragments with normal saline using irrigation, and have the patient rinse his mouth with warm water.

■ Inspect the oral cavity and dentition, assessing for concurrent lacerations, foreign bodies, or other dental trauma. Observe dental alignment for bite disturbances caused by the fractured tooth or additional trauma.

■ Consider using dental or orthodontal wax placement over the fractured tooth as a temporary measure to protect the pulp.

## Postprocedure patient teaching

■ Refer the patient to a professional dentist for follow-up care; in the case of tooth avulsion, emphasize that this should occur as soon as possible.

■ Advise the patient that the prognosis for tooth salvage remains dependent upon pretreatment time and tooth storage factors as well as pretrauma dentition health, and that despite treatment, nonviability of the tooth may result.

■ Recommend analgesics for pain relief.

■ Recommend a soft diet and careful, diligent oral hygiene.

## Complications

■ Bacterial endocarditis and bacteremia are rare and may be avoided with penicillin prophylaxis.

■ Necrosis of the root may result in nonviable repair and complete loss of tooth.

■ Root (nerve) damage may necessitate root canal.

## Special considerations

■ An avulsed tooth that has dried due to lack of proper storage, or that has remained out of its socket for more than 1 hour, is nonviable, and temporary replacement shouldn't be attempted. Explain its nonviability to the patient, inspect the oral cavity and clean the socket as noted above, prescribe analgesics, and refer the patient for dental follow-up.

## Documentation

- Record trauma history and storage method and duration (if avulsed), as reported by patient.
- Record physical examination findings, including concurrent facial, neck, or neurologic trauma; dental trauma; and general condition of the teeth.
- Document treatment provided, patient tolerance, medications given or prescribed (if any), and instructions given to the patient for posttreatment follow-up recommendations.

# *T*OPICAL HEMOSTASIS

*CPT code*
*No specific code has been assigned.*

## Overview

Topical hemostatic agents are used to rapidly control and stop bleeding from capillaries and small surface vessels. Application of a hemostatic agent is a quick, easy, and typically painless procedure that can be performed in the health care provider's office or in an acute care setting without the use of electrocautery.

Various hemostatic agents are available; your selection will depend on product availability, the area of the body involved, the patient's sensitivity to the product,

and the degree of tissue staining possible.

Products commonly used to control bleeding include silver nitrate, aluminum chloride 30%, Monsel's solution (ferric subsulfate), and epinephrine (topical and injectable). All are fast-acting, very effective, and inexpensive. However, the likelihood of staining and necrosis is low to moderate with aluminum chloride 30%, moderate with Monsel's solution, high with larger doses of epinephrine (topical or injectable), and highest with silver nitrate.

## Indications

- To stop bleeding from skin lesions, superficial tissue lacerations, broken capillaries, or small blood vessels

## Contraindications

**RELATIVE**

- History of cardiovascular disease
- Highly visible area (if staining likely)
- Potential for development of ischemia and necrosis resulting from vasoconstriction of a finger or toe

## Preprocedure patient preparation

- Advise the patient that bleeding should stop immediately after application of the hemostatic agent. Assure him that he should feel little to no pain or discomfort. Explain that the site may be red for the first 24 to 48 hours.
- Clean or irrigate the wound as necessary.

## Equipment

Topical hemostatic agent of choice ◆ field drape ◆ gloves ◆ sterile 4″ × 4″ gauze pads ◆ large cotton-tipped applicator ◆ tape

## Procedure

- Verify that the patient isn't allergic to topical medications.
- Explain all steps to the patient to ensure cooperation and relieve anxiety. Address any questions or concerns he may have.

✓ **OBTAIN INFORMED CONSENT**

- Prepare the field and set up the equipment.
- Place the patient in a comfortable position that fully exposes the site.
- Assess the type of lesion or laceration, direct and surrounding skin tissue responses, estimated blood loss, and the patient's mental status.
- Select an appropriate hemostatic product based on your assessment of the wound site and the advantages and disadvantages of the product to the skin site and surrounding tissue area.
- Drape the area.
- Put on gloves.
- Apply direct pressure to the site with 4″ × 4″ sterile gauze pads; blot the site.
- Apply the topical hemostatic product, using direct pressure with a cotton-tipped applicator or sterile gauze (depending on the wound site) for approximately 15 seconds.
- Clean off excess blood at the site and surrounding tissue.

- Repeat the application, if necessary, to complete hemostasis.
- Assess the wound site.
- Apply sterile 4″ × 4″ gauze and tape, if necessary.
- If appropriate, give a tetanus immunization before the patient leaves the office. Administer tetanus prophylaxis for a deep, dirty wound if the patient hasn't had one in the past 5 years and for a clean, superficial wound if the patient hasn't had one in the past 10 years.

## Postprocedure patient teaching

- Tell the patient to call you if he experiences recurrence of bleeding, increased pain or discomfort, or signs of infection, such as fever, red surrounding tissue, swelling, and colored drainage from the site.
- Advise the patient to use a mild analgesic such as ibuprofen, if necessary, for site pain or discomfort.
- Inform him that site tissue staining may not resolve and could be permanent.

## Complications

- Tissue staining is possible, depending on the hemostatic agent used.

## Special considerations

- Evaluate potentially negative cosmetic effects that could occur when using a particular agent with staining possibilities.
- Because of its high vasoconstrictive potential with epinephrine, don't use topical hemostasis on

body appendages, such as the fingers and nose; permanent damage can occur from ischemia or necrosis.

## Documentation

■ Before performing this procedure, document any abnormal physical findings on the consent form. Have the patient initial the comments and sign the form to signify acknowledgment of preprocedural abnormalities. In the chart, the preprocedural and postprocedural notes must include an evaluation of potentially affected function, range of motion, and sensation.

■ Note that informed consent was received, if necessary; consent should indicate that options and risks (specifically for staining and necrosis) were discussed and that the patient agreed to treatment.

■ Record the results of the site assessment before and after the procedure, the type of hemostatic agent used, the patient's response to the procedure, and the patient's understanding of your instructions.

### *T*RANSCUTANEOUS *ELECTRICAL NERVE STIMULATION*

***CPT code***
64550  *Application of surface (transcutaneous) neurostimulator*

## Overview

Transcutaneous electrical nerve stimulation (TENS) is based on the gate theory of pain, which proposes that painful impulses pass through a "gate" in the spinal cord.

A portable, battery-powered device transmits painless electrical current to peripheral nerves or directly to a painful area over relatively large nerve fibers. This treatment effectively alters the patient's perception of pain by blocking painful stimuli traveling through smaller fibers. A TENS device reduces the need for analgesic drugs and may allow the patient to resume normal activities. Typically, a course of TENS treatments lasts 3 to 5 days. Some conditions, such as phantom limb pain, may require continuous stimulation; other conditions, such as a painful arthritic joint, require shorter periods (3 to 4 hours).

## Indications

■ To alleviate postoperative or chronic pain

## Contraindications

**ABSOLUTE**
■ Cardiac pacemakers
■ Pregnant patients
■ Senility

**RELATIVE**
■ Cardiac disorders
■ Vascular disorders or seizure disorders (TENS electrodes shouldn't be placed on the head or neck.)

(See *Positioning TENS electrodes,* page 494.)

## Preprocedure patient preparation

■ Tell the patient that TENS involves placement of small electrodes on his body, usually near the pain site. The electrodes are connected to a small, battery-powered generator, which electrically stimulates nerve fibers, inhibiting or blocking pain sensations. Add that TENS treatments also help stimulate endorphin production. Mention, too, that they help to distract the patient from his pain.

■ Advise the patient that he may feel varying degrees of pain relief. Some patients report relief only when the unit is on; others report prolonged pain relief.

■ Inform the patient that TENS effectively treats both acute and chronic pain. In particular, it may benefit the patient concerned about adverse effects of drug therapy for such conditions as headache syndromes, chronic or acute musculoskeletal disorders, or menstrual cramps. Add that TENS is most effective for localized mild to moderate pain. It's contraindicated only in patients with pacemakers or loss of sensation. Tell the patient that it can be used indefinitely (without adverse effects) to control pain. However, skin breakdown is possible either from prolonged use or an allergic reaction to the adhesive on the electrodes.

## Equipment

TENS device ◆ alcohol pads ◆ electrodes ◆ electrode gel ◆ warm water and soap ◆ lead wires ◆ charged battery pack ◆ battery recharger ◆ adhesive patch or nonallergenic tape (optional: commercial TENS kit that includes the stimulator, lead wires, electrodes, spare battery pack, battery recharger, and sometimes the adhesive patch)

### Equipment preparation

■ Before beginning the procedure, always test the battery pack to make sure that it's fully charged.

## Procedure

■ Explain the procedure to the patient, and address any questions or concerns he may have. If the patient has never seen a TENS unit before, show him the device.

■ Wash your hands and maintain aseptic technique. Provide privacy.

■ With an alcohol pad, thoroughly clean the skin where the electrode will be applied. Then dry the skin.

■ Apply electrode gel to the bottom of each electrode.

■ Place the electrodes on the proper skin area, leaving at least 2″ (5 cm) between them. Then secure them with the adhesive patch or nonallergenic tape. Tape all sides evenly so the electrodes are firmly attached to the skin.

■ Plug the pin connectors into the electrode sockets. To protect the cords, hold the connectors, not the cords themselves, during insertion.

## Positioning TENS electrodes

In transcutaneous electrical nerve stimulation (TENS), electrodes placed around peripheral nerves (or an incisional site) transmit mild electrical pulses to the brain. Health care providers think the current may block pain impulses. The patient can influence the level and frequency of his pain relief by adjusting the controls on the device.

Typically, electrode placement varies even though patients may have similar complaints. Electrodes may be placed to cover the painful area or surround it (as with muscle tenderness or spasm or painful joints). They may also be placed to capture the painful area between the electrodes (as with incisional pain).

In peripheral nerve injury, electrodes should be placed proximal to the injury (between the brain and the injury site) to avoid increasing pain. Placing electrodes in a hypersensitive area also increases pain. In an area lacking sensation, electrodes should be placed on adjacent dermatomes.

The illustrations below show combinations of electrode placement (black squares) and areas of nerve stimulation (shaded) for lower back and leg pain.

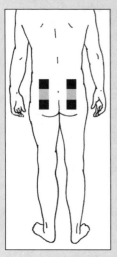 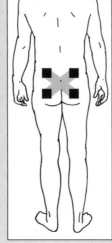 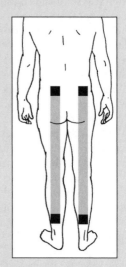

- Turn the channel controls to the "off" position or to the position recommended in the operator's manual.
- Plug the lead wires into the jacks in the control box.
- Turn the amplitude and rate dials slowly, as the manual directs. (The patient should feel a tingling sensation.) Then adjust the controls on the device to the pre-

scribed settings or to settings that are most comfortable. Most patients select stimulation frequencies of 60 to 100 Hz.
- Attach the TENS control box to part of the patient's clothing, such as a belt, pocket, or bra.
- To make sure the device is working effectively, monitor the patient for signs of excessive stimulation (such as muscular twitch-

es) or inadequate stimulation (the patient's inability to feel a mild tingling sensation).

### *After TENS treatment*

- Turn off the controls and unplug the electrode lead wires from the control box.
- If another treatment will be given soon, leave the electrodes in place; if not, remove them.
- Clean the electrodes with soap and water and clean the patient's skin with alcohol sponges. (Don't soak the electrodes in alcohol because it will damage the rubber.)
- Remove the battery pack from the unit and replace it with a charged battery pack.
- Recharge the used battery pack so it's always ready for use.

## Postprocedure patient teaching

- Explain that treatment will begin with a TENS trial of at least 1 week, usually conducted by a physical therapist, a nurse, a nurse practitioner, a physician assistant, or a physician. The trial will help determine the best placement of the electrodes and the optimal settings for amplitude frequency and pulse width. It will also give the patient practice in using the TENS unit at home.
- If appropriate, allow the patient to study the operator's manual. Teach him how to place the electrodes properly and how to take care of the TENS unit.

## Complications

- None known

## Special considerations

- If you must move the electrodes during the procedure, turn off the controls first. Incorrect placement of the electrodes will result in inappropriate or inadequate pain control.
- Setting the controls too high can cause pain; setting them too low will fail to relieve pain.
- Never place the electrodes near the patient's eyes or over the nerves that innervate the carotid sinus or laryngeal or pharyngeal muscles to avoid interference with critical nerve function.
- If TENS is used continuously for postoperative pain, remove the electrodes at least daily to check for skin irritation and provide skin care.

## Documentation

- Before performing this procedure, document any abnormal physical findings on the consent form. Have the patient initial the comments and sign the form to signify acknowledgment of preprocedural abnormalities. In the chart, the preprocedural and postprocedural note must include an evaluation of function, range of motion, and neurosensory testing (such as 2-point discrimination).
- On the patient's medical record, note the electrode sites and control settings used, document the patient's tolerance of the procedure, and evaluate the effectiveness of pain control.

# TRIGGER POINT INJECTIONS

### CPT codes
20552  *Injection; trigger point(s); one or two muscle groups*
20553  *Injection; trigger point(s); three or more muscle groups*

## Overview

A trigger point is a highly localized sensitive spot in a taut band of myofascial muscle fibers. It produces local and referred pain when pressure is applied. Trigger point injections interrupt the pain cycle, allowing other pain relief measures, such as dry needling, stretch and spray, and transcutaneous electrical nerve stimulation, and the body's natural healing process a chance to work. Trigger point injections cause the release of chemicals that dilate local arterioles and restore circulation to the trigger point, relax the motor end plates, release calcium and thus decrease muscle rigidity, and extend the peripheral nerve refractory period. This is referred to as insertional activity.

## Indications

■ To treat myofascial pain syndromes of cervical, thoracic, and lumbar back and extremities; fibromyalgia syndrome; and temporomandibular disorders
■ To alleviate chronic pelvic pain (rare)

## Contraindications
### ABSOLUTE
■ Cellulitis or broken skin at injection site
■ Anticoagulant therapy or coagulapathy
■ Septicemia or suspected bacteremia
■ Unavailability of emergency equipment

### RELATIVE
■ Lack of response to two to three previous injections

## Preprocedure patient preparation

■ Inform the patient that he may feel a burning sensation for a few seconds as the medication is injected. Explain that the area may become numb for up to 3 hours and that pain relief generally lasts for several days.

## Equipment

Alcohol wipes ◆ gloves ◆ drape ◆ marking pen ◆ 0.5% to 1% lidocaine (without epinephrine) or bupivacaine 0.125% to 0.25% (single-dose vials to avoid preservative or precipitation problems) ◆ methylprednisolone ◆ 25G or 27G 1¼″ needles ◆ 3-, 5-, and 10-ml syringes ◆ emergency resuscitation equipment

## Procedure

■ Explain the procedure to the patient, and address any questions or concerns he may have.

## ☑ OBTAIN INFORMED CONSENT

- Wash your hands. Lay all equipment on a tray within easy reach.
- Put on gloves.
- Position and drape the patient for privacy, comfort, and safety.
- Expose the area surrounding the injection site.
- Identify the exact location of the trigger point by palpating the maximal point of tenderness with your thumb or forefinger.
- Mark the area by drawing a circle around your finger.
- Clean the area with alcohol wipes.
- Draw up the desired amount of lidocaine or bupivacaine, depending on the site to be used. If using methylprednisolone, draw the local anesthetic first and change the needle to prevent dulling or contamination; then draw up the proper amount of the steroid.
- Proceed with the trigger point injection, using one of two techniques:
– Insert the needle at a 90-degree angle until it reaches the trigger point. Aspirate for blood. Inject the solution, withdraw slightly but not totally from the skin, and then reinject at a 60-degree angle both to the left and to the right of the original injection. (See *Choosing an angle for trigger point injection*.)
– Insert the needle at a 50- to 70-degree angle into the subcutaneous tissue adjacent to the trigger point region. Aspirate for blood. Using about three needle insertions, inject the desired amount of solution with each insertion into the trigger

## Choosing an angle for trigger point injection

When injecting trigger points, you'll commonly use either a 90-degree angle or a 50- to 70-degree angle, depending on your preference and the depth and location of the trigger point.

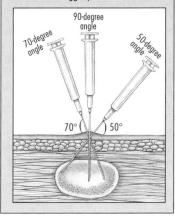

point without removing the needle from the skin.

- If the procedure is done correctly, the patient will experience immediate relief.
- Remove the needle and place an adhesive bandage over the injection site.

**◄ CLINICAL TIP**
*Observe for reactions to the local anesthetic: light-headedness, tinnitus, peripheral numbness, slurring of speech, drowsiness, or seizure activity. Treatment includes general supportive measures and drug discontinuation. Maintain a patent airway and carry out other respiratory support measures immediately. Administer diazepam or thiopental to treat seizures. Administer vasopressors (including dopamine and*

*norepinephrine) to treat significant hypotension.*

## Postprocedure patient teaching

■ Tell the patient he can apply heat to the site before exercising the muscle.

■ Ask him to move the muscles passively or actively to enhance the effectiveness of the injection and to begin restoring normal function and range of motion (ROM) to the area. Within 4 hours of injection, he can start working on ROM and stretching exercises; then gradually add weight-bearing exercises over the following days to weeks. Encourage him to progress to exercising at least 5 times daily (frequency is crucial to symptom relief).

■ Urge the patient to avoid isometric exercises such as weightlifting and excessively quick, jerky movements because these tend to exacerbate pain and injury.

■ Advise the patient not to constrict his muscles in the trigger point area — for example, as occurs when carrying a heavy knapsack.

■ Tell him to observe for edema and ecchymosis, which may indicate bleeding into the muscle. Instruct him to apply ice to the site to minimize these symptoms, which will resolve over a few days.

■ Tell the patient to report signs and symptoms of infection, such as increased pain after 24 hours, elevated temperature, redness, swelling, yellow or green discharge, and foul odor.

## Complications

■ Vasovagal syncope or a reaction to the local steroid may require use of emergency equipment.

■ Skin infection can be treated with topical or oral antibiotics.

■ Hematoma formation can be treated by applying ice to the affected site for 15 to 20 minutes.

■ Neuritis may require supportive care and physical therapy.

## Special considerations

■ Patients with myofascial pain are likely to experience pain reduction and increased ROM.

■ Patients with fibromyalgia may initially experience increased ROM without pain relief, and pain relief may be delayed up to 2 weeks after the injection.

■ Trigger point injections with a local anesthetic can be repeated every 3 to 4 days; if steroids are used, injections should be 6 weeks apart. Research suggests that the specific medication injected is less important than the actual piercing of the muscle with a needle.

■ Apply heat for 20 to 30 minutes after the injection to increase permeability into the trigger point area.

## Documentation

■ Before performing this procedure, document any abnormal physical findings on the consent form. Have the patient initial the comments and sign the form to signify acknowledgment of preprocedural abnormalities. In the chart, the preprocedural and postprocedural note must include an evaluation of function, ROM, and neurosensory testing (such as two-point discrimination).

■ Record an accurate history of the trigger point area, the patient's ROM, and strength of affected muscles.

■ Specify the type and amount of local anesthetic and steroid used, the exact location of the injection (draw a picture of the muscle group area), and the appearance of the injection site.

■ Note the patient's pain perception before and after the injection.

# TUBERCULIN SKIN TESTS

## CPT codes
86580 *Skin test, tuberculosis, intradermal*
86585 *Skin test, tuberculosis, tine test*

## Overview

Tuberculin skin tests are used to screen patients for previous infection by the tubercle bacillus. They are routinely performed in children, young adults, and people with radiographic findings that suggest this infection.

In both the old tuberculin (OT) and the purified protein derivative (PPD) tests, intradermal injection of the tuberculin antigen causes a delayed hypersensitivity reaction in patients with active or dormant tuberculosis (TB); sensitized lymphocytes gather at the injection site, causing erythema, vesiculation, and induration that peaks within 24 to 48 hours and persists for at least 72 hours.

The most accurate tuberculin test method, the Mantoux test, uses a single-needle intradermal injection of PPD, which permits precise measurement of dosage. Multipuncture tests, such as the tine test, Mono-Vacc test, and Aplitest, involve intradermal injections using tines impregnated with OT or PPD. Because multipuncture tests require less skill and are more rapidly administered than the Mantoux test, they're generally used for screening. However, a positive multipuncture test usually requires a Mantoux test for confirmation.

## Indications

■ To distinguish TB from blastomycosis, coccidioidomycosis, and histoplasmosis
■ To identify persons who need diagnostic investigation for TB because of possible exposure

## Contraindications
### ABSOLUTE
■ History of allergic reaction to acacia (don't perform an OT test because this product contains acacia)
■ Active TB
■ A current reaction to smallpox vaccination
■ Presence of a rash or skin disorder

### RELATIVE
■ Don't perform a skin test in ar-

eas with excessive hair, acne, or insufficient subcutaneous tissue, such as over a bone or tendon

## Preprocedure patient preparation

- Explain to the patient that this test helps detect TB. Tell him the test requires an intradermal injection, which may cause him transient discomfort.

## Equipment

Alcohol swabs ◆ vial of PPD (intermediate strength) — 5 tuberculin units (TU) per 0.1 ml and 1-ml tuberculin syringe with ½″ or ⅝″ 25G or 26G needle for the Mantoux test ◆ commercially available device (tine, Mono-Vacc, or Aplitest) for multipuncture tests ◆ epinephrine (1:1,000) and 3-ml syringe (for emergency use)

## Procedure

- Explain the procedure to the patient, and address any questions or concerns he may have.
- Wash your hands.
- Assist the patient to a sitting position with his arm extended and supported on a flat surface. Clean the volar surface of the upper forearm with alcohol, and let the area dry completely.
- For the Mantoux test, draw up 0.1 ml (5 TU) of PPD into the syringe and administer an intradermal injection. (See "Injection, intradermal," page 270.)

**➤ CLINICAL TIP**
*If the patient is known to be hypersensitive to skin tests, use a first-strength dose to avoid necrosis at the puncture site.*

- For multipuncture tests, remove the protective cap on the injection device to expose the four tines. Hold the patient's forearm in one hand, stretching the skin of the forearm tightly. Then, with your other hand, firmly depress the device into the patient's skin (without twisting it). Hold the device in place for at least 1 second before removing it. If you've applied sufficient pressure, you'll see four puncture sites and a circular depression made by the device on the patient's skin.
- Tuberculin skin tests are generally read 48 to 72 hours after injection; however, the Mono-Vacc test can be read 48 to 92 hours after the test. (See *Reading tuberculin test results*.)

## Postprocedure patient teaching

- Instruct the patient to return at the specified time so that test results can be read. Inform him that a positive reaction to a skin test appears as a red, hard, raised area at the injection site. Although the area may itch, instruct him not to scratch it. Stress that a positive reaction doesn't always indicate active TB.

## Complications

- Ulceration or necrosis may develop at the injection site; apply cold soaks or a topical steroid.
- Have epinephrine available to treat an anaphylactic or acute hypersensitivity reaction.

## Special considerations

■ Normal findings are:
– for Mantoux test — induration less than 5 mm in diameter or no induration
– for tine test and Aplitest — no vesiculation; no induration or induration less than 2 mm in diameter
– for Mono-Vacc test — no induration.

■ A positive tuberculin reaction indicates previous infection by tubercle bacilli. It doesn't distinguish between an active and dormant infection, nor does it provide a definitive diagnosis. If a positive reaction occurs, sputum smear and culture and chest X-rays are necessary to provide more information.

■ In the Mantoux test, induration of 5 to 9 mm in diameter indicates a borderline reaction; larger induration, a positive reaction. Because patients infected with atypical mycobacteria other than tubercle bacilli may have borderline reactions, repeat testing is necessary.

■ In the tine test or Aplitest, vesiculation indicates a positive reaction; induration of 2 mm in diameter without vesiculation requires confirmation by the Mantoux test. Any induration in the Mono-Vacc test indicates a positive reaction but requires confirmation by the Mantoux test.

## Documentation

■ Record where the test was given, the date and time, and when it's to be read.

---

## Reading tuberculin test results

You should read the Mantoux, tine, and Aplitest skin tests 48 to 72 hours after injection; the Mono-Vacc test, 48 to 96 hours afterward.

In a well-lighted room, flex the patient's forearm slightly. Observe the injection site for erythema and vesiculation, then gently rub your finger over the site to detect induration. If induration is present, measure the diameter in millimeters, preferably using a plastic ruler marked in concentric circles of specific diameter.

In multipuncture tests, you may find separate areas of induration around individual punctures or induration involving more than one puncture site. If so, measure the diameter of the largest single area of induration or coalesced induration.

---

# *T*YMPANOMETRY

### *CPT codes*
92567 *Tympanometry (impedance testing)*
92568 *Acoustic reflex testing*

## Overview

The purpose of tympanometry is to objectively assess the air pressure within the middle ear and the mobility of the tympanic membrane. This provides an objective analysis of middle ear function. Using a tympanometer, positive, normal, and negative air pressures are introduced into the external meatus of the ear to measure the sound energy flow. The sound energy flow is then traced on a graph called a tympanogram.

This procedure is useful in determining resolution of otitis media and serous otitis media through the assessment of middle ear function and in identifying dysfunction that could result in hearing loss or repeated infections.

## Indications

- To determine eustachian tube patency
- To evaluate hearing loss or ear pain
- To detect perforations of the tympanic membrane
- To determine mobility of the tympanic membrane
- To evaluate persistent middle ear effusions
- To evaluate patency of pressure-equalization tubes
- To assess middle ear function when patient is unable to cooperate with audiometry
- To verify middle ear abnormalities

## Contraindications

ABSOLUTE
- Canal totally obstructed by cerumen
- External otitis media

RELATIVE
- Age younger than 7 months

## Preprocedure patient preparation

- If the patient is a child, show him and allow him to hold the

tympanometer to lessen anxiety and promote cooperation.

## Equipment

Tympanometer tool with 220 to 226 Hz probe tone and air pressure range of − 400 decaPascals (daPa) to +200 daPa ◆ otoscope ◆ various size ear tips

## Procedure

- Explain the procedure to the patient or parent and describe how the patient should indicate hearing the tone. Answer any questions.
- Seat the patient in a comfortable, upright position or allow the patient to sit independently or in a parent's lap.
- Using an otoscope, inspect the ear canal for cerumen obstruction or evidence of infection.
- Select the proper ear tip that provides a tight seal of the ear canal, insert it snugly, and activate the tympanometer.
- Gently apply traction to the pinna, pulling up and back on an older child and adult or pulling back on an infant or child under age 3, to produce a good seal.
- When an appropriate seal is achieved, the tympanometer will automatically transmit the sound, measure the air pressures, record readings, and print out results.
- Interpret the results of tympanometer reading. Low compliance measurements indicate a stiff or obstructed middle ear, while high compliance measurements indicate flaccid or highly mobile tympanic membrane.

■ Review results with the patient or parents.

## Postprocedure patient teaching

■ Explain the results, and if a problem is identified, explain the epidemiology.
■ Discuss choices for therapeutic interventions and expected resolution timetable.
■ Discuss any environmental factors, such as allergies, smoking, and loud noises that may be contributing to the problem and appropriate avoidance measures.
■ Instruct the patient or parent of the need for follow-up care and evaluation and specify the date for each.
■ Provide instructions verbally and in written form. Any referrals should include the provider's name, address, and phone number.
■ Instruct the patient or parents to call you if the symptoms continue after 72 hours or if they worsen in any way.

## Complications
■ None known

## Special considerations
■ If problems are indicated, consult with an ear, nose, and throat specialist and consider immediate referral.
■ If external otitis media is present and the ear canal is occluded with purulent material, consult with a physician about treatment options.

■ If the tympanic membrane is occluded with cerumen, order cerumen softener and have patient return in 48 to 72 hours for cerumen removal and tympanogram.

## Documentation
■ Note the reason for tympanometry.
■ Document the number, type, and frequency of problems.
■ Record previous treatment modalities.
■ Include a copy of the tympanogram on the chart and document findings and the care plan.

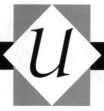

## Unna's Boot Application

***CPT code***
29580 *Strapping with Unna's boot*

### Overview

Unna's boot is a commercially prepared, medicated gauze compression dressing that wraps around the foot and leg. It's used to treat uninfected, nonnecrotic leg and foot ulcers. Alternatively, a preparation known as Unna's paste (gelatin, zinc oxide, calamine lotion, and glycerin) may be applied to the ulcer and covered with lightweight gauze. The boot's effectiveness results from compression applied by the bandage combined with moisture supplied by the paste.

### Indications

- To treat leg and foot ulcers resulting from venous insufficiency or stasis dermatitis

### Contraindications

**ABSOLUTE**
- Allergy to any ingredient (gelatin, zinc oxide, calamine lotion, and glycerin) used in the paste
- Presence of arterial ulcers, weeping eczema, cellulitis, suspected infection, or necrosis
- Deep vein thrombosis, phlebitis, or arterial insufficiency

### Preprocedure patient preparation

- Advise the patient that the amount of discomfort varies with the degree of neurovascular compromise. Assure him that discomfort will lessen over time.

### Equipment

Scrub sponge with cleaning agent ◆ normal saline solution ◆ commercially prepared gauze bandage saturated with Unna's paste (or Unna's paste and lightweight gauze) ◆ bandage scissors ◆ gloves ◆ elastic bandage to cover Unna's boot ◆ metal clips or tape ◆ extra gauze for excessive drainage (optional) ◆ mineral oil (optional)

## Procedure

- Explain the procedure to the patient, and address any questions or concerns he may have.
- Verify that the patient isn't allergic to topical medications.
- Wash your hands and put on gloves.
- Assess the ulcer and the surrounding skin. Evaluate ulcer size, drainage, and appearance. Perform a neurovascular assessment of the affected foot.

◢➤ **CLINICAL TIP**
*If pulses are undetectable, order Doppler studies immediately. Depending on the patient's condition, consider referring to a physician or surgeon.*

- Clean the affected area gently with the sponge and cleaning agent. Rinse with normal saline solution.
- Some health care providers use mineral oil on the unaffected areas that will be covered with the dressing to decrease pruritus. Don't allow mineral oil onto any compromised skin.
- If a commercially prepared gauze bandage isn't available, spread Unna's paste evenly on the leg and foot. Then cover the leg and foot with the lightweight gauze. Apply three to four layers of paste interspersed with layers of gauze. In a prepared bandage, the bandage is impregnated with the paste.
- Apply gauze or the prepared bandage in a spiral motion, from just above the toes to the knee. Be sure to cover the heel. The wrap should be snug but not tight. To cover the area completely, make sure each turn overlaps the previous one by half the bandage width. (See *How to wrap Unna's boot,* page 506.)
- Continue wrapping the patient's leg up to the knee, using firm, even pressure. Stop the dressing 1″ (2.5 cm) below the popliteal fossa. Mold the boot with your free hand as you apply the bandage.
- Cover the boot with an elastic bandage, using the same technique.
- Secure the bandage with metal clips or tape.
- Instruct the patient to remain with his leg outstretched and elevated until the paste dries (approximately 30 minutes). Observe the patient's foot for signs of impairment, such as cyanosis, loss of feeling, and swelling. These signs indicate that the bandage is too tight and must be removed.
- Leave the boot on for 3 to 14 days (with an average of 5 to 7 days), depending on the amount of exudate.
- Change the boot as indicated to assess the underlying skin and ulcer healing. Remove the boot by unwrapping the bandage from the knee, back to the foot.

## Postprocedure patient teaching

- Explain to the patient that resolution of the ulcer can vary, depending on the ulcer's size and on the coexistence of other conditions, such as diabetes, peripheral vascular disease, and infection.
- Emphasize the need to keep the affected leg clean and dry. Remind him to wrap it in plastic to a point

## How to wrap Unna's boot

After cleaning the patient's skin thoroughly, flex his knee. Then, starting with the foot positioned at a right angle to the leg, wrap the medicated gauze bandage firmly — not tightly — around the patient's foot. Make sure the dressing covers the heel. Continue wrapping upward, overlapping the dressing slightly with each turn. Make sure that the dressing circles the leg at an angle to avoid compromising the circulation. Smooth the boot with your free hand as you go, as shown below.

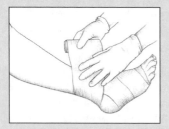

Stop wrapping about 1″ (2.5 cm) below the knee, as shown below. If necessary, make a 2″ (5-cm) slit in the boot just below the knee to relieve constriction that may develop as the dressing hardens.

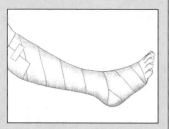

If drainage is excessive, you may wrap a roller gauze dressing over the Unna's boot. As the final layer, wrap an elastic bandage in a figure-eight pattern.

above the knee before bathing, and caution him not to submerge the affected leg.

■ Advise him not to put anything inside the boot or to scratch under the dressing; doing so increases the risk of infection and additional skin breakdown.

■ If the patient can change his own dressing, review the proper technique to use, and answer any questions he has.

■ Instruct the patient to walk on and handle the wrap carefully to avoid damaging it. Tell him the boot will stiffen but won't be as hard as a cast.

■ Instruct the patient to notify you promptly if he experiences severe itching or signs and symptoms of neurovascular compromise (change in color or temperature, numbness or tingling, swelling, or increased pain) or infection (increasing redness, swelling, drainage, odor, or pain).

■ Have the patient schedule weekly follow-up appointments so you can evaluate progress.

### Complications

■ Contact dermatitis may result from hypersensitivity to Unna's paste; treat by immediately removing the Unna's boot.

■ Vascular compromise is minimized by promptly removing and reapplying the boot, as indicated, and by teaching the patient to detect and report signs and symptoms of vascular compromise.

## Special considerations

■ If the boot is applied over a swollen leg, it must be changed as the edema subsides — if necessary, more frequently than every 5 days.
■ Don't make reverse turns while wrapping the bandage. This could create excessive pressure areas that may cause discomfort as the bandage hardens.
■ For bathing, instruct the patient to cover the boot with a plastic kitchen trash bag sealed at the knee with an elastic bandage to avoid wetting the boot. A wet boot softens and loses it effectiveness. If the patient's safety is a concern, instruct him to take a sponge bath.

## Documentation

■ Record the date and time of application, indications, and the presence of a pulse in the affected foot.
■ Specify which leg you bandaged.
■ Describe the appearance of the patient's skin before and after boot application.
■ Name the equipment used (a commercially prepared bandage or Unna's paste and lightweight gauze).
■ Describe any allergic reaction.
■ Note instructions given to the patient and the patient's tolerance for the procedure.

# UREA BREATH TEST

**CPT codes**
83013 Helicobacter pylori; *breath test analysis*

83014 H. pylori; *breath test analysis; drug administration and collection*

## Overview

The urea breath test is used to diagnose *Helicobacter pylori* infection of the stomach. It's a noninvasive test based on the hydrolysis of urea by *H. pylori* to produce carbon dioxide ($CO_2$) and ammonia. A carbon isotope is labeled and given to the patient by mouth; the *H. pylori* then releases the tagged $CO_2$, which is collected in a breath sample.

The American College of Gastroenterology recommends a urea breath test as the best nonendoscopic test for documenting *H. pylori* infection. Other noninvasive tests to confirm *H. pylori* infection include serology testing, which uses enzyme-linked immunosorbent assay testing to detect immunoglobulin G antibodies. Stool antigen assay is also used.

## Indications

■ To diagnose suspected *H. pylori* infection
■ To screen patients with active peptic ulcer disease or a history of documented peptic or duodenal ulcer or of mucosa-associated lymphoid tissue lymphoma
■ To document eradication in patients who have undergone treatment for *H. pylori*

## Using a PYtest balloon

A PYtest balloon and straw are needed to collect the exhaled specimen. Instruct the patient to inhale deeply, hold his breath for 10 seconds, then blow into the straw until the balloon is fully inflated. Reinforce that he doesn't need to fully exhale and shouldn't overinflate the balloon.

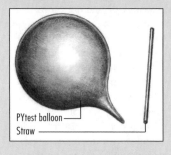

PYtest balloon

Straw

## Contraindications

**ABSOLUTE**

- Use of bismuth or antibiotics within 30 days of testing (can produce a false-negative result)
- Use of sucralfate or proton-pump inhibitors within 14 days (can suppress *H. pylori* and produce false-negative result)
- Patient's failure to fast for 6 hours before testing
- Pregnancy

◥ **CLINICAL TIP**

*Although the dose of radiation contained in the 14C–urea breath test is small, it isn't currently recommended for use in children or pregnant women. A nonradioactive 13C test may be used instead.*

## Preprocedure patient preparation

- Inform the patient that the test will help confirm the presence or absence of *H. pylori* infection, which will help determine whether treatment is necessary. Reassure him that he won't experience discomfort or adverse reactions from the procedure.
- Confirm that the patient hasn't had bismuth or antibiotics in the past 30 days, sucralfate or proton-pump inhibitors in the past 14 days, and food in the past 6 hours.
- Tell him he may leave when the test is complete.

## Equipment

PYtest capsule ◆ two 30-ml medicine cups ◆ timer ◆ collection balloon ◆ straw

## Procedure

- Explain the procedure to the patient, and address any questions or concerns he may have. Perform a dry run of the test to ensure his understanding.
- Wash your hands.
- Give him one PYtest capsule and 20 ml of water. Instruct him to swallow the capsule without chewing, using the 20 ml of water to wash down the capsule.
- After he swallows the capsule, begin timing for 10 minutes.
- After 3 minutes, refill the medicine cup with 20 ml of water and instruct the patient to swallow this additional water to ensure that the

capsule has passed completely into the stomach.

■ Label the collection balloon with the patient's name and date of birth. Insert a straw into the balloon opening in preparation for the collection.

■ After 10 minutes have elapsed, give the balloon with the straw in place to the patient. (See *Using a PYtest balloon.*)

■ Instruct him to inhale deeply, hold his breath for 10 seconds, and then fully inflate the balloon through the straw. Tell him not to overinflate the balloon.

■ Process the sample following the manufacturer's guidelines or forward it to the laboratory for processing.

### Postprocedure patient teaching

■ Review and give the patient preprinted patient-teaching supplements from the manufacturer.

■ Tell him to schedule a follow-up in 1 week to discuss test results and necessary treatments, if any.

### Complications

■ None known

### Special considerations

■ Testing for *H. pylori* in patients with nonulcer dyspepsia and without a history of peptic ulcer disease is controversial, although some health care providers examine the patient for infection. In general, testing should be done

only in the patient who will be treated if the test result is positive.

### Documentation

■ Record the test date, the time the sample was collected, and the patient's name, date of birth, and identification number.

■ Note the patient's referring health care provider, if appropriate.

■ Document your confirmation that the patient didn't have bismuth or antibiotics in the past 30 days, sucralfate or proton-pump inhibitors in the past 14 days, and food in the past 6 hours.

■ Note the patient's history of partial gastrectomy, if applicable.

■ Record test results, whether positive, negative, or indeterminate.

# *U*RINALYSIS

***CPT codes***
81002  *Urinalysis, by dipstick or tablet reagent, without microscopy*
81007  *Urinalysis, bacteriuria screen, nonculture, non-dipstick technique*
81015  *Urinalysis, microscopic*

### Overview

Routine urinalysis is important in screening for urinary and systemic disorders. These tests evaluate color, odor, and opacity (odor, though not usually documented on laboratory reports, may be noted under specimen comments); determine specific gravity and pH;

detect and measure protein, glucose, and ketone bodies; and examine sediment for blood cells, casts, and crystals.

Diagnostic laboratory methods include visual examination, reagent strip screening, refractometry for specific gravity, and microscopic inspection of centrifuged sediment.

## Indications

■ To screen urine for renal or urinary tract disease
■ To help detect metabolic or systemic disease unrelated to renal disorders

## Contraindications

■ None known

## Preprocedure patient preparation

■ Explain that this test, which requires a urine specimen, aids diagnosis of renal or urinary tract disease and helps evaluate overall body function.
■ Tell the patient he needn't restrict food or fluids but should avoid strenuous exercise before the test.
■ Check the medication history for drugs that may affect test results.

## Equipment

Gloves ◆ graduated container ◆ three sterile 2″ × 2″ gauze pads ◆ povidone-iodine solution ◆ sterile specimen container with lid ◆ urinometer or refractometer ◆ reagent strips with color-coded chart ◆ centrifuge and appropriate specimen tube ◆ glass microscope slide with coverslip ◆ microscope (Commercial clean-catch urine kits containing antiseptic towelettes, sterile specimen container with lid and label, and instructions for use in several languages are widely used.)

## Procedure

■ Because the goal is a virtually uncontaminated specimen, explain the procedure to the patient carefully. Provide illustrations to emphasize the correct collection technique, if possible.
■ Have the patient collect a clean-catch midstream urine specimen. Tell the patient to remove all clothing from the waist down and to stand in front of the toilet as for urination or, if female, to sit far back on the toilet seat and spread her legs. Then have the patient clean the periurethral area (tip of the penis or labial folds, vulva, and urinary meatus) with soap and water and wipe the area three times, each time with a fresh 2″ × 2″ gauze pad soaked in povidone-iodine solution or with the wipes provided in a commercial kit. Instruct the female patient to separate her labial folds with the thumb and forefinger. Tell her to wipe down one side with the first pad and discard it, to wipe the other side with the second pad and discard it and, finally, to wipe down the center over the urinary meatus with the third pad and dis-

card it. Stress the importance of cleaning from front to back to avoid contaminating the genital area with fecal matter. For the uncircumcised male patient, emphasize the need to retract his foreskin to effectively clean the meatus and to keep it retracted during voiding.

■ Tell the female patient to straddle the toilet to allow labial spreading and to keep her labia separated while voiding.

■ Instruct the patient to begin voiding into the toilet. Then, without stopping the urine stream, the patient should move the collection container into the stream, collecting 30 to 50 ml at the midstream portion of the voiding. He can then finish voiding into the toilet.

■ Put on gloves and take the sterile container from the patient. Be sure the cap is on securely. If the outside of the container is soiled, clean it and wipe it dry. Proceed to the designated area in your facility for urine testing. Remove the cap.

■ Examine the physical appearance of the urine, noting color, turbidity, and odor. Measure the specific gravity with a urinometer or refractometer.

■ Detect and measure protein, glucose, and ketone bodies. Dip the reagent strip into the urine for time specified by manufacturer, remove it, and tap off the excess urine from the strip. Hold the strip horizontally to avoid mixing reagents from adjacent test areas on the strip. Then compare the colors on the strip with the standardized color chart on the strip package. The manufacturer provides the time in seconds for each measurement.

■ Perform microscopic examination — centrifuged urine sediment contains cells, casts, crystals, bacteria, yeasts, and parasites. Place 10 to 15 ml of urine in a centrifuge tube and centrifuge for 5 minutes at a centrifugal force of 400. After the urine is spun down, remove most of the supernate fluid (clear fluid that will be on top of the sediment), leaving about 1 ml in the tube. Gently mix, or resuspend, the urine sediment in the remaining supernate fluid. Place one drop of the resuspended sediment on a glass microscope slide and apply a cover slip. Place the slide under the microscope and examine first with the low-power lens, viewing at least 10 different fields. Low-power lenses are used to detect and count the number of casts. Then switch to a high-power lens and view at least 10 different fields. High-power lenses are used to detect and count white blood cells (WBCs), red blood cells, and bacteria.

■ Discard the remaining urine, container, and your gloves, and wash your hands.

■ Evaluate your results. (See *Normal findings in routine urinalysis,* page 512.)

## Postprocedure patient teaching

■ Explain the results of the test to the patient, and provide teaching and treatment and recommend follow-up care as necessary.

## Normal findings in routine urinalysis

Refer to the table below when evaluating urinalysis results.

| ELEMENT | FINDINGS |
| --- | --- |
| **MACROSCOPIC** | |
| Color | Straw to dark yellow |
| Odor | Slightly aromatic |
| Appearance | Clear |
| Specific gravity | 1.005 to 1.035 |
| pH | 4.5 to 8.0 |
| Protein | None |
| Glucose | None |
| Ketones | None |
| Bilirubin | None |
| Urobilinogen | Normal |
| Hemoglobin | None |
| Red blood cells | None |
| Nitrite (bacteria) | None |
| White blood cells | None |
| **MICROSCOPIC** | |
| Red blood cells | 0 to 2/high-power field |
| White blood cells | 0 to 5/high-power field |
| Epithelial cells | 0 to 5/high-power field |
| Casts | None, except 1 to 2 hyaline casts/low-power field |
| Crystals | Present |
| Bacteria | None |
| Yeast cells | None |
| Parasites | None |

## Complications

- None known

## Special considerations

- If the patient is being evaluated for renal colic, strain the specimen to catch stones or stone fragments. Place an unfolded 4″ × 4″ gauze pad or a fine-mesh sieve over the specimen container, and carefully pour the urine through it.
- If analysis will be delayed longer than 1 hour, refrigerate the specimen.
- Nonpathologic variations in normal values may result from diet, use of certain drugs, non-pathologic conditions, specimen collection time, and other factors. (See *Drugs that influence routine urinalysis results.*)

## Documentation

- Record the time of specimen collection and the appearance, odor, and color as well as any unusual characteristics of the specimen. Also record the tests performed.
- If a microscopic examination was done, record the number of casts as number per low-power field and the number of cells as number per high-power field (hpf). For example, 10 WBCs/hpf.
- Record patient teaching, treatment prescribed, and follow-up care as necessary.

# Drugs that influence routine urinalysis results

Following is a list of variations in urinalysis results and drugs that can account for such non-pathologic changes.

## URINE COLOR CHANGES

Amitriptyline (blue-green)
Anthraquinone laxatives (reddish brown)
Chloroquine (rusty yellow)
Chlorzoxazone (orange to purple-red)
Deferoxamine mesylate (red)
Fluorescein sodium I.V. (yellow-orange)
Furazolidone (brown)
Iron salts (black)
Levodopa (dark)
Methylene blue (blue-green)
Metronidazole (dark)
Nitrofurantoin (brown)
Oral anticoagulants (orange)
Phenazopyridine (orange, red, or orange-brown)
Phenolphthalein (red to purple-red)
Phenolsulfonphthalein (pink or red)
Phenothiazines (dark)
Phenytoin (red to reddish brown or pink)
Quinacrine (deep yellow)
Riboflavin (yellow)
Rifabutin (red-orange)
Rifampin (red-orange)
Sulfasalazine (orange-yellow)
Sulfobromophthalein (red)
Triamterene (blue-green)

## URINE ODOR

Antibiotics
Paraldehyde
Vitamins

## INCREASED URINE SPECIFIC GRAVITY

Albumin
Dextran
Glucose
Radiopaque contrast media

## DECREASED URINE PH

Ammonium chloride
Ascorbic acid
Diazoxide
Methenamine compounds
Metolazone

## INCREASED URINE PH

Acetazolamide
Amphotericin B
Carbonic anhydrase inhibitors
Mafenide
Potassium citrate
Sodium bicarbonate

## FALSE-POSITIVE RESULTS FOR PROTEINURIA

Acetazolamide (Combistix)
Aminosalicylic acid (sulfosalicylic acid or Exton's method)
Captopril
Cephalothin in large doses (sulfosalicylic acid method)
Dichlorphenamide
Fenoprofen
Methazolamide
Nafcillin (sulfosalicylic acid method)
d-Penicillamine
Sodium bicarbonate
Tolbutamide (sulfosalicylic acid method)
Tolmetin (sulfosalicylic acid method)

## TRUE PROTEINURIA

Aminoglycosides
Amphotericin B
Bacitracin
Cephalosporins
Cisplatin
Etretinate
Gold preparations
Isotretinoin
Nonsteroidal anti-inflammatory drugs
Phenylbutazone
Polymyxin B
Sulfonamides
Trimethadione

## EITHER TRUE PROTEINURIA OR FALSE-POSITIVE RESULTS

Penicillin in large doses (except with Ames reagent strips); some penicillins cause true proteinuria
Sulfonamides (sulfosalicylic acid method)

## FALSE-POSITIVE RESULTS FOR GLYCOSURIA

Aminosalicylic acid (Benedict's test)
Ascorbic acid (Clinistix, Diastix, Tes-Tape)
Ascorbic acid in large doses (Clinitest tablets)
Cephalosporins (Clinitest tablets)
Chloral hydrate (Benedict's test)
Chloramphenicol (Clinitest tablets)
Isoniazid (Benedict's test)

*(continued)*

# Drugs that influence routine urinalysis results *(continued)*

**FALSE-POSITIVE RESULTS FOR GLYCOSURIA** *(continued)*

Levodopa (Clinistix, Diastix, Tes-Tape)
Levodopa in large doses (Clinitest tablets)
Methyldopa (Tes-Tape)
Nalidixic acid (Benedict's test or Clinitest tablets)
Nitrofurantoin (Benedict's test)
Penicillin G in large doses (Benedict's test)
Phenazopyridine (Clinistix, Diastix, Tes-Tape)
Probenecid (Benedict's test, Clinitest tablets)
Salicylates in large doses (Clinitest tablets, Clinistix, Diastix, Tes-Tape)
Streptomycin (Benedict's test)
Tetracycline (Clinistix, Diastix, Tes-Tape)
Tetracyclines, due to ascorbic acid buffer (Benedict's test, Clinitest tablets)
Unasyn (ampicillin/sulbactam)

**TRUE GLYCOSURIA**

Ammonium chloride
Asparaginase
Carbamazepine
Corticosteroids
Dextrothyroxine
Estrogens
Lithium carbonate
Nicotinic acid (large doses)
Phenothiazines (long-term)
Phenytoin
Thiazide diuretics

**FALSE-POSITIVE RESULTS FOR KETONURIA**

Bromosulfophthalein
Isoniazid
Isopropanolol
Levodopa (Ketostix, Labstix)
Phenazopyridine (Ketostix or Gerhardt's reagent strip shows atypical color)
Phenolsulfonphthalein (Rothera's test)
Phenothiazines (Gerhardt's reagent strip shows atypical color)
Salicylates (Gerhardt's reagent strip shows reddish color)
Sulfobromophthalein (Bili-Labstix)

**TRUE KETONURIA**

Ether (anesthesia)
Insulin (excessive doses)
Isoniazid (intoxication)
Isopropyl alcohol (intoxication)

**INCREASED WHITE BLOOD CELL COUNT**

Allopurinol
Ampicillin
Aspirin (toxicity)
Kanamycin
Methicillin

**HEMATURIA**

Amphotericin B
Aspirin
Bacitracin
Caffeine
Coumadin derivatives
Gold
Indomethacin

**HEMATURIA** *(continued)*

Methenamine in large doses
Methicillin
Para-aminosalicylic acid
Phenylbutazone
Sulfonamides

**CASTS**

Amphotericin B
Aspirin (toxicity)
Bacitracin
Ethacrynic acid
Furosemide
Gentamicin
Griseofulvin
Isoniazid
Kanamycin
Neomycin
Penicillin
Radiographic agents
Streptomycin
Sulfonamides

**CRYSTALS (IF URINE IS ACIDIC)**

Acetazolamide
Aminosalicylic acid
Ascorbic acid
Nitrofurantoin
Theophylline
Thiazide diuretics

# URINE CULTURE

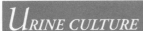

## Quick centrifugation test

The quick centrifugation test is used to determine the source of a urinary tract infection (UTI): the lower tract (bladder) or the upper tract (kidneys). The test involves centrifugation of urine in a test tube, followed by staining of the sediment with fluorescein. If at least one-fourth of the bacteria fluoresce when viewed under a fluorescent microscope, an upper-tract UTI is present; if bacteria don't fluoresce, a lower-tract UTI is present.

## CPT codes

87086 *Culture, bacterial, urine; quantitative, colony count*
87088 *Culture, bacterial, urine; with isolation and presumptive identification of isolates*

## Overview

Laboratory examination and culture of urine are necessary for evaluation of urinary tract infections (UTIs) — most commonly bladder infections. Although urine in the kidneys and bladder is normally sterile, a small number of bacteria are usually present in the urethra and, consequently, may pass into the urine. Nevertheless, bacteriuria generally results from prevalence of a single type of bacteria. Indeed, the presence of more than two distinct bacterial species in a urine specimen strongly suggests contamination during collection. However, a single negative culture does not always rule out infection, as in chronic, low-grade pyelonephritis. Urine cultures also identify pathogenic fungi such as Coccidioides immitis.

Many laboratories perform a quick and easy screen on urine submitted for culture. A common screening test used is the leukocyte esterase-nitrate dipstick. The purpose of the screen is to determine if the urine contains high bacteria or white blood cell (WBC) counts. Only the urine with bacteria or WBCs is processed for culture; urine that doesn't contain either of these is classified as negative by urine screen.

Significant results of urine culture are possible only after quantitative examination. To distinguish between true bacteriuria and contamination, it's necessary to know the number of organisms in a milliliter of urine, estimated by a culture technique known as a "colony count." In addition, a quick centrifugation test can determine where a UTI originates. (See *Quick centrifugation test.*)

Clean-voided midstream collection, rather than suprapubic aspiration or catheterization, is now the method of choice for obtaining a urine specimen.

## Indications

- To diagnose UTI
- To monitor microorganism colonization after urinary catheter insertion

## Contraindications

■ A contaminated specimen

## Preprocedure patient preparation

■ Explain to the patient that this test helps detect UTI. Advise him that it requires a urine specimen and that he needn't restrict food or fluids.

■ Teach him how to collect a clean-voided midstream specimen, and emphasize the importance of cleaning the external genitalia thoroughly. Or, if appropriate, explain catheterization or suprapubic aspiration to the patient, and inform him that he may experience some discomfort during specimen collection.

■ Tell the patient with suspected urogenital tuberculosis that specimen collection may be required on three consecutive mornings.

■ Check the patient history for current use of antimicrobial drugs.

## Equipment

Gloves ◆ sterile specimen cup ◆ premoistened, antiseptic towelettes (Commercial clean-catch urine kits are available; many include instructions in several languages.)

## Procedure

■ Explain the procedure to the patient, and address any questions or concerns he may have.

■ Instruct the patient to obtain a clean-catch midstream urine specimen. (See "Urinalysis," page 509.)

If necessary, perform suprapubic bladder aspiration (see "Suprapubic bladder aspiration," page 451) or urinary catheterization (see "Straight catheterization," page 425) to obtain the specimen. Put on gloves, take the specimen container from the patient, and be sure the sterile lid is on securely. Record the suspected diagnosis, the collection time and method, current antimicrobial therapy, and fluid- or drug-induced diuresis on the laboratory request.

■ Send the specimen to the laboratory immediately. If transport is delayed for more than 30 minutes, store the specimen at 39.2° F (4° C) or place it on ice, unless a urine transport tube containing preservatives is used.

## Postprocedure patient teaching

■ Advise the patient as to when the test results will be available. Provide teaching and treatment and recommend follow-up as appropriate.

## Complications

■ None known

## Special considerations

■ Collect at least 3 ml of urine, but don't fill the specimen cup more than halfway.

■ Culture results of sterile urine are normally reported as "no growth," which usually indicates the absence of UTI.

- Bacterial counts of 100,000 or more organisms of a single microbe species per milliliter indicate probable UTI. Counts under 100,000/ml may be significant, depending on the patient's age, sex, history, and other individual factors; however, these counts typically suggest that the organisms are contaminants, except in symptomatic patients or those with urologic disorders.
- All growths from catheterized urine or suprapubic aspirations are considered significant and are investigated by using susceptibility tests to identify the causative organism.
- A special test for acid-fast bacteria can isolate Mycobacterium tuberculosis, indicating tuberculosis of the urinary tract.
- Isolation of more than two species of organisms or of vaginal or skin organisms usually suggests contamination and requires a repeat culture.
- Antimicrobials are the treatment of choice (single-dose or 3- to 5-day regimens) to kill the pathogen and render the urine sterile.

## Documentation

- Record the indications for the procedure, method of specimen collection, and the appearance, color, odor, and amount of urine obtained.
- Document patient teaching, treatment prescribed, and follow-up care as necessary.

# UTERINE CONTRACTION PALPATION

**CPT code**
*No specific code has been assigned.*

## Overview

Periodic, involuntary uterine contractions characterize normal labor and cause progressive cervical effacement and dilation, impelling the fetus to descend. Uterine palpation can tell you the frequency, duration, and intensity of contractions as well as the relaxation time between them. The character of contractions varies with the stage of labor and the body's response to labor-inducing drugs, if administered. As labor advances, contractions become more intense, occur more often, and last longer. (See *Quick guide to stages of labor,* page 518.)

## Indications

- To assess labor and patient's response to interventions

## Contraindications

- None known

## Preprocedure patient preparation

- Advise the patient that uterine contraction palpation involves placing fingertips lightly on the edge of the uterus farthest from

## Quick guide to stages of labor

Normal labor advances through the four stages summarized below. Offer your patient encouragement and progress reports throughout the stages.

### FIRST STAGE
Regular contractions, which repeat at 15- to 20-minute intervals and last between 10 and 30 seconds, signal the onset of labor's first stage. This stage has three phases: latent, active, and transitional. In primiparous patients, the first stage of labor may range from 3.3 to 19.7 hours; in multiparous patients, it may range from 0.1 to 14.3 hours.

In the latent phase (characterized by irregular, brief, and mild contractions), the cervix dilates to 3 or 4 cm. Other signs and symptoms include abdominal cramping and backache. The patient may expel the mucus plug during this phase. This phase averages 8.6 hours in primiparous patients and 5.3 hours in multiparous patients.

During the active phase, cervical dilation increases to between 5 and 7 cm. Contractions occur every 3 to 5 minutes, last 30 to 45 seconds, and become moderately intense. In primiparous patients, this phase averages 5.8 hours; in multiparous patients, this phase averages 2.5 hours.

In the transitional phase, the cervix dilates completely (8 to 10 cm). Uterine contractions grow intense, last between 45 and 60 seconds, and repeat at least every 2 minutes. The patient may thrash about, lose control of breathing techniques, and experience nausea and vomiting. This phase typically lasts less than 3 hours in primiparous patients and less than 1 hour in multiparous patients.

### SECOND STAGE
In the second stage of labor, contractions occur every $1\frac{1}{2}$ to 2 minutes and last up to 90 seconds. This stage commonly ends within 1 hour for a primiparous patient and possibly 15 minutes for a multiparous patient.

Signs and symptoms signaling onset of the second stage include increased bloody show, rupture of membranes (if they're still intact), severe rectal pressure and flaring, and reflexive bearing down with each contraction. The fetal head approaches the perineal floor and emerges at the vaginal opening. The second labor stage concludes with birth.

### THIRD STAGE
Strong but less painful contractions expel the placenta, which normally emerges within 30 minutes after the neonate emerges. Signs indicating normal separation of the placenta from the uterine wall include lengthening of the umbilical cord, a sudden gush of dark blood from the vagina, and a palpable change in uterine shape from disclike to globular.

### FOURTH STAGE
This stage begins with placental expulsion and extends through the next 4 hours, while the patient's body rests and begins adjusting to the postpartum state.

the vaginal opening, and feeling the changes in muscle tension that occur with contractions. Normal uterine contractions are like waves, with the muscle hardness slowly building to a peak (also called an acme), and then subsiding.

## Equipment

Watch with a second hand ◆ sheet (for draping)

## Procedure

■ Review the patient's admission history to determine the onset, frequency, duration, and intensity of contractions. Also, note where contractions feel strongest or exert the most pressure.

■ Wash your hands and provide privacy.

■ Describe the palpation procedure to the patient and answer any questions she may have. Because she may be ticklish or sensitive to touch, forewarn her that you'll palpate her abdominal area over the uterus.

■ Assist the patient to a comfortable side-lying position to relieve pressure on the inferior vena cava and promote uteroplacental circulation. This position also relieves direct pressure on the sacral area from the fetal head and eases backache.

■ Drape the patient with a sheet.

■ Plant the palmar surface of your fingers on the uterine fundus, and palpate lightly to assess contractions. Note the uterine tightening and abdominal lifting that occur with contractions. Each contraction has three phases: increment (rising), acme (peak), and decrement (letting down or ebbing).

■ Palpate several contractions. Simultaneously, use the second hand on your watch to assess and measure such contraction qualities as frequency, duration, and intensity.

■ To assess frequency of the contraction, time the interval between the beginning of one contraction and the beginning of the next. In normal labor, contractions begin slowly and gradually occur more frequently with briefer relaxation intervals.

■ To assess duration of the contraction, time the period from when the uterus begins tightening until it begins relaxing. As labor progresses, contractions typically last longer.

■ To assess intensity of the contraction, press your fingertips into the uterine fundus when the uterus tightens. During mild contractions, the fundus indents easily and feels like a chin; during moderate contractions, the fundus indents less easily and feels like a nose; and during strong contractions, the fundus resists indenting and feels like a forehead.

■ Determine how the patient copes with discomfort by assessing her breathing and relaxation techniques, if any. This may help guide your intervention choices. Provide ongoing emotional support.

■ Observe the patient's response to contractions to evaluate whether she needs an analgesic, anesthetic, or other appropriate measures, such as repositioning and back massage.

■ Assess contractions at least hourly during the latent phase of first-stage labor and every 30 minutes throughout the active phase. During second-stage labor, assess contractions every 15 minutes.

## Postprocedure patient teaching

■ Tell the patient that her uterine contractions will be assessed periodically to determine their interval, character, and duration. This information is helpful in the assessment of how labor is progressing and permits early intervention if there isn't an adequate interval between contractions. The interval between contractions is important, not only to allow her respite, but also to permit a return of full blood flow to the fetus.

## Complications
- None known

## Special considerations
- Because the patient may become irritable or anxious during the transitional phase of first-stage labor — when the cervix dilates fully — and because abdominal palpation may aggravate her distress, assess contractions only as necessary. If appropriate, teach her support person to palpate and record contractions.
- If any contraction lasts longer than 90 seconds and isn't followed by uterine muscle relaxation, further evaluate maternal and fetal well-being. Also, evaluate a brief relaxation period between contractions because inadequate relaxation intervals increase the risk of fetal hypoxia and exhaust the patient.
- Be aware that false labor (or Braxton Hicks) contractions occur at irregular intervals and vary in intensity. They're felt over the abdomen and are often relieved by walking. During false labor, membranes remain intact, and there is no show of blood or progressive cervical dilation or effacement.

## Documentation
- Record the frequency, duration, and intensity of contractions.
- Keep track of the relaxation time between contractions, and describe the patient's response to contractions.

## VAGINAL EXAMINATION

**CPT code**
*No specific code has been assigned.*

### Overview

Vaginal examination is performed during first-stage labor to assess cervical dilation, effacement, membrane status, and fetal presentation, position, and engagement.

Important considerations during the examination include respecting the patient's privacy, providing simple explanations for her and her support person, maintaining eye contact when possible, and using aseptic technique. This enables the examination to proceed precisely and efficiently.

### Indications

- To check for cervical changes before ruling out labor
- To perform routine assessment during labor
- To check for rupture of membranes (ROM)
- To exclude the presence of cord prolapse following spontaneous rupture of membranes
- To evaluate cervical changes prior to the administration of analgesics

### Contraindications

**RELATIVE**
- Premature labor (prior to the completion of 37 weeks' gestation)
- Premature ROM (prior to the completion of 37 weeks' gestation)
- Active genital herpes
- Known placenta previa
- Less than 4 hours since the last vaginal examination
- Excessive vaginal bleeding, which may signal placenta previa or abruptio placentae

### Preprocedure patient preparation

- Give the patient an opportunity to empty her bladder because a distended bladder may interfere with accurate examination findings.

# Step-by-step vaginal examination

Begin the vaginal examination—usually in early labor—by inserting your gloved index and middle fingers palm side down into the vagina. Use your nondominant hand to gently but firmly press on the uterus to steady the fetal presenting part against the cervix for examination, as shown below.

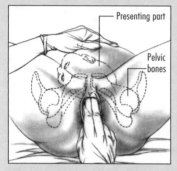

Presenting part

Pelvic bones

## CONFIRM THE PRESENTING PART AND POSITION

Rotate your fingers to palpate and confirm the fetal presenting part (a fetal head feels firm, the buttocks soft) and position (left, right, anterior, posterior, or transverse), identified by using Leopold's maneuvers, as shown below.

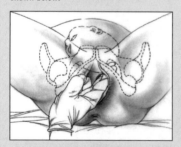

## ASSESS CERVICAL EFFACEMENT AND DILATION

Estimate cervical dilation by palpating the internal os. Each fingerbreadth of dilation averages 1.5 to 2 cm, depending on the width of the examiner's finger.

Next, determine the percentage of effacement by palpating the ridge of tissue around the cervix. Assign a low percentage of effacement to defined and thick cervical tissue. Indistinct, wafer-thin cervical tissue scores 100%.

## ASSESS FETAL ENGAGEMENT AND STATION

Estimate the extent of fetal engagement (descent of the fetal presenting part into the pelvis). Then palpate the presenting part and grade the fetal station (where the presenting part lies in relation to the ischial spines of the maternal pelvis). A zero grade indicates that the presenting part lies level with the ischial spines.

Station grades range from −3 (3 cm above the maternal ischial spines) to +4 (4 cm below the maternal ischial spines, causing the perineum to bulge), as shown below.

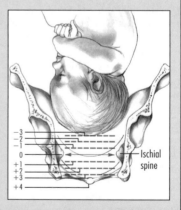

Ischial spine

## EVALUATE MEMBRANE STATUS

If appropriate, also check amniotic membrane status. If you feel a bulging, slick surface over the presenting fetal part, you know the membranes remain intact.

## Equipment

Sterile gloves ◆ sterile water-soluble lubricant or sterile water ◆ linen-saver pads ◆ sterile gauze

## Procedure

■ Explain the procedure to the patient and address any questions she may have.

■ Use Leopold's maneuvers to identify the fetal presenting part and position. Then help the patient into a lithotomy position for the vaginal examination.

■ Wash your hands. Place a linen-saver pad under the patient's buttocks, and put on sterile gloves.

■ Inform the patient when you are about to touch her to avoid startling her.

■ Apply sterile lubricating gel to your index and middle finger.

■ Spread the labia with the thumb and ring finger of your examining hand.

■ Ask the patient to relax by taking several deep breaths and slowly releasing the air. Then insert your lubricated fingers (palmar surface down) into the vagina. Keep your uninserted fingers flexed to avoid the rectum. Be mindful of where your thumb is; it should be in a tucked position. Flexing the thumb or even resting it against the clitoris can cause the patient undue discomfort. (See *Step-by-step vaginal examination.*)

■ Palpate the cervix, keeping in mind that it may assume a posterior position in early labor and be difficult to locate. When you find the cervix, note its consistency.

The cervix gradually softens throughout pregnancy, reaching a buttery consistency before labor begins. (See *Cervical effacement and dilation,* page 524.)

■ Gently withdraw your fingers after identifying the presenting fetal part and position, evaluating dilation and effacement, assessing fetal engagement and station, and verifying membrane status. Let the patient clean her perineum herself with sterile gauze if she can walk to the bathroom. If she's confined to bed, you can clean her perineum and change the linen-saver pad.

■ To encourage the patient and help reduce her anxiety, describe how labor is progressing, and define the stage and phase if appropriate.

## Postprocedure patient teaching

■ Notify the patient of the degree of dilation. Be certain to emphasize that the cervix opens very slowly until it's about halfway dilated, then it opens fully very quickly.

## Complications

■ None known

## Special considerations

■ Patients with immunoglobulin A deficiency are at increased risk for an anaphylactic reaction.

■ In early labor, perform the vaginal examination between contractions, focusing primarily on the

## Cervical effacement and dilation

As labor advances, so do cervical effacement and dilation, thereby facilitating birth. During effacement, the cervix shortens and its walls become thin, progressing from 0% effacement (palpable and thick) to 100% effacement (fully indistinct—or effaced— and paper thin). Full effacement obliterates the constrictive uterine neck to create a smooth, unobstructed passage for the fetus.

At the same time, dilation occurs. This progressive widening of the cervical canal—from the upper internal cervical os to the lower external cervical os—advances from 0 to 10 cm. As the cervical canal opens, resistance decreases. This further eases fetal descent.

NO EFFACEMENT
OR DILATION

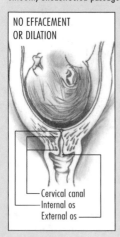

Cervical canal
Internal os
External os

EARLY EFFACEMENT
AND DILATION

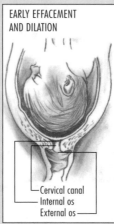

Cervical canal
Internal os
External os

FULL EFFACEMENT
AND DILATION

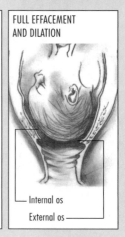

Internal os

External os

extent of cervical dilation and effacement. At the end of first-stage labor, perform the examination during a contraction, when the uterine muscle pushes the fetus downward. This examination will focus on assessing fetal descent.

■ If the amniotic membrane ruptures during the examination, record the fetal heart rate. Then note the time, and describe the color, odor, and approximate amount of fluid. Determine fetal station, and check for umbilical cord prolapse. After the membranes rupture, perform the vaginal examination only when labor changes significantly to minimize the risk of introducing intrauterine infection.

### Documentation

■ After each examination, record the percentage of effacement, centimeters dilated, the station of the presenting fetal part, amniotic membrane status, and the patient's tolerance of the procedure.

# VENIPUNCTURE

## CPT code
36415 *Routine venipuncture or finger, heel, or ear stick for collection of specimen(s)*

## Overview
Venipuncture involves piercing a vein with a needle, then collecting blood in a syringe or evacuated tube. Typically, venipuncture is performed using the antecubital fossa. If necessary, however, it can be performed on a vein in the wrist, the dorsum of the hand or foot, or another accessible location.

## Indications
■ To obtain a venous blood sample

## Contraindications
■ Distorted (from trauma or surgery) or infected local anatomy

## Preprocedure patient preparation
■ Tell the patient that you're about to collect a blood sample.
■ Tell the patient he will feel a "pinch" when the needle is inserted. Ask him if he's ever felt faint, sweaty, or nauseated when having blood drawn.

## Equipment
Tourniquet ◆ gloves ◆ syringe or evacuated tubes and needle holder ◆ alcohol or povidone-iodine pads ◆ 20G or 21G needle for the forearm or 25G needle for the wrist, hand, and ankle, and for children ◆ color-coded collection tubes containing appropriate additives (See *Guide to color-top collection tubes,* page 526.) ◆ 2″ × 2″ gauze pads ◆ adhesive bandage ◆ labels ◆ laboratory request forms

### Equipment preparation
■ If you're using evacuated tubes, open the needle packet, attach the needle to its holder, and select the appropriate tubes.
■ If you're using a syringe, attach the appropriate needle to it. Be sure to choose a syringe large enough to hold all the blood required for the test.
■ Label all collection tubes clearly with the patient's name and the date and time of collection.

## Procedure
■ Explain the procedure to the patient, and address any questions or concerns he may have.
■ Wash your hands and put on gloves.
■ Ask the patient to sit in a chair and support his arm securely on an armrest or table.
■ Assess the patient's veins to determine the best puncture site. (See *Common venipuncture sites,* page 527.) Observe the skin for the vein's blue color, or palpate the vein for a firm rebound sensation.

## Guide to color-top collection tubes

Refer to this table when selecting color-coded collection tubes before venipuncture.

| TUBE COLOR | DRAW VOLUME | ADDITIVE | PURPOSE |
|---|---|---|---|
| Red | 2 to 20 ml | None | Serum studies |
| Lavender | 2 to 10 ml | EDTA | Whole-blood studies |
| Green | 2 to 15 ml | Heparin (sodium, lithium, or ammonium) | Plasma studies |
| Blue | 2.7 or 4.5 ml | Sodium citrate and citric acid | Coagulation studies on plasma |
| Black | 2.7 or 4.5 ml | Sodium oxalate | Coagulation studies on plasma |
| Gray | 3 to 10 ml | Glycolytic inhibitor, such as sodium fluoride, powdered oxalate, or glycolytic-microbial inhibitor | Glucose determinations on serum or plasma |
| Yellow | 12 ml | Acid-citrate-dextrose (ACD) | Whole-blood studies |

■ Tie a tourniquet 2″ (5 cm) proximal to the area chosen. By impeding venous return to the heart while still allowing arterial flow, a tourniquet produces venous dilation. If arterial perfusion remains adequate, you'll be able to feel the radial pulse. (If the tourniquet fails to dilate the vein, have the patient open and close his fist repeatedly. Then ask him to close his fist as you insert the needle and to open it again when the needle is in place.)

■ Clean the venipuncture site with an alcohol or a povidone-iodine pad. Don't wipe off the povidone-iodine with alcohol because alcohol cancels the effect of povidone-iodine. Wipe in a circular motion, spiraling outward from the site to avoid introducing potentially infectious skin flora into the vessel during the procedure. If you use alcohol, apply it with friction for 30 seconds or until the final pad comes away clean. Allow the skin to dry before performing venipuncture.

■ Immobilize the vein by pressing just below the venipuncture site with your thumb and drawing the skin taut.

■ Position the needle holder or syringe with the needle bevel up and the shaft parallel to the path of the vein and at a 30-degree angle to the arm. Insert the needle into the

## Common venipuncture sites

The illustrations below depict the anatomic locations of veins commonly used for venipuncture. The most commonly used sites are on the forearm, followed by those on the hand.

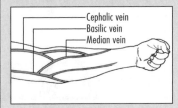

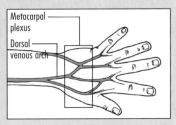

vein. If you're using a syringe, venous blood will appear in the hub; withdraw the blood slowly, pulling the plunger of the syringe gently to create steady suction until you obtain the required sample. Pulling the plunger too forcibly may collapse the vein. If you're using a needle holder and an evacuated tube, grasp the holder securely to stabilize it in the vein, and push down on the collection tube until the needle punctures the rubber stopper. Blood will flow into the tube automatically.

■ Remove the tourniquet as soon as blood flows adequately to prevent stasis and hemoconcentration, which can impair test results. If the flow is sluggish, leave the tourniquet in place longer, but always remove it before withdrawing the needle.

■ Continue to fill the required tubes, removing one and inserting another. Gently rotate each tube as you remove it to help mix the additive with the sample.

■ After you've drawn the sample, place a gauze pad over the puncture site and slowly and gently remove the needle from the vein. When using an evacuated tube, remove it from the needle holder to release the vacuum before withdrawing the needle from the vein.

■ Apply gentle pressure to the puncture site for 2 to 3 minutes or until bleeding stops. This prevents extravasation into the surrounding tissue, which can cause a hematoma.

■ After bleeding stops, apply an adhesive bandage.

■ If you've used a syringe, transfer the sample to a collection tube. Detach the needle from the syringe, open the collection tube, and gently empty the sample into the tube, being careful to avoid foaming, which can cause hemolysis.

■ Finally, check the venipuncture site to see if a hematoma has developed. If it has, apply warm soaks to the site.

■ Discard syringes, needles, and used gloves in the appropriate containers.

## Postprocedure patient teaching

■ Advise the patient as to when his test results will be available. Provide treatment, teaching, and follow-up care as appropriate.

## Complications

■ A hematoma at the needle insertion site is the most common complication of venipuncture.
■ Infection may result from poor technique.

## Special considerations

■ Don't collect a venous sample from an infection site because this may introduce pathogens into the vascular system. Likewise, avoid collecting blood from edematous areas, arteriovenous shunts, and sites of previous hematomas or vascular injury.
■ If the patient has large, distended, highly visible veins, perform venipuncture without a tourniquet to minimize the risk of hematoma formation. If the patient has a clotting disorder or is receiving anticoagulant therapy, maintain firm pressure on the venipuncture site for at least 5 minutes after withdrawing the needle to prevent hematoma formation.
■ Avoid using veins in the patient's legs for venipuncture, if possible, because this increases the risk of thrombophlebitis.

## Documentation

■ Record the date, time, and site of the venipuncture; the name of the test; the time the sample was sent to the laboratory; the amount of blood collected; the patient's temperature; and any adverse reactions to the procedure.

# VISION EVALUATION

*CPT code*
*No specific code has been assigned. The procedure is usually charged as part of the clinical examination.*

## Overview

The purpose of this procedure is to assess visual acuity, visual field defects, and color vision and to determine the presence or absence of strabismus — all of which must be detected early for intervention to be most effective. Visual acuity is best assessed using the Snellen eye chart if the patient is able to read or the Illiterate E chart if the patient can't read. Defects of the visual fields are best identified through confrontation testing, and color vision is best assessed using Ishihara's book. To determine and identify the presence or absence of strabismus, the cover/uncover test, corneal light reflex test, or extraocular muscle movement tests are usually performed.

## Indications

■ To perform routine screening as part of wellness visit
■ To evaluate visual function and acuity
■ To detect visual defects
■ To assess visual complaints
■ To determine level of ocular trauma
■ To screen for school or employment

## Contraindications

■ None known

## Preprocedure patient preparation

■ Inform the patient that no pain or discomfort is associated with this procedure.

## Equipment

Penlight ◆ Snellen chart, Illiterate E chart (also called the tumbling E), or a standard near-vision pocket chart ◆ color vision book such as Ishihara's (optional)

## Procedure

■ Obtain a complete history and physical examination.
■ Explain the procedure to the patient or parent, and address any questions or concerns they may have.
■ Perform the screening in a well-lit area where the patient can stand 20′ (6 m) from the Snellen chart. If using the near-vision pocket chart, the chart should be 14″ (35.6 cm) from the patient's eyes.

### Visual acuity

■ Have the patient cover one eye and ask him to identify all the letters beginning at any line.
■ Determine the smallest line in which he can identify all the letters, and record the visual acuity.
■ Repeat this step with the opposite eye and then perform the screening with both of the patient's eyes open.
■ Alternatively, if the patient can't read, use the Illiterate E chart and have him point his finger in the direction of the E on the chart.

### Visual fields, confrontation

■ Standing 2′ (0.6 m) away from the patient, have him cover one eye and look into your uncovered eye. For example, if the patient covers his left eye, you should cover your right eye.
■ Move an object, such as a pen or penlight, into each of the visual fields and have the patient tell you when he can see the object in each area. The examiner's view and the patient's view should match.

### Color vision

■ Using a color vision book, have the patient describe the number he sees on each page. The numbers or figures in the color vision book are distorted by color variances and are unreadable to the person who has abnormal color discrimination ability.

*Strabismus*

■ Carefully observe both eyes for any obvious deviation.

■ Standing directly in front of the patient at a distance of 2', shine a light into his eyes and inspect the reflections of the light in each cornea. Then ask the patient to follow the light as you move through the six cardinal fields of gaze (making a large H in the air, guide the patient's gaze to the extreme right, to the upper right, to the lower right, to the extreme left, to the upper left, and to the lower left).

■ Looking directly at the patient's eyes, cover one of his eyes for a brief time. Unveil the eye and observe for any movement of the uncovered eye indicating it had strayed while covered. Repeat the procedure with the opposite eye.

## Postprocedure patient teaching

■ Explain the results of the testing and the epidemiology, if there is a problem. Discuss choices for therapeutic interventions and expected resolution timetable. Instruct the patient or parent on the need for follow-up care and evaluation, and specify the date for each. If deviations from the norm are elicited, refer him to the appropriate professional.

■ Provide verbal and written instructions. Any referrals should include the provider's name, address, and phone number. Explain the need for prompt evaluation by an ophthalmologist and provide a specific time frame for further evaluation.

■ If a prescription is written, instruct the patient to take all of the medication that's prescribed and administer it as ordered.

■ Instruct the patient to call you if any vision problems develop.

## Complications

■ None known

## Special considerations

**COLLABORATION**
*If a vision problem is detected, consult with a vision specialist or consider immediate referral.*

## Documentation

■ Note the reason for vision testing.

■ Record the number, type, and frequency of problems.

■ List any previous treatment modalities.

■ Record findings of all visual tests performed, and whether the patient was wearing corrective eyeglasses or contact lenses for the testing.

■ Document referral recommendations, including contact information given and risks of not being further evaluated or treated.

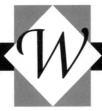

## WOOD'S LIGHT EXAMINATION

**CPT code**
*No specific code has been assigned.*

## Overview

The Wood's light is used in many observational assessments, ophthalmologic procedures, and dermatologic presentations to enhance visibility and aid diagnosis. The lamp converts ultraviolet light into visible light. A fluorescein stain and a magnifying lens are sometimes used to help increase visibility of the area being examined. In ophthalmologic procedures, the fluorescein stain allows the injured area in the cornea or sclera to present as a bright yellow-green color. In dermatologic presentations, the light allows the health care provider to see many lesions and parasites that might otherwise go undetected.

## Indications

■ To aid differential diagnosis of bacterial, fungal, and pigmented skin lesions and to delineate borders of suspicious lesions
■ To enhance visualization of corneal abrasions, ulcers, and foreign objects in the cornea and conjunctiva
■ To detect porphyria

## Contraindications

■ None known

## Preprocedure patient preparation

■ Explain the purpose of the Wood's light examination.
■ Assure the patient that the procedure is painless.

## Equipment

Wood's light apparatus ◆ magnifying lens, if necessary, for increased visibility ◆ fluorescein stain (optional)

## Procedure

■ Explain the procedure to the patient, and address any questions or concerns he may have.
■ Wash your hands.

## Understanding Wood's light findings

A Wood's light is commonly used with a fluorescein stain and a magnifying glass to aid in the differential diagnosis of dermatologic problems (such as fungal infections) and ophthalmologic conditions (such as corneal abrasions). Make your diagnosis only after reviewing the patient's history and physical findings; the following table can help you narrow your focus. The listed findings pertain to the skin, unless otherwise noted.

| WOOD'S LIGHT FINDINGS | POTENTIAL DIAGNOSES |
| --- | --- |
| Cold bright white | Albinism or loss of pigmentation |
| Blue-white | Tuberous sclerosis (genetic), hypopigmentation, leprosy, vitiligo |
| Blue-green to green | Pseudomonas |
| Pale green to brilliant green | Dermatophytosis (tinea) |
| Off-white or yellow to deep green | Tinea versicolor |
| Bright yellow to green (conjunctiva) | Corneal abrasion |
| Darker, sometimes a purple brown | Hyperpigmentation |
| Orange red to pink red (urine) | Porphyria (genetic) |
| Pink to coral red | Erythrasma (bacteria) |
| Bright red | Squamous cell carcinoma |
| Enhanced visualization of tunneling beneath the skin and mites | Scabies (parasite) |
| Enhanced visualization of lice | Pediculosis (parasite) |

■ Place him in a comfortable position that fully exposes the area to be examined.
■ Stain the area, if indicated.
■ Darken the room.
■ Turn on the Wood's light to examine the area. Use a magnifying lens if necessary. Hold the light approximately 6″ to 8″ (15 to 20 cm) away for maximum effectiveness.

■ Note findings. (See *Understanding Wood's light findings*.)

### Postprocedure patient teaching

■ Explain the results of the examination to the patient, and provide treatment, teaching, and follow-up care as appropriate.

## Complications

■ None known

## Special considerations

■ Question the patient about any treatments, lotions, or ointments previously applied to the skin. Use of these items could confound your findings.

## Documentation

■ Include in your procedural documentation the use of the Wood's light in aiding and establishing your diagnosis.

# *WOUND DRESSING*

### CPT codes

16020 *Dressing and debridement, initial or subsequent, without anesthesia, office or hospital (small)*
16025 *Dressing and debridement, initial or subsequent, without anesthesia, office or hospital (medium)*
16030 *Dressing and debridement, initial or subsequent, without anesthesia, office or hospital (large)*

## Overview

Several considerations are involved in determining the type of dressing that will promote the optimal moist wound healing environment. First, assess the wound to determine: the timing of the injury (chronic or acute); the mechanism of the injury (surgical excision, burn, or other); the depth and size of injury; and the need for debridement.

The health care provider must also understand and recognize the phases of wound healing and tailor the wound dressing approach accordingly. A familiarity with the wide array of dressings available and their proper indications will aid in promoting the best healing environment for the patient's wound. (See *Tailoring wound care to wound color,* page 534.)

## Indications

■ To dress partial-thickness burns that extend no deeper than the mid-dermal level and involve less than 15% of total body surface area (TBSA)
■ To dress abrasions, skin tears, lacerations, and surgical wounds
■ To dress pressure ulcers, leg ulcers, and foot ulcers

## Contraindications

### ABSOLUTE

■ Partial-thickness burns that involve more than 15% TBSA
■ Full-thickness burns involving more than 2% TBSA
■ Any significant burn involving the face, perineum, hands, fingers, or toes

### RELATIVE

■ Significant wounds in children less than age 2 or adults age 75 or older, or in patients who are otherwise debilitated or immunologically compromised
■ Wounds that will require extensive surgical debridement

## Tailoring wound care to wound color

With any wound, promote healing by keeping it moist, clean, and free of debris. For open wounds, use wound color to guide the specific management approach and to assess how well the wound is healing.

### RED WOUND

Red, the color of healthy granulation tissue, indicates normal healing. When a wound begins to heal, a layer of pale pink granulation tissue covers the wound bed. As this layer thickens, it becomes beefy red. Cover a red wound, keep it moist and clean, and protect it from trauma. Use a transparent dressing (such as Tegaderm or Op-site), a hydrocolloid dressing (such as DuoDerm), or a gauze dressing moistened with sterile normal saline solution or impregnated with petroleum jelly or an antibiotic.

### YELLOW WOUND

Yellow is the color of exudate produced by microorganisms in an open wound. When a wound heals without complications, the immune system removes microorganisms. However, if there are too many microorganisms to remove, exudate accumulates and becomes visible. Exudate usually appears whitish yellow, creamy yellow, yellowish green, or beige. Dry exudate appears darker.

If your patient has a yellow wound, clean it and remove exudate, using high-pressure irrigation; then cover it with a moist dressing. Use absorptive products (for example, Debrisan beads and paste) or moist gauze dressing with or without an antibiotic. You may also use hydrotherapy with whirlpool or high-pressure irrigation.

### BLACK WOUND

Black, the least healthy color, signals necrosis. Dead, avascular tissue slows healing and provides a site for microorganisms to proliferate.

You should debride a black wound. After removing dead tissue, apply a dressing to keep the wound moist and guard against external contamination. Use enzyme products (such as Elase or Travase), surgical debridement, hydrotherapy with whirlpool or high-pressure irrigation, or a moist gauze dressing.

### MULTICOLORED WOUND

You may note two or even all three colors in a wound. In this case, you would classify the wound according to the least healthy color present. For example, if your patient's wound is both red and yellow, classify it as a yellow wound.

---

■ Wounds that are thought to be the result of nonaccidental trauma

## Preprocedure patient preparation

■ Administer tetanus toxoid if it has been more than 5 years since the patient last received a booster.
■ For burns, cover the wound with sterile gauze saturated with sterile iced saline while prepara-

tions for the procedure are being made.
■ For other wounds, apply a sterile pressure dressing and elevate the injured body part to promote hemostasis.
■ Assess the wound and discuss the treatment options with the patient.

# Equipment

Clean and sterile gloves ◆ sterile normal saline solution ◆ large syringe (20- or 60-ml) ◆ scalpel with #15 blade, scrub brush, or iris scissors ◆ topical antibiotic or 1% silver sulfadiazine (optional) ◆ sterile nonadherent dressing ◆ sterile 4″ × 4″ gauze ◆ flexible dressing wrap (such as Kling) ◆ equipment for local anesthesia (optional)

# Procedure

■ Explain the procedure to the patient, and address any questions or concerns he may have.

### ✔ OBTAIN INFORMED CONSENT

■ Wash your hands and put on gloves.

■ Gently wash the wound using sterile 4″ × 4″ gauze pads and mild soap (avoid hydrogen peroxide and other harsh cleansers because these may cause further tissue damage).

■ Remove gloves and put on a sterile pair.

■ Irrigate the wound with sterile normal saline solution and a 20- or 60-ml syringe and remove any foreign material, such as gravel and nonviable tissue. If the wound is grossly contaminated or requires extensive debridement, you may need to provide local anesthesia to the area. (See "Anesthesia: Topical, local, and digital nerve block," page 20.)

■ Further irrigate and debride the wound as needed using a scrub brush, scalpel, or scissors.

### ➤ CLINICAL TIP

*Creating a proper wound bed is essential to healing. If extensive debridement is necessary, consider referring the patient to a health care provider who specializes in wounds.*

■ For burns, remove blisters by using the scalpel if they're broken, tense and about to break, or in areas where breakage is inevitable, such as the soles of the feet or palms of the hands.

■ Apply a topical antibiotic or 1% silver sulfadiazine to the wound as necessary and cover with a nonadherent dressing such as a Telfa pad. Extend the gauze at least 1″ (2.5 cm) beyond the wound in each direction, and cover the wound evenly with enough dressing to absorb all drainage until the next dressing change.

### ➤ CLINICAL TIP

*There are a large number of specialty dressings that can be used for a variety of wound conditions. Familiarize yourself with these to greatly enhance your ability to effectively treat a wider spectrum of wounds.*

■ Apply several layers of absorbent dressing such as sterile 4″ × 4″ gauze pads.

■ Secure the wound site with a flexible dressing wrap and tape.

# Postprocedure teaching

■ Instruct the patient to keep the dressing clean and dry and to elevate the affected area whenever possible.

■ If the patient will be doing the dressing changes, provide him with a list of materials he'll need and teach him the proper technique. Instruct him to watch for signs of infection, such as redness, yellow or green drainage, a foul odor from the wound, or an increase in temperature. Tell him to notify your facility if he experiences any of these.

■ If pain medication is prescribed, provide the patient with instruction on proper usage.

■ Openly discuss with the patient the possibility of scarring to minimize unrealistic expectations.

■ Instruct the patient to return to the office for follow-up care in 24 to 48 hours.

## Complications

■ Infection can be avoided by maintaining strict aseptic technique throughout the procedure and treating contaminated wounds prophylactically with antibiotics.

■ Failure of the wound to heal or tissue necrosis should be referred to a health care provider with expertise in wounds.

## Special considerations

**COLLABORATION**

*Because wound care can be complex, some health care providers have expertise in treating wounds. Seek consultation early and often in cases that you aren't comfortable treating. Surgical consultation should be offered in all complex cases or anytime when scarring is a concern.*

■ Special precautions should be taken with the very young and the very old as well as with debilitated, malnourished, or immunocompromised patients.

■ Blood glucose control is essential to good healing in diabetic patients.

■ Ulcers must be "off-loaded" to accomplish healing — for example, non–weight bearing for foot ulcers.

## Documentation

■ Record the details of your initial wound assessment (size, condition of margins, presence of necrotic tissue, and odor), evidence of informed consent, the details of the procedure (including irrigation and debridement as necessary and a description of the dressing applied), and medications prescribed.

■ Document after-care instructions given and teaching provided.

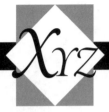

## X-RAY INTERPRETATION, ABDOMINAL

### CPT codes
74000 *Radiologic examination, abdomen; anteroposterior view*
74020 *Radiologic examination, abdomen; including decubitus and erect views*

### Overview

Abdominal X-rays can provide preliminary diagnostic information for problems originating in the abdomen. Because it allows for evaluation of the gastrointestinal, hepatobiliary, and genitourinary systems, it's one of the most common X-rays used. Although abdominal X-ray is less accurate than other imaging studies, such as ultrasound or computed tomography, it may aid the direction further, more specific testing may take. It also provides specific information regarding bowel gas pattern and the presence of stones or calcifications.

### Indications

■ To evaluate abdominal pain, distension, vomiting, diarrhea, and abdominal trauma
■ To detect kidney stones or other calcifications

### Contraindications
**ABSOLUTE**
■ Pregnancy

### Preprocedure patient preparation

■ Advise the patient that he must remain still to produce the best image as possible and that he may be asked to hold his breath while the X-ray is taken.

### Equipment
Abdominal X-rays ◆ X-ray view box or bright light to examine specific areas of the X-ray

### Procedure

■ Before reading the film, verify patient information and the position of left and right markers on the film.

## Right renal staghorn calculus

This plain X-ray film of a 70-year-old woman who hadn't received I.V. contrast shows a branching staghorn calcification, indicated by the arrows, filling the right renal collecting system.

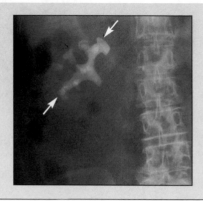

- Place the films on the illuminated view box.
- Judge the technical quality of the film, especially the adequacy of penetration (vertebral bodies should appear clear).
- Look briefly at films for obvious abnormalities. Then systematically evaluate the structures in the abdomen.
- Identify the skeletal landmarks in the abdomen, such as the pelvis, sacrum, and lumbar vertebrae. Evaluate for the presence of demineralization, pathologic calcifications, or fractures.
- Assess the diaphragm. Look below it to detect the presence of free air. Free air in the peritoneal cavity is a classic sign of perforation and appears as collections of air beneath the diaphragm. Look above the diaphragm for a good view of the lower lobes of the lungs.
- Evaluate the stomach and determine the presence of a gastric bubble, which is a normal finding that

appears about the size of a golfball in the fundus of the stomach.
- Evaluate the soft tissue contours of the liver, spleen, kidneys, and the psoas muscles. The spleen may be hidden by the gastric bubble; the uterus of the female patient and the pancreas generally aren't visible. The bladder may be visualized as a smooth, round mass if full. Assess for the enlargement of any organ (which may make it visible when it isn't usually seen) or for abdominal masses.
- Assess for the presence of calcifications. Gallstones and renal calculi are readily visible and may appear as bright white spots that are round, smooth, or jagged. Rapidly growing stones tend to branch and form staghorn shapes. (See *Right renal staghorn calculus.*) Assess for the presence of renal calculi in both kidneys, down the length of both ureters, and in the bladder. Vascular calcification refers to a widened, tortuous aorta or any of

## Ileus

The bowel-gas pattern in this 76-year-old man's postoperative abdominal X-ray reveals a diffuse, gas-filled dilation of the small bowel and colon, characteristic of an ileus.

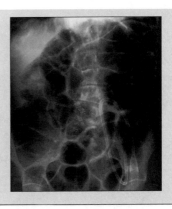

its branches (such as the renal arteries).

■ Observe the intestinal gas pattern, which is usually random and nonspecific. The small intestine has a lumen of about 1″ (2.5 cm); it extends in coils from the pyloric sphincter to the ileocecal valve and is encircled and framed by the large intestine. No air is typically seen in the small intestine, however a small amount may be considered normal. The large intestine extends from the ileocecal valve to the anus. Observe for disturbed or abnormal gas patterns. Radiographic findings of a patient with an ileus include retention of large amounts of gas and fluid in a dilated small and large bowel. The small and large bowels appear almost uniformly dilated, and no point of obstruction can be seen. (See *Ileus.*) Small-bowel obstruction may appear with dilated, gas-filled bowel loops and a lack of

colon gas. (See *Small-bowel obstruction*, page 540.)

■ Scan the entire peritoneum for signs of free air or fluid.

## Postprocedure patient teaching

■ Discuss the results of the X-ray finding with the patient.

## Complications

■ None known

## Special considerations

■ Contrasting agents such as barium may be administered to the patient to better outline the structures being studied.

■ Always interpret a patient's abdominal X-ray in light of his history and physical examination.

■ Compare any X-ray film with previous films.

■ Establish a pattern for evaluat-

## Small-bowel obstruction

A 73-year-old woman with breast cancer presented with abdominal pain and vomiting. A plain abdominal X-ray shows dilated, gas-filled bowel loops, indicated by the arrows, and lack of colon gas, indicating a small-bowel obstruction.

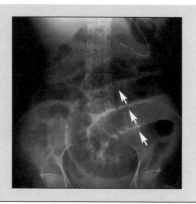

ing abdominal films to make it less likely to miss a pathology.

■ Remember that plain films have limitations; they aren't extremely sensitive so they may miss pathologies. Know when to move to further studies such as a computed tomography scan.

### Documentation

■ Document the details of your X-ray analysis, comparisons with previous films, and the correlation with clinical findings.

## X-RAY INTERPRETATION, BONE

### CPT codes
*Codes for X-ray examinations of major anatomic sites are listed here. For more options, refer to a CPT coding manual.*

| | |
|---|---|
| 70250 | *Skull* |
| 71015 | *Chest* |
| 71101 | *Ribs* |
| 72010 | *Spine* |
| 73020 | *Shoulder* |
| 73110 | *Wrist* |
| 73120 | *Hand* |
| 73500 | *Hip* |
| 73590 | *Lower leg* |
| 73600 | *Ankle* |
| 73650 | *Heel* |

### Overview
Plain X-rays are the most common initial screening technique and the most useful diagnostic tool for evaluating structural or functional changes in musculoskeletal diseases and injuries. X-rays obtained in multiple views, for example, will reveal most dislocations and fractures. They're also the main technique for detecting and monitoring scoliosis. X-rays record levels of brightness or shadow that reveal details about internal structures. (See *Brightness levels on*

## Brightness levels on X-ray

As emitted photons (commonly called X-rays) pass through the patient, they are deflected by body tissues and absorbed into film on the opposite side. The film is darkened by interaction with the X-rays. Therefore, darker areas indicate less X-ray absorption by the body and more film exposure.

X-rays are deflected and absorbed to different degrees by different body tissue types. The amount of absorption depends on the tissue composition. For example, dense bone tissue absorbs many more X-rays than soft tissues, such as muscle, fat, and blood. The amount of deflection depends on the density of electrons in the tissues. Tissues with high electron density cause more X-ray scattering than those of lower density. The table below shows levels of brightness associated with specific density levels.

| SHADE | GROSS IDENTIFICATION | EXAMPLES |
|---|---|---|
| Bright white | Metal | Jewelry, teeth fillings |
| Almost as white as metal | Bone tissue | Bone |
| Medium brightness | Fluid and muscle tissue | Organs, blood vessels |
| Gray black | Adipose tissue | Breast tissue, fat deposits |
| Black (radiolucent) | Air | Air in lungs, emphysema |

*X-ray.*) They also assist in identifying pathologic processes, such as arthritis, bone lesions, and fractures.

Bones — classified by shape and location — may be long (humerus, radius, femur, and tibia), short (carpals and tarsals), flat (scapula, ribs, and skull), irregular (vertebrae and mandible), or sesamoid (patella). There are two basic types of bone tissue: compact and spongy (cancellous). Compact bone is dense and looks smooth and uniform. Spongy bone is composed of small needlelike or flat pieces of bone called trabeculae. Spongy bone has large amounts of open space.

The long axis of a bone, called the shaft or diaphysis, is made of a thick collar of compact bone that surrounds a medullary cavity. In adults, the medullary cavity contains fat (yellow marrow) and is called the yellow bone marrow cavity. This long shaft merges into a broader, necklike portion called the metaphysis, composed of spongy bone. The end of the bone, the epiphysis, has a thin layer of compact bone on the outside and red marrow on the inside. In young bones, cartilage at the end of the shaft, where the metaphysis and the epiphysis meet, allows space for the long bone to lengthen as the body grows. (See *Internal structures of bone,* page 542.)

The periosteum helps protect the bone. The outer layer of the periosteum is made of dense, irreg-

## Internal structures of bone

To interpret X-ray studies accurately, you must have a thorough understanding of gross and microscopic anatomy. This illustration identifies the internal structures of bone.

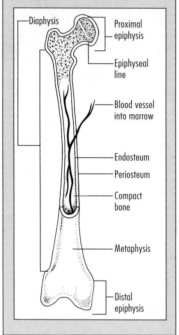

### Indications

- To confirm suspicion of bone injury, deformity, or disease
- To investigate pain of unknown etiology
- To evaluate multiple trauma or any laceration, hematoma, angulation, or edema in long bone or joint

### Contraindications
**RELATIVE**
- Pregnancy, particularly in the first trimester

### Preprocedure patient preparation

- Advise the patient that he may feel slight discomfort or pain, either from touching cold metal surfaces or from positioning the body part to be X-rayed. Reassure him that any discomfort should resolve within minutes after the procedure is completed.
- Emphasize the importance of following directions closely to avoid adversely affecting the quality of the X-ray.
- Explain that radiation from individual X-ray studies is minimal and that the reproductive organs are covered with lead shields.

### Equipment
X-ray view box or bright light to examine specific areas of the X-ray

### Procedure
- Verify the patient's name as well

ular connective tissue; the inner layer, abutting the bone surface, consists primarily of bone-forming cells, or osteoblasts. The periosteum is densely laced with nerve fibers, lymphatic vessels, and blood vessels, which enter the bone. The junctions of long bones that articulate, or move, are covered with a smooth articular cartilage that cushions the bone ends and absorbs stress during joint movement.

## Rheumatoid arthritis of the hands

This is the X-ray film of a mature male with rheumatoid arthritis. The X-ray reveals periarticular soft tissue swelling (as indicated by ➤➤) and many erosions involving the distal ulna, carpals, metacarpals, and phalanges (as indicated by ➤). Narrowing of the joint spaces is also apparent. Also, note the periarticular osteoporosis around the metacarpal and phalangeal joints (as indicated by ✳).

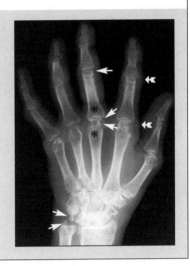

as the date and time of the X-ray study.

■ Complete a thorough history and physical examination, focusing on the suspected mechanism of injury. Any suspected fracture requires complete evaluation of adjacent joints.

■ Verify that a female patient isn't pregnant before ordering X-rays.

■ If you're unsure about the best X-ray view to order, write the site to be X-rayed and identify what you expect to find or rule out.

■ Request that the patient's previous films be retrieved for comparison.

■ Verify the position of the X-ray in the view box: check right and left markers to ensure that your view is as if you were facing the patient (your left should be the X-ray study's right).

■ Confirm that the view is unobstructed — for example, by jewelry or a medication patch.

■ Follow a system for viewing that reduces the risk of missing abnormal findings. For example, consistently view the film from left to right, top to bottom, or external to internal.

■ Verify anatomic alignment and positioning. Knowledge of normal anatomy is essential to X-ray interpretation.

■ Evaluate bone age. Epiphyseal growth plates (called epiphyseal lines on X-ray film) may be visible in females younger than age 20 and males younger than age 23. These plates can be seen as thin, dark lines between the epiphysis and the metaphysis. In mature adults, decreased density associated with osteoporosis may be visible.

## Osteoarthritis of the knee

This is the X-ray film of a mature male with pain in his right knee. The X-ray reveals medial joint space narrowing (as indicated by ➤) and mild osteophyte formation (as indicated by ➡).

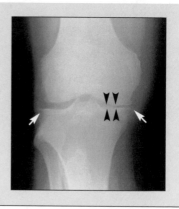

■ Assess bone density. This is generally consistent over the entire bone; inconsistencies indicate fractures, tumors, and sclerosis. In addition, loss of joint spaces, kyphosis, and stress fractures may be incidental findings. A common finding in mature adults is the degenerative changes and calcifications that bridge the joint spaces between bones associated with arthritis.

■ Evaluate continuity. Assess the entire perimeter of the bone and then the internal bone structures for disruption in continuity that would reveal fractures or soft tissue inflammation. Check the bone perimeter and then the outer layer (also called the cortex or periosteum) for discontinuities or increased opacity. Increased opacity associated with a fracture may be due to bone impaction, fragment rotation, or callus formation. While cortex thickness decreases with age, loss of 50% of the cortex or a bony lesion greater than 1″

(2.5 cm) in diameter warrants referral to an orthopedic surgeon. Conversely, thickening indicates stress fractures or inflammation.

■ Look for lucency in a linear fashion that's common between bone fragments after a fracture. Mottled areas that have lucent and dense areas suggest neoplasms with metastasis, congenital disorders, infection, or metabolic diseases.

■ Examine the periosteum. Check the size and shape of bones. Contour abnormalities or excess calcification may indicate either a chronic disorder (such as metabolic disease) or a congenital disorder.

### Postprocedure patient teaching

■ Discuss the results of the X-ray study with the patient.

### Complications

■ None known

## Bone tumor

This is the leg X-ray film of an adolescent female. The X-ray reveals a well-defined, eccentric, bubbly expansile lesion, indicated by the arrows, in the distal femoral diaphysis.

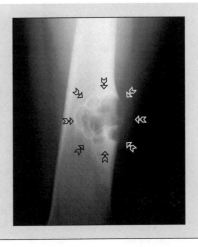

### Special considerations

■ In children, the epiphysis may be evident if bones haven't finished growing. Order films of bilateral extremities so you can compare the patient's injured extremity to the uninjured one.

■ When viewing cervical spine X-rays, be sure to count the vertebrae for proper identification of abnormalities. Follow each rib to its lateral edges to detect subtle fractures.

■ A pelvic fracture can be hard to detect because it's commonly nondisplaced and because its appearance differs only slightly from a normal pelvis.

■ In advanced rheumatoid arthritis, the bone atrophies and the joint becomes misaligned, deformed, and fused, resulting in fibrous ankylosis. X-rays reveal:
– loss of joint space and cartilage, periarticular bone erosion, and

joint subluxation (See *Rheumatoid arthritis of the hands,* page 543.)
– soft tissue swelling
– bones appearing as osteoporotic and more radiolucent before erosion can be seen, with malalignment of the affected joints often apparent as the disease progresses
– joint fusion in advanced disease.

■ Plain X-ray findings that indicate osteomyelitis include:
– erosions
– aggressive bone destruction
– periostitis
– soft-tissue swelling
– osteosclerosis (chalky or opaque appearance with obliteration of distinct borders between cortex and trabeculae [outer and inner layers])
– bone fragmentation
– fractures
– subluxation
– ill-defined bone contours.

■ Plain X-ray findings that indicate osteoarthritis include:

## Leg fractures

This is the X-ray film of a young adult male involved in a motor vehicle accident. The X-ray reveals an oblique, comminuted fracture of the tibia (as indicated by ➤) with lateral displacement of distal parts. It also reveals a comminuted avulsion-type fracture of the medial malleolus (as indicated by ➻).

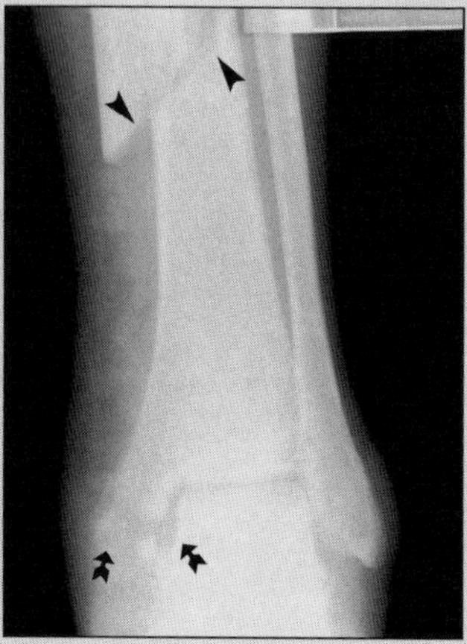

– joint narrowing and bone sclerosis (See *Osteoarthritis of the knee,* page 544.)
– presence of osteophytes
– bony overgrowths that give the bone a lumpy or irregular contour, a hallmark of osteoarthritis
– cystlike lesions in the subarticular area, which appear as small, radiolucent, circular, or piriform areas that may extend to the joint surface.

▪ Plain X-ray findings that indicate skeletal tumor include:
– osteopenia (scarcity of bone substance), which appears as bone more radiolucent than normal
– lytic lesions, which may appear as radiolucent, "punched out" areas of bone destruction
– pathologic fractures, common in the ribs and vertebrae
– an area of destroyed bone that appears to have been eaten by moths
– indistinct borders merging into normal tissue
– abundant periosteal reaction appearing as irregular new bone growth on bone edges (See *Bone tumor,* page 545.)
– ragged, irregular bone defects that are mottled or radiolucent
– absence of sclerosis along the margin
– foci of dense areas or a diffuse density involving a large area in the bone.

▪ Plain X-ray findings that indicate fracture include:
– displacement of bone fragments
– radiolucent breaks in bone continuity
– malalignment of joints
– associated soft tissue edema. (See *Leg fractures.*)

**COLLABORATION**
*Because X-ray interpretation is a skill that requires much experi-*

*ence, have your collaborating physician and radiologist review X-rays.*

## Documentation

■ Record the purpose of the X-ray study.

■ Compare clinical findings with current and previous radiologic findings.

■ Record any referrals made or collaborative communication with other health professionals.

■ Note any instructions you gave to the patient, including when to follow up with you.

# X-RAY INTERPRETATION, CHEST

### CPT codes

71010  *Radiologic exam, chest, frontal*
71020  *Radiologic exam, chest, frontal and lateral*

## Overview

Used in conjunction with patient history and physical examination, chest X-rays can help a health care provider arrive at a more accurate diagnosis of conditions, such as cardiomegaly, pulmonary edema, heart failure, and broken ribs. For a chest X-ray to provide the most useful information, the health care provider needs a basic knowledge of how X-rays work and how to read films to detect the pathologies that chest X-rays can reveal. (See *X-ray terminology,* page 548.)

To produce a chest X-ray film, the X-ray machine sends a stream of X-rays (or photons) through the chest. Structures in the chest then absorb these X-rays to a greater or lesser degree. Denser structures, such as bone, absorb more X-rays; less dense structures, such as soft tissue and fat, allow more X-rays to pass through; and the least dense structures, such as air, allow the most X-rays to pass through. X-rays that pass through the chest strike a film, turning it darker. The areas of film behind the densest structures (such as bone) appear the lightest because the dense structure absorbed most of the X-rays before they could reach the film. As a result, a typical chest X-ray film shows ribs and other bones as white against a darker background.

The patient typically stands or lies supine for a chest X-ray and requires no special preparation. Basic chest views include the posterior-anterior and lateral views (for a standing patient) and the anterior-posterior view (for a supine patient). During the procedure, the patient is exposed to approximately 20 milliroentgens of radiation. (See *Chest X-ray case studies,* pages 549 to 552.)

## Indications

■ To assess chest trauma
■ To detect and assess lung disease
■ To verify the placement of devices

## X-ray terminology

To evaluate a chest X-ray, you need to understand the terminology involved:
- *Density:* brightness or any area of whiteness on an image
- *Lucency:* blackness or any area of blackness on an image
- *Shadow:* anything visible on an image; any specific density or lucency
- *Edge:* any visible demarcation between a density on one side and a lucency on the other
- *Line:* a thin density with lucency on both sides, or a thin lucency with density on both sides
- *Stripe:* any edge or line
- *Silhouette:* another term for edge; the ability to see an edge is the silhouette sign

## Contraindications

**ABSOLUTE**
- Pregnancy

## Preprocedure patient preparation

- Tell the patient he'll feel only minimal discomfort from the position he must maintain and the cold metal of the X-ray table touching his body.

## Equipment

X-ray films ◆ photographic light box

## Procedure

- Before reading the film, verify patient information and the position of left and right markers on the film.
- Place the films on the illuminated photographic light box.
- Judge the technical quality of the film, especially the adequacy of penetration (vertebral bodies should appear clear).
- Look briefly at films for obvious abnormalities.

### Scanning the frontal view

- Study the lungs, looking both up and down and side to side. Include lung volume and symmetry of markings.
- Check the periphery of the lungs for pneumothorax and effusions.
- Evaluate the edges and shape of the mediastinal contour; note the diaphragm.
- Evaluate heart size and location.
- Follow the trachea to the carina and main stem bronchi.
- Look at both hili for enlargement and abnormal bulges.
- Begin at the neck and review the periphery of chest — include the shoulders, ribs, and clavicle.
- Check the upper abdomen for free air and abnormal air collection.

### Scanning the lateral view

- Follow the airway from the neck to the hilum. Note lung markings and look for fissures.
- Look down to the heart and up the anterior mediastinum to the neck.
- Follow the spine and posterior ribs to the costophrenic angle.
- Judge the shape of the diaphragm and the upper abdomen.

(*Text continues on page 553.*)

# Chest X-ray case studies

These eight chest X-rays can help you recognize what various pathologies look like on film. The first shows the structures you'll see in a normal chest X-ray, and the next seven show pathology ranging from lobar pneumonia to lung cancer

## NORMAL POSTEROANTERIOR CHEST X-RAY
This X-ray shows certain normal, soft, and bony structures in the chest and upper abdomen.

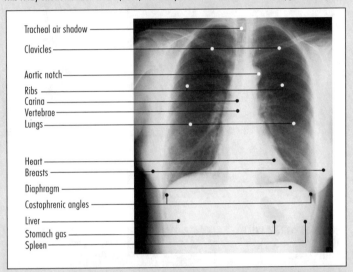

Tracheal air shadow

Clavicles

Aortic notch

Ribs
Carina
Vertebrae
Lungs

Heart
Breasts
Diaphragm
Costophrenic angles
Liver
Stomach gas
Spleen

## LOBAR PNEUMONIA
This chest X-ray of a 79-year-old woman shows classic findings of lobar pneumonia involving the left lower lobe (as indicated by ➤). These signs include the silhouette sign, in which the left hemidiaphragm and heart shadow borders can't be seen, mild atelectasis (note the smaller left lung), and depressed left hilum with mediastinal shift to the left (as indicated by ➤➤).

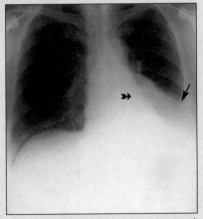

*(continued)*

## Chest X-ray case studies (continued)

### PULMONARY CHANGES WITH ASTHMA

In this posteroanterior chest X-ray of a young woman with asthma, note the hyperinflated lungs (as indicated by ➤), small heart (as indicated by ➤➤), and depressed diaphragm (as indicated by ➤).

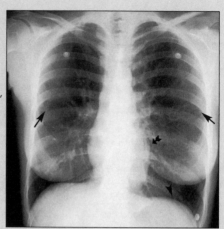

### PNEUMOTHORAX WITH SUBCUTANEOUS EMPHYSEMA

In this posteroanterior chest X-ray of a patient with a pneumothorax, the chest tube (as indicated by ➤) has migrated outside of the pleural space. As a result, the patient has a larger pneumothorax (as indicated by ➤➤) than he originally had. He has also developed subcutaneous and mediastinal emphysema (as indicated by ➤➤).

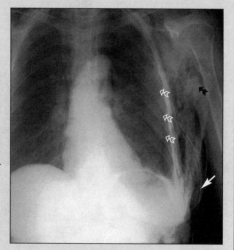

# Chest X-ray case studies *(continued)*

**PLEURAL EFFUSION**

This is a posteroanterior chest X-ray of a 58-year-old man with a history of heart failure. The patient has right-side pleural fluid blunting the right costophrenic angle due to the pleural fluid. Note the concavity of the upper border of the pleural fluid (as indicated by the ➤ ).

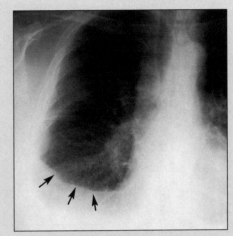

**RIB FRACTURES**

This anteroposterior chest X-ray of a trauma patient after a motor vehicle accident shows left fifth (as indicated by ➤➤) and sixth (as indicated by ⧐⧐) lateral rib fractures. Note the separation at fracture sites from displacement and associated left clavicle (as indicated by ➝ ) and left scapula fractures (as indicated by ➤ ).

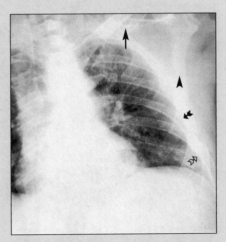

*(continued)*

## Chest X-ray case studies *(continued)*

### LUNG CANCER

This is a chest X-ray of a 67-year-old woman with bronchogenic lung cancer. Note the large mass (as indicated by ➤) with cavitation at the center (as indicated by ➤➤) in the right hilum area. The right lower lobe is opaque, which indicates atelectasis caused by the tumor.

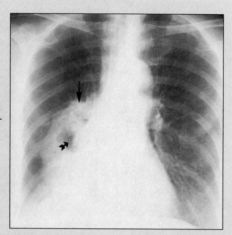

### FOREIGN BODY

This is a classic inspiratory and expiratory anteroposterior chest X-ray of a 17-month-old child with a ball-valve-type foreign body in the left bronchus. Inspiratory film is essentially normal, but expiratory film shows the left lung hyperinflated (as indicated by ➤) because air is being trapped by the foreign body. You can also see a shift of the mediastinum to the right (as indicated by ➤) and relative increased lucency, or dark air-filled area, on the left.

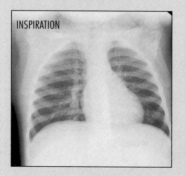

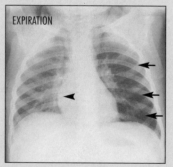

■ Check the anterior chest wall and sternum.

### *Evaluating the frontal view*
■ Evaluate lung markings (vessels) and minor fissures. Specifically, evaluate the:
– mediastinum
– airways (trachea, carina, and main bronchi)
– hili (left and right pulmonary arteries)
– soft tissues (in the neck and chest walls, breast shadows, diaphragms, and intestinal gas)
– bones (ribs, clavicles, scapulae, humerus, spine, vertebral bodies, and disk spaces).

### *Evaluating the lateral view*
■ Evaluate the airways, including the trachea and main and left bronchi. Also evaluate:
– hili (left and right pulmonary arteries)
– lung (major and minor markings and fissures)
– left ventricle of the heart.
■ On the posterior chest view, evaluate the spine, ribs, diaphragms, and intestinal gas.
■ Evaluate the anterior chest.
■ Evaluate the chest wall and sternum.

## Postprocedure patient teaching
■ Discuss the results of the X-ray study with the patient.

## Complications
■ None known

## Special considerations
■ Always interpret a patient's chest X-rays in light of his history and physical examination.
■ Compare any X-ray film with previous films, particularly when assessing the progression of a disorder, such as pneumonia or a pneumothorax. Keep in mind the position in which the film was taken; a structure on an anterior-posterior view may appear to be a different size than on a posterior-anterior view because of the distance from the X-ray source. For instance, the heart may appear enlarged in an anterior-posterior projection because it was closer to the X-ray tube (and farther from the film) when exposed.
■ Establish a pattern for evaluating chest films to make it less likely to miss a pathology.
■ Include both frontal and lateral views in most evaluations.
■ Remember that plain films have limitations; they aren't extremely sensitive so they may miss many pathologies. Know when to move to further studies such as a computed tomography scan.
■ Four general patterns of pulmonary disease can be seen on a chest X-ray: a distinct mass, consolidative (alveolar) pattern, interstitial pattern, and vascular pattern.

## Documentation
■ Document the details of your X-ray analysis, comparisons with previous films, and the correlation with clinical findings.

# APPENDIX A
# MEDICAL ENGLISH-SPANISH TRANSLATIONS

## POSITIONING AND PREPARATION

| | |
|---|---|
| Bend over backward. | Dóblese Ud. hacia atrás. |
| Bend over forward. | Dóblese Ud. hacia adelante. |
| Lean backward. | Recuéstese Ud. |
| Lean forward. | Inclínese Ud. hacia adelante. |
| Lie down. | Acuéstese Ud. |
| Lie on your back. | Acuéstese Ud. boca arriba. |
| Lie on your:<br>  –side<br>  –left side<br>  –right side. | Acuéstese Ud.:<br>  –de lado.<br>  –del lado izquierdo<br>  –del lado derecho. |
| Lie on your stomach. | Acuéstese boca abajo. |
| Roll over. | Dé Ud. una vuelta. |
| Sit down. | Siéntese Ud. |
| Sit up. | Enderécese Ud. |
| Stand up. | Párese Ud. |
| Turn to the side. | Voltéese Ud. hacia un lado. |
| Keep your feet together. | Mantenga Ud. los pies juntos. |
| Tighten your muscle. | Tense Ud. el músculo. |
| Turn to the right. | Voltéese Ud. hacia la derecha. |
| Turn to the left. | Voltéese Ud. hacia la izquierda. |
| Lift up your arms. | Levante Ud. los brazos. |
| Make a fist. | Cierre Ud. el puño. |
| Don't move. | No se mueva. |
| When I tell you, hold your breath. | Cuando le diga, contenga Ud. el aliento. |
| Don't breathe (hold your breath). | No respire (contenga el aliento). |
| Breathe. | Respire Ud. |
| Once more. | Una vez más. |
| Are you pregnant? | ¿Está Ud. embarazada? |
| Don't talk. | No hable Ud. |
| Say "AAHH." | Diga Ud. "AAAA." |
| Whisper. | Murmure Ud. |

## *POSITIONING AND PREPARATION (continued)*

| | |
|---|---|
| I need to put a tourniquet on your arm. | Tengo que ponerle un torniquete en el brazo. |
| You'll feel pain like a pinprick. | Ud. sentirá un dolor como un alfilerazo. |
| You must drink this liquid before the test. | Ud. tiene que tomarse este líquido antes de la prueba. |
| You must drink this liquid during the test. | Ud. tiene que tomarse este líquido durante la prueba. |
| We must give you an enema before the test. | Tenemos que ponerle una enema (lavativa) antes de la prueba. |
| You must hold the enema in until we're finished with the test. | Ud. tiene que retener la enema (la lavativa) hasta que terminemos con la prueba. |
| You may go to the bathroom when we tell you. | Ud. puede ir al baño cuando le digamos. |
| Is your bladder very full? | ¿Tiene Ud. la vejiga muy llena? |
| You can't empty your bladder until the test is finished. | Ud. no puede vaciar la vejiga hasta que la prueba se termine. |

## *PHYSICAL EXAMINATION*

I'm going to examine your:
- –skin.
- –hair.
- –nails.
- –head and neck.
  - *head.*
  - *nose.*
  - *mouth.*
  - *throat.*
  - *neck.*
- –eyes.
- –ears.
- –respiratory system.
  - *chest.*
  - *lungs.*
- –cardiovascular system.
  - *heart.*
  - *pulse.*
- –gastrointestinal system.
  - *abdomen.*
  - *rectum.*
- –urinary system.
  - *bladder.*
  - *kidneys.*

Le voy a reconocer:
- –la piel.
- –el cabello.
- –las uñas.
- –la cabeza y el cuello.
  - *la cabeza.*
  - *la nariz.*
  - *la boca.*
  - *la garganta.*
  - *el cuello.*
- –los ojos.
- –los oídos.
- –el sistema respiratorio.
  - *el pecho.*
  - *los pulmones.*
- –el sistema cardiovascular.
  - *el corazón.*
  - *el pulso.*
- –el sistema gastrointestinal.
  - *el abdomen.*
  - *el recto.*
- –el sistema urinario.
  - *la vejiga.*
  - *los riñones.*

## PHYSICAL EXAMINATION (continued)

| | |
|---|---|
| –reproductive system. | –el sistema reproductivo. |
| *breasts.* | *las mamas or los senos.* |
| *pelvis.* | *la pelvis.* |
| *penis.* | *el pene.* |
| *testicles.* | *los testículos.* |
| –nervous system. | –el sistema nervioso. |
| *reflexes.* | *los reflejos.* |
| –musculoskeletal system. | –el sistema musculoesquelético. |
| *arms.* | *los brazos.* |
| *legs.* | *las piernas.* |
| –immune system. | –el sistema inmunológico. |
| –endocrine system. | –el sistema endocrino. |

| | |
|---|---|
| I'm going to take your: | Voy a medirle: |
| –vital signs. | –los signos vitales. |
| –blood pressure. | –la presión sanguínea. |
| –pulse. | –el pulso. |
| –temperature. | –la temperatura. |

| | |
|---|---|
| I'm going to take a blood sample. | Voy a tomarle a Ud. una muestra de sangre. |
| You need to provide a urine specimen. | Tiene Ud. que darnos un espécimen de orina. |
| I'm going to inspect your _____. | Le voy a examinar _____. |
| I'm going to auscultate (listen to) your _____. | Le voy a auscultar _____. |
| I'm going to palpate your _____. | Le voy a palpar _____. |
| I'm going to percuss your _____. | Le voy a percutir _____. |
| Are you comfortable? | ¿Está Ud. confortable? |
| Does this hurt? | ¿Le duele a Ud. esto? |
| –Where does it hurt? | –¿Dónde le duele a Ud.? |

## EXAMINATION WITH INSTRUMENTS

| | |
|---|---|
| I'm going to use: | Voy a usar: |
| –a measuring tape to measure your: | –una cinta métrica para medirle: |
| *arm.* | *el brazo.* |
| *leg.* | *la pierna.* |
| *belly.* | *el vientre.* |
| *hand.* | *la mano.* |
| *head.* | *la cabeza.* |
| *chest.* | *el pecho.* |
| –an ophthalmoscope to examine your eyes. | –un oftalmoscopio para examinarle los ojos. |
| –an otoscope to examine your ears. | –un otoscopio para examinarle los oídos. |

## EXAMINATION WITH INSTRUMENTS (continued)

| | |
|---|---|
| —a penlight to look in your eyes. | —una linterna de bolsillo para examinarle los ojos. |
| —a scale to weigh you. | —una báscula (balanza) para medir su peso. |
| —a sphygmomanometer to take your blood pressure. | —un esfigmomanómetro para medirle la tensión sanguínea arterial. |
| —a stethoscope to listen to your: | —un estetoscopio para escuchar: |
| *lungs and breathing.* | *sus pulmones y su respiración.* |
| *heart.* | *su corazón.* |
| —a syringe to take a blood sample. | —una jeringa para obtener una muestra de sangre. |
| —a thermometer to take your temperature. | —un termómetro para tomarle la temperatura. |
| —a tongue blade to examine your mouth and throat. | —un depresor de lengua para examinarle la boca y la garganta. |
| —a tuning fork to test your hearing. | —un diapasón para examinarle el oído. |
| —a vaginal speculum to perform a pelvic examination and examine your vagina. | —un espéculo vaginal para hacerle un examen de la pelvis y de la vagina. |
| —a visual acuity chart to test your sight. | —gráfica simplificada para medir su agudeza visual. |

## TESTING

### General tests

| | |
|---|---|
| I have ordered: | Yo he pedido que se le haga: |
| —a biopsy. | —una biopsia. |
| —a blood test. | —un análisis de la sangre. |
| —a blood culture. | —un cultivo de la sangre. |
| —a computed tomography scan. | —una tomografía computerizada. |
| —an endoscopy. | —una endoscopia. |
| —a magnetic resonance imaging scan. | —una resonancia magnética. |
| —an ultrasound. | —un ultrasonido. |
| —a urinalysis. | —un urinálisis (or un análisis de orina). |
| —an X-ray. | —una radiografía. |
| —allergy tests. | —pruebas de alergia. |
| —a neck X-ray. | —una radiografía del cuello. |
| —a nose culture. | —un cultivo de la nariz. |
| —a skull X-ray. | —una radiografía del cráneo. |
| —a throat culture. | —un cultivo de la garganta. |
| —a glaucoma test. | —un examen de glaucoma. |
| —a vision test. | —un examen de la vista. |
| —a hearing test. | —un examen de la audición. |

## TESTING *(continued)*

### Respiratory tests

I have ordered:
   –an arterial blood gases test.
   –a bronchoscopy.
   –a chest X-ray.
   –a lung scan.
   –pulmonary function tests.

   –a pulse oximetry.

Yo he pedido que se le haga:
   –gases de la sangre arterial.
   –una broncoscopia.
   –una radiografía del tórax.
   –un ultrasonido pulmonar.
   –una prueba de la función pulmonar.
   –una oximetría del pulso.

### Cardiovascular tests

I have ordered:
   –an arteriogram.
   –a blood test for:
      *cardiac enzymes.*
      *cholesterol.*
      *partial thromboplastin time.*
      *prothrombin time.*
      *triglycerides.*
   –a cardiac catheterization.
   –an electrocardiogram.
   –a Holter monitor.
   –a stress test.
   –a venogram.

Yo he pedido que se le haga:
   –un arteriograma.
   –un análisis de la sangre para:
      *enzimas cardiacas.*
      *colesterol.*
      *tiempo de tromboplastina parcial.*
      *tiempo de protrombina.*
      *triglicéridos.*
   –un cateterismo cardiaco.
   –un electrocardiograma.
   –monitoreo Holter.
   –un examen de estrés.
   –un venograma.

### Gastrointestinal tests

I have ordered:
   –an abdominal ultrasound.
   –a barium enema.
   –a barium swallow.
   –a blood test for:
      *amylase.*
      *liver enzymes.*
   –a cholangiogram.
   –a cholecystogram.
   –a colonoscopy.
   –a gastric analysis.
   –a gastroscopy.
   –a liver biopsy.
   –a sigmoidoscopy.
   –a spleen scan.

   –a stool culture.
   –an upper GI series.

Yo he pedido que se le haga:
   –un ultrasonido abdominal.
   –una enema de bario.
   –tragar bario.
   –un análisis de la sangre para:
      *amilasa.*
      *enzimas del hígado.*
   –un colangiograma.
   –un colecistograma.
   –una colonoscopia.
   –un análisis gástrico.
   –una gastroscopia.
   –una biopsia del hígado.
   –una sigmoidoscopia.
   –una visualización del bazo por ecos de ultrasonidos.
   –un cultivo de la defecación.
   –una serie gastrointestinal superior.

## TESTING *(continued)*

### Renal and urologic tests

I have ordered:
  –a blood test for:
    *blood urea nitrogen.*
    *creatinine.*
    *electrolytes.*
  –a cystoscopy.
  –an excretory urography.
  –a renal biopsy.
  –a retrograde pyelogram.
  –a urine culture.

Yo he pedido que se le haga:
  –un análisis de la sangre para:
    *nitrógeno y urea sanguínea.*
    *creatinina.*
    *electrolitos.*
  –una cistoscopia.
  –una urografía excretora.
  –un cultivo renal.
  –un pielograma retrógrado.
  –un cultivo de la orina.

### Genitourinary tests

I have ordered a:
  –breast biopsy.
  –breast examination.
  –cervical biopsy.
  –mammogram.
  –Papanicolaou test.
  –pelvic examination.
  –pregnancy test.
  –prostate examination.
  –prostatic biopsy.
  –rectal examination.
  –semen analysis.
  –vaginal culture.

Yo he pedido que se le haga:
  –una biopsia de la mama.
  –un reconocimiento de los senos.
  –una biopsia cervical.
  –un mamograma.
  –una prueba Papanicolaou.
  –un reconocimiento pélvico.
  –un análisis de embarazo.
  –un reconocimiento de la próstata.
  –una biopsia de la próstata.
  –un reconocimiento del recto.
  –un análisis del semen.
  –un cultivo vaginal.

### Neurologic tests

I have ordered:
  –a brain scan.
  –a cerebral arteriogram.
  –a computed tomography scan of the brain.
  –an electroencephalogram.
  –a lumbar puncture.
  –a myelogram.

Yo he pedido que se le haga:
  –un ultrasonido cerebral.
  –un arteriograma cerebral.
  –una tomografía computerizada del cerebro.
  –un electroencefalograma.
  –una punción lumbar.
  –un mielograma.

### Musculoskeletal tests

I have ordered:
  –an arthroscopy.
  –a bone biopsy.
  –an electromyogram.
  –a muscle biopsy.

Yo he pedido que se le haga:
  –una artroscopia.
  –una biopsia del hueso.
  –un electromiograma.
  –una biopsia del músculo.

## Musculoskeletal tests *(continued)*

—an X-ray of the:
  ankle.
  arm.
  back.
  elbow.
  foot.
  hand.
  hip.
  knee.
  leg.
  shoulder.
  wrist.

—una radiografía de:
  el tobillo.
  el brazo.
  la espalda.
  el codo.
  el pie.
  la mano.
  la cadera.
  la rodilla.
  la pierna.
  el hombro.
  la muñeca.

## Hematologic blood tests

I have ordered a:
  —blood test for:
    blood cell count.
    differential blood cell count.

    red blood cell count.

    white blood cell count.

    clotting times.
    hematocrit.
    hemoglobin level.
    hepatitis B.
    human immunodeficiency virus (HIV).
    platelet count.
  —bone marrow biopsy.

Yo he pedido que se le haga:
  —un análisis de la sangre para:
    recuento sanguíneo.
    recuento diferencial de las células de sangre.
    recuento de los glóbulos rojos de la sangre.
    recuento de los glóbulos blancos de la sangre.
    el tiempo de coagulación.
    hematócrito.
    el nivel de hemoglobina.
    hepatitis tipo B.
    virus de inmunodeficiencia humana (VIH).
    recuento de plaquetas.
  —una biopsia de la médula ósea del hueso.

## Endocrine tests

I have ordered:
  —an analysis of:
    adrenal function.
    ovarian function.
    parathyroid function.
    pancreatic function.
    pituitary function
    testicular function.
    thyroid function.

Yo he pedido que se le haga:
  —un análisis de:
    la función adrenal.
    la función ovárica.
    la función paratiroidea.
    la función pancreática.
    la función de la pituitaria.
    la función testicular.
    la función de la tiroides.

## *TESTING* (continued)

### **Endocrine tests** (continued)

–a blood test for:
  *serum calcium level.*
  *serum glucose level.*
  *fasting glucose level.*
  *glucose tolerance.*
  *glycosylated hemoglobin level.*

  *2-hour postprandial glucose level.*

  *serum hormone levels.*
  *serum phosphorus concentration.*

–un análisis de sangre para revisar:
  *el nivel de calcio.*
  *el nivel de glucosa.*
  *el nivel de glucosa en abstención.*
  *la tolerancia a la glucosa.*
  *el nivel de hemoglobina glucosilata-
  da.*
  *el nivel de glucosa dos-horas pos-
  prandial.*
  *niveles hormonales.*
  *niveles de fósforo.*

## *MEDICATION INSTRUCTIONS*

Don't eat or drink anything after midnight before the test.

No coma ni beba nada después de medianoche antes de la prueba (del examen).

Don't eat or drink anything after _____ a.m.

No coma ni beba nada después de las _____ de la mañana.

Don't eat or drink anything after _____ p.m.

No coma ni beba nada después de las _____ de la tarde (or la noche).

You may take your usual medicine in the morning with a small amount of water.

Ud. puede tomarse todas sus medicinas habituales en la mañana con una cantidad pequeña de agua.

You may take all of your usual medicine in the morning with a small amount of water except _____.

Ud. puede tomarse todas sus medicinas habituales en la mañana con una cantidad pequeña de agua con la excepción de _____.

# APPENDIX B
## OBTAINING INFORMED CONSENT

Being adequately informed about proposed treatment, procedures, surgery, or research in order to properly give consent is a patient's legal right. It isn't surprising, therefore, that the topic of informed consent appears in all current medical texts, and must be evidenced in the patient's records where invasive or experimental procedures, treatment, or surgery is contemplated.

In the 1960s, physicians were primarily responsible for obtaining the patient's consent. Since then, other health care providers, such as nurse practitioners and physician assistants, have also played a role in obtaining informed consent. Generally, it's a basic rule that the responsibility for obtaining a patient's informed consent rests with the person who will carry out the procedure or who is recommending a course of treatment. This procedure may be delegated to an appropriate person under certain circumstances; for example, to the nurse practitioner or physician assistant working with the physician who will participate in the procedure.

Informed consent involves the patient, or someone acting on his behalf, having enough information to know what the patient is risking should he decide to undergo the proposed treatment or surgery or the anticipated consequences should consent to the treatment be refused or withdrawn. The health care provider has the legal responsibility to give the patient such information and must not use coercion to obtain the consent.

Under certain circumstances, persons with mental disorders may be held competent to consent. When there's a question about an individual's capacity to give consent, a legal determination may be sought from the appropriate court (for example, probate court) or an ethics committee of the facility.

The bottom line in determining capacity must be whether the person giving consent is impaired in his capacity or judgment so as not to know what he's getting into before the treatment begins.

To assess capacity to consent, you may need to rely on your instincts as well as professional judgment. If you believe the patient doesn't understand, you should reassess the patient's understanding of the treatment and discuss the consent issue with the patient, his guardian if applicable, and the collaborating physician before the treatment begins.

## INFORMED CONSENT STANDARDS

Generally, informed consent can be viewed legally from two different perspectives. The first is known as the majority rule or malpractice model: what a reasonable medical practitioner would have disclosed to his patient regarding the proposed treatment, under the same or similar circumstances. Consider *Nathanson v. Kline* (1960), a case in which the physician allegedly failed to inform the patient of the adverse effects of cobalt radiation therapy. The court ruled that the physician had a duty to disclose information "which a reasonable medical practitioner would disclose under the same or similar circumstances." Therefore, under the majority rule, the information is viewed from what a reasonable health care provider would tell a patient or patient's family about the procedure.

The second perspective, known as the minority rule, looks at the disclosure of the material information that a reasonable patient in the same or similar situation would deem important to know in making a decision to undergo the proposed treatment.

## NEGLIGENT NONDISCLOSURE

Consider *Canterbury v. Spence* (1972). In this case, a patient had a laminectomy and then fell and developed paralysis. The patient sued the physician for failing to warn him of the inherent risks. The court ruled that the physician had a duty to disclose as much information as he knew, or should have known, a reasonable patient would need to make an informed decision.

What should the patient be told? First, it's well accepted that a reasonable disclosure of risks inherent to the particular medical diagnosis and treatment is required. Information should be provided regarding the likelihood of success of the treatment as well as viable alternatives, if any exist. The patient must be given an opportunity to evaluate the recommended treatment, alternatives, and risks, and then exercise his choice. In medical malpractice cases involving consent issues, expert testimony is commonly required to establish whether the information given to the patient was reasonable, understandable, presented at a time when the patient was functionally able to process the information (as opposed to being sedated or medicated), and complete enough to allow the patient to knowledgeably agree to proceed. It's generally agreed that it isn't necessary to address every possible risk or benefit; however, discussions with the patient or his decision maker must include those risks and benefits that arise frequently or regularly. In addition, if there are specific consequences known to the health care provider to be particularly significant to this patient, they must be discussed before true informed consent may be obtained. All health care providers involved at this point must exercise professional judgment. There should also be time given for a discussion on what the consequences may be if the treatment or procedure is refused.

A landmark case, *Karp v. Cooley* (1998), is a good example of how informed consents are added to other allegations in malpractice cases. Mr. Karp was offered a mechanical heart transplant when it was obvious that his medical condition was deteriorating, and he was near death. Many consultants evaluated Mr. Karp. One, Dr. Beasley, wrote in Mr. Karp's chart that he didn't recommend the procedure because he thought the patient wasn't a suitable candidate for the surgery. Dr. Cooley, the surgeon, admitted at trial that he didn't tell Mr. Karp of Dr. Beasley's note, which was made during initial work-ups and, actually, was directed and related to Dr. Beasley's reservation about the patient's psychological or emotional acceptance of a less-than-perfect outcome.

Mrs. Karp testified to what Mr. Karp's physicians said in her presence. However, Mr. Karp also spoke with his physicians on several occasions about the proposed treatment when his wife wasn't present, and it was Mr. Karp who signed the consent form. The consent form matched the details Dr. Cooley testified to as being the basis of discussions with Mr. Karp before he signed the form. No expert testimony was offered to indicate that what Dr. Cooley discussed with Mr. Karp was inadequate or breached Dr. Cooley's duty to obtain informed consent.

The court dismissed the informed consent issue on that basis and also raised the issue that the plaintiff, the estate of Mr. Karp, didn't present substantial evidence that there was any causal connection between their claimed lack of informed consent and Mr. Karp's death. To address this proximate cause relationship, the court looked at Texas case law (previous cases on this issue) and noted that for a finding of proximate causation between the alleged omissions of informed consent and injury (in this case death), the following criteria must exist:

- a hidden risk that should have been made known, but wasn't, must materialize
- the hidden risk must be harmful to the patient
- causality exists only when disclosures of significant risks incidental to treatment would have resulted in the patient's decision against the treatment.

What the court relied upon in discussing the case on the proximate cause issue was testimony that Mr. Karp was near death prior to the wedge excision operation, to which he gave consent. There was no dispute by Mrs. Karp about the validity of that consent. After the operation, Mr. Karp was also near death. Therefore, no one testified that to a reasonable degree of medical certainty the mechanical heart caused Mr. Karp's death. Finally, there was no proof offered at trial that Mr. Karp wouldn't have agreed to proceed with the mechanical heart surgery had alleged undisclosed material risks been disclosed. On appeal, the dismissal on the informed consent issue was upheld.

Another scenario: Suppose a patient is scheduled for surgery. He has talked to his physician and signed the consent form. However, the day before surgery, he doesn't seem to understand the implications of the procedure. If you're the health care provider caring for this patient and preparing him for surgery, what would you do?

## Basic elements of informed consent

The basics of informed consent should include:
■ a description of the treatment or procedure
■ a description of inherent risks and benefits that occur with frequency or regularity or specific consequences known by the health care provider to be particularly significant to this patient or his designated decision maker
■ an explanation of the potential for death or serious harm (such as brain damage, stroke, paralysis, or disfiguring scars) or for discomforting adverse effects during or after the treatment or procedure
■ an explanation and description of alternative treatments or procedures
■ the name and qualifications of the person who will perform the treatment or procedure

■ a discussion of the possible effects of not having the treatment or procedure.

Patients must also be told that they have a right to refuse the treatment or procedure without having other care or support withdrawn and that they can withdraw consent after giving it.

If you witness a patient's signature on a consent form, you attest that:
■ the patient voluntarily consented
■ the signature of the patient or the patient's designated decision maker is authentic
■ the patient appears to be competent to give consent.

There are many consent issues now, especially due to such procedures as human immunodeficiency virus (HIV) testing, drug and alcohol treatment, and sterilization. Your facility's risk manager should define your responsibilities, your employer's policies, and your state's legal requirements. Each state has specific statutes governing informed consent that are subject to change as tort reform evolves and as case law interprets existing statutes or legal concepts.

### INFORMED CONSENT UNDER STATE LAW

Many state legislatures have passed laws supporting the standards of informed consent set by the courts. States have procedural laws on informed consent — laws that describe, for example, the tort of negligent nondisclosure. A few states have laws that are substantive, meaning they actually define what must be present for informed consent to have been established. These laws define who is able to give consent and for what and what type of documentation is required. They also define exemptions to documented consent and when consent becomes invalid.

**INABILITY TO CONSENT**

Informed consent relies on an individual's capacity, or ability, to make decisions at a particular time under specific circumstances. To make decisions about his medical care, the patient must possess the capacity and the competence to make such decisions. He must possess three critical elements of decision making:

- the ability to understand and communicate information relevant to the decision
- the ability to reason and deliberate concerning the decision
- the ability to apply a set of values to the decision.

If you have reason to believe that a patient is incompetent to participate in giving informed consent because medication or sedation is affecting his decision-making capacity, you have an obligation to refrain from obtaining consent at that time (or to seek a guardian or family member to obtain the consent, if appropriate). You should return when the patient can adequately and legally provide informed consent. Why? If you fail to provide adequate information for consent because of the patient's medicated status, the patient may sue you for lack of informed consent due to temporary

incapacitation. The courts might hold you responsible if you knowingly didn't provide adequate information to a patient. It's better to delay a procedure than to become a defendant in a battery lawsuit because you didn't obtain informed consent.

**INCOMPETENT PATIENTS**

A patient is deemed mentally incompetent if he can't understand the explanations or can't comprehend the results of his decisions. When the patient is incompetent, the health care provider has two alternatives. He may seek consent from the patient's next of kin, usually a spouse. (Legal definition of next of kin varies from state to state.) Alternatively, other interested family members, the physician, or the hospital may petition the court to appoint a legal guardian for the patient. Sometimes, a Probate Court may decide who the proper legal guardian should be after reviewing petitions and taking testimony. This works well if there's time to appoint a proper guardian. However, that isn't always possible in the case of a potentially dangerous or deadly medical condition. Under those circumstances, the courts will look to the reasonableness of the actions by the health care providers, before they proceeded with the treatment, in determining if there was informed consent by a proper party or whether the informed consent requirement was properly waived.

Mental illness isn't the same as incompetence. Persons suffering from mental illness have been found competent to consent because they're alert and, above all, able to understand the proposed treatment, risks, benefits, and alternatives, as well as the consequences of refusing the treatment. Consider a patient with mental illness who has been hospitalized involuntarily but who remains alert and oriented. His mental status and education enable him to understand the information presented by the health care provider, despite his incarceration. Should this patient be allowed to make medical decisions affecting his life or future health? Why should a court-appointed person assume this authority? On the other hand, shouldn't the patient have the right to refuse treatment even if it might ease his mental illness (for example, electroconvulsive shock therapy)?

Since the late 1980s, health care providers have had to resolve medical restraint issues that involve elderly, confused, and infirm patients. It's now well established that a confined patient, mentally or physically disabled, may be forcibly medicated only in an emergency when he may cause harm to himself or others. In such cases, documentation in the patient record is critical regarding the actual mental status of the patient and competency to give consent.

## MINORS

Over the last 25 years, health care providers have witnessed a great social and legal challenge involving the rights of minors, especially

their right to seek health care. As concerns for the rights of minors regarding consent to health care have arisen, all states have looked at the issue of just who can give consent for minors to receive what care and what information a minor may keep confidential in regard to that care. Certain rules have evolved.

Generally, the person giving consent for the care and treatment of a minor is a parent or other designated adult. However, this isn't always the case. The health care provider still must disclose all relevant information to the person giving consent to ensure that the consent is informed.

The patchwork of rights and limitations of the various state laws governing when minors can and can't consent give us alternating perceptions of teenagers. They're viewed as adultlike and childlike, and there's a desire to protect and respect these qualities. For example, although a teenage mother must give consent before her baby can receive treatment, she generally isn't permitted to determine the course of her own health care. Under federal law, adolescents can be tested and treated for HIV without parental involvement; however, in most cases, parental consent is required to set an adolescent's broken arm.

Every state will allow an emancipated minor to consent to his own medical care and treatment. So far, state definitions of emancipation vary, but it's generally recognized that to be emancipated, the individual must be a minor by state definition (less than the legal age of majority in that state) and must have obtained a legal declaration of freedom from the custody, care, and control of his parents. In doing so, emancipated minors forgo the right to financial support from their parents as well as any protection from lawsuits. Once declared emancipated, minors gain the right to enter binding contracts, to sue, and to consent to medical, dental, or psychiatric care without parental approval. They also assume all the financial obligations for this care, just as an adult would, if an adult had entered into such contracts. In granting emancipated status to minors, the courts will look for employment, demonstrated fiscal responsibility, other evidence of support systems the minor has available, and the individual circumstances that underlie the request for legal determination of emancipation.

Most states will allow teenagers to consent to treatment, even though they haven't been determined emancipated, in situations involving pregnancy or sexually transmitted disease. Because privacy issues are involved, the health care provider must understand the specific circumstances that allow a minor to consent as well as the circumstances under which he should contact the parent or legal guardian. Your risk manager should be able to help you. Contact with a parent or legal guardian and disclosure of confidential information have resulted in lawsuits for breach of confidentiality.

An unemancipated minor, in mid-to-late teens, who shows signs of intellectual and emotional maturity, is considered a "mature minor." In some cases, a mature minor is allowed to exercise some of the rights regarding health care that are generally reserved for adults. Because there's no consensus about when maturity occurs, and thus, no clear guidelines for those who must make such assessments, the issue of maturity must be decided on a case-by-case basis.

It's an accepted practice to allow children, to the extent they may participate, to be involved in the decision-making process regarding life-sustaining medical treatment. In making the ultimate decisions, there must be a weighing of "the best interests" standards, which involves considering the benefits and the burdens to the child. Some benefits to be considered are prolonging life and improving the quality of life following treatment. Some of the burdens of the proposed treatment may be intractable pain, irremediable disability or helplessness, emotional suffering, and invasiveness of the procedure, which could severely detract from the quality of life. Keep in mind that the quality of life to be considered is from the child's perspective, not that of the parent or decision maker, or even the health care providers. Without evidence to the contrary, the assumption is that life-sustaining medical treatment will be provided in accordance with existing medical, ethical, and legal norms.

**RIGHT TO REFUSE TREATMENT**

It's generally held that parents have the right to refuse life-sustaining medical treatment for unemancipated children who lack the capacity or statutory criteria for maturity to make such decisions for themselves.

Decisions to limit, withhold, discontinue, or forgo treatment must be very carefully documented and must be very specific in nature. The collaborative process must occur between patient, parent (or parent's surrogate), and health care provider. Young children deserve to hear the general conclusions of a decision that will affect their survival, especially when the clinician believes treatment no longer will benefit the patient and should be withdrawn.

Emancipated or mature minors are presumed to have the capacity to give consent. Regarding younger children, it might be helpful to consider what a Tennessee State Supreme Court did in a 1987 case, utilizing the "Rule of Sevens." The court presumed that up to age 7 the child lacked capacity to consent. From age 7 to 14, the presumption of incapacity can be rebutted (by evidence to demonstrate that the child, in fact, possesses maturity); over age 14, we should presume capacity.

Remember that informed consent is a process, not a document. Hospitals generally address informed consent in policy and procedure manuals to ensure consistency and thorough implementation and documentation. Current "hot spots" of the Joint Commission on Accreditation of Healthcare Organizations (JCAHO) include issues of informed consent, advance directives, and confidentiality. Regarding informed consent issues, evidence is required that the consent is voluntary and that sufficient information regarding the treatment was given. This includes an explanation of the risks and benefits, alternatives, differences in effectiveness of alternatives, consequences of not having the proposed treatment, impact on daily living, likelihood of success, responsible health care providers, and any possible conflicts of interest. In addition, this information must be presented in a manner that the patient understands, including appropriate language, reading level, cognitive ability, and ethnic orientation. Lastly, the appropriate documentation must be completed properly.

**EVIDENCE OF CONSENT**

Consent can be demonstrated by a signed, witnessed document; a note in the medical record detailing communications between the physician and patient; or the patient willfully undergoing the procedure by appearing at the appointed time and place. Some states have statutes stating that a signed consent form disclosing the treatment in general terms is deemed conclusive proof of a valid consent. Georgia's law is such a statute. Of course, the validity of the signature may be challenged. However, if the patient is legally competent to sign the form, and does so, he waives the right to a later claim that he didn't. He also waives the right to a later claim that he didn't understand the medical treatment or that the physician didn't explain information presented in the consent form.

Other states take the position that a signed consent form is evidence of informed consent but may be refutable, if the patient offers sufficient evidence to the contrary. The patient may challenge his consent by attacking the substance of the consent form. He may claim that the health care provider didn't explain medical terms in a manner that a patient could understand or (given the medical diagnosis, the patient's condition, or the surgery contemplated) that relevant information significant to the patient wasn't provided.

A signed consent form may not be required in your state. However, there must still be evidence that the patient has been provided with the required information and has given his consent to proceed. This may be done by a notation in the progress notes indicating that the patient has been told of specific risks, benefits, and alternatives; has had an opportunity to have questions answered; and understands and agrees to the procedure. The evidence of informed consent is further enhanced if the medical record documents other family members who were present with the patient when the consent was obtained such as "Wife present and concurs in patient's decision to proceed with surgery."

If you work in an institution that uses investigational drugs or engages in research, your policies and procedures must state that the patient or surrogate receives a clear explanation of experimental treatment. This includes the procedures to be followed, a clear description of potential discomforts and risks, a list of alternative treatments, and a clear explanation that the patient may refuse to participate in the research project without compromising access to care or treatment.

Most of JCAHO Type 1 Recommendations concerning informed consent result from inadequate or incomplete documentation. (Health care organizations must resolve insufficient or unsatisfactory compliance with standards in a specific performance area within a specific time to maintain accreditation.) It's easier to comply with JCAHO standards if forms are user-friendly and include the required criteria, if an audit system is in place to validate that forms are consistently completed appropriately, and if the forms are included in the medical records.

## Exceptions to obtaining informed consent first

Emergency treatment to save a patient's life or to prevent loss of an organ, a limb, or a function may be done without first obtaining consent in specific circumstances. If the patient is unconscious (or is a minor who can't give consent), emergency treatment may be performed. The presumption is that the patient would have consented if he had been able, unless there's reason to believe otherwise. For example, to sustain the life of unconscious patients in the emergency department (ED), intubation has been held to be appropriate even if there's no one to consent to the procedure. Children brought to the ED following a serious injury in school, whose parents can't be located in time, may be provided with emergency medical care without consent while attempts are made to locate the parents. Although consent is presumed in such cases, lawsuits may still occur. For example, giving blood to a severely injured unconscious person may be a lifesaving procedure, but the patient or a family member may sue if such action is against their religious convictions. Courts will uphold emergency medical treatment as long as reasonable effort was made to obtain consent and no alternative treatments were available to save life or limb. The courts won't uphold treatment in the absence of informed consent if the health care provider has had prior contact and has been told that such treatment would be refused. The courts will require the health care provider to locate family members or obtain proper consent from the patient, if time and the circumstances allow him to do so.

Before proceeding, a prudent health care provider will make certain that the precise medical emergency has been documented in the medical record, along with all attempts to obtain proper consent and any information that has been conveyed to the patient.

Patients may also waive their rights to additional information by appointing someone else as their medical decision maker. Advance directives are one way to have another person participate and be responsible for one's medical care and treatment. If this has been decided beforehand, proper documentation must appear in the medical record.

## WHEN INFORMED CONSENT BECOMES INVALID

Informed consent can become invalid if the change in the patient's medical status alters the risks and benefits of treatment. In such situations, the health care provider must explain the new risks and benefits to make sure the patient will consent to the treatment.

To summarize, the controversy over informed consent centers on medical and surgical treatments and procedures that are invasive, risky, or experimental or that have low likelihood for a successful outcome. We've come a long way since the concept of silence or therapeutic privilege. In that situation, the physician was allowed to withhold information from a patient at the sole discretion of the physician and the patient's family, who believed that the information would jeopardize the patient's health. In some instances, patients weren't told that they were dying or that the treatment would have no benefit. Now, therapeutic privilege is viewed narrowly; withholding of significant information from patients or their designated decision makers is frowned upon by the courts because of a patient's right to self-determination, a right that the health care provider is charged with protecting.

# Right to consent: From birth to adulthood

A person attains more medical rights as he reaches the age of majority, defined as the age when a person is considered legally responsible for his activities and becomes entitled to the legal rights held by citizens generally.

### BIRTH
From birth, everyone has medical rights to:
- confidentiality concerning medical records
- privacy during treatment
- reasonable and prudent medical care.

### MINORS
Anyone under age 18 or 21 (depending on the state in which he lives) has the right to consent to treatment for sexually transmitted diseases, serious communicable diseases, and drug or alcohol abuse (although state law may require that the minor's parents be notified).

### MATURE MINORS
In certain instances, a physician or judge may decide that a minor is sufficiently mature (has a sufficiently developed awareness and mental capacity) to consent to

medical treatment. If so, the minor has the right to make decisions about medical care.

### ADULTS
Anyone who has reached the age of majority or who is legally emancipated has the right to:
- consent to or refuse medical treatment
- consent to or refuse medical treatment for his children (in most cases).

# APPENDIX C
## 12-LEAD ECG INTERPRETATION

The most common test for evaluating cardiac status, the 12-lead, or standard, electrocardiogram (ECG) helps identify various pathologic conditions — most commonly, acute myocardial infarction (MI).

## BASIC COMPONENTS AND PRINCIPLES

The 12-lead ECG provides 12 views of the heart's electrical activity. (See *12 views of the heart,* page 574.) The 12 leads include:
■ three bipolar limb leads (I, II, and III)
■ three unipolar augmented limb leads ($aV_R$, $aV_L$, and $aV_F$)
■ six unipolar precordial, or chest, leads ($V_1$, $V_2$, $V_3$, $V_4$, $V_5$, and $V_6$).

## Leads

The six limb leads record electrical potential from the frontal plane, and the six precordial leads record electrical potential from the horizontal plane. Each waveform reflects the orientation of a lead to the wave of depolarization passing through the myocardium. Normally, this wave moves through the heart from right to left and from top to bottom.

**BIPOLAR LEADS**
Bipolar leads record the electrical potential difference between two points on the patient's body, where you place electrodes.
■ Lead I goes from the right arm (–) to the left arm (+).
■ Lead II goes from the right arm (–) to the left leg (+).
■ Lead III goes from the left arm (–) to the left leg (+).

Because of the orientation of these leads to the wave of depolarization, the QRS complexes typically appear upright. In lead II, these complexes are usually the tallest because this lead parallels the wave of depolarization.

**UNIPOLAR LEADS**
Unipolar leads (the augmented limb leads and the precordial leads) have only one electrode, which represents the positive pole. The ECG computes the negative pole. Lead $aV_R$ typically records negative QRS complex deflections because the wave of depolarization moves away from it. In the $aV_F$ lead, QRS complexes are positive; in the $aV_L$ lead, they're biphasic.

Unipolar precordial leads $V_1$ and $V_2$ usually have a small R wave because the direction of ventricular activation is left to right initially. That's because conduction time is normally faster down the left bundle branch than down the

## 12 views of the heart

The electrocardiogram's six limb leads view the heart from six different angles. This chart shows the direction of each lead relative to the wave of depolarization and lists the six views of the heart revealed by these leads.

| PLANES OF THE HEART | LEADS | VIEW OF THE HEART |
|---|---|---|

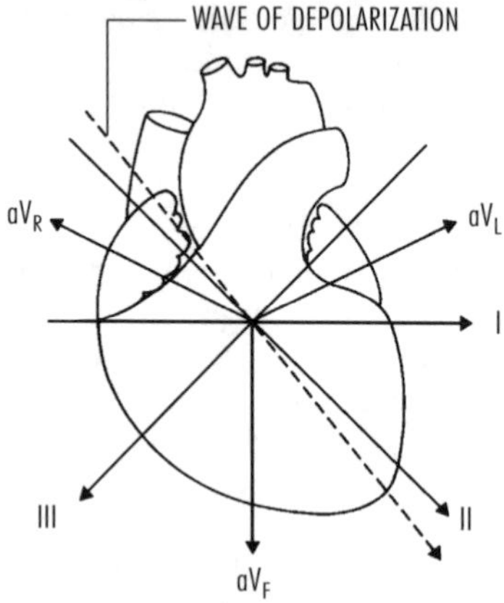

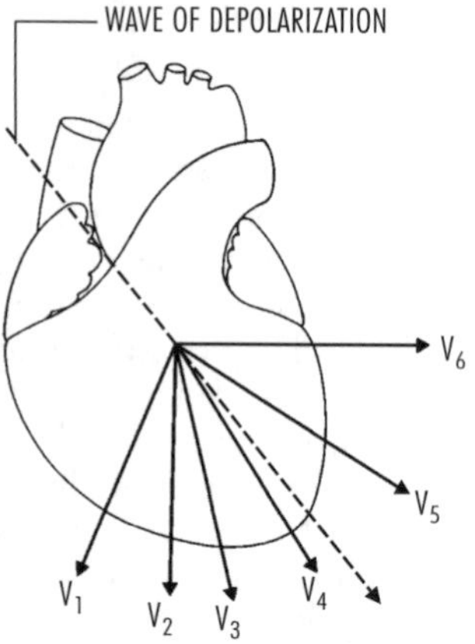

| LEADS | VIEW OF THE HEART |
|---|---|
| **Standard limb leads (bipolar)** | |
| I | Lateral wall |
| II | Inferior wall |
| III | Inferior wall |
| **Augmented limb leads (unipolar)** | |
| $aV_R$ | Provides no specific view |
| $aV_L$ | Lateral wall |
| $aV_F$ | Inferior wall |
| **Precordial, or chest, leads (unipolar)** | |
| $V_1$ | Anteroseptal wall |
| $V_2$ | Anteroseptal wall |
| $V_3$ | Anterior and anteroseptal walls |
| $V_4$ | Anterior wall |
| $V_5$ | Anterolateral wall |
| $V_6$ | Anterolateral wall |

right. However, the wave of depolarization moves toward the left ventricle and away from these leads, causing a low S wave.

In leads $V_3$ and $V_4$, the R and S waves may have the same amplitude, and you won't see a Q wave. In leads $V_5$ and $V_6$, the initial ventricular activation appears as a small Q wave; the following tall R wave represents the strong wave of depolarization moving toward the left ventricle. These leads record a small or absent S wave.

## DETERMINING ELECTRICAL AXIS

As electrical impulses travel through the heart, they generate small electrical forces called instant-to-instant vectors. The mean of these vectors represents the direction and force of the wave of depolarization, also known as the heart's electrical axis.

In a healthy heart, the wave of depolarization (or the direction of the electrical axis) originates in the sinoatrial (SA) node, travels through the atria and the atrioventricular (AV) node, and on to the ventricles. The normal movement is downward and to the left — the direction of a normal electrical axis.

In an unhealthy heart, the wave of depolarization varies. That's because the direction of electrical activity swings away from areas of damage or necrosis.

A simple method for determining the direction of your patient's electrical axis is the quadrant method. Before you use this method, you'll need to understand the hexaxial reference system — a schematic view of the heart that uses the six limb leads.

As you know, these leads include the three standard limb leads (I, II, and III), which are bipolar,

and the three augmented limb leads ($aV_R$, $aV_L$, and $aV_F$), which are unipolar. Combined, these leads give a view of the wave of depolarization in the frontal plane, including the right, left, inferior, and superior portions of the heart.

## HEXAXIAL REFERENCE SYSTEM

The axes of the six limb leads also make up the hexaxial reference system, which divides the heart into six equal areas. To use the hexaxial reference system, picture in your mind the position of each lead: lead I connects the right arm (negative pole) with the left arm (positive pole); lead II connects the right arm (negative pole) with the left leg (positive pole); and lead III connects the left arm (negative pole) with the left leg (positive pole). The augmented limb leads have only one electrode, which represents the positive pole. As a result, lead $aV_R$ goes from the heart toward the right arm (positive pole); $aV_L$ goes from the heart toward the left arm (positive pole); and $aV_F$ goes from the heart to the left leg (positive pole).

Now, take this mental picture one step further and draw an imaginary line to illustrate the axis of each lead. For example, for lead I, you would draw a horizontal line between the right and left arms; for lead II, between the right arm and left leg; and so on. All the lines should intersect near the center, somewhere over the heart. If

## Understanding the hexaxial reference system

The hexaxial reference system consists of six bisecting lines, each representing one of the six limb leads, and a circle, representing the heart. The intersection of these lines divides the circle into equal 30-degree segments.

Note that 0 degrees appears at the 3 o'clock position. Moving counterclockwise, the degrees become increasingly negative, until reaching ±180 degrees at the 9 o'clock position. The bottom half of the circle contains the corresponding positive degrees. A positive-degree designation doesn't necessarily mean that the pole is positive.

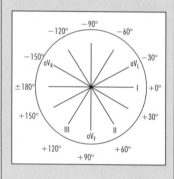

+180 degrees indicates right axis deviation; one between 0 degrees and −90 degrees, left axis deviation; and one between −180 degrees and −90 degrees, extreme axis deviation (sometimes called the northwest axis). Some experts, however, feel that the portion from 0 degrees to −30 degrees has no clinical significance.

## QUADRANT METHOD

A simple, rapid method for determining the heart's axis is the quadrant method, in which you observe the main deflection of the QRS complex in leads I and $aV_F$. The QRS complex serves as the traditional marker for determining the electrical axis because the ventricles produce the greatest amount of electrical force when they contract. Lead I indicates whether impulses are moving to the right or left; lead $aV_F$, whether they're moving up or down. (See *Using the quadrant method.*)

On the waveform for lead I, a positive main deflection of the QRS complex indicates that the electrical impulses are moving to the right, toward the positive pole of the lead, which is at the 0-degree position on the hexaxial reference system. Conversely, a negative deflection indicates that the impulses are moving to the left, toward the negative pole of the lead, which is at the +180-degree position on the hexaxial reference system. On the waveform for lead $aV_F$, a positive deflection of

you draw a circle to represent the heart, you would end up with a rough pie shape, with each wedge representing a portion of the heart monitored by each lead. (See *Understanding the hexaxial reference system.*)

This schematic representation of the heart allows you to plot your patient's electrical axis. If his axis falls in the right lower quadrant, between 0 degrees and +90 degrees, it's considered normal. An axis between +90 degrees and

## Using the quadrant method

This chart can help you quickly determine the direction of a patient's electrical axis, which is indicated by the gray arrow. First, observe the deflections of the QRS complexes in leads I and aV$_F$. Next, plot the deflections on the diagram. (Positive deflections are on the side that has positive degrees for that lead, and negative deflections are on the side that has negative degrees.) Then check the chart to determine if the patient's axis is normal or whether it has a left, right, or extreme deviation.

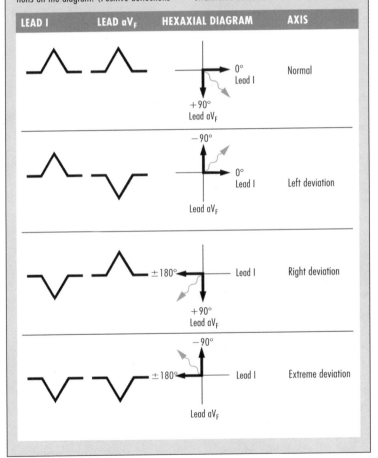

| LEAD I | LEAD aV$_F$ | HEXAXIAL DIAGRAM | AXIS |
|---|---|---|---|
| | | 0° Lead I / +90° Lead aV$_F$ | Normal |
| | | −90° / 0° Lead I / Lead aV$_F$ | Left deviation |
| | | ±180° Lead I / +90° Lead aV$_F$ | Right deviation |
| | | −90° / ±180° Lead I / Lead aV$_F$ | Extreme deviation |

the QRS complex indicates that the electrical impulses are traveling downward, toward the positive pole of the lead, which is at the +90-degree position of the hexaxial reference system. A negative deflection indicates that impulses are traveling upward, toward the negative pole of the lead, which is at the +90-degree position in the hexaxial reference system.

Plotting this information on the hexaxial reference system (with the horizontal axis representing lead I and the vertical axis representing lead $aV_F$) will reveal the patient's electrical axis. For example, if lead I shows a positive deflection of the QRS complex, darken the horizontal axis between the center of the hexaxial reference system and the 0-degree position. If lead $aV_F$ also shows a positive deflection of the QRS complex, darken the vertical axis between the center of reference system and the +90-degree position. The quadrant between the two axes you have darkened indicates the patient's electrical axis. In this case, it's the left lower quadrant, which indicates a normal electrical axis.

## CAUSES OF AXIS DEVIATION

Determining a patient's electrical axis can help confirm a diagnosis or narrow the range of clinical possibilities. Many factors influence the electrical axis, including the position of the heart within the chest, the size of the heart, the conduction pathways, and the force of electrical generation.

As you know, cardiac electrical activity swings away from areas of damage or necrosis. More specifically, electrical forces in the healthy portion of the heart take over for weak, or even absent, electrical forces in the damaged portion. For instance, after an inferior-wall MI, portions of the inferior wall can no longer conduct electricity. As a result, the major electrical vectors shift to the left, resulting in a left axis deviation.

Typically, the damaged portion of the heart is the last area to be depolarized. For example, in a left anterior hemiblock, the left anterior fascicle of the left bundle branch can no longer conduct electricity. Therefore, the portion normally served by the left bundle branch is the last portion of the heart to be depolarized. This shifts electrical forces to the left; consequently, the ECG shows left axis deviation.

An opposite shift occurs with right bundle-branch block. In this condition, the wave of impulse travels quickly down the normal left side but much more slowly down the damaged right side. This shifts the electrical forces to the right, causing a right axis deviation.

An axis shift also takes place when the right or left ventricle is artificially paced or when the ventricles are depolarizing abnormally such as occurs in ventricular tachycardia. Both of these conditions can cause a left axis deviation or, occasionally, an extreme axis deviation.

Axis deviation may also result from ventricular hypertrophy. For example, an enlarged right ventricle generates greater electrical forces than normal and would consequently shift the electrical axis to the right. Wolff-Parkinson-

White syndrome may produce a right, left, or extreme axis deviation, depending on which part of the ventricle is activated early. Sometimes axis deviation may be a normal variation, as in infants and children, who normally experience right axis deviation. It may also stem from noncardiac causes. For example, if the heart is shifted in the chest cavity because of a high diaphragm from pregnancy, expect to find a left axis deviation. In addition, if a patient's heart is situated on the right side of the chest instead of the left (a condition called dextrocardia), expect to find right axis deviation.

## HOW TO INTERPRET A 12-LEAD ECG

You can use various methods to interpret a 12-lead ECG. Here's a logical, easy-to-follow, seven-step method that will help ensure that you're interpreting it accurately.

**1.** Find the lead markers and note the leads.

**2.** Note whether there are full or half standardization marks.

**3.** Using the four-quadrant method, observe the waveforms for leads I and $aV_F$, and determine the heart's axis. This can provide an early clue to a possible problem.

**4.** Note the R-wave progression through the six precordial leads. Normally, in the precordial leads, the R wave (the first positive deflection of the QRS complex) appears progressively taller from lead

$V_1$ to lead $V_6$. Conversely, the S wave (the negative deflection after an R wave) appears extremely deep in lead $V_1$ and becomes progressively smaller through lead $V_6$. (See *Normal findings,* pages 580 and 581.)

**5.** Next, look at the T wave, which normally goes in the same direction as the QRS complex. If the main deflection of the QRS complex is positive, the T wave should be positive, too. If the main deflection of the QRS complex is negative, the T wave should be negative. The two exceptions to this are leads $V_1$ and $V_2$, in which a negative QRS complex with a positive T wave is normal.

If a T wave deflects in the opposite direction from the QRS complex, it's considered abnormal (except, as mentioned, in leads $V_1$ and $V_2$). Such a deflection is commonly referred to as an inverted T wave — a term that can be confusing when the QRS complex is negative and the T wave is actually positive. Keep in mind that in this case, inversion signifies that the T wave deflects in the direction opposite the QRS complex. It doesn't necessarily mean that the T wave is negative, as the word inverted suggests.

**6.** If you suspect an MI, start with lead I and continue through to lead $V_6$, observing the waveforms for changes in ECG characteristics that can indicate an acute MI, such as T-wave inversion, ST-segment elevation, and pathologic Q waves. Note the leads in which you see such changes and describe the changes. When first learning

*(Text continues on page 582.)*

## Normal findings

LEAD I

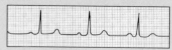

P wave: upright
Q wave: small or none
R wave: largest wave
S wave: none present, or smaller than R wave
T wave: upright
U wave: none present
ST segment: may vary from +1 to −0.5 mm

LEAD II

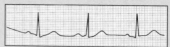

P wave: upright
Q wave: small or none
R wave: large (vertical heart)
S wave: none present, or smaller than R wave
T wave: upright
U wave: none present
ST segment: may vary from +1 to −0.5 mm

LEAD III

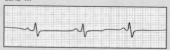

P wave: upright, diphasic, or inverted
Q wave: usually small or none (a Q wave must also be present in aV$_F$ to be considered diagnostic.)
R wave: none present to large wave
S wave: none present to large wave, indicating horizontal heart
T wave: upright, diphasic, or inverted
U wave: none present
ST segment: may vary from +1 to −0.5 mm

LEAD aV$_R$

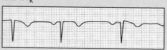

P wave: inverted
Q wave: none, small wave, or large wave present
R wave: none or small wave present
S wave: large wave (may be QS)
T wave: inverted
U wave: none present
ST segment: may vary from +1 to −0.5 mm

LEAD aV$_L$

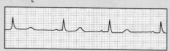

P wave: upright, diphasic, or inverted
Q wave: none, small wave, or large wave present (A Q wave must also be present in lead I or precordial leads to be considered diagnostic.)
R wave: none, small wave, or large wave present (A large wave indicates horizontal heart.)
S wave: none present to large wave (A large wave indicates vertical heart.)
T wave: upright, diphasic, or inverted
U wave: none present
ST segment: may vary from +1 to −0.5 mm

LEAD aV$_F$

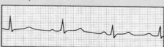

P wave: upright
Q wave: none, or small wave present
R wave: none, small wave, or large wave present (A large wave suggests vertical heart.)
S wave: none to large wave present (A large wave suggests horizontal heart.)
T wave: Upright, diphasic, or inverted
U wave: none present
ST segment: may vary from +1 to −0.5 mm

LEAD V₁

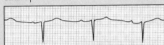

P wave: upright, diphasic, or inverted
Q wave: deep QS pattern may be present
R wave: none present or less than S wave
S wave: large (part of QS pattern)
T wave: usually inverted but may be upright and diphasic
U wave: none present
ST segment: may vary from 0 to +1 mm

LEAD V₂

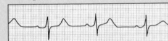

P wave: upright
Q wave: deep QS pattern may be present
R wave: none present or less than S wave (wave may become progressively larger)
S wave: large (part of QS pattern)
T wave: upright
U wave: upright, lower amplitude than T wave
ST segment: may vary from 0 to +1 mm

LEAD V₃

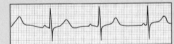

P wave: upright
Q wave: none or small wave present
R wave: less than, greater than, or equal to S wave (Wave may become progressively larger.)
S wave: large (greater than, less than, or equal to R wave)
T wave: upright
U wave: upright, lower amplitude than T wave
ST segment: may vary from 0 to +1 mm

LEAD V₄

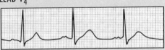

P wave: upright
Q wave: none or small wave present
R wave: progressively larger wave; R wave greater than S wave
S wave: progressively smaller (less than R wave)
T wave: upright
U wave: upright, lower amplitude than T wave
ST segment: may vary from +1 to −0.5 mm

LEAD V₅

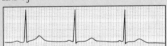

P wave: upright
Q wave: small
R wave: progressively larger but less than 26 mm
S wave: progressively smaller; less than the S wave in V₄
T wave: upright
U wave: none present
ST segment: may vary from +1 to −0.5 mm

LEAD V₆

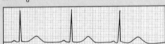

P wave: upright
Q wave: small
R wave: largest wave but less than 26 mm
S wave: smallest; less than the S wave in V₅
T wave: upright
U wave: none present
ST segment: may vary from +1 to −0.5 mm

## Locating myocardial damage

| WALL AFFECTED | LEADS | ECG CHANGES | ARTERY INVOLVED | RECIPROCAL CHANGES |
|---|---|---|---|---|
| Inferior (diaphragmatic) | II, III, $aV_F$ | Q, ST, T | Right coronary artery (RCA) | I, $aV_L$ and, possibly, $V_4$ through $V_6$ |
| Posterolateral | I, $aV_L$, $V_5$, $V_6$ | Q, ST, T | Circumflex or branch of left anterior descending (LAD) artery | $V_1$, $V_2$, or II, III, and $aV_F$ |
| Anterior | $V_1$, $V_2$, $V_3$, $V_4$ | Q, ST, T, loss of R-wave progression across precordial leads | Left coronary artery | II, III, $aV_F$ |
| Posterior | $V_1$, $V_2$ | None | RCA or circumflex, either of which supplies posterior descending artery | R greater than S in $V_1$ and $V_2$, ST-segment depression, T-wave elevation |
| Right ventricular | $V_{4R}$, $V_{5R}$, $V_{6R}$ | Q, ST, T | RCA | None |
| Anterolateral | I, $aV_L$, $V_4$, $V_5$, $V_6$ | Q, ST, T | LAD and diagonal branches, circumflex and obtuse marginal branches | II, III, $aV_F$ |
| Anteroseptal | $V_1$, $V_2$, $V_3$ | Q, ST, T, loss of R wave in $V_1$ | LAD | None |

to interpret the 12-lead ECG, ignore lead $aV_R$, because it won't provide clues to left ventricular infarction or injury.

**7.** Determine the site and extent of myocardial damage. To do so, use the chart *Locating myocardial damage,* and follow these steps:
■ Identify the leads recording pathologic Q waves. Look at the second column of the chart for those leads. Then look at the first column to find the corresponding myocardial wall, where infarction has occurred. Keep in mind that this chart serves as a guideline only. Actual areas of infarction may overlap or be larger or smaller than listed.

■ Identify the leads recording ST-segment elevation (or depression for reciprocal leads), and use the chart to locate the corresponding areas of myocardial injury.

■ Identify the leads recording T-wave inversion, and locate the corresponding areas of ischemia.

## ACUTE MYOCARDIAL INFARCTION

An acute MI can arise from any condition in which the myocardial oxygen supply can't meet the oxygen demand. Starved of oxygen, the myocardium suffers progressive ischemia, leading to injury and, eventually, to infarction.

In most cases, an acute MI involves the left ventricle, although it can also involve the right ventricle or the atria, and is classified as either Q wave or non–Q wave.

In an acute transmural MI, the characteristic ECG changes result from the three I's — ischemia, injury, and infarction.

■ Ischemia results from a temporary interruption of the myocardial blood supply. Its characteristic ECG change is T-wave inversion, a result of altered tissue repolarization. ST-segment depression also may occur.

ISCHEMIA

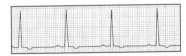

Ischemia produces T-wave inversion

■ Injury to myocardial cells results from a prolonged interruption of blood flow. Its characteristic ECG

change, ST-segment elevation, reflects altered depolarization. Usually, an elevation greater than 0.1 mV is considered significant.

INJURY

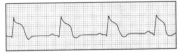

Injury produces ST-segment elevation

■ Infarction results from an absence of blood flow to myocardial tissue, leading to necrosis. The ECG shows pathologic Q waves, reflecting abnormal depolarization in damaged tissue or absent depolarization in scar tissue. The characteristic of a pathologic Q wave is a duration of 0.04 second or an amplitude measuring at least one-third the height of the entire QRS complex.

INFARCTION

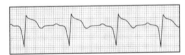

Infarction produces pathologic Q waves

Besides these three characteristic ECG changes, you may see reciprocal (or mirror image) changes. Reciprocal changes — most commonly, ST-segment depression or tall R waves — occur in the leads opposite those reflecting the area of ischemia, injury, or infarction.

## Acute MI phases

To detect an acute MI, look for ST-segment elevation first, followed by T-wave inversion and pathologic Q waves.

Serial ECG recordings yield the best evidence of an MI. Normally, an acute MI progresses through the following phases.

### HYPERACUTE PHASE
This phase begins a few hours after the onset of an acute MI. You'll see ST-segment elevation and upright (usually peaked) T waves.

### FULLY EVOLVED PHASE
This phase starts several hours after the onset of an acute MI. You'll see deep T-wave inversion and pathologic Q waves.

### RESOLUTION PHASE
This appears within a few weeks of an acute MI. You'll see normal T waves.

### STABILIZED CHRONIC PHASE
After the resolution phase, you'll see permanent pathologic Q-waves revealing an old infarction.

With an acute non–Q-wave MI, you may see persistent ST-segment depression, T-wave inversion, or both. However, pathologic Q waves may not appear. To differentiate an acute non–Q-wave MI from myocardial ischemia, cardiac enzyme tests must be performed.

It's important to remember that for a true clinical diagnosis of an acute MI, a patient must have symptoms, ECG changes, and elevated cardiac enzyme levels. If the patient shows such signs and symptoms as chest pain, left arm pain, diaphoresis, and nausea, proceed as if he's had an acute MI until this possibility has been ruled out.

## RIGHT-SIDED ECG, LEADS $V_{1R}$ TO $V_{6R}$

A right-sided ECG provides information about the extent of damage to the right ventricle, especially during the first 12 hours of an MI. Right-sided ECG leads, placed over the right side of the chest in similar but reversed positions from the left precordial leads, are called unipolar right-sided chest leads.

### PLACING ELECTRODES
Right-sided ECG leads are precordial leads designated by the letter V, a number representing the electrode position, and the letter R, indicating lead placement on the right side of the chest. Lead positions are:
- $V_{1R}$: fourth intercostal space, left sternal border
- $V_{2R}$: fourth intercostal space, right sternal border
- $V_{3R}$: midway between $V_{2R}$ and $V_{4R}$, on a line joining these two locations
- $V_{4R}$: fifth intercostal space, right midclavicular line
- $V_{5R}$: fifth intercostal space, right anterior axillary line
- $V_{6R}$: fifth intercostal space, right midaxillary line.

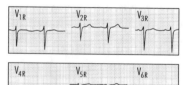

## Understanding polarity

The right-sided chest ECG leads measure the difference in electrical potential between a right-sided chest electrode and a central terminal. The chest electrode used in each of the right V leads is positive. The negative electrode is obtained by adding together leads I, II, and III, whose algebraic sum equals zero.

## Viewing the heart

Chest leads, whether on the left or the right side of the chest, view the horizontal plane of the heart. The placement of left precordial leads gives a good picture of the electrical activity within the left ventricle. Because the right ventricle lies behind the left ventricle, the ability to evaluate right ventricular electrical activity when using only left precordial leads is limited. Right-sided ECG leads provide a better picture of the right ventricular wall. This may be especially useful when evaluating a patient for a right ventricular MI.

Leads $V_{1R}$ and $V_{2R}$ provide limited visualization of the right ventricle. Leads $V_{3R}$ through $V_{6R}$ are the most useful right ventricular leads. A decrease in the R wave with an increase in the S wave is normally seen from $V_{1R}$ through $V_{6R}$, the reverse of the standard left precordial leads. $V_{3R}$ to $V_{6R}$ (particularly $V_{4R}$) are the most commonly used and the most helpful leads when looking for ECG changes indicating right ventricular ischemia and infarction.

## Left bundle-branch block

In left bundle-branch block, a conduction delay or block occurs in both the left posterior and the left anterior fascicles of the left bundle. This delay or block disrupts the normal left-to-right direction of depolarization. As a result, normal septal Q waves are absent. Because of the block, the wave of depolarization must move down the right bundle first and then spread from right to left. (See *Characteristics and interpretation: Left bundle-branch block,* page 586.)

This arrhythmia may indicate underlying heart disease such as coronary artery disease. It carries a more serious prognosis than right bundle-branch block because of its close correlation with organic heart disease and because it requires a large lesion to block the thick, broad left bundle branch.

**INTERVENTION**

When left bundle-branch block occurs along with an anterior-wall MI, it usually signals complete heart block, which requires insertion of a pacemaker.

## Right bundle-branch block

In the conduction delay or block associated with right bundle-branch block, the initial left-to-right direction of depolarization isn't affected. The left ventricle depolarizes on time, so the intrinsicoid deflection in leads $V_5$ and $V_6$ (the left precordial leads) takes place on time as well. However,

## Characteristics and interpretation: Left bundle-branch block

**Rhythm:** regular atrial and ventricular rhythms
**Rate:** atrial and ventricular rates within normal limits
**P wave:** normal size and configuration
**PR interval:** within normal limits
**QRS complex:** duration that varies from 0.10 to 0.12 second in incomplete left bundle-branch block (It's at least 0.12 second in complete block. Lead $V_1$ shows a wide, entirely negative rS complex [rarely a wide rS complex]. Leads I, $aV_L$, and $V_6$ show a wide, tall R wave without a Q or S wave.)
**T wave:** deflection opposite that of the QRS complex in most leads
**QT interval:** may be prolonged or within normal limits
**Other:** several changes paralleling the magnitude of the QRS complex aberration, with normal axis or left axis deviation; delayed intrinsicoid deflection over the left ventricle (lead $V_6$)

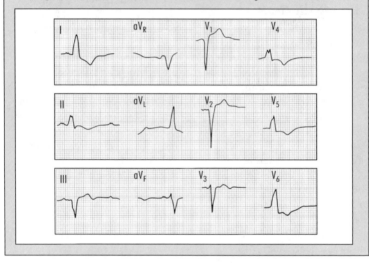

the right ventricle depolarizes late, causing a late intrinsicoid deflection in leads $V_1$ and $V_2$ (the right precordial leads). This late depolarization also causes the axis to deviate to the right. (See *Characteristics and interpretation: Right bundle-branch block*.)

**INTERVENTION**

One potential complication of an MI is a bundle-branch block. Some blocks require treatment with a temporary pacemaker. Others are monitored only to detect progression to a more complete block.

## PERICARDITIS

An inflammation of the pericardium, the fibroserous sac that envelops the heart, pericarditis can be acute or chronic. The acute form may be fibrinous or effusive, with a purulent serous or hemor-

## Characteristics and interpretation: Right bundle-branch block

**Rhythm:** regular atrial and ventricular rhythms
**Rate:** atrial and ventricular rates within normal limits
**P wave:** normal size and configuration
**PR interval:** within normal limits
**QRS complex:** duration of at least 0.12 second in complete block and 0.10 to 0.12 second in incomplete block (In lead $V_1$, the QRS complex is wide and can appear in one of several patterns: an rSR' complex with a wide S and R' wave; an rS complex with a wide R wave; and a wide R wave with an M-shaped pattern. The complex is mainly positive, with the R wave occurring late. In leads I, $AV_L$, and $V_6$, a broad S wave can be seen.)

**T wave:** in most leads, deflection opposite that of the QRS-complex deflection
**QT interval:** may be prolonged or within normal limits
**Other:** in the precordial leads, occurrence of triphasic complexes because the right ventricle continues to depolarize after the left ventricle depolarizes, thereby producing a third phase of ventricular stimulation

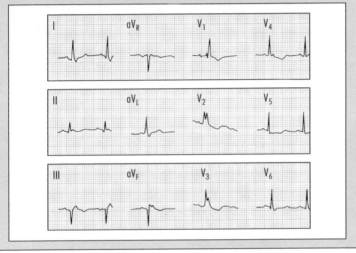

rhagic exudate. Chronic constrictive pericarditis causes dense fibrous pericardial thickening. Regardless of the form, pericarditis can cause cardiac tamponade if fluid accumulates too quickly. It can also cause heart failure if constriction occurs. (See *Characteristics and interpretation: Pericarditis,* page 588.)

In pericarditis, ECG changes occur in four stages. Stage 1 coincides with the onset of chest pain. Stage 2 begins within several days. Stage 3 starts several days after stage 2. Stage 4 occurs weeks later.

**INTERVENTION**
Pericarditis is usually treated with aspirin or nonsteroidal anti-inflammatory drugs. A last resort is prednisone, quickly tapered over 3 days.

## Characteristics and interpretation: Pericarditis

**Rhythm:** usually regular atrial and ventricular rhythms
**Rate:** atrial and ventricular rates usually within normal limits
**P wave:** normal size and configuration
**PR interval:** usually depressed in all leads except $V_1$ and $aV_R$, in which it may be elevated
**QRS complex:** within normal limits, but with a possible decrease in amplitude

**ST segment:** in stage 1, elevated 1 to 2 mm in a concave pattern in leads I, II, and III and the precordial leads
**T wave:** flattened in stage 2, inverted in stage 3 (lasting for weeks or months), and returning to normal in stage 4 (although sometimes becoming deeply inverted)
**QT interval:** within normal limits
**Other:** possible atrial fibrillation or tachycardia from sinoatrial node irritation

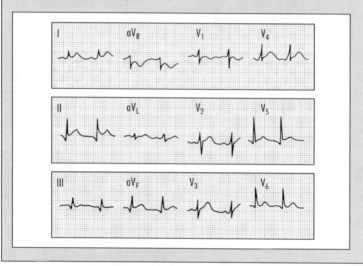

## DIGOXIN: ECG EFFECTS

Digoxin increases the force of myocardial contraction, decreases conduction velocity through the AV node to slow the heart rate, and prolongs the effective refractory period of the AV node by direct and sympatholytic effects on the SA node. Excess amounts of this drug can slow conduction through the AV node and cause irritable ectopic foci in the ventricles. (See

*Characteristics and interpretation: Digoxin.*)

ECG changes only indicate that the patient is receiving a form of digoxin. If an arrhythmia develops, these ECG changes can help identify the cause of the arrhythmia as digoxin toxicity.

Virtually any type of arrhythmia can be caused by an excess of digoxin. The most common ones include premature ventricular contractions (especially bigeminy), paroxysmal atrial tachycardias with

## Characteristics and interpretation: Digoxin

**Rhythm:** regular atrial and ventricular rhythms
**Rate:** atrial and ventricular rates are usually within normal limits, but bradycardia is possible
**P wave:** decreased voltage; may be notched
**PR interval:** within normal limits or prolonged
**QRS complex:** within normal limits
**ST segment:** gradual sloping, causing ST-segment depression in the direction opposite that of the QRS deflection

**T wave:** may be flattened and inverted in a direction opposite that of the QRS-complex deflection
**Other:** QT interval commonly shortened; ST-segment sloping and depression and QT-interval shortening from digoxin use but not necessarily signs of digoxin toxicity; ST-segment depression and T-wave inversion in leads with negatively deflected QRS complexes, possibly indicating a need to reduce the digoxin dose

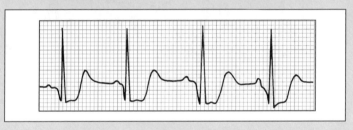

or without a block, second-degree heart block, and sinus arrest.

**INTERVENTION**
Monitor the patient for noncardiac symptoms of digoxin toxicity. Withhold digoxin for 1 to 2 days before performing electrical cardioversion.

## QUINIDINE: ECG EFFECTS

An antiarrhythmic that decreases sodium transport through cardiac tissues, quinidine slows conduction through the AV node. It also prolongs the effective refractory period and decreases automaticity. (See *Characteristics and interpretation: Quinidine,* page 590.)

Although ECG changes occur as a result of quinidine use, they aren't necessarily a sign of quinidine toxicity. At toxic levels, however, quinidine can cause SA and AV block and ventricular arrhythmias.

**INTERVENTION**
Prolongation of the QT interval is a sign that the patient is predisposed to developing polymorphic ventricular tachycardia. Preventing ventricular tachyarrhythmias involves administering a cardiac glycoside for atrial tachyarrhythmias before quinidine.

## Characteristics and interpretation: Quinidine

**Rhythm:** regular atrial and ventricular rhythms
**Rate:** atrial and ventricular rates within normal limits
**P wave:** may be widened and notched, especially in leads I and II
**PR interval:** within normal limits

**QRS complex:** widens slightly (Abnormal widening may be an early sign of developing quinidine toxicity.)
**ST segment:** commonly depressed
**T wave:** may be flattened or inverted
**QT interval:** may be prolonged
**U wave:** may be visible

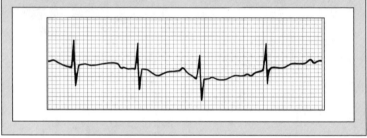

# SELECTED REFERENCES

Barker, L.R., et al. *Principles of Ambulatory Medicine,* 6th ed. Philadelphia: Lippincott Williams & Wilkins, 2002.

Braunwald, E., et al., eds. *Harrison's Principles of Internal Medicine,* 15th ed. New York: McGraw-Hill Book Co., 2001.

Burns, C.E., et al. *Pocket Reference for Pediatric Primary Care,* 2nd ed. Philadelphia: W.B. Saunders Co., 2001.

Fitzpatrick, T.B., et al. *Color Atlas and Synopsis of Clinical Dermatology,* 4th ed. New York: McGraw-Hill Book Co., 2001.

Goldman, L., and Bennett, J.C. *Cecil Textbook of Medicine,* 21st ed. Philadelphia: W.B. Saunders Co., 2000.

*Guidelines for Cardiopulmonary Resuscitation and Emergency Cardiovascular Care.* Dallas: American Heart Association, 2000.

Hoekelman, R.A., et al. *Primary Pediatric Care,* 4th ed. St. Louis: Mosby–Year Book, Inc., 2001.

Jarvis, C. *Physical Examination and Health Assessment,* 3rd ed. Philadelphia: W.B. Saunders Co., 2000.

Lookingbill, D.P., and Marks, J.G. *Principles of Dermatology,* 2nd ed. Philadelphia: W.B. Saunders Co., 2000.

Mengel, M.B., and Schwiebert, L.P. *Ambulatory Medicine: The Primary Care of Families,* 3rd ed. Norwalk, Conn.: Appleton & Lange, 2000.

Pfenninger, J.L., and Fowler, G.C. *Procedures for Primary Care Physicians,* 2nd ed. St. Louis: Mosby–Year Book, Inc., 2002.

*Procedures for Nurse Practitioners.* Springhouse, Pa.: Springhouse Corp., 2001.

*Professional Guide to Diseases,* 7th ed. Springhouse, Pa.: Springhouse Corp., 2001.

Rakel, R., and Bope, E.T., eds. *Conn's Current Therapy.* Philadelphia: W.B. Saunders Co., 2002.

Ridgeway, N.A., et al. "An Efficient Technique for Communicating Reports of Laboratory and Radiographic Studies to Patients in a Primary Care Practice," *American Journal of Medicine* 108(7):575-77, May 2000.

Robinson, D.L., and McKenzie, C.L. *Procedures for Primary Care Providers.* Philadelphia: Lippincott Williams & Wilkins, 2000.

Seltzer, V.L., and Pearse, W.H. *Women's Primary Health Care: Office Practice and Procedures,* 2nd ed. New York: McGraw-Hill Book Co., 2000.

Tierney, L.M., et al. *Current Medical Diagnosis and Treatment,* 41st ed. New York: Lange Medical Books/McGraw-Hill Book Co., 2002.

Tintinalli, J.E., et al., eds. *Emergency Medicine: A Comprehensive Study Guide,* 5th ed. New York: McGraw-Hill Book Co., 2000.

# INDEX

i refers to an illustration; t refers to a table.

i refers to an illustration; t refers to a table.

---

i refers to an illustration; t refers to a table.

---

i refers to an illustration; t refers to a table.

---

i refers to an illustration; t refers to a table.